PERSPECTIVES IN LIFE CYCLE IMPACT ASSESSMENT

A Structured Approach to Combine Models of the Technosphere, Ecosphere and Valuesphere

PERSPECTIVES IN LIFE CYCLE IMPACT ASSESSMENT

A Structured Approach to Combine Models of the Technosphere, Ecosphere and Valuesphere

by

Patrick Hofstetter
Swiss Federal Institute of Technology, Zurich

KLUWER ACADEMIC PUBLISHERS
Boston / Dordrecht / London

Distributors for North, Central and South America:
Kluwer Academic Publishers
101 Philip Drive
Assinippi Park
Norwell, Massachusetts 02061 USA
Telephone (781) 871-6600
Fax (781) 871-6528
E-Mail <kluwer@wkap.com>

Distributors for all other countries:
Kluwer Academic Publishers Group
Distribution Centre
Post Office Box 322
3300 AH Dordrecht, THE NETHERLANDS
Telephone 31 78 6392 392
Fax 31 78 6546 474
E-Mail <services@wkap.nl>

Electronic Services <http://www.wkap.nl>

Library of Congress Cataloging-in-Publication Data

Hofstetter, Patrick, 1965-
Perspectives in life cycle impact assessment : a structured approach to combine models of the technosphere, ecosphere, and valuesphere / by Patrick Hofstetter.
p. cm.
Includes bibliographical references and index.
ISBN 0-7923-8377-X (alk. paper)
1. Environmental risk assessment. 2. Life cycle, Human--Environmental aspects. 3. Environmental engineering. I. Title.
GE145.H45 1998
333.7'14--dc21 98-46060
CIP

Printed on acid-free paper.

Printed in the United States of America

OVERVIEW OF CONTENT

LIST OF CONTENT

ACRONYMS

APHEA	short term effects of AIr Pollution on HEAlth
BaP	Benzo(a)Pyrene
BCF	BioConcentration Factor
BCME	Bis(ChlorMethyl)Ether
BUWAL	Bundesamt für Umwelt, Wald und Landschaft (Swiss EPA)
CML	Centrum voor Milieukunde Universiteit Leiden (The Netherlands)
COD	Chemical Oxygen Demand
COI	Costs Of Illness
COPD	Chronic Obstructive Pulmonary disease
CT	Cultural Theory
DALYs	Disability Adjusted Life Years
DEHP	Di(2-EthylHexyl)Phthalate
DtT	Distance to Target
E	Egalitarian
E-R slope	Exposure-Response slope
ECU	European Currency Unit (new name = EURO)
EI	Eco-Index
EI'95	Eco-Indicator'95
EIA	Environmental Impact Assessment
ELU	Environmental Load Unit
EMEP	European Monitoring and Evaluation Programme
EPA	Environmental Protection Agency of the United States of America
EPS	Environmental Prioritising System
ERV	Emergency Room Visit
ESEERCO	Empire State Electric Energy Research Corporation
ETHZ	Eidgenössische Technische Hochschule Zürich (Swiss Federal Institute of Technology)
F	Fatalist
GWP	Global warming potential
H	Hierarchist
I	Individualist
IARC	International Agency for Research on Cancer
IPCC	Intergovernmental Panel on Climate Change
ISO	International Organization for Standardization
LCA	Life Cycle Assessment
LCI	Life Cycle Inventory Analysis
LCIA	Life Cycle Impact Assessment
MADs	Manageability Adjusted Damages
MIPS	Material Intensity Per Service Unit
NMVOC	Non Methane Volatile Organic Compound
NoMADs	Normalised Manageability Adjusted Damages
NoUDs	Normalised Unknown Damages
PCBs	Polychlorinated Biphenyls
PM_{10}	Particulate matter less than 10 microns in diameter
POCP	Photochemical Ozone Creation Potential
POM	polycyclic organic matter
QALY	Quality Adjusted Life Years
QSARs	Quantitative Structure-Activity Relationships
RA	Risk Assessment
SETAC	Society of Environmental Toxicology and Chemistry
SEYLL	Standard Expected Years of Life Lost
SFA	Substance Flow Analysis
TCDD	Tetrachlor-Dibenzo-p-Dioxin
TSP	Total suspended particulates
UBA	Umweltbundesamt (German EPA)
UR	Unit Risk
USEPA	Environmental Protection Agency of the United States of America
VOCs	Volatile Organic Compounds
VSL	Value of a Statistical Life
WHO	World Health Organisation
WTA	Willingness-To-Accept
WTP	Willingness To Pay
YLD	Years Lived Disabled
YLL	Years Life Lost

SYMBOLS

A	Area
a	age
B	world-wide anthropogenic and geogenic emissions
C	Correction factor to calculate DALYs/ concentration
D	known Damage
DT50	half life time
E	Effect factor
EH	Ecological Health
F	Fate factor
H	Height of mixing layer
HH	Human Health
I	environmental Intervention
K	degree of age-weighting
K_{ow}	Octanol-water coefficient
L	standard expected years of life Lost
LT	Life Time
M	Manageability/ mass flow
m	manageability factor, specific mass flow
N	impact due to present environmental interventions in a fixed area during a fixed time-span (Normalisation value)
p	proxy equivalency factor
PEF	Potential Extrapolation Factor
R	ease of damage Reduction/ respiratory disease factor/ Resources
r	discount rate
S	Success of regulation
T	Target level/ Tumour incidence factor
τ	residence time
U	Unknown damage
V	dilution Volume
w	weighting factor
X	eXcess of long-term policy targets
β	parameter to calculate the shape of the age-weighting/of the population density
ρ	population density
σ_g	geometric standard deviation

INDICES

c	cultural perspective (individualists, egalitarians, hierarchists)
i	substances
j	compartment
k	exposure path
m	endpoint/cause
p	environmental problem

PREFACE

The development of advanced methods for Life Cycle Assessment has been my core interest for the last ten years. After having contributed to developments in Life Cycle Inventory Analysis, this book presents my propositions towards a second generation framework and method for Life Cycle Impact Assessment. Many of the suggested and operationalised elements are either based on other tools for environmental analysis, e.g., risk assessment, or may well be used in such other tools and concepts like, e.g., industrial ecology, technology assessment, environmental impact assessment. The reach of the presented framework goes therefore beyond the scope of presently used methods for Life Cycle Impact Assessment and may stimulate new developments in more than this area.

The research towards this aim has benefited from a twofold structure. At ETH Zurich I have greatly profited from the freedom provided me by Prof. Dr. Peter Suter (Energy Systems Laboratory, ETHZ), a professor with insightful perspectives who had supported the foundation of a research group in Life Cycle Assessment (ESU), and by Prof. Dr. Wolfgang Kröger (Chair of Safety Technology, ETHZ) and Prof. Dr. Roland W. Scholz (Chair of Environmental Sciences: Natural and Social Science Interface, ETHZ) who both made possible the continued existence of ESU even after Prof. Dr. Peter Suter's retirement. I would like to thank them for the confidence they placed in my research activities, the provided freedom that was necessary to develop the framework, the scientific support given whenever needed, and the motivation to bring this project with this book to a successful end. The ESU-group itself has, of course, been a great stimulus for the development of my thinking. Since 1993 I have also profited from close collaboration with Dr. Arthur Braunschweig and Prof. Dr. Ruedi Müller-Wenk from the Institute of Economy and Ecology (IWÖ) at the University of St. Gall and with Ruth Förster from EMPA St. Gall. Our common research projects on Life Cycle Impact Assessment have provoked many of the research questions that I address in this book and the discussions in that circle were a valuable source for the ideas and arguments used here.

Besides the many unnamed experts who answered my questions presented to them by e-mail and phone, I want to explicitly express my gratitude to Dr. Ch. Braun Fahrländer (University of Basle), Stephan Brunner (ex-ETHZ), Gabor Doka (consultant, Zürich), Dr. Rolf Frischknecht (ex-ETHZ, now ESU-services, Uster), Verena Gelpke (ETHZ), Christian Grasser (Kiefer & Partners, Zurich), Dr. Gunnar Grendstad (University of Bergen), Stefanie Hellweg (ETHZ), Dr. Olivier Jolliet (EPFL), Niels Jungbluth (ETHZ), Prof. Dr. Florian Kaiser (ETHZ), Dr. A. Kappos (Behörde für Arbeit, Gesundheit und Soziales, Hamburg), Dr. Detlef Keller (ITA-FhG, Hannover), Dr. Wolfram Krewitt (IER, University of Stuttgart), Annick Lalive d'Epinay (ETHZ), Dr. Peter Maier (ETHZ), Thomas Mettier (ETHZ), José Potting (DTU, Copenhagen), Dr. Ari Rabl (Ecole des Mines, Paris), Dr. Regula Rapp (University of Basle), Dr. Martin Scheringer (ETHZ), Dr. Georges Schüler (Cancer Register of the District Zurich), Dr. Johannes Schlatter (BAG, Zürich), Dr. Joseph Spadaro (Ecole des Mines, Paris), Prof. Dr. Michael Thompson (Musgrave Institute, London/University of Bergen), Dr. Olaf Tietje (ETHZ), Alfred Trukenmüller (IER, University of Stuttgart), Marjoleine van Asselt (ICIS, University of Maastricht), Dr.

Olaf Weber (ETHZ), Dr. André Weidenhaupt (ex-ETHZ, now Centre de Ressources des Technologies pour l'Environnement (Lux)), Dr. Sybille Wölfling (University of Berne), Dr. Nicoline Wrisberg (CML, Leiden), Dr. Devrim Yetergil Kiefer (ETHZ), my colleagues from the Dutch EcoIndicator-team headed by Mark Goedkoop (Pré, Amersfoort), and the colleagues from the SETAC-Europe working group on Life Cycle Impact Assessment for their detailed information and review comments on various parts of this book.

Many thanks go to Anton Küchler who made sure that the list of references is complete and looks as it does.

I will forever be grateful for Christine Weilenmann's support – for understanding the countless short weekends and for her assistance when it all came together and a great many things had to be taken care of at once.

The work on this book has profited from a number of different research projects close to the book's topic. They have been supported financially by the Swiss Priority Programme Environment (Swiss Science Foundation), the Daimler-Benz AG, and the research fund of the Swiss electricity utilities (PSEL). I would like to thank them for both the funding and the freedom they provided me within these projects.

Last but not least, I gratefully thank Dr. Thomas Baumgartner (CREATO/ETHZ) who has always tried his best to turn my drafts into something that sounded more like English and thus improved their understandability. Without his help I would not have been able to gain access to the potential readership provided by the large English-speaking community. Finally, Daniela Urbatzka looked through the final document through the glasses of an American. Many thanks go to her for pragmatically improving the language within a very short time.

From all this it is clear that the presented book has been supported and influenced by many colleagues. However, the sole responsibility for the content is mine.

Patrick Hofstetter

Chair of Environmental Sciences: Natural and Social Science Interface
Swiss Federal Institute of Technology (ETH Zurich)

ABSTRACT

Environmental Life Cycle Assessment (LCA) is a tool used to compare the environmental impacts along the life cycle of products. It thus supports the design of products which cause less harm to the environment. ISO separates distinguishes between four phases within LCA: the goal and scope definition, the inventory analysis, the impact assessment (LCIA), and the interpretation. The impact assessment phase as well as some aspects of the interpretation phase are the subject of this book.

LCA is a young tool which is still under development. In the course of its international standardisation ,*two main problems* have been identified: (1) LCA is full of subjectivity and does not properly separate objective from subjective elements, and (2) the impact assessment records phantoms rather than actual damages. This book suggests a new framework for LCA designed to master these two problems.

The new structure represents a radical departure from past attempts in LCA methodology development to distinguish clearly between so-called objective and subjective elements and to assign them to distinct process phases. It builds instead on the acceptance of the view that *LCA is the art of modelling and combining the valuesphere, the ecosphere, and the technosphere*. This basic structure is then particularised with the use and combination of elements developed independently in many different research fields in the natural, social, and medical sciences. The book's focus is on problems rather than disciplinary research questions that highlights the interface between natural and social sciences. The careful review and combination of these existing elements in the new structure results in a partly operationalised framework organised around a number of hypotheses. These have a high level of explanatory power for past developments and new trends and seem to offer a fruitful base for further validation.

The book offers concrete and pragmatic operationalisations of many of the hypotheses demonstrating that a consistent realisation of the framework is feasible in principle even though central elements remain in the status of hypotheses. The following elements are fully worked out in this book:

- The *valuesphere* is explicitly accepted as a sphere of its own and not seen as making up the undesired subjective elements which somehow have to be circumvented. The valuesphere therefore has to be modelled as such. An evaluation of models which characterise societal groups and their world views revealed that Cultural Theory serves well to model the valuesphere. Cultural Theory claims: (i) that people can be classified according to the degree that they organise themselves in groups and the degree to which individual lives are circumscribed by externally imposed prescriptions; (ii) that cultural biases can be understood as shared values and beliefs; and (iii) that there are five viable ways of life which combine different social relations and cultural biases. This theory serves to model value choices inherent in LCA in a way that is compatible with the values and beliefs of archetypes identified as viable ways of life. Only *three of the five archetypes* (hierarchists, individualists, and egalitarians) are considered because they are the only ones that actively take part in decision making. Consequently, this book offers not just one but three assessment systems. Each one is compatible with one of three active perspectives.

- The *ecosphere* is modelled by three submodels: a model for the known damage, a model for the unknown damage, and a model for the manageability of the damage.

  The model of the *known damage* includes causal effects by environmental interventions on safeguard subjects representing the environment. The model is operationalised for carcinogenic and respiratory effects in human beings and includes fate, exposure, effect, and damage analyses for a selection of more than 150 substances contributing to these effects. Damage to human health is measured in terms of disability adjusted life years (DALYs), a unit that is already used internationally and which is adapted here for use in LCA. The best estimate for the steady-state health damages in Europe due to actual emissions of carcinogenic substances resulted in a share of about 3% compared to all health damages (including all risk factors) and is dominated by the heavy metals and persistent organics. The same share for substances causing respiratory effects is estimated to be about 6% and is fully dominated by primary and secondary particles.

  The model of the *unknown damage* acknowledges that little is known so far on causal relationships in a system which is best characterised as overcomplex. The proxy index combines bioconcentration factors and world-wide emissions in order to consider the accumulating behaviour of, and the relative knowledge that is available on, a substance.

  The *manageability of damage* considers the dynamic aspects of the damages and is quantified by indicators for the ease of damage reduction, the excess of target damage, and the success of regulation.

- The *combination of the three spheres* is relatively easy because the outcome of the inventory analysis, i.e., the model of the *technosphere*, is already well known and presented in so-called inventory tables which are the direct input for the three submodels of the ecosphere. The ecosphere's submodels are chosen in such a way that their outcomes fulfil the requirements from all those archetypes considered to be active decision makers and that are characterised in the valuesphere. The interface between the valuesphere and the technosphere is described on the basis of two examples.

- A *graphical dominance analysis* is presented in order to improve the interpretation of the modelling results. Decisive rankings between alternatives can be made thanks to this new tool with as little weighting as necessary. This avoids the need to offer in all cases a full aggregation with a fixed weighting set which is the direction taken by several proposals to valuate environmental impacts in LCA.

This ambitious framework for LCA is partly operationalised and partly complemented with suggestions for a pragmatic operationalisation of those elements left inoperable. The framework is open for adjustments and the elements can be made operable by use of adequate models from the different disciplines concerned. A fourfold meaning of perspectives is worked out in this book: the LCA perspective of the world addressing the life-cycle view and its implications; the perspective of understanding LCA as a model of three spheres; the cultural perspectives leading to models that depend on world views; and finally the perspective of future developments supported by the openness of the framework.

Keywords: *Life Cycle Assessment, impact assessment, Cultural Theory, damage assessment, unknown damage, manageability, carcinogenic effects, respiratory effects, graphical dominance analysis*

1 Introduction to Life Cycle Assessment and its Positioning

The book's contribution is twofold: first to unveil the relationship between subjective and objective elements in Life Cycle Impact Assessment and to propose ways to deal with the natural and social science interface; and second to enhance the state-of-the art in modelling the ecosphere, i.e., to improve the predictions of impacts and other characteristics that are relevant in decision making supported by Life Cycle Assessment.

There are many ways we can model and analyse man-environment relations. Life Cycle Assessment (LCA) is just one of them. The purpose of this introduction is: to show how this tool can be viewed in comparison to the many other instruments for modelling and analysing man-environment relations and to make the reader familiar with the author's own understanding of what Life Cycle Assessment is.

The theme of this book is likely to be of interest to a wide range of people from different scientific disciplines and both to LCA specialists – developers of the instrument as well as the practitioners – and those interested in the topic for one reason or another with most likely only a general knowledge of the rapidly evolving field of LCA. That is to say that the readers will approach this book with widely different backgrounds, uneven familiarity with LCA, and possibly very specific interests. Given the broad array of questions and fields of sciences coming together under the umbrella of Life Cycle Impact Assessment, the likely reader of this book will be faced with theories and information from many different fields of research and with new elements concerning many – but by far not all – open questions.

The following overview of the book's structure sets forth out the main line of argumentation and suggests sequences of chapters that might be best suited for one or the other of the readers. This overview should enable each reader to find her or his optimal path through the book and to skip over those sections whose theme or arguments are already familiar or that do not address aspects that she or he might consider as central to the further development of LCA.

1.1 Reader's guide

The subject matter dealt with in this book can be seen as belonging to one of four parts:

Part I: *The Discussion Setting.* Chapters 1 and 2 introduce the state of the art of Life Cycle Assessment, identify the questions that are still open and the problems that remain as yet unresolved. A set of propositions are formulated with respect to these problems that will be in part verified within this book.

Part II: *Framework and Methods.* Chapters 3 to 5 are the methodological heart of the book. Here we introduce:

- a method to model the valuesphere (Chapter 3),
- a new framework to model environmental impacts based on the three pillars 'damage', 'unknown damage', and 'manageability of damage' (Chapter 4), and
- a method to aggregate damages to human health (Chapter 5)

Part III: *Case Studies.* This part contains two case studies which operationalise the framework and methods proposed and introduced in Part II. The two cases concern carcinogenic and respiratory effects on human beings due to environmental pollution. Damage factors are calculated for 55 carcinogenic substances (Chapter 6) and for about 120 substances causing respiratory effects (Chapter 7).

Part IV: *Results, Consequences and Conclusions.* A graphical dominance analysis helps to interpret the framework's results (Section 8.1). The universality of the framework presented in Part II allows its use both as a meta-method and within all other phases of LCA (Sections 8.2&8.3). A critical discussion of the approach in Chapter 9 leads to the identification of further research needs. The final Chapter, 10, unveils the meaning of 'perspectives' used in the book's title, reflects critically on the support for the propositions set out in Chapter 2, summarises the new findings, discusses the contribution made in this book to solve the identified problems, and gives an outlook for each of the broad group of readers.

This book's main audience will be the LCA community:

- LCA commissioners may be interested in Chapter 1, where the tool is positioned and the commissioner can check whether other tools may be more appropriate. Section 8.1 may be interesting to get an idea about what kind of decision support they can expect from LCA.
- LCA practitioners and analysts may turn directly to the operationalised parts of the impact assessment for carcinogenic and respiratory effects in human beings in Chapters 6 and 7 respectively. It should also be possible to use or adapt these damage assessments to other methods for LCIA.
- Purely methodology-oriented developers of Life Cycle Impact Assessment methodology are referred to Chapters 2.2, 3.2, 3.4, 4, 5.4, 8 and 9.

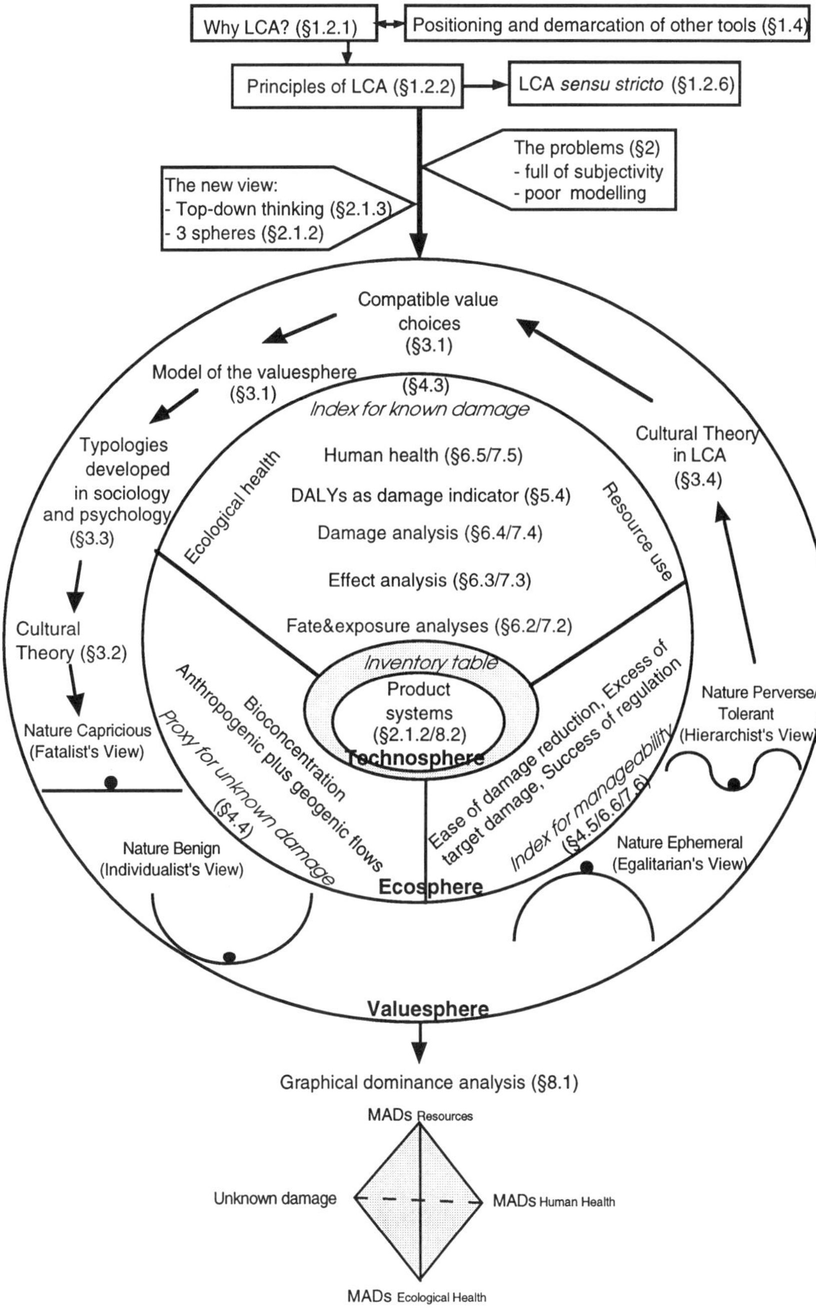

Fig. 1.1: Visualisation of the book's content, numbers after the sign "§" indicate the chapter, section, or subsection where the element is described.

- Researchers specialised in the subjective and weighting steps within Life Cycle Impact Assessment will find Chapters 3, 4 and 8 valuable.

- Software developers are primarily referred to Chapters 4 and 8 to get a feeling for the flexibility needed from the software (concerning structure and computing functions) and the possibilities of graphic presentation in the weighting triangle or tetrahedron.

However, parts of the book may well be relevant for other scientists, i.e.:

- Researchers familiar with environmental tools other than LCA may be attracted by Chapter 1 to learn more about LCA and its positioning within the area of modelling of and accounting for man-environment relations and by Chapters 3, 4, and 8 in order to profit from the methods presented there, which are able to be generalised and therefore can be used for other environmental tools as well.
- Researchers in the field of calculating externalities by the damage cost approach or in the fields of risk assessment may profit in addition from the quantitative data provided in Chapters 6 and 7, which may also serve as a first screening.
- Modelers which are looking for more meaningful ways to construct scenarios compatible with cultural perspectives are referred to Chapter 3.
- Scientists in public health will profit from the fully quantified causal chains from emission to exposure, to effects, and to damage on human health. These are provided for 55 carcinogenic substances (Chapter 6) and about 120 substances contributing to respiratory effects (Chapter 7).

Figure 1.1 tries to help at this point to be more specific about the book's structure. Based on the introduction, characterisation and positioning of LCA in the first chapter, Chapter 2 elaborates on the two problems of subjectivity and poor modelling that have been identified in Chapter 2 and suggests how a new view towards LCA could help to overcome them. It is suggested that LCA be understood as a tool to model and combine three spheres: the valuesphere, the ecosphere, and the technosphere. The visualisation of the book in Figure 1.1 represents this structure of the three spheres. The largest concentric circle symbolises the valuesphere, the middle one the ecosphere and the two small ellipses the technosphere and its interface to the ecosphere. The ecosphere is divided into three submodels which will be introduced in Section 4.2.

The interpretation phase of LCA can be located within the interface of the ecosphere and valuesphere. But it is drawn here outside the circles to keep the drawing simpler. Its graphical representation – shown here as a weighting tetrahedron – will be introduced in Section 8.1.

The figure's aim is to help orient the readers and guide them in focusing on those specific elements within the framework that might be of special interest.

1.2 LCA – a short introduction

Introducing LCA requires a book in itself. But this is not our main purpose. Here we will focus only on the basics of LCA and those aspects that are relevant for the subsequent developments which are the focus of this book. Good introductions to LCA can be found in, e.g., Heijungs *et al.* (1992), SETAC (1993b), Lindfors *et al.* (1995), ISO (1997), and ISO (1998). The terminology used here draws on Udo de Haes (1996) and ISO (1997/98).

We do not go into the motivations that led to the development of LCA nor do we provide a history of this development. However, one can make the observation that the tools to provide information along the life cycle of a product are only needed if the economy is organised based on the principle of the division of labour. Therefore, first attempts at LCA can be traced as far back as the 19th century with Jevons (1965) and his coal question (1865) and with the accounting system proposed by Geddes (1884). Renewed interest in LCA-like tools emerged at the end of the sixties and in the seventies in connection with packaging wastes and the energy crisis (Jansen *et al.* 1972, Hunt *et al.* 1974, Basler & Hofmann 1974, Müller-Wenk 1978). A generalisation of these instruments and attempts to standardise them have been the hallmark of the nineties and we will focus here exclusively on these most recent developments.

1.2.1 The place of LCA

At least since the beginning of industrialisation, the specie *homo sapiens* is the source of observed, expected and predicted environmental damages for which the culprits are both increasing population and increasing needs. Formula (1.1) makes explicit the thinking behind this last sentence[1] (adapted from Basler (1971:86), Daly (1991:78)).

$$WD = \underset{(P)}{\text{population}} \cdot \left(\underset{(S)}{\frac{\text{service gained}}{\text{person}}} \cdot \underset{(C)}{\frac{\text{consumption}}{\text{service gained}}} \cdot \underset{(T)}{\frac{\text{throughput}}{\text{consumption}}} \cdot \underset{(I)}{\frac{\text{envir. impact}}{\text{throughput}}} \cdot \underset{(D)}{\frac{\text{envir. damage}}{\text{envir. impact}}}\right) \quad (1.1)$$

where: WD = Total world-wide environmental damages

This formula also underlies the approach chosen by LCA. LCA is neither concerned with a regulation of the size of population (factor P) nor does it question the demand for services by this population (factor S). LCA is concerned only with the environmentally efficient provision of these services. Its aim is to provide the information that makes three things possible:

- to generate as many services as possible with the least amount of products, i.e., to have intelligently conceived products with a long life and that can be shared (factor C),

[1] Basler (1971) introduced a similar formula to identify the different "knobs" we can turn to reduce environmental damages. Daly (1991) uses only the four last ratios of the formula. The rationale behind this simplified world model is the possibility to separate growth from development. Daly states that it is essential for a steady-state economy to keep constant at least the four ratios. For development he postulates that a decrease in these ratios is necessary.

- to produce these products with a minimal material flow, i.e., the production efficiency is maximised (factor T),
- to reduce, as much as possible, environmental interventions per industrial throughput, i.e., to apply clean technology and to minimise wastes (factor I).

The final factor (D) describes the environmental consequences of doing this in terms of damage from the environmental interventions emanating from the industrial metabolism. LCA models the environmental damage per service gained in order to either compare this ratio for alternative ways to provide the given service or to identify those processes that dominate environmental interventions.

This characterisation of LCA should make it clear from the outset that LCA will not be the tool with which to check the conformity of processes, products or consumption styles with sustainable development. It is only one of the tools that can be used to minimise the environmental impacts per service unit[2]. Meadows *et al.* (1992) suggest policies to influence all the factors contained in Equation (1.1). The population growth factor (P) could be influenced according to Meadows *et al.* (1992) through family planning, the schooling of women, the provision of social care systems, the improvement of the socio-economic position of women, and access to, and ownership of, land. The factor (S), the services demanded per capita, could be influenced by complete cost accounting and setting prices accordingly, but also by focusing on societal goals, value changes, and a discussion of 'how much is enough'.

The aim of LCA is to integrate environmental goods in the accounting frame and thus to attribute damages to environmental goods to service units in the same way that all service units have economic values expressed in monetary terms. Once damages to environmental goods are accountable, they become explicit and transparent and can be considered in the decision making process of consumers, managers and politicians[3].

1.2.2 Basic principles of LCA and attempts towards its epistemological foundation

According to SETAC (1993b:7) LCA "... is an objective process to evaluate the environmental burdens associated with a product, process or activity by identifying and quantifying energy and materials used and wastes released to the environment, to assess the impact of those energy and material uses and releases to the environment, and to evaluate and implement opportunities to affect environmental improvements. The assessment includes the entire life cycle of the product, process or activity, encompassing extracting and processing raw materials, manufacturing, transportation and distribution; use, re-use, maintenance; recycling and final disposal." LCA is a young tool and almost all the methodological developments have occurred within the last decade. Therefore, ISO (1997) defines LCA in already a slightly different manner

[2] LCA is not the tool that prevents the "ship" from sinking. It can only help the "ship" do this at the latest point in time possible.

[3] This aim to make LCA into a powerful tool for decision making leads to problems in its standardisation because some industry representatives do not want the instrument to have this integrative force (see, e.g., Owens 1995, Barnthouse *et al.* 1997, ISO 1998)

as: "Compilation and evaluation of the inputs, outputs and the potential environmental impacts of a product system throughout its life cycle."

Both definitions confirm to some extent the following basic principles of LCA:

- Full life cycles from cradle to grave are analysed.
- All relevant environmental interventions along the life cycle are reported and their impacts assessed.
- Environmental interventions are attributed to products which can consist of goods, processes, services or activities.
- LCA supports decisions.

The objectivity of the process as claimed by the definition from SETAC (1993b) is discussed nowadays more critically and one separates today explicitly subjective from objective elements (see next subsection). LCA combines normative with descriptive elements. This makes LCA a prescriptive tool appropriate for real world decision support (Jungermann 1976, Keeney 1992, Raiffa 1994) (see also Section 1.5).

Heijungs (1997) claims that LCA is still premature due to its lack of an epistemological foundation. Traditional validation by experiment fails because the dimensions of time and of place are not considered in the description of the product system and its interventions while they are essential to the observation of environmental damages. In addition, observed environmental effects cannot be attributed unambiguously to economic activities (Heijungs 1997).

Heijungs (1998) offers a first insight into how he would like to epistemologically ground LCA. For this purpose he makes use of the notions of *definitions, axioms*, and *theorems*[4]. The starting point for his axiomatic is reproduced here in the same order as in Heijungs (1998:180ff) but without giving the proofs provided in that text:

Definition 1: LCA is a process to evaluate the environmental burdens associated with deriving utility[5] from a product, whereby the entire life cycle of the product is included.

Axiom 1: Deriving less utility with the same product should give an environmentally preferable result.

Axiom 2: Producing less environmental burdens for deriving the same utility should give an environmentally preferable result.

Theorem 1: LCA is a quantitative method, and there exists a mathematical function which maps the amount of utility derived from a product to an assessment.

Definition 2: The mathematical function which maps an amount of utility derived from a product to a quantitative assessment is defined as:

$$\mathbf{LCA}: \alpha_x \rightarrow \mathbf{LCA}(\alpha_x) \tag{1.2}$$

[4] Both definitions and axioms cannot be proven, while theorems are proven by the use of definitions, axioms and logic. Definitions, as distinct from axioms, do not imply the existence of the concepts thus defined.

[5] In the language of LCA one would speak from function measured by the functional unit rather than from utility.

where α_X represents the fulfilment of a specified utility α by a certain product x, and **LCA** represents the vector-valued function.

Theorem 2: The function $\mathbf{LCA}(\alpha_x)$ is a monotonous function of α_x, the amount of utility derived.

Axiom 3: If α_x and $\alpha'_{x'}$ represent two utilities derived from two products x and x', the sum of $\mathbf{LCA}(\alpha_x)$ and $\mathbf{LCA}(\alpha'_{x'})$ is equal to $\mathbf{LCA}(\alpha_x + \alpha'_{x'})$.

Theorem 3: $\mathbf{LCA}(\alpha_x)$ is a linear function of the utility derived:

$$\mathbf{LCA}(y \cdot \alpha_x) + \mathbf{LCA}(z \cdot \alpha'_{x'}) = y \cdot \mathbf{LCA}(\alpha_x) + z \cdot \mathbf{LCA}(\alpha'_{x'}) \quad (1.3)$$

where y and z represent real coefficients.

Theorem 4: LCA is based on modelling of the burdens of flows from the life cycle, and not on *in situ* measurements of burdens.

Theorem 5: LCA cannot predict actually occurring burdens.

Theorem 6: LCA cannot answer the question whether a standard or a threshold is exceeded.

If one agrees with the stated definitions and axioms, the theorems describe additional characteristics of LCA. Important characteristics are the inherently quantitative nature of the modelling approach, the prediction of potential rather than of actually occurring burdens, and the incapacity of LCA to control the overshooting of a threshold. By varying the definitions and axioms one can create other types of LCA (see subsection 1.2.5 and Heijungs (1998)) or even other environmental tools (Heijungs 1997). However, an axiomatic epistemological foundation will necessarily highlight the normative elements of a tool. It follows that the prescriptive strength of LCA necessary for a robust decision support cannot be grounded in an axiomatic way alone.

1.2.3 The structure of LCA

The internationally co-ordinated debate on the features and the structure of LCA began in 1990 when the Society for Environmental Toxicology and Chemistry (SETAC) started with its activities in the field of LCA. The structure of LCA has been refined and the definition of terms internationally harmonised through a series of documents from SETAC (1991/1992/1993a/b) and Heijungs *et al.* (1992). ISO, the international standardisation organisation, started in 1994 an initiative to establish standards in environmental management (ISO 14000ff). LCA (ISO 14040ff) is one of the management instruments thus standardised. We present in Figure 1.2 the current proposal (early 1998) for the structure of LCA and its terminology, relying for this on ISO (1997/98).

Succinctly described, LCA is an iterative procedure made up the four phases in Figure 1.2 that are executed for several rounds and which serves as a decision support. Only the phase of 'Impact Assessment' in Figure 1.2 is here subdivided in substeps because this phase is of special relevance for this book. But all the other phases can be similarly divided into substeps.

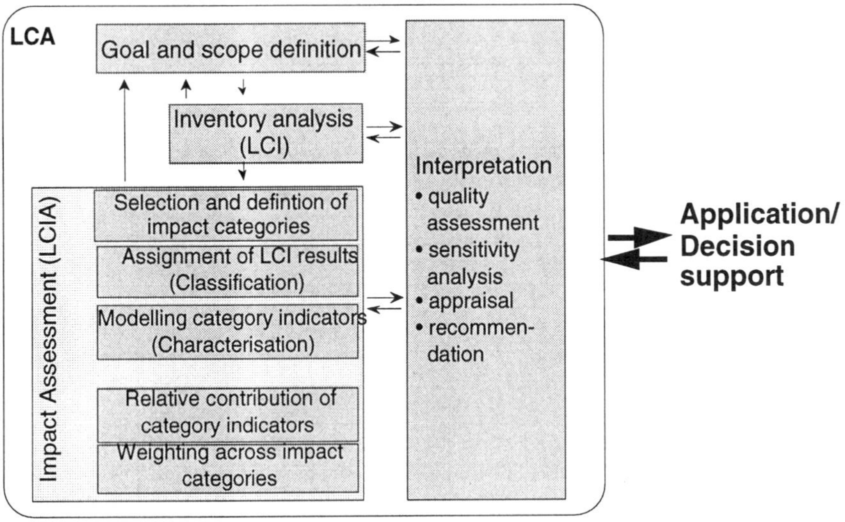

Fig. 1.2: Structure and terms of LCA (adapted from ISO (1997) and ISO (1998))

The phases can be described as follows :

- In the phase of the goal and scope definition one defines the functional unit, selects the product systems to be analysed, defines the scope of the analysis including the setting of system boundaries. It is primarily a normative phase where value choices dominate.
- The life cycle inventory analysis (LCI) describes the product system with all the processes that are considered to contribute in a relevant way to those environmental interventions that have been prioritised in the scope definition. The consideration of all relevant processes is a difficult task for practical reasons and thus some selection is almost always necessary. And especially the process of allocating environmental interventions to the functional unit is partly based on value choices. The outcome of the inventory analysis is an inventory table listing environmental interventions per functional unit.
- The phase of life cycle impact assessment (LCIA) "assists in the understanding of LCI results, making these results more manageable in relation to the natural environment, human health, and resources and may identify the relative significance of the LCI results" (ISO 1998). In a first step, the impact categories are selected in accordance with the goal and scope definition and then unambiguously defined. The environmental interventions listed in the inventory table are in a next step classified according to these impact categories (some of the interventions belong to more than one category). In the characterisation step one models the indicator for each category ('category indicator') for the different interventions that cause environmental impacts. E.g., the radiative forcing of gases contributing to global warming are modelled or the potential to acidify soil and water is assessed. The steps of relative contribution of category indicators and weighting allow for comparisons across impact categories in order to add information on the environmental priorities. The relative contribution of category indicators is calculated by the division through the score of the same category indicator for a

specified area during a specified time duration, e.g., for Europe during one year. Methods for the weighting across impact categories will be presented in the next section. The first and the last of these five steps are considered to be fully subjective and their determination therefore has to follow a transparent procedure.

- The phase of 'interpretation' has been introduced by ISO and acknowledges the fact that all phases provide information relevant for the decision maker, that uncertainty plays a major role in all phases and has to be assessed, and that LCA results should be prepared in a balanced way for the decision making process.

The final application of the LCA results as decision support lies outside the scope of LCA (see next subsection).

The structure presented in Figure 1.2 is the product of ISO's aim to distinguish between subjective and objective elements in LCA – and – to make LCA as objective as possible. The 'goal and scope definition', the 'selection and definition of impact categories', the 'weighting across impact categories', elements of the 'interpretation' phase, and allocation in the inventory analysis are considered as value-laden choices which should be separated as much as possible from the more value-free, i.e., objective elements. Such a division is understandable and has many advantages in the operationalisation and communication of the tool. However, such separations have been questioned in other tools (Hyman *et al.* 1988). In this book we will develop another approach to take care of the subjective elements than the one chosen by ISO (see Section 2.1 and Chapters 3ff).

The first iteration in an LCA, i.e., the first execution of all the four phases identified in Fig. 1.2, is sometimes called a screening. Special methods are under development to reduce the effort that has to be put into such an exercise and yet to improve the quality of insights than can be expected from such a shortened procedure (Christiansen 1997).

1.2.4 Typical applications

The applications of LCA sometimes decisively influence the structure of the procedure, the way value choices can be made, and the type of model which is used (see, e.g., Braunschweig *et al.* 1996:16ff). Typical applications are (see, e.g., Udo de Haes (1993), ISO (1997)):

- Product development and improvement, including eco-design and the identification of weak points (optimisation)
- Strategic planning
- Public policy-making
- Marketing and product information to consumers to support product comparisons

In addition LCA can assist in:

- Environmental management systems
- Environmental performance evaluation
- Environmental labelling

The applications in product development, weak-point identification, product comparisons, and consumer information are those foremost in mind in this book whenever reference is made to decision-makers or to the requirements of operationalisation[6].

1.2.5 There is more than one type of LCA

The previous subsection mentioned applications such as weak-point identification, product information, or environmental labelling, for which primarily information on the present status quo is required. Public policy-making or product development and improvement are, in contrast, much more change-oriented.

The first set of applications can be called the *attribution case.* The central question here is which share of environmental impacts has to be attributed to which process or product. The second set is the *change-oriented case.* Here the question is how much the environmental impacts will increase or decrease if in the future product (A) will be produced according to an alternative design. The first case is the static case, which aims to attribute all environmental impacts to all provided services. The second is the dynamic one where the marginal changes are of interest. Such different applications of LCA will lead to different scope definitions, and to different models in the inventory analysis and in the impact assessment (see, e.g., Frischknecht 1997/1998, Heijungs 1997). Heijungs *et al.* (1992) have already addressed these different cases and they recommended the use of long term marginal data in the second instance. In addition, the important notion of *ceteris paribus* has been introduced in the context of this discussion. This notion says that the functional unit at hand, with its product system, will be analysed assuming that all other processes will stay as they are, i.e., the millions of decisions on processes and products that are made at the same time (world-wide) and their consequences will be left unconsidered.

Other differences between LCAs concern the degree of information on release time, release and receptor site, and further specific characteristics like source strength and release temperature. Most known LCAs disregard time and space. Environmental interventions of the same type are added up independent of the exact place where the emissions occur or of their temporal profile or the season during which they happen. There are a few approaches to LCA that are more site-specific or at least site-dependent (Giegrich 1994, Potting *et al.* 1994, Potting *et al.* 1997, Hogan *et al.* 1996, Udo de Haes 1996, Assies 1997, Hillier *et al.* 1997). The main aim of these latter approaches is to consider more accurately the receptors that are really exposed and their sensitivity to the substances to which they are exposed. In the case of substance emissions showing a threshold behaviour, additional information on background concentrations may help to decide whether any effects are to be expected at all. In this context, White *et al.* (1995) introduced another distinction: *'less is better'* versus *'only above threshold approach'.* 'Less is better' follows the precautio-

[6] It is not possible to go further into the consequences of this distinction here. However, strategic planning has a very long time horizon and this causes special problems (see Subsection 1.4.4). Public policy making, in contrast, is a very special application because politicians are the decision-makers. They can decide in place of societal interests; they have little knowledge about the ecosphere; but they are quite able to weigh alternatives and therefore want to weight themselves across impact categories. The requirements for the tools that use LCA in an assisting role only may differ from those that are considered important in LCA.

nary principle and is based on the epistemological foundation suggested by Heijungs (1998) (see Subsection 1.2.2). The 'only above threshold approach' focuses instead on environmental interventions that will cause effects at the point of the receptor, i.e., contribute to exposure concentrations or doses which surpass thresholds.

The terms *foreground and background system* have been introduced in order to reflect more specific information in the model for the inventory analysis and the impact assessment for the foreground system. Foreground processes consist of processes which are within the control or freedom of choice of the decision maker commissioning the LCA study (Frischknecht 1998:57). Control, in this instance, means that all other decisions relevant for the system are known, can be influenced, and their impacts can be considered (i.e., the *ceteris paribus* assumption is no more valid here), that the temporal and spatial resolution of information is maximal for this system, and that a dynamic modelling is possible. The background system – in contrast – is largely under the control of others and cannot be shifted into a state that might be desired by those commissioning the LCA. Although the formal procedure for making such a distinction between systems does not yet exist, many case studies have used this distinction automatically by adding more details of, and calculating several scenarios for, those processes that are well known while sticking to average data gained from perusing the literature for all other processes.

1.2.6 "Our" LCA *sensu stricto*

Due to the many differences identified in LCA methods, it makes sense to specify more exactly what we mean when we speak of LCA. SETAC (1993b) and Hofstetter (1996b:127ff) have created the term of "LCA *sensu stricto*" to designate one specific approach to LCA[7]. Subsequent discussions have suggested the need to become even more specific in stating the conditions and requirements. When we refer in this book to an LCA *sensu stricto,* we refer therefore to an LCA, which:

- only considers the dimension "environment", i.e., the dimensions society and economy are not analysed and also, e.g., occupational health is disregarded[8],
- includes no detailed information on the time pattern of releases and it can be assumed consequently that all environmental interventions occur today,
- includes no detailed information on the site of releases and it can be assumed therefore that all environmental interventions occur in places with meteorological conditions, eco-system sensitivities, and densities of receptors that are typical for, e.g., Western Europe,
- analyses functional units that are small enough to cause incremental changes only,
- relies on fully quantitative information on a ratio scale,
- is based on simple linear or linearised models,
- allows for trade-offs between different kinds of environmental impacts, i.e., they have a compensatory character (additive disutility function),

---

[7] Which does not mean that the other approaches to LCA will loose their claim to also be LCA.

[8] This last exclusion is currently still disputed (see, e.g., Udo de Haes *et al.* 1997). It is excluded here based on the criterion that the dimension environment concerns damage which is exerted via the ecosphere, which is not fulfilled in the case of working places (Müller-Wenk 1997:9).

- refers to the change-oriented approach, i.e., is interested in marginal environmental interventions and environmental damages,
- respects *ceteris paribus*, i.e., assumes that all other processes will stay as they are,
- follows the 'less is better' approach, and
- consists only of a background system, i.e., the special case of foreground systems with all the modelling parameters known is not considered.

The consequence of all these restrictions is that one can assess, at best, potential damages with an LCA *sensu stricto*. In Chapters 4, 6, and 7, methodological elements are sometimes mentioned that would make it possible to carry out less restricted kinds of LCA. In one respect, this definition of LCA *sensu stricto* goes beyond the requirement of the established methodology; the change-oriented view requires a modelling of marginal changes, at least within the phase of impact assessment. A detailed discussion of the consequences stemming from this requirement for the inventory analysis can be found in Frischknecht (1998).

The restrictions mentioned above imply that LCA *sensu stricto* makes use of a very simple model to represent a dynamic anthroposphere and very complex ecosphere. The limited aspiration to model only small changes due to single functional units justifies these simplifications. Tools based on less restrictive modelling assumptions are discussed in Section 1.5.

1.3 Overview of methods for Life Cycle Impact Assessment

A comprehensive introduction to, and discussions of, methods that are available for Life Cycle Impact Assessment (LCIA) can be found in Braunschweig *et al.* (1994/1996), Finnveden (1996), Giegrich *et al.* (1995), Lindfors *et al.* (1995), Udo de Haes (1996), and Hertwich *et al.* (1997). The purpose of this section is to just provide a typology for comparing weighting methods and a set of references for each type of LCIA method[9].

1.3.1 A typology for weighting methods

In Table 1.1 we classify the weighting methods used and known to us according to two criteria (Hofstetter 1996b:135ff):

- Firstly we ask if the principle used more follows a bottom-up approach by weighting directly environmental interventions, or a top-down approach by looking to environmental problems and effects in the environment. This distinction is not exclusive because, e.g., authoritative goals[10] on an intervention level also take the different effects and environmental problems (mostly implicit) into account. But from an LCA perspective, this distinction is defensible because the starting point for the weighting method lies in the first (intervention-based) case after the inventory analysis, and in the second (effect-oriented) case after the characterisation step.
- The second criterion for the typology differentiates partly between the different ways to express preferences, and partly between the extents to which the weighting principles model the environmental damages.

  Proxy indicators are indicators which are, once they are normatively selected, easy to measure or calculate with a low level of subjectivity. The indicators are strongly non-identical[11], i.e., they do not model but stand as a proxy for an environmental damage.

  Methods which use the *characteristics of abatement technology and of the market mechanism* to derive weights are classified on a higher level. The weights derived are still non-identical, i.e., they do not directly address an environmental damage, but assume an indirect relation with it (revealed preferences).

  Panel methods are used to derive perceptions of the importance of environmental damages. The weights derived are therefore partly identical or even identical (expressed preferences).

  Using *authoritative goals and targets* as a weighting principle does not represent an even higher level or a more explicit formulation of weights than the panel

---

[9] This overview is a shortened version of Hofstetter (1996b:135ff) that has been updated with some more recent references.

[10] These are goals that have been implicitly defined through, or explicitly stated in, environmental policy documents and laws.

[11] In system analysis, we can distinguish between identical, partly-identical, and non-identical indicators. In this order, the descriptive character of the indicators decreases and the tendency to act as a proxy increases.

methods do. But many weighting methods use this principle. This justifies a separate listing for this method. In principle, it would be possible to derive an identical index from environmental policy and from panels if environmental policy was based on negotiated weighting sets. But this is not the case and so we are compelled to base the weights on authoritative targets and goals. The resulting methods work therefore with partly identical indices only.

Weighting principle	Intervention-based methods	Effect-oriented methods
Proxy indicator(s)	Relation of man-made to natural interventions Energy demand MIPS Dilution space and environmental lifetime	
Characteristics of abatement technology and of the market mechanism	Abatement energy/exergy Abatement (prevention, avoidance) costs Ecological footprint (resource oriented)	Damage costs Abatement costs at actual level Abatement costs at target level
Panel	Expert panel	Expert panel Non-expert panel Willingness to pay/sell
Authoritative goals and targets	Ecological footprint (emission oriented) Critical surface time Distance to policy targets	Distance to policy targets Distance to sustainability levels

Tab. 1.1: Typology of weighting principles used in weighting methods

1.3.2 Approaches using proxy indicators

These approaches are based on the observation that environmental mechanisms are overcomplex. It is impossible to ever understand all the mechanisms involved in eco-system behaviour (Berg *et al.* 1994). These methods therefore make use of proxies in place of directly modelling complexity. A proxy is easier to derive while it is assumed to still show the right direction of impact development.

Several popular methods represent this philosophy. *Cumulated* (direct and indirect) *energy demand* was seen as a good approximation for system optimisation at the end of the sixties and in the seventies (IFIAS 1974, Boustead *et al.* 1979, Schaefer 1982). Only recently, a new standard has been formulated to formalise the calculation of cumulated energy demand (VDI 1995)[12].

The concept of mass intensity per service unit (MIPS) uses *displaced materials* measured in mass units as proxy (Schmidt-Bleek 1992). Scheringer *et al.* (1994a) calculate the dilution space and the environmental lifetime of emissions. Through a formalised procedure they derive two indicators which are not combined further. The use of undisturbed nature as a baseline partly can be classified as a proxy method. *Geogenic flows or concentrations* are used as an evaluation base in material flow analysis (e.g., Baccini *et al.* 1991) and proposed for life cycle impact assessment by Hofstetter (1991). In Section 4.4 we will develop our own proxy indicator as an element of the framework proposed in this book.

[12] Frischknecht *et al.* (forthcoming) discuss, in detail, the foundation for and the positioning of different approaches using energy as a proxy indicator.

1.3.3 Characteristics of abatement technology and of the market mechanism

These methods use the efforts made to abate or displace environmental interventions or impacts as an indicator of their relevance. The strength and originality of these methods lie in their self-regulating and improvement-oriented nature. Something will become subject to action because the need to reduce or abate is judged to be relevant on the basis of its need for a lot of energy, money or land. As a consequence, less interventions can be expected in the future and this will reduce the effort required for control. It is also likely that one response to the problem will be spending resources on technical developments that ultimately will reduce abatement costs for such interventions, thus making control of them relatively less important.

Bauer (1992) and Cramer *et al.* (1993), for example, propose to account for the *energy or exergy effort required for the abatement* of environmental interventions. *Abatement costs*, sometimes also referred to as *prevention and avoidance costs*, are used widely in energy planning, e.g., by Destribats (1990) and Putta (1991). Tellus (1992) and Hofstetter (1991) use them as an intervention-based approach in LCA. They are developed in a more effect-oriented approach by, e.g., Krozer (1992) and, in some aspects, in Tellus (1992). Krozer (1992) differentiates between two approaches.: In one of them, he determines abatement costs given the actual level of pollution and existing technology; in the other, by using the target levels defined in the Dutch National Environment Plan as political targets (leading to much higher abatement costs). (This second approach is a method that belongs also to those discussed in Subsection 1.3.5.) The use of damage costs to infrastructure and economic goods can also be seen as belonging to this class of methods. Steen *et al.* (1992) use this type of costs but only in a minor number of cases.

Steen *et al.* (1992) use alternative ways of resource production or the land surface required for the renewable production of consumed resources to weight resource depletion. The ecological footprint approaches used by Wackernagel *et al.* (1993) and Krotschek *et al.* (1994) also make use of these two principles.

The weighting principles presented here mix economic, technical, and environmental mechanisms and information in order to derive weighting factors. The damage-oriented approaches which analyse damages to endpoints like human health and ecosystems health are not subsumed here under market mechanisms (see, e.g., ExternE 1995, ESEERCO 1995, Rabl *et al.* 1996a/b/1997a/b, Krewitt *et al.* 1996/1997, Goedkoop *et al.* 1997). However, the valuation of the endpoints themselves can be based on market mechanisms or panel methods (see next subsection). The damage-oriented analysis will be extensively used in this book in Chapters 4 to 7.

1.3.4 Panel-oriented approaches

Panels applied within LCA are so far mostly expert panels and are in most cases just one element within the whole impact assessment. Brunner (1998) provides an introduction to panel methods and their application in LCA weighting.

Wilson *et al.* (1994) is the only instance known to us where the panel method has been applied as part of an intervention-based approach to LCA. The authors used the Delphi method with experts. Several institutes have worked on effect-oriented approaches using panel methods. UBA (1994) has used qualitative weights determined by an expert panel in an LCA for beverages. Other methods have so far been just proposed or executed as a pilot. Volkwein *et al.* (1996a/b) use a case-by-case approach similar to the one used by UBA (1994), but follow a more structured procedure. Expert panels were used in this case to link three pre-defined criteria with the results of the case. Christiansen *et al.* (1990) have developed a completely expert-based qualitative weighting system. This system is designed to be applied separately for each case and for the different steps of the life cycle. McKinsey has developed a scheme for valuation by a panel that uses a kind of cost and damage matrix adapted from management sciences (reported in VNCI (1991)). To our knowledge, this scheme has never been fully applied. Kortman *et al.* (1994) have used a small group of 20 experts and stakeholders to perform several weighting exercises based on an adapted Delphi method. After a first round, the panel was confronted with additional information and results from another weighting method. The panellists were also asked to explicitly state the criteria they used for weighting. Nagata *et al.* (1995) have used several different reference groups and three related weighting procedures (ranking method, score allocation method, and the analytical hierarchy process method). Further methods, like the iso-utility approach, have been proposed in the recent past for the weighting step in LCA by Heijungs (1994a/b), Tukker (1994), and Weidema (1994b).

Herbert *et al.* (1992) organised a panel study outside of LCA in Germany with about 400 experts and stakeholders from different societal groups. This interesting work concentrated on a mixture of effect-oriented and intervention-based environmental topics.

The contingent valuation methods used in economics can be seen as a more formal variant of panel methods. Many different approaches are made use of in this context such as 'willingness to pay', 'willingness to accept', 'willingness to sacrifice', 'willingness to sell', 'hedonic prices', and 'travel costs'. Pearce *et al.* (1994) is a good source for more details concerning the economic theory behind all of them. Steen *et al.* (1992) partly use such information within their method. The main difference to the above mentioned panel methods is that the weighting is determined in relation to other monetary expenditures or incomes instead of a relative weighting between environmental problems. Next to the problems of all panel methods, the problem of systematic overestimation of selling prices is added to boot (Pearce *et al.* 1994, Spash *et al.* 1995).

Hofstetter (1996b:139f) contains a critical analysis of panel methods as used within LCA. Chapter 4 and 9 in this book will show that a prescriptive approach can be chosen to design a new framework, but that many of the choices required still need to be subjected to more empirical validation applying panel methods.

1.3.5 Authoritative goals and targets

One can differentiate between two groups of methods that fall within this principle. One of them uses national regulations on single substances that limit their concentrations or their freights. The other makes use of effect-oriented targets that are formulated as short or long term goals by national governments or international bodies.

To the first group belong developments of the critical volume approach developed in Jansen *et al.* (1972) and Basler & Hofmann (1974) which became widely known after the publication of BUWAL (1984). These developments concern the introduction of the equivalency principle to add up critical volumes of air, water, and land use (Thalmann-Graf 1991, Hofstetter 1991/1993, Schaltegger *et al.* 1992, Gebler 1992, Jolliet 1993a). The equivalency principles used refer mostly to some physical or natural effects and the results are, in our view, rather arbitrary.

The Swiss ecoscarcity approach applies policy targets on total loads of single substances and additional statements from Swiss environmental policy (Müller-Wenk 1978, Braunschweig 1988, Ahbe *et al.* 1990, BUWAL 1998). This target level is interpreted in such a way that the ratio formed by the actual and the target load should reflect the importance of the environmental threat caused by a substance. This system has since also been applied in Sweden (Baumann *et al.* 1992), Norway (Baumann *et al.* 1993), the Netherlands (SIMA-PRO 1993), and Belgium (S.G.P 1994).

CML and others have proposed to apply the principles of the ecoscarcity method to the effect scores after CML had developed an operable effect-oriented characterisation method (Heijungs *et al.* 1992). These methods are called distance-to-target methods and use different calculation algorithms and target levels (see Braunschweig *et al.* 1996). Adriaanse (1993), Müller-Wenk (1994b), Kortman *et al.* (1994), Corten *et al.* (1994), Kalisvaart *et al.* (1994), Guinée (1995) and Goedkoop (1995) all provide further details and calculated weighting sets.

The ratio between present flows and target flows is used within the approach presented here in Section 4.5, albeit in a different context, i.e., in order to show the need for flow reductions.

1.3.6 Outlook

The overview presented here concerns mainly the fifth step within the phase of impact assessment, i.e., 'weighting across impact categories', as defined by the LCA-procedure proposed by ISO (see Fig. 1.2). ISO designates both the relative contribution and the weighting step as voluntary, but the problem is not that simple as the execution of these two steps determines, to a large extent, the shape of the other preceding steps. Many of the weighting methods mentioned in this section cannot be fitted into the suggested five-step procedure. Principles that will be suggested later in Section 2.1 may make obsolete the steps of the selection and definition of impact categories, and of classification, and replace them instead with additional steps within the goal and scope definition. Damage-oriented approaches – extensively used in Chapters 4 through 7 – will probably challenge the meaning of the characterisation step.

It seems that in the ongoing methodology development of LCIA panel methods are acquiring increasing importance as elements therein and that there exists a tendency to reflect more accurately the emission-to-effect relation as well. The observation of developments outside the field of LCA suggests that the proxy indicators 'energy' and 'mass displacement', on the one hand, and monetarisation methods based on damage costs, on the other, acquire a relatively greater importance. Synergies between panel methods and monetarisation methods are obvious and it might well be that a closer look at both of them together could stimulate their future developments.

1.4 Positioning of LCA

This section's aim is to position LCA within the decision making process. This requires making explicit the characteristics and dimensions of decision making which the current design of LCA do meet. The other side of this coin is that one can then decide which of the other available instruments may be preferable if other features of decision making have to be satisfied. The number of tools, procedures, and concepts to support or make decisions with respect to environmental questions has become quite large within a short time and has created a situation in which it is almost impossible to gain an overview that is both complete and up-to-date. Attempts to present such overviews – mostly from an LCA point of view – can be found in Hyman *et al.* (1988), OECD (1995), Beck *et al.* (1995), UNEP (1996), Scholz *et al.* (1996), de Smet *et al.* (1997), Heijungs (1997), Cowell *et al.* (1997), and Wrisberg *et al.* (1998).

The positions assigned to the different instruments and the figures to illustrate these judgements are based on Beck *et al.* (1995) and Hofstetter (1996c). They are used to position LCA and not to introduce the other tools and concepts. Such introductions and references to the introductory literature can be found in the overviews referred to above.

1.4.1 Decision support or decision making?

Rational decision making always considers all aspects related to a decision at hand, i.e., economical, societal and environmental aspects[13,14]. LCA is a tool to support rational decision making within the dimension environment. Figure 1.3 illustrates the conceptualisation of the decision making process that is used in systems analysis (see, e.g., Miser *et al.* 1985). The decision is supported by a set of more specific decisions concerned more exclusively with the economic, social and environmental aspects. The many tools developed to support decisions look at the decision problem from different angles and each one of them can therefore be placed accordingly in one of three "pillars". The decision making itself is a procedure which encompasses the single tools, i.e., the decision making process first identifies a problem and then selects – as support for the decision – the tools that are oriented toward the different dimensions to generate the appropriate information on the consequences of a set of alternative courses of action. This information will be evaluated in a subsequent step – either in an intuitive fashion or according to a formalised procedure – and leads to a decision or policy. Further important phases of this process are the implementation of the decision or policy and the evaluation of the new state of the system. This last phase often leads to the identification of new problems, thus turning decision making into an ongoing, iterative process.

---

[13] Sometimes the additional dimensions of 'technology' and of 'safety' are mentioned. However, we assume here that the decision making is judging a given functional unit which can be fulfilled by different techniques which influence the three dimensions 'economy', 'society', and 'environment' to differing extents. The same holds for safety. A higher level of safety in a system will lead to lower effects within the three main dimensions.

[14] This provocative statement should make clear that also if only one dimension is finally decisive for the decision making, there preceded a scoping which set the other dimensions to an importance of zero or found that the other dimensions are not discriminating for the alternatives at hand.

Two observations have to be made here in order to justify claims that will be made later in Chapter 2:

- The decision support tools are an embedded part of the decision process. They therefore have to correspond with the decision maker's problem definition and personal value frame in all those instances where value choices are necessary. Therefore, LCA can not be established fully isolated from the decision making process.
- Decision makers that follow the rational procedure sketched out here[15] are confronted with decision support in all three dimensions, resulting, in most cases, from an even larger number of tools. Often, it seems therefore an unrealistic hope therefore that decision makers know all those tools in detail and that they will be willing, capable and interested in personally making value choices that might be required by these tools. The conclusion is that the tools, including LCA, have to offer highly aggregated information and yet not violate the observation made in the preceding point, i.e., the aggregation has to reflect the decision makers value frames.

A way to deal with these problems will be outlined in Section 2.2 and worked out in the rest of this book.

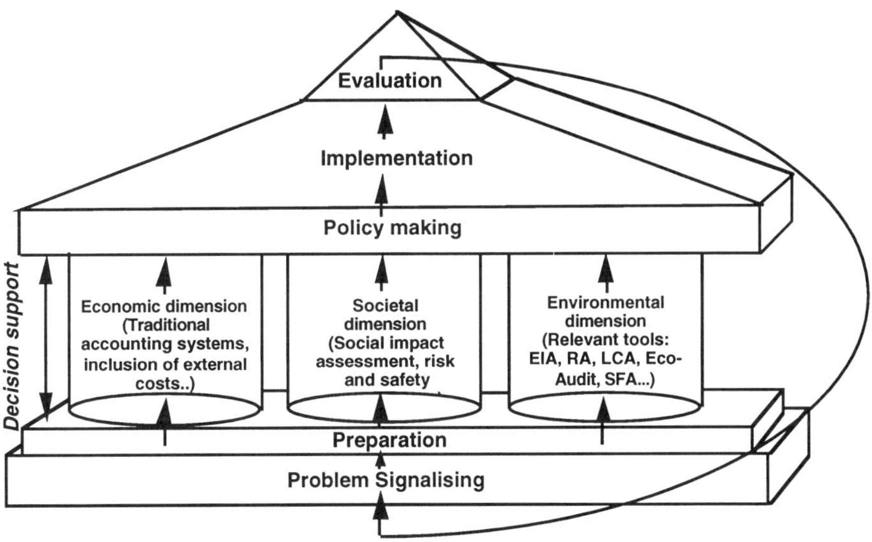

Fig. 1.3: General set-up for a policy making process with the most important phases. (EIA = Environmental Impact Assessment, SFA = Substance Flow Analysis, RA = Risk Assessment)

[15] Many decisions are not made on a rational basis. This is the case in most everyday decisions of a routine character (i.e., they are a replication of what was done earlier), in decisions where there is no time waiting for the generation of decision support, or if decision makers are unfamiliar with rational decision making or explicitly favour more holistic approaches.

1.4.2 The level of analysis

The decision support tools are not only specific with respect to their position within the decision making process and to the dimension they help to analyse. One can also distinguish them according to different levels of analysis: tools may be developed for applications on the micro level (i.e., products, services, or production plants), on the meso level (i.e., projects or technologies) or even on the macro level, where whole countries or even the whole world are modelled.

Figure 1.4 is one proposal for such a positioning exercise. The main aim of this picture is to make it clear that LCA is mainly positioned on the micro level and within the environmental dimension[16]. Other tools cover other levels of analysis or/and other dimensions, or they may compete head-on with LCA.

Why should LCA be restricted to the micro level? This is one of the most obvious questions from someone who looks for a tool with the most general application possible. Here, some arguments are given to justify this restriction and make it become more fundamental, as has been the case so far:

- Decision support systems on a macro level need a predictive element. Predictions on the macro level are only possible if all three dimensions can be analysed simultaneously because they strongly influence each other. A world model for only one dimension fails to support rational decision making. This argument implies that if LCA should cover the meso and macro levels as well, then it would have to be extended to include all dimensions17.
- Modelling on the micro level needs a high level of resolution and great detail, but may remain valid despite the use of simple linear and static models. Models on the macro level should make use of dynamic modelling that allows for non-linearity. Practically, this requires that the model includes only a few highly relevant parameters which are then modelled accurately. This may be thought to be an all too pragmatic argument, but decision making in real situations has to be made in a comparatively short time and the system to be described is always changing. A more fundamental argument for this restriction of LCA to the micro level is that we are here facing something like a "MicMac-effect", i.e., the more detailed information one adds on the micro level, the less predictive the model will become on the macro level; and the better a macro model predicts future system behaviour and system states, the less it will be able to deliver detailed information on the micro level (see also Jørgensen 1994:12, Mayer 1992:23ff).
- If the object of a decision at hand can be located on the micro to macro scale, it does not make sense to apply a meta model which needs a large volume of information which is of no relevance for the decision at hand. This would make the tool unnecessarily costly, slow, complex and maybe even intransparent.

To restrict LCA to the micro level can therefore be justified by the need to have a tool which is suited to answer micro level environmental questions and the know-

[16] A survey among actors involved in 10 LCA case studies revealed that they prefer to include all dimensions in decision making, but to keep the other dimensions 'economy' and 'society' apart from LCA (Huybrechts *et al.* 1996).

[17] Note that this statement reveals an obvious lack of appropriate instruments. The young tool of Integrated Assessment (Rotmans *et al.* 1997) may fill some of the gaps implied here.

ledge that the tool would increase in complexity if we wanted it to answer other kinds of questions too.

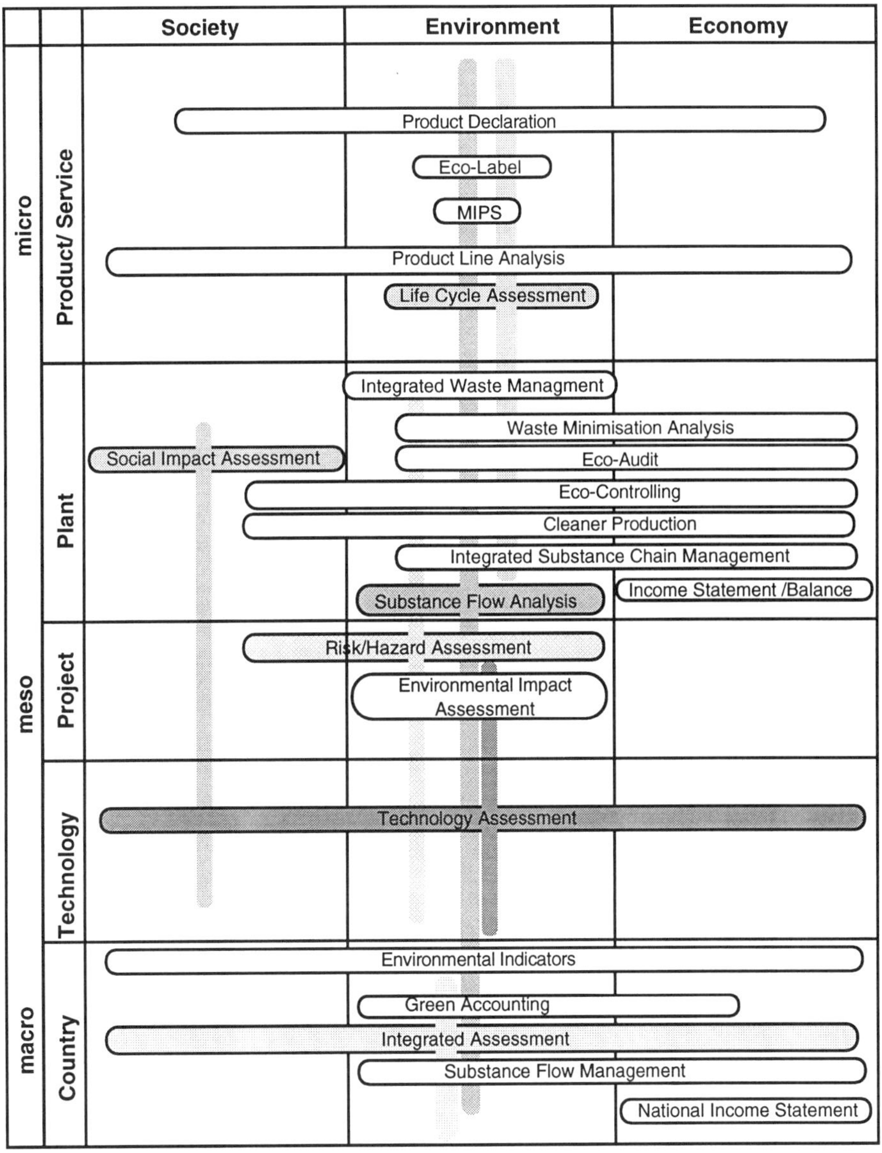

Fig. 1.4: Positions of a selected number of decision support tools in the two dimensions "level of analysis" (from micro to macro) and "dimension of analysis" (from 'society' to 'economy') (further developed based on Baumgartner (1987) and Rubik *et al.* (1992:15).
Readers guide: The vertical bars indicate that some tools cover more than one level or dimension of analysis. The vertical bars can be attributed to the tools by looking for the same shading.

Vester (1988) developed principles which are clearly located on a macro level and which therefore cover system aspects which are out of the range of LCA. Two examples of Vester's principles shall illustrate this different type of recommendations:

> *"The principle of negative feedback: Negative feedback has to dominate positive feedback.*
>
> *The principle of independence of growth: The functioning of the system has to be independent of growth."*

The consequence of this different modelling level is, on the one hand, that the dynamic modelling used by Frederic Vester (1983/1984/1985/1988) to gain insights into anthropogenic systems and to make predictions on a meso or macro level are outside the scope of LCA. On the other hand, Vester's models fail to compare two single product alternatives which fulfil the same function or to advice a company in eco-design, i.e., they do not provide quantitative decision support on the micro level.

1.4.3 LCA measures pressure

The OECD has developed the so-called pressure-state-response (PRS) framework as a part of its work on environmental indicators (OECD 1991/1994). *Pressure* stands for stresses in the environment caused by human beings. *State* refers primarily to the quality of the environment, measured as air, water, and soil quality and as the diversity of fauna and flora. *Response* summarises the actions and social measures taken to protect or manage the environment. Information on all three levels is important to describe the present environmental situation and the direction of change[18].

LCA is mainly concerned with the pressure-step of this PRS-framework. It fails to measure the state of the environment because only changes are looked at and because only one human activity is analysed at any one time. Its impact is normally too insignificant to produce visible changes. Responses, however, can be a consequence of the use of LCA in decisions, but they are not analysed within the framework of LCA. LCA is a change-oriented tool on the micro level.

1.4.4 Time and space

Tools can also be positioned with respect to their treatment of the very important dimensions of *space* and *time*. The space dimension has at least two separate aspects to it:

- Which geographical area is considered to be within the system boundaries of the analysis?
- Which spatial information and details are considered with which degree of resolution?

As suggested in Section 1.2, LCA covers world-wide the environmental interventions and damages caused by the product system at hand. The limitations of LCA *sensu stricto* (Subsection 1.2.6) are explicitly concerning the second question. The

[18] If the responses are not strong enough to reduce the stressors, then the state of the environment will become worse.

impacts of all world-wide environmental interventions are assessed on the basis of the fiction that the meteorological conditions and ecosystems world-wide are the same as the average conditions in Western Europe. That is, impacts are assessed site-independent. The vertical axis in Figure 1.5 reflects this second aspect of the spatial dimension and a number of the decision-support tools are arranged accordingly. Site-independent tools such as LCA and other product-oriented tools which make no spatial differences within the system are located below the 'zero'-point of the ordinate. Site-specific tools are listed correspondingly along the positive axis of the ordinate. Total cost assessment, environmental accounting, and environmental indicators consider spatial differences to a limited extent. But tools such as EIA and occupational health indicators evaluate impacts in a completely site-specific manner.

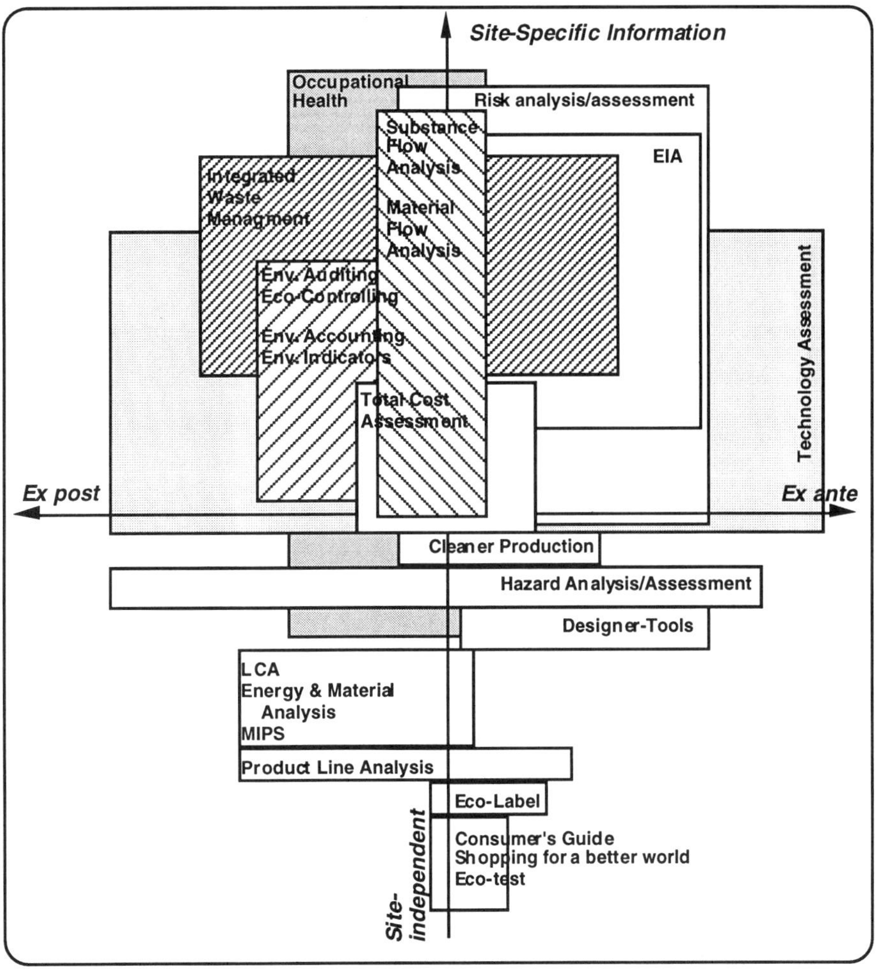

Fig. 1.5: The location of environmental tools in the time-space area. 'Time' addresses the descriptive or predictive power of the tools and 'space' addresses the spatial differentiation within the tool. All tools in the lower half of the figure are site-independent (ordinal scale), EIA = Environmental Impact Assessment

Many time-aspects are relevant for environmental tools (see Hofstetter (1996a) for an overview). For Figure 1.5, we selected the *ex post/ex ante* differentiation as the aspect structuring the tools. The power to describe a system after things have already happened (*ex post*) places a tool to the left side. If a tool predicts future states of the system (*ex ante*), it is placed towards the right. Tools that describe things that are presently happening are placed more towards the centre. Predictive tools are, e.g., technology assessment, EIA, or risk assessment. LCA, substance and material flow analysis, or environmental audits are descriptive rather than predictive, i.e., they model the present system as accurately as possible in order to get information about the system at hand and to make short term predictions. These tools are therefore sited near the centre.

To make predictions it is necessary to take into account all the dimensions that are relevant for (societal) decision making. If one wants to know how the anthroposphere will look like in 20 or 50 years from now, it is important to know how society and societal values will evolve, the development of the size of the population, the change in economic structures and in the economy's size. This information cannot be derived from just an analysis of the environmental dimension. The upshot of this argument is that the predictive tools have to analyse all dimensions in order to generate sensible scenarios for the future. Technology Assessment and Integrated Assessment fulfil these requirements to some extent and are therefore the tools of choice for prospective studies.

A further characteristic of the treatment of time in LCA is that time is looked at in a compressed way. Processes and their interventions in the past, present and future are added up without correcting for calendar time, e.g., without applying a discount factor. In many cases, one even makes the simplifying assumption of a steady-state situation. The number of years during which the service is provided and how long it will last are set with the definition of the functional unit that takes place in the phase of the goal and scope definition. In principle, it is possible to increase the time resolution in LCA. However, this increases the amount of data that is required and thus increases considerably the complexity of the model.

1.4.5 Summary

The aim of this section was to position LCA within the decision making process and in relationship to other decision support tools. This overview makes it clear that LCA is only one of the perspectives that can be used when assessing human activities. There exists a large number of competing tools, each with its own characteristics that differ from those of LCA. LCA's main characteristics (in comparison to other tools) as determined here are:

- LCA is a tool used to model the environmental dimension.
- LCA is used as part of a decision support process and does not in itself encompass the whole decision making procedure.
- LCA is designed to support decisions on a micro level, i.e., products and plants are the objects of analysis.
- LCA assesses changes in single human activities (pressure) and cannot describe the state of the environment or societal responses to environmental stress.

- LCA assesses global environmental interventions and damages by assuming a unit world with average meteorological and ecological conditions.
- LCA compresses the time dimension and therefore does not discount the future nor the past.

Any of the other tools may therefore be more appropriate than LCA, depending on the problem to be solved and the question to be answered.

A last remark has to be added here with respect to the frequently made claim that LCA is a tool to assess the sustainability of products or processes. The list of characteristics given above makes it quite obvious that LCA in its present form cannot fulfil this claim for a number of reasons:

- it covers only a part of *one* of the dimensions relevant for sustainability,
- it analyses only single human activities while sustainability can only be defined on the macro level, i.e., the level of all activities together,
- it does not predict, and consequently cannot be used to control, the state of the environment, and
- it lacks the appropriate time and space resolution to control the overshooting of any level of sustainability.

LCA is only about the optimisation of the subsystems of the anthroposphere with respect to their environmental dimensions. It can therefore help only to make them more sustainable in their environmental dimension, not globally so. Once LCA is understood in the way described here, the expectations from this tool will become more realistic and consequently will end the present situation that too much is expected from LCA methodology.

1.5 Life Cycle Impact Assessment revisited by decision theory

Subsection 1.4.1 and Figure 1.3 already positioned LCA with respect to its place as decision support tool. The questions raised by decision theory and the questions faced within the development of LCIA and LCA cover some of the same ground. It is therefore useful to define LCIA in terms of decision theory. Hofstetter (1996b:142-164) gives an overview of decision theory and of multi criteria analysis and their relationship to LCA. Here, we chose a different approach. Zionts (1997:233f) presented ten myths of decision making and himself added arguments for or examples of why they are sometimes nothing more than myths. Three of these myths are as quite relevant for LCA and are discussed here:

"The myth of a decision maker. We think of a decision maker making a decision, like a wise person in isolation. What is a more accurate scenario is that often a group rather than an individual makes a decision. Even where there is not a group, many people normally influence the decision maker."

This myth can be transposed to LCA and would mean that several decision contexts should be considered when LCA is used to support decisions. In addition, this complicates the question of whose values should be considered if more than one person acts as a decision maker (see Subsection 3.1.2).

"The myth of a fixed set of alternatives. We tend to think as the set of alternatives as being fixed. More likely the set is dynamic, and changes over time."

In a comparative assertion, the alternatives to be analysed are fixed in the phase of goal and scope definition. If the functional unit is defined in terms of a service, this allows for the to extension of the set of alternatives. The generation of new alternatives is one of the aims of LCA in product improvement and eco-design. Therefore, it is important that LCIA is not dependent on the number and kind of alternatives[19].

"The myth of a utility or value function. Though a utility or value function may be a useful construct for decision makers, it seems more important to analysts than to decision makers."

LCIA is very much concerned by this myth and it is assumed that decision makers not interested in the disutility function would discard LCA as such. Finnveden (1997) pointed out the ethical notion of deontological and teleological theories (see, e.g., Frankena 1963). Translated to the LCIA context, a deontological view would mean that, e.g., certain elements in the environment have an absolute right of protection. As long as such a right is not met, none of the alternatives is acceptable. The requirements are mostly based on ethical, religious or international demands. LCA is clearly not concerned with this type of view because such protection requires regulations or instruments at the macro level. The teleological theories look to the

[19] The discussion of generic *versus* case-by-case LCIA will not be added here. Hofstetter (1996b:144ff) concluded that a generic LCIA is most appropriate but more than one 'version' has to be provided while, e.g., Volkwein *et al.* (1996b) pleads for a case-by-case approach.

consequences of an act and utilitarianism is one school within this group of theories. Trade-offs between attributes are therefore possible.

Within decision theory, one differentiates between compensating and non-compensating criteria. The Anglo-American school of decision making is primarily concerned with a clear overall objective which allows for the building of a utility function. These methods aim at *multicriteria decision making* (MCDM), and a hierarchisation, ranking or scoring is assumed to always be possible. The francophone school of decision making is concerned with *multicriteria decision aid* (MCDA) and it allows that more than one alternative rates best. Outranking procedures are often used in these situations and incommensurable elements are not combined, i.e., certain criteria can have a non-compensating nature (Pictet 1995).

To conclude, LCIA can start with the claim that there is a disutility function built on the foundation of compensating disutilities due to the use of different impact categories. LCIA can therefore be labelled as an element belonging to the teleological theories and the Anglo-American school of multicriteria decision making.

The myths of Zionts make explicit both the purely normative and the descriptive or behavioural bases of decision theory. As set out in Subsection 1.2.2 LCA has many elements of a normative theory and tends therefore to be congruent with these myths[20]. However, the short discussion above shows that it is quite possible to take into account the critique from the perspective of descriptive theory in order to prepare LCA for actual decision making environments, i.e., to make it a prescriptive tool. In this book we will follow the lines of bounded rational decision making by accepting that cultural bias and social relations influence the expression of rationality (see Chapter 3).

Next to the clarification above, the valuation problem of LCIA can be characterised as follows (structure partly from Tietje *et al.* 1996):

- What is the intended meaning? Anthropogenic impacts on the environment can be reduced by influencing single decisions contributing to the impacts. Anthropogenic impacts are assessed according to the degree that they cause damage on pre-defined safeguard subjects.
- What will be valued? The relative environmental impact of a product system distinguishing different phases in the life cycle or comparing it to other product systems.
- Who values? The decision maker is either a single person or a group of persons. They themselves are only partly concerned by the environmental impacts because the environment is a public good.
- Which scale? The model used in LCIA is quantitative in its nature, uses where possible a ratio scale, and defines the valuation problem in terms of a multi criteria decision making problem.

[20] Prof. Dr. Rainer Züst (ETHZ) suggested describing LCA as well in terms of myths which concern normative settings of LCA, as well, e.g., the myth of linearity, the myth of additivity, the myth of independence, etc. Such an exercise may help to open the eyes for decisive assumptions made years ago and are close to the axiomatic suggested by Heijungs (1998). However, standards for LCA methodology should first become more settled as a point of reference before a mythology is developed (ISO 1997/1998).

- Which kind of decision making process? An analytical rather than an intuitive decision making process is assumed. Therefore, the LCIA model has to provide not just a single disutility function, but also its constituting factors.
- How to validate? The quality of the assessment will not be a matter of empirical validation. There will be no feedback loop which mirrors the effects of the decision made. The quality assessment therefore needs other criteria. Four criteria are mentioned here:
  - The LCIA is able to include latest findings of the sciences concerned.
  - Decision makers feel comfortable relying on LCIA as a decision support system because it is at the same time complete, transparent, and practicable.
  - The value choices are made explicit and compatible with the values relevant for the decision making.
  - Differences to other methods and tools for LCIA are either small or explainable.

The valuation structure and its functions will be specified in Chapter 4.

This large array of statements, requirements, criteria, and assumptions represents an integration of elements from the dominant normative and from the descriptive decision theory. This bridging of approaches is one of the particularities offered by this book.

2 Shift of Paradigm – Propositions – Objectives

In Chapter 1 we situated LCA within the decision making process and in relationship to other decision support tools. LCA has been identified as only one of the perspectives that can be used when assessing human activities from an environmental perspective. There exists a large number of competing tools, each with its own characteristics, that differ from those of LCA. Therefore, LCA *sensu stricto* as used in this book was defined in Subsection 1.2.6. However, the two following main criticisms towards LCA have not been answered with this clarification of what LCA *sensu stricto* is and what it can and cannot do (see, e.g., Barnthouse *et al.* 1997): (1) LCA cannot strictly separate objective and subjective elements, and (2) LCA does not have an acceptable way to model impacts.

This second chapter takes up these two points and shows how this book will deal with them. The position on the first criticism is that it is in principle impossible to keep objective facts and subjective choices apart. All that can be hoped for is that the value choices everywhere in LCA are made in a mutually compatible and coherent way. Subsection 2.1.1 identifies the sources of this unease and Subsections 2.1.2 and 2.1.3 suggest a way to overcome it. The later chapters will then suggest explicitly how this can be done. The practicality of this proposal will be shown in the course of this book, but verification of this claim will have to wait for another time.

Subsection 2.1.4 takes up the second criticism and suggests that the problem can be dealt with by shifting the focus of LCA from impacts to damages and safeguard subjects. It is this shift which will allow the building of better models. This shift, best described as a change from a bottom-up to a top-down methodology, is used to identify and specify needs for further methodological developments and to suggest some lines along which these developments could be pursued. These considerations are used in Section 2.2 to formulate and justify a number of propositions. Working out solutions to the problems underlying them and verifying their practicality makes up the heart of this book (Section 2.3).

2.1 LCA – the art to combine three spheres

2.1.1 The limits of the bottom-up approach

Historically, LCAs have been dominated by the inventory analysis and the pragmatic limitations placed on them by the data that has been available. There were, of course, always thoughts given on the definition of the functional unit and some reflections made on appropriate system boundaries. However, the heart of the analysis was considered to be the inventory analysis. Yet, the goal to be fulfilled by the analysis has rarely been made explicit.

The development of the LCA tool has been mainly influenced by the idea that the modelling of a product system from cradle to grave and the calculation of environmental interventions would provide the insights that had been missing so far and whose availability would make for better decisions. And indeed, the analysis of processes with respect to their inputs and outputs, including the environmental interventions, has given us a different perspective on a process or a plant and that change of perspective has been responsible for many improvements in environmental as well as other respects.

However, this gathering of information did not just lead to improvements, but also to more and more extensive databases (see, e.g., Frischknecht *et al.* 1994). The information contained in them is presumably of relevance, but so far we have not been able to ascertain if this is true. The problem is that, if in the phase of goal definition, one does not explicitly determine according to which criteria the optimisation should be made, one cannot determine the relevance of single environmental interventions gathered during the inventory analysis.

The definition of LCIA already cited in Subsection 1.2.3 and which has been taken from ISO (1998) reflects that bottom-up way of thinking when it is stated that LCIA should make the LCI results "more manageable" and "may identify the relative significance of the LCI results". This way of thinking makes it necessary to model all the inputs and the outputs of a product system[1]. This leads to a very large effort in data gathering and computing which may exceed the benefit provided in support of a decision. The criterion of *relevant interventions* is inoperative in such situations unless "relevance" is defined in an explicit and applicable manner.

[1] This statement is not very helpful because all processes that have occurred in the world so far are directly or indirectly causally related to any product system, e.g., the wood cut for the production of the chair sat on by the worker who produced the pencil with which Henry Ford started to design cars is causally related to all of today's industrial activities. Only rules on the setting of system boundaries and on the cutting-out of processes that are only of minor relevance makes it possible to restrict the analysis to a subset of processes representative of the product system.

2.1.2 Paradigm shift - three spheres and their combination

Tackling this problem of "relevance" requires a new look at LCA. This new understanding of LCA encompasses the traditional modelling of the product system which we call here *technosphere* (it could also be called *anthroposphere*). As has been the case so far in the practice of LCA, the environmental interventions, which span the border between the technosphere and the *ecosphere* are taken into consideration. But the new perspective recognises explicitly an ecosphere in which the technosphere is embedded and they in turn are embedded in the *valuesphere* (Figure 2.1). It is the valuesphere that enables us to perceive both the eco- and the technosphere and that shapes the way we see them. This view states that the ecosphere and the technosphere are, to some extent, constructs of the valuesphere, i.e., the ecosphere and technosphere are not entities *per se*. Our perception of them is shaped in distinct ways.

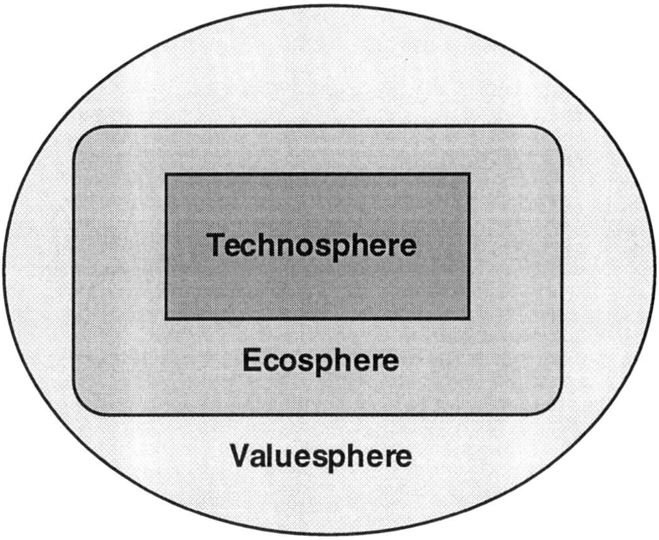

Fig. 2.1: The three spheres modelled and linked by LCA

Figure 2.1 is just one way to visualise the position of the three spheres. The chosen presentation illustrates that the values also are understood as a sphere which can be modelled. The technosphere and the ecosphere are not just perceived, but influence themselves again the valuesphere[2].

If LCA is understood as a model born out of the three spheres, then the tool has to be designed in such a way that it can model adequately the three spheres and then also *link* these models together. The respective sciences provide us with plenty of modelling approaches for any one of these three spheres. There are sociological and psychological models for the valuesphere, models from the ecosphere provided by the different natural sciences and environmental science, and the model of the

[2] While the mechanisms within the ecosphere can only be altered to a limited extent by human beings, the technosphere is strongly influenced by them.

technosphere that is primarily provided by economists and engineers. However, LCA is the art of *combining* these models, i.e., to select the appropriate disciplinary models, to develop bridges that model the interfaces between thc sphere-specific models, and to link them in such a manner that they provide support for the decision making at hand.

LCA is seen as the art of combining the three spheres by focusing on the interface problems.

In this book we will model the valuesphere in Chapter 3 and suggest in Chapters 4 and 5 a model for the ecosphere, paying special attention to the interfaces between it and the valuesphere. The modelling of the technosphere is only touched upon in Section 8.2 and is not the focus of this book.

2.1.3 Top-down modelling

One immediate consequence of the view presented in Figure 2.1 is that the traditional bottom-up perspective embedded in LCA has to be given up. Instead of starting with the modelling of the product system, we have to clarify first a set of questions such as:

A) What exactly is the aim of LCA?

B) If the aim is to reduce environmental impacts through product improvements and comparative assertions, then one has to ask: What is the environment and what are the impacts which should be reduced?

C) Once the environmental impacts to be reduced are specified, one has to ask: Which kind of environmental interventions cause these impacts?

Answering all these questions will result in a list of input and output parameters which have to be modelled in the inventory analysis. If question (C) is answered quantitatively by assigning numerical weights to single environmental interventions, one is able to limit the number of processes within the product system that have to be looked at and can restrict the analysis to the relevant environmental interventions. Relevant are all environmental interventions which, together, make up, for example, 95% of the known impacts. Braunschweig (1996) describes an algorithm to allow for an efficient inventory analysis thanks to this top-down approach.

This shift in the modelling philosophy will influence all phases within LCA. However, the consequences will not be dramatic because:

- the bottom-up approach was also implicitly guided by the environmental relevance of single substances,
- the bottom-up thinking of past years and the experiences so far will influence the realisation of the top-down approach, and
- the bridges to link the spheres will only be optimal if both "river banks" are known and carefully looked at.

This combination of top-down thinking and bottom-up knowledge is further discussed in Section 4.1 and Subsection 4.3.6 and practised in Chapters 6 and 7.

2.1.4 Safeguard subjects in LCA

The new core of LCA is the identification of what exactly should be its objective. What is meant by environment, what are its constituent factors, and which of the changes occurring in it have to be considered as adverse, adding to the disutility? The environment is too complex to be modelled *per se*. One has to define what is understood by the "environment" and which elements are considered as its constituent factors:

- The notion of top-down thinking introduced above is not new in LCA. Hofstetter (1991) discussed already the need to identify the safeguard subjects first and the "environmental factors" which damage them afterwards. In essence, it was a plea to protect human beings from direct and indirect damages, i.e., an anthropocentric world view. However, it was concluded there that this can be achieved only if the whole ecosphere is protected because changes in the ecosphere may well harm human beings. It was argued there that knowledge about the causal relationships between environmental interventions and damages to safeguard subjects is very limited and that one should therefore aim for an aggregation at the level of the environmental factors[3].
- Within LCA, the Environmental Prioritising System (EPS) was the first method that consequently observed the top-down procedure (Steen *et al.* 1992, Steen 1996). The authors defined five safeguard subjects based on the Rio Declarations: biological diversity, human health, production of biomass and freshwater, resource use, and aesthetic values. These safeguard subjects were not only precisely defined, but also valued with a mix of different monetarisation approaches. Subsequently, they identified pathways to emissions and resource extraction which damage one or several of the safeguard subjects. The causal relationships were constructed through a 6-step procedure including fate, effect, and damage analysis. Only a small number of causal relationships were known at the time this work was undertaken. Therefore, only a limited set of environmental interventions was considered to causally and relevantly damage the five safeguard subjects.

  At that time this structurally interesting approach was mainly used by Swedish industry and poorly understood by the LCA community. An attempt to explain and discuss this method in more detail was made by Braunschweig *et al.* (1994). The damage assessment introduced in Section 4.3 is close to the EPS-method. EPS therefore may be seen as an early attempt to summarise the knowledge on causal relationships between emissions and damage to safeguard subjects.
- SETAC (1993b) and ISO (1997) mention human health, ecological health, and resources as main categories or areas in need of protection. However, this selection is poorly reasoned and specified. Other definitions are also in use within SETAC itself (SETAC 1993a).
- Goedkoop (1995) developed EcoIndicator'95, a method which assesses damage to three safeguard subjects: human fatalities, human health impairment, and

[3] Nowadays they are called impact categories or environmental problems. A set of about two dozens of such factors was suggested in Hofstetter (1991). However, only a few of them were operationalised there.

ecosystem impairment. The latter two damages were only weakly defined. The link between category indicators and the damage to safeguard subjects was made by a distance-to-target method. The target was set in such a way that the damage at target level is equal for all impact categories, i.e., one premature death per million inhabitants per year, no health impairments, and 5% long-term ecosystem impairment. Resources were not considered as a safeguard subject.

- Volkwein et al (1996a) argued that the safeguard subjects should be based on international treaties, rights, and declarations. They listed many relevant paragraphs but did not make a selection among the possible subjects nor did they operationalise them.
- Hofstetter (1996b:170ff) has argued that the widely understood anthropocentric view corresponds best to the position of human beings in the decision process and that this view will indirectly protect ecological health as well. Human welfare as a meta-safeguard-subject was considered to be "comprehensive and empty at the same time". Therefore the use of human health, ecological health and/or biodiversity was argued for. Resource depletion was rejected as a safeguard subject due to the lack of a convincing concept to include it.
- Müller-Wenk (1997) acknowledges the safeguard subjects as the core element of LCIA and suggests that *life* merits protection. Based on that, he distinguishes between human health and ecosystems as the most obvious safeguard subjects. Concerning resources, he suggests that resources may be treated like impact categories, thus requiring modelling of the consequences for 'life' if they are depleted. Müller-Wenk discusses the precise meaning of these terms and offers several interpretations especially for the safeguard subject 'ecosystems', focusing either on the diversity of species or of habitats. Müller-Wenk (1998) subsequently shows that the destructive use of resources in the specific case of fossil energies may well be considered as a safeguard subject while the dissipative or even accumulating use of abiotic resources should rather be considered as impact categories. Worst-case calculations for a set of metal ores suggest that the decrease in ore concentrations will lead to small increases of the environmental impacts of mining and beneficiation in the future.
- The selection and definition of safeguard subjects involves, to a large extent, value choices that depend on the valuesphere. It is therefore obvious that different schools of thinking approach the problem setting from different angles. One such attempt is documented in Hofstetter *et al.* (1997). Scientists from ethics, theology, philosophy, economy, and law were confronted with the problems of identifying safeguard subjects and were asked to prioritise them. As one of the outcomes one can state that representatives from ethics and the science of religion are able to identify or normatively define safeguard subjects; some of the subjects are close to basic values while the choice of others depends on the moral or religious position of the scientists. Economists and legal scholars, on the other hand, try to reflect the present societal position (descriptive). In addition, it was made clear that representatives of the humanities will not define safeguard subjects in isolation which then can be adopted by LCA. A more intensive exchange between these disciplines is necessary if one wants to find those safeguard subjects which are operational in terms of LCA and yet reflect the moral meaning intended by ethical and religious considerations.

This lengthy description of the state-of-the-art can be summarised as follows:

- The importance of clear-cut definitions of the safeguard subjects is acknowledged by a growing number of scientists.
- The justification, specification, and operationalisation of them is still going on. It may be necessary to do this by working directly together with scientists from philosophy, ethics, and religious sciences.
- The selection and prioritisation of safeguard subjects is seen as a value choice and is therefore inherently dependent on a model of the valuesphere.

In Section 3.2 we will introduce a model for the valuesphere. In Sections 4.1 and 4.3 we will further discuss the selection of safeguard subjects made within this book.

2.1.5 First consequences

The shift postulated here in the way LCA is looked at will challenge several elements of LCA that have been considered as sacrosanct so far:

- The statement that the ecosphere can only be defined by means of a clear model of the valuesphere can be seen as an attempt at relativism. However, natural *laws* will not be violated by this way of modelling the ecosphere. All natural laws are respected, but some of them become more important than others because they describe the elements of the ecosphere that are considered to be particularly relevant for a given value perspective.
- The careful *separation* between the so-called objective and subjective phases or steps within LCA (see, e.g., Heijungs *et al.* 1992, SETAC 1993b, ISO 1997/1998) is *abandoned.* It is accepted that all steps are embedded in the valuesphere. However, the step 'goal definition' now becomes the most value-laden element of the LCA procedure. Here the value structure that will be the basis of the valuesphere has to be determined and used to derive the safeguard subjects. All subsequent steps within LCA can then be based on these settings. They will still be subjective in their nature, but compatible with the goal definition and the valuesphere.
- Instead of just modelling the technosphere within the inventory analysis and assessing some of the consequences for the environment, we suggest modelling the three spheres – technosphere, ecosphere, and valuesphere – and their interfaces. This will lead to a more comprehensive and structured modelling effort. This then, leads *to a need for more steps* within the LCA process, something already claimed by Huppes (1997) and suggested in Hofstetter (1996b).
- The established *policy themes* approach (Adriaanse 1993, Heijungs *et al.* 1992, SETAC 1993b) is abandoned. The clear-cut definition of the safeguard subjects makes it possible to group the impact classes in a different way. The formation of the groups can alternatively be based on *common mechanisms* or *common endpoints* (Udo de Haes 1998). A mixture of the two alternatives best reflects the way science is organised. The two examples given in Chapters 6 and 7 follow the approach of the 'common mechanisms' and both of them concern the same endpoint, i.e., human health.

The subsequent Chapters 3 to 5 will show how the consequences of LCA outlined here are approached in this book.

2.2 Propositions and their motivation

Because the objectives of this book can not be classified within the classical line of research 'hypothesis-experiment-falsification', five propositions are offered for consideration or acceptance which will guide the procedure in the further chapters:

1. *The combination of models for the three spheres – technosphere, ecosphere and valuesphere – and their interfaces form the LCA tool.*

This proposition is the basis for all the others. It makes possible the structured inclusion of knowledge from different fields of science and makes clear that the way of integration and combination will determine the quality of LCIA.

2. *The potential damages due to substances causing carcinogenic and respiratory effects in human beings can be assessed by a structured multi-step approach. The damage can be expressed in the same unit for all substances and can be assessed in a site-independent manner.*

As suggested by Figure 2.1 and Subsection 2.1.4 the ecosphere can only be adequately modelled if – based on a model of the valuesphere – one is able to identify safeguard subjects which represent the relevant elements of the ecosphere. Once the safeguard subjects are identified, it is possible, in principle, to assess damages to safeguard subjects by environmental interventions. This second proposition claims that this is indeed possible and that it can be exemplified by two examples damaging the safeguard subject of human health.

3. *Decision makers like to be informed not only about results of the damage assessment, but prefer to get complementary information through other indices for attributes of known and unknown damage.*

From the discussion in Subsection 1.3.2, it is clear that only a limited number of causal relations between damages to safeguard subjects and environmental interventions of the technosphere can be quantified. This small number of so-called damage functions should therefore be complemented by an element addressing the unknown damage. Next to that the damage assessment is based on a static view, i.e., a steady-state situation is assumed without consideration of possible developments. Further damage attributes may therefore increase the informative content of the assessment.

4. *The plurality of methods in LCIA and the attitude towards LCA in decision making are caused by different properties of the value perspectives and are due to different intentions in modelling.*

The model of the valuesphere will not just help to define the ecosphere, but may also be used to position different approaches and tools which have, in principle, the same aim and explain why they are – or even have to be – different. Therefore, Proposition (4) suggests in addition that the attitude towards LCA in decision making has to be analysed from different viewpoints.

5. *If LCA is developed and performed based on distinctly different value perspectives, this will significantly influence its recommendations for product development and improvement as well as comparative assertions.*

If the valuesphere shapes the perception of the ecosphere and the technosphere as suggested in Section 2.1.2, then we have to allow for different models for the eco- and technosphere. If we use different models, or at least different model parameters, then it is obvious that the model outcomes may well lead to different outcomes which in turn, may lead to different recommendations. The motivation behind this proposition is that decision makers who disagree on the values and the relevant life support functions of the ecosphere each need their own LCA and may well draw other conclusions.

Proposition (2) will be worked out in Chapters 5 to 7 to an extent that one could claim that it is verified. The other propositions will not be verified, but it will be shown that paying attention to them will help to understand, structure, and perform LCIA.

These propositions will be revisited in Section 10.2.

2.3 Objectives and the book's contribution

The main objective of this book is to approach new frontiers in LCIA, i.e., to pay attention to the perspectives within LCIA and contribute by this to the next generation of methods for LCIA. The full meaning of perspectives – also used as a label in the book's title – will be unveiled in Section 10.1.

In addition to the propositions discussed here and their motivation, one can ask what is the book's contribution, its message, and what are the results that can be expected.

The core of the book's message is the need to consider and to model the valuesphere in LCA to a degree that is equal to what is done for the ecosphere and the technosphere. The consequence of this view is that subjective elements are no longer thought to be undesirable and separated from the objective elements, but are constitutive factors of the decision support tool.

The book's main contribution is the development of a framework which allows not only to operationalise this new view of LCA and LCIA, but to do this in such a way that the framework's structure functions as a kind of umbrella or meta-structure that makes it possible to position LCIA in a manner that is compatible with widely differing world views. LCIA is a comprehensive and very broad task which incorporates information and models from many sciences. The adaptation of these disciplinary elements, the addition of models that have not been used so far, and the combination of all these elements to an interdisciplinary tool is the concrete manifestation of this book's contribution. Section 10.3 will summarise the new elements that are added in this book.

The expected results are partly suggested by the propositions listed here and by the two main points of criticism towards LCIA, i.e., that it cannot strictly separate objective from subjective elements, and that it is poor in modelling impacts (see, e.g., Barnthouse *et al.* 1997). These results can be summarised as follows:

- A new framework will be developed which allows the inclusion of those elements that are judged to be relevant by decision makers holding different world views and which considers values and subjective elements as essential, rather than undesired or non-scientific, parts of the tool.
- The components of the new framework will be worked out to an extent that permits demonstrating its operationability.
- The damage assessment, one of the main element of the framework, will be worked out to such a level of detail that it can be shown that there exist within LCIA reliable and scientific models to calculate potential damages.

Chapters 9 and 10 will discuss these results and offer the final conclusions.

3 Modelling the Valuesphere by Cultural Theory

Chapter 2 claimed that many elements within life cycle assessment are, by their nature, subjective settings, i.e., value choices. It was stated that at the highest level at which disutility is to be measured are the safeguard subjects which themselves reflect a certain world view. This chapter explains the need for a model of the valuesphere, introduces a heuristic, and discusses its application within LCA. Section 3.1 highlights the problem at hand and specifies the requirements such a heuristic should fulfil. The chosen heuristic, called Cultural Theory, is introduced and discussed in Section 3.2. A short overview on other typologies is provided in Section 3.3 in order to position Cultural Theory. First, consequences of the use of Cultural Theory within LCA are highlighted in Section 3.4. Cultural Theory is not uncontroversial and is introduced here as just *one* useful heuristic and not as the key for the rationalisation of all subjective elements.

3.1 Introduction

3.1.1 Problem setting

As introduced in Section 2.1, LCA is a tool covering three spheres: the techno-, eco-, and valuesphere (see Figure 2.1). It is therefore necessary to model the three spheres separately as well as – and this is one of the major added values provided by LCA – to integrate and make the link between these spheres. In fact, many models developed by the different sciences are available for single spheres. What is often missing is the linkage between spheres and the models of the different sciences. These interfaces make LCA unique, useful, and comprehensive. The scope of this task is complicated by the fact that, e.g., the ecosphere cannot be modelled independently from the valuesphere when not just changes, but undesired changes – called damages – are the centre of interest in the modelling. The ecosphere is understood here as a human construct, i.e., the perception of human beings guides the definition and the description of 'environment' and selects the functions it fulfils for us[1]. Human beings have to identify which elements of nature have to be protected, i.e., to define the safeguard subjects and their desired states. Without such settings we cannot identify adverse effects in the environment. Without differentiating between

[1] This works also the other way around: the available information and definitions influence perception. For the differentiation between perception on a individual and on a societal level, see Weber (1995) and Fuhrer *et al.* (1995).

adverse and intended changes in the ecosphere, it is neither possible to develop nor to select models that represent the ecosphere.

In the past, the strategy in LCA methodology development has been to keep apart, as much as possible, the so-called objective parts of LCA (inventory analysis, characterisation) and the more subjective 'goal definition' and 'valuation' (see, e.g., BUWAL 1991, Heijungs *et al.* 1992, SETAC 1993b). One reason for this distinction is the pragmatic need to limit data requirements and modelling efforts in the analysis of both the technosphere and the ecosphere[2]. Such distinctions have been suggested and applied already earlier in systems analysis and in other tools for environmental decision support. However, a closer look at the respective debates shows that the real problems concerned the proper link of facts and values (see, e.g., Miser *et al.* 1985/1988, Hyman *et al.* 1988).

The formulation of the problem setting in this chapter is therefore not directed at the identification of the largest possible areas where purely objective and value-free modelling can be performed. The aim is rather to describe and operationalise the valuesphere in order to make it possible to describe and to model the ecosphere and the technosphere.

3.1.2 Whose valuesphere?

As long as human beings develop LCA methods and practitioners are asked to perform case studies, the required value choices will be made in one way or another. Consequently, the problem is not whether or not to consider values in LCA, but to do this in an adequate and coherent way. The following requirements may guide the search for the answer to the question of whose valuesphere it is that should be described and operationalised:

1) All the value choices – from goal definition through inventory analysis and impact assessment up to interpretation – should be based on the same set of values, i.e., the value choices that have to be made during the different steps of an LCA should form a coherent whole.
2) Designing LCA as a decision support tool makes it obvious that the values held or represented by the decision maker(s) should be the basis for the value choices.
3) The modelling effort necessary for the application of an LCA in a case study should be affordable by those actors commissioning the study.

Requirement (3) has been the driving force so far in the development of LCA methodology. The existing LCA methodologies therefore incorporate the values of the LCA methodology developers wherever value choices are necessary for the formulation of methodology. Values of LCA analysts enter wherever the methodology developers leave open value choices, e.g., allocation rules, that are not closed by specifications given by the decision maker. Finally, the decision maker's values may enter in the goal definition, choice of impact assessment method, of impact categories and of valuation weights; choices that are, by design, left by the developers to the decision maker. This description makes obvious that the first and second

[2] Keeping the analysis of the technosphere and the ecosphere as so-called objective parts makes it possible to build up databases with only one set of data (see, e.g., Heijungs *et al.* 1992, Frischknecht *et al.* 1994, Goedkoop 1995).

requirements mentioned above are not met today by the current designs of LCA methodology.

Requirements (1) and (2) can only be fulfilled simultaneously if the decision maker's values[3] are the basis for all the choicess that have to be made in an LCA. As a consequence, LCA methodology development, as well as undertaking an LCA, and its interpretation, have to be done in close co-operation and exchange of views between methodology developers, LCA practitioners, and the decision maker concerned. Either that, or the values to be considered have to be known beforehand. It is clear that in most cases the effort to develop and undertake an LCA anew for each decision maker separately will be larger than the expected benefit from the LCA. Simultaneity will therefore not be assured as a rule.

In order to fulfil requirement (3), besides requirements (1) and (2), two lines of development can be followed:

A) It can be argued that the environment is a collective good. Therefore the collective or societal values should be the basis for defining what the environment is, its safeguard subjects, etc. I.e., decision makers do have to bear in mind that their decisions should be based on societal values. These are reflected in, for example, environmental policy.

B) It is understood and accepted that the valuesphere is made up of about six billion different value sets (the number of human beings). A number of representative subsets can be identified and characterised and will form the bases for developing few distinct LCA methods.

Track B) has been followed in the course of the approach proposed here for the following reasons:

- LCA is still a voluntary tool positioned at the micro level and used for the environmental optimisation and the selection of products. Someone asking for LCA results as a decision support in order to be able to consider environmental criteria should be allowed to make decisions based on her view of the environment and her perception of what should and should not be safeguarded.
- Determining the present set of societal values is a difficult task due to the limited extent to which these values have been negotiated and incorporated explicitly in policy by making reference to attributes of the environment. Environmental policy and its decisions are a patchwork of historical decisions whose outcomes have been dominated by changing sets of different interest groups. These decisions therefore hardly reflect a stable and uniform set of values.
- The optimisation of the technosphere in order to reduce the burden on the environment is done with the goal of improving the future environmental situation. It may therefore be justified to look at single world views that incorporate a consistent picture of how the desired future should be instead of looking at the current mix of world views.
- Track B) is the more attractive approach both from a scientific and a decision maker's point of view. Scientists will understand the three spheres much better once they have learned to look at them from different angles. Decision makers

[3] A decision maker may well consider values in addition to his own that are held by society as a whole or by a specific interest group.

get additional insights from the information on what the outcomes are by applying different value sets[4].

- Finally, track B) can be transformed into track A) if the distinct value sets are integrated. The opposite transformation would be impossible.

It is clear that track B) has flaws of its own and that the effort required to develop methodology is larger than in the case of track A) (although not necessarily in its application).

The consequence from the discussion in this subsection is that a limited number of value sets from among the whole valuesphere should be identified and modelled in order to allow for compatibility between LCA method, choices made by the LCA analyst, and the values held or represented by the decision maker.

3.1.3 Do value judgements alter the perceived relevance of environmental problems?

In the previous subsection it was assumed that the eco- and the technosphere are perceived and therefore modelled differently depending on the value set adopted by the actor. Jäggi (1997) has confirmed the reality of this assumption with his analysis of different religions and their relation to the environment (see also Jäggi 1993, Jäggi 1994, Krieger 1994). From an ethical point of view, there is also more than one world view, e.g., anthropocentrism, pathocentrism, and biocentrism. Each of them would result in a different selection of safeguard subjects that have to be considered or, at a minimum, would differ in the weights assigned to the different subjects in one and the same selection (Stern 1992, Stern *et al.* 1992, Schaber 1997, Beltrani 1997).

The societal reference system influences risk judgements and management styles, a point that is more fully developed in Hofstetter (1996b:148ff), using findings of Karpowicz-Lazreg *et al.* (1993) and Hofstede (1991). Dunlap *et al.* (1993a/b) have found that people all over the world are, in general, concerned by environmental problems and that they do agree on their major causes. However, the data in their comprehensive coverage of countries reveal some significant differences between countries. These are sometimes due to different preconditions (e.g., population density, climate, GNP), but in some cases they depend on cultural differences.

A large body of literature on the perception of risks points in the same direction. Fischhoff *et al.* (1978) and Slovic *et al.* (1980/1983) can be taken as representative for all those studies of the question why experts rank risks differently than lay persons. They showed that this difference is mainly due to a different definition of 'risk'. Risk experts try to estimate the number of fatalities as accurately as possible while lay persons use a much richer definition of risk. They found that such persons include the following criteria – the so-called psychometric paradigm – in their conceptualisation of risk (Fischhoff *et al.* 1978):

- voluntariness of risk
- immediacy of effect (delayed effect)

---

[4] Decision makers do not like to be told what is best, but like to know which effects do occur if input parameters are changed.

- knowledge about risk by the persons who are exposed to those risks
- knowledge about risk by science
- chronic *versus* catastrophic risk
- common dread
- severity of consequences
- control over risk
- newness

The last two items have been replaced in later studies by (see Marris *et al.* 1996b):

- harm to future generations
- unfairness (unequal distribution of risk and benefit)

Risk experts and lay persons obviously seem to differ fundamentally in their perception of the importance of these criteria. This difference explained to a large extent the variation in the rating given to risky technologies by experts and lay persons. However, no progress was made in the question of why different persons perceive risks differently, i.e., why they use different sets of criteria.

These few examples of arguments and of references to empirical work support the notion that judgements do alter the perceived relevance of environmental problems. The much more interesting question of how they alter this relevance will be addressed in Subsection 3.2.2.

3.1.4 The different levels from behaviour to culture

From what has been said so far and in order to solve the problem identified in Subsection 3.1.1 the following questions have to be answered:

- What exactly is the valuesphere?
- How can we distinguish between different value sets? Can this distinction be based on existing proposals?
- If there exist useful proposals, do they refer to the values and at the same time link them to characteristics of the eco- and the technosphere?
- And finally, do we look for value sets which are necessarily expressed in behaviour?

The fuzzy term of valuesphere can be described as the entirety of all wills, beliefs, attitudes, and convictions held by people. Rapoport (1976) characterises the valuesphere as one particular level of abstraction between the highly abstract concept of culture and the concrete activities of people (see Figure 3.1). The further down we go along these levels the more the values are expressed in behaviour, i.e., in activities. The description on the level of culture, world view or values focuses still very much on the belief system and is thus a rather theoretical or ideal construct free from obvious contradictions. Such a construct, though, does not necessarily reflect the lifestyles and activities observed. Lifestyles and activities are concepts belonging to the level of behaviour and do not just depend on the so-called subjective factors, e.g., the underlying cultures, world views and values, but also on objective factors such as income, education, professional background, etc. Activities and lifestyles are therefore much more dependent on the concrete limitations individuals are faced with than are the values making up their cultural background. Socio-demographic characteristics, i.e., objective factors, tend to change during an individual's life. It is therefore to be expected that the stability in the level of activities and lifestyles is smaller than in the level of world view or culture.

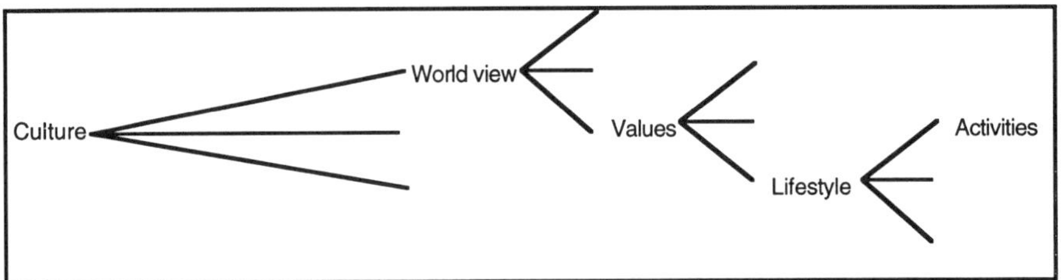

Culture	World View	Values	Life-Style	Activities
At the very least (there are many definitions in anthropology), it is in some way about a group of people who share a world view, beliefs, values etc. which are learned and transmitted. These create a system of rules and habits which are consistent and related (at least theoretically).	This is related to choices, and reflects an ideal.	Values are frequently embodied in images.	This consists of manners, rules, choices, role allocations, allocation of resources, etc.	These are the single bricks of the visible behaviour.

Fig. 3.1: The different levels of abstraction between culture and activities, adapted from Rapoport (1976)

Groups consisting of individuals defined by similar patterns of constitutive factors can be described at most of the different levels of abstraction identified in Figure 3.1. These levels also have the particularity that they are the object of different sciences:

- Anthropologists (e.g., Douglas *et al.* 1982), scientists of religion (Krieger 1994, Kinsley 1995, Jäggi 1993/1994/1997), and also ethnologists (Bargatzky 1986) are concerned with the level of culture[5].
- The intermediate levels of world views and values are mostly addressed by psychologists and sociologists. A frequently addressed research theme here is the mechanism at both an individual and a societal level that lead to changes in values (see, e.g., Inglehart 1977/1979, Hillmann 1989, Klages 1992, Alheit *et al.* 1994, Klein 1995, Laszlo *et al.* 1996).
- Empirical social scientists and marketing research are very much interested in differentiating society according to life and consumption styles. A large body of approaches exists in this area and is applied to specific questions (Bourdieu 1987a/b, Lüdtke 1989, Prose *et al.* 1991, Schulze 1992, Müller 1992, Vester *et al.* 1993, Stern 1993, Reusswig 1994, GfK o.J.)

It was shown that (1) there exist a large number of proposals to distinct lifestyles or cultures and that (2) these characterisations can be found at different levels. As a next step we have to select an adequate approach for the purpose at hand.

The question raised earlier in this subsection, whether or not existing proposals enable one to link values to characteristics of the eco- and the technosphere, should

[5] Only a small and non-representative number of references is given to studies which analyse culture with respect to ecology and the environment. The scientific disciplines mentioned are concerned with research on the subsequent "lower" levels as well.

be reformulated rather as a criterion for the choice of a heuristic. Adequate approaches have to be theoretically founded and/or be subject to verification through empirical work in the area of the perception and the characterisation of the environment. In any case, the approach has to make, for each perspective (i.e., class or group), explicit predictions about how the world is viewed and how it works.

A second major criterion for the selection of an approach is the question of whether the classification of society should be related more to attitudes or to behaviour as expressed by activities and consumption patterns. Environmental psychology has shown that the causal link between attitude and environmental behaviour is sometimes moderate, i.e., attitude cannot be used as valid predictor supported by a high significance[6] (Hines *et al.* 1987, Diekmann *et al.* 1992, Gardner *et al.* 1996). This insight points to the importance of choosing the appropriate level of abstraction. The selection of one perspective from the valuesphere determines the perception, description and the modelling of the eco-sphere and to some extent even of the technosphere. This perspective therefore should be based on a consistent system of culture, world view, and values. It should have some stability and remain unchanged even if some of the objective factors do change. These considerations suggest that the level of culture or of world view is optimal for the purpose of identifying a classification, but the selection of this level brings with it at least two disadvantages:

- The prediction of the behaviour of a group defined at the level of world view or culture is possible to a limited extent only. Certain activities will be typical but others not, and these then cannot be predicted.
- The assignment of individuals to groups of specific world views through empirical studies can not be based solely on data about the objective factors and activities.

The first objection is meaningless for our purpose: The biocentric world view itself is not invalidated just because someone holding it gives, in everyday decisions, much more importance to human beings than to the rest of the biosphere. LCA based on a biocentric world view would offer support for decisions aimed at an optimisation with respect to the minimisation of effects on biocentric safeguard subjects. And again, whether the individual with a biocentric world view will consider this decision support or not is not decisive for the decision support system as such. Zwick (1996) confirms this view by mentioning that values and world view are better predictors of environmental attitude than environmental behaviour[7].

---

[6] Most studies have found an association between attitude and behaviour but the correlations were often weak. Schultz *et al.* (1995) show that the correlation coefficient is higher in older studies. They adduce two reasons for this finding: first, most new studies are only published if they do not confirm a high correlation between attitude and behaviour, and second, prior to 1980, the recycling industry and the supporting infrastructure for collecting wastes had just begun to be set up (at least in USA). Recycling, the case for which these correlations were determined, therefore required a high effort from the individual. Several studies show that the relationship between attitudes and behaviour that needs high effort is significant.
Kraus (1995) shows in a meta-analysis of 88 attitude-behaviour studies that attitudes significantly and substantially predict future behaviour. Kaiser *et al.* (in press) show that responsibility is even a better predictor for behaviour than attitudes.

[7] One has to take into account many situative factors in order to be able to capture environmentally relevant behaviour.

The second disadvantage becomes relevant as soon as empirical work is done in order to determine who belongs to which group. Therefore, questionnaires have to collect subjective factors as well as objective factors.

We claim now that Cultural Theory, introduced in the next section, will meet most of the requirements and criteria identified here. This claim is based on an evaluation of alternative typologies that are described later in Section 3.3. We prefer first to describe Cultural Theory as such in the next section because this gives us the possibility to evaluate the other typologies by identifying commonality with and differences to Cultural Theory.

3.2 Cultural Theory – an overview

This section serves to introduce Cultural Theory (CT) as a heuristic to be used later in LCA. In order to be short but yet provide more than a commented bibliography, we focus here on the points most relevant for its later application, i.e., the theoretical basis (Subsection 3.2.1), the characteristics of the archetypes that make them operational (Subsection 3.2.2), the stability of the archetypes (Subsection 3.2.3), an overview of the theory's empirical validation (Subsection 3.2.4), the quantitative presence in some European countries of the different archetypes (Subsection 3.2.5), and finally some answers to questions that will arise in the course of this presentation and a discussion of the theory's weak points (Subsection 3.2.6).

3.2.1 Introduction to Cultural Theory

The basis of Cultural Theory (CT) was laid by an anthropologist, Mary Douglas (Douglas 1982, Douglas *et al.* 1982), and further developed and adapted to other contexts by a group of methodologists (see, e.g., Thompson *et al.* 1990, Schwarz *et al.* 1990, Rayner 1987/1991, Rayner *et al.* 1987, O'Riordan *et al.* 1991).

There are many ways to understand and define culture, as suggested in Subsection 3.1.4. Thompson *et al.* (1990) roughly differentiate between the view of political scientists who understand culture as mental products, i.e., as a composition of values, beliefs, norms, rationalisations, symbols, and ideologies and the view of anthropologists who refer to culture as a person's total way of life – their interpersonal relations as well as attitudes. One can describe CT without having to opt for one of these views by making instead a distinction between the three concepts of cultural bias, social relations, and ways of life. *Cultural bias* refers to shared values and beliefs. *Social relations* addresses the pattern of interpersonal relations. Combinations of cultural biases and social relations which appear to be viable are called a *way of life* (Thompson *et al.* 1990:1). It is an essential element of the theory that cultural bias and social relations condition each other without giving causal priority to one of them in the formation of ways of life.

A way of life is subject to the *compatibility condition*, that is, "the viability of a way of life depends upon a mutually supportive relationship between a particular cultural bias and a particular pattern of social relations" (Thompson *et al.* 1990:2). The full name for CT is *sociocultural viability theory* which does not only refer to the combinations of social relations and cultural biases but also infers that the combinations have to be sustainable (hence viable).

Douglas has proposed a grid-group theory to help identify and compare ways of life (Douglas *et al.* 1982). She argues that the variety of an individual's involvement in social life can be adequately captured by the two dimensions of sociality: group and grid. "*Group* refers to the extent to which an individual is incorporated into bounded units. The greater the incorporation, the more individual choice is subject to group determination. *Grid* denotes the degree to which an individual's life is circumscribed by externally imposed prescriptions. The more binding and extensive the scope of the prescriptions, the less of life that is open to individual negotiation." (cited from Thompson *et al.* (1990:5))

Each combination of the extremes of these two dimensions results in an *archetype* (or a *way of life* or a *cultural perspective*; all these terms will be used as synonyms). These four archetypes based on different characteristics of social relations are complemented by a fifth, called "autonomy", devoid of social interactions. This archetype is placed in the centre of the grid and group dimensions as shown in Figure 3.2, but in reality is meant to be in a third dimension where no social interactions at all occur.

Thompson *et al.* (1990:7) illustrate their proposal with flesh-and blood vignettes of the following type: "A high caste Hindu villager and a member of a self-sufficient Western commune both have strongly positive group contexts. At the other end of the scale, a self-made Victorian manufacturer and an ununionised weaver employed at his mill both have strongly negative group contexts. What separates the Hindu villager from the Western communard, and the mill owner from his hired hand, is the extent of prescriptions: the grid dimension. The high-caste Hindu villager and the ununionised mill worker both have strongly positive grid contexts in that their freedom is everywhere constrained by a socially imposed gridiron of things they cannot do and moves they cannot make. At the other extreme, the self-made Victorian manufacturer and the self-sufficient communard both have strongly negative grid contexts in that each rejects coercion; they both consider themselves free to act as they please - the one to hire and fire as he sees fit, the other to act as the equal in all respects of his fellow communards." A more precise description of the five archetypes taken from Thompson *et al.* (1990:6f) is given below. It is essentially based on Douglas (1982:202ff).

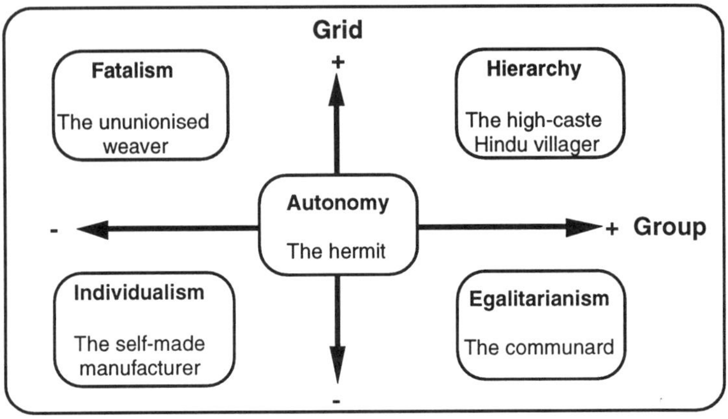

Fig. 3.2: Proposal for a constructed division of society into five cultures or life-styles according to the group - grid theory (Thompson *et al.* 1990)

"Strong group boundaries coupled with minimal prescriptions produce social relations that are *egalitarian*. Because such groups lack (as a consequence of their low grid position) internal role differentiation, relations between group members are ambiguous. And since no individuals are granted the authority to exercise control over others by virtue of their position, internal conflicts are difficult to resolve. Individuals can exercise control over one another only by claiming to speak in the name of the group, hence the frequent resort to expulsion from the group in resolving intragroup differences. The drastic nature of these solutions, however, tends to drive disagreements underground, hence the presence of covert factions vying for control.

When an individual's social environment is characterised by strong group boundaries and binding prescriptions, the resulting social relations are *hierarchical*. Individuals in this social context are subject both to the control by other members in the group and to the demands of socially imposed roles. In contrast to egalitarianism, which has few means short of expulsion for controlling its members, hierarchy has an armoury of different solutions to internal conflicts, including up-grading, shifting sideways, downgrading, resegregating, redefining. The exercise of authority (and inequality more generally) is justified on the ground that different roles for different people enable people to live together more harmoniously than under alternative arrangements.

Individuals who are bound by neither group incorporation nor prescribed roles inhabit an *individualistic* social context. In such an environment all boundaries are provisional and subject to negotiation. Although the individualist is, by definition, relatively free from control by others, that does not mean the person is not engaged in exerting control over others. On the contrary, the individualist's success is often measured by the size of the following the person can command.

People who find themselves subject to binding prescriptions and are excluded from group membership exemplify the *fatalistic* way of life. Fatalists are controlled from without. Like the hierarchist, their sphere of individual autonomy is restricted. they may have little choice about how they spend their time, with whom they associate, what they wear or eat, where they live and work. Unlike hierarchists, however, fatalists are excluded from membership in the group responsible for making the decisions that rule their life.

For a few individuals there is a fifth possible way of life, one in which the individual withdraws from coercive or manipulative social involvement altogether. This is the way of life of the *hermit,* who escapes social control by refusing to control or to be controlled by others."

Using the grid-group dimensions it is possible to sharpen the compatibility condition by stating an *impossibility theorem*: Five and only five ways of life – hierarchy, egalitarianism, fatalism, individualism, and autonomy – satisfy the conditions of viability (Thompson *et al.* 1990:3). Thompson *et al.* (1990) acknowledge that this theorem is ambitious and that only five ways of life may seem an impossibly small number. However, they show that the great social theorists of the past[8] rarely went beyond a development that went from hierarchy to individualism. By omitting fatalism, egalitarianism, and autonomy, many of their theories are limited in the explanation of the variety actually observed. However, the claim that CT doubles the number of ways of life in comparison to other theories is a weak argument in support of the impossibility theorem. One additional dimension besides grid and group would increase the number of ways of life to nine. Subsection 3.2.4 will show that empirical validations suggest that the majority of human beings belong to ways of life that combine the five archetypes, i.e., there are many more than just five ways of life. Nevertheless, the impossibility theorem is important in the sense that it enables one to identify only five extreme archetypes in such a way that everybody is able to position her-/himself with respect to them.

A further basic element of CT is the condition of *requisite variety*. The five ways of life compete on the one hand for adherents and on the other hand are depending on

[8] In an analysis of the "masters" Thompson *et al.* (1990) analyse Montesquieu, Compte, Spencer, Durkheim, Marx, Weber, Malinowski, Radcliff-Brown, Parsons, Merton, Stinchcombe and Elster. Another example would be Inglehart's materialism/postmaterialism dichotomy (Inglehart 1977, 1979).

each other. The existence of other ways of life is necessary either to profit from them or to be forced to demarcate oneself from the other groups and to define one's own identity. Without the existence of hierarchists and individualists, the egalitarians would lack a target to oppose and their strong group boundary would fail to make sense any longer, which would then weaken their way of life. Similarly the individualist needs the hierarchist as an extra-market authority to ensure that the basic instruments of markets, such as contracts, are provided for and protected. That is why CT claims that each way of life depends on the existence of each of the other four rival ways of life for survival. However, this condition should not be over-interpreted. The five ways of life do not necessarily have to be equally represented at a given point in time and place. Autonomy is, as a rule, the way of life with the lowest share of adherents. This can be explained by the fact that humans are social beings that, by nature, look for interaction, but the other four ways of life are also distributed unevenly and their shares change over time and place (see Section 3.2.5).

3.2.2 The many predictions by Cultural Theory

CT and its archetypal ways of life are made operational by the above descriptions of cultural bias and the grid-group dimensions. However, we can sharpen the understanding of the archetypes if many more attributes are causally linked with the five ways of life. The more attributes that can be identified, the easier will be the theory's application to concrete situations. Knowledge on the characteristics inherent to the five viable ways of life will enable one to make predictions about how representatives of a way of life will think about a decision-making problem and how they will deal with it. "Like rational choice models, CT generates a large number of explanations and predictions from a few simple theoretical assumptions"[9] (Thompson *et al.* 1990:106).

This subsection presents the attributes, both those identified by the proponents of CT and those found by empirical studies using CT. This collection of attributes serves as a heuristic in order to facilitate the application of CT to LCA and LCIA in particular. For a beginning we are interested in how the representative members of the archetypes perceive the environment.

Thompson *et al.* (1990) – based on Holling (1986) and Timmermann (1986b) – have introduced the concept of the social construction of nature. The starting point is with four myths of nature – nature benign, nature ephemeral[10], nature perverse/tolerant, and nature resilient – as postulated by ecologists in their attempt to explain the behaviour of agencies managing ecosystems (see, e.g., Holling 1977/1979/1986, Timmermann 1986a/b).

Nature benign refers to the equilibrium-centred view. In Figure 3.3 "a landscape with a bowl-shaped valley within which a ball moves in a way determined by its own acceleration and direction and by the forces exerted by the bowl and gravity. If the bowl was infinitely large, or events beyond its rim meaningless, this would be an example of global stability" (Holling 1986:294). In such a world, trials and mistake of any scale can be made, i.e., recovery is assured once the disturbance is removed.

[9] Subsection 3.2.6 addresses the fact that this belief in functionalism, which is inherent to CT, is one of the criticism coming from sociologists.
[10] I.e., nature is fragile and its state therefore fleeting and passing.

Nature ephemeral or the *myth of instability* can be seen as the obverse of the myth of nature benign. "In natural systems, the best example of this may be a simple closed predator-prey relationship-a proliferation of prey leads to a proliferation of predators who eventually consume all the prey and then starve to death" (Timmermann 1986b:439). Only if the ecosystems are treated with great care and the fragility of nature is respected can the complete collapse be prevented. Both, *nature perverse/tolerant* and *nature resilient* assume that multiple equilibrium states are possible or even necessary. In the case of nature perverse/tolerant it is expected that nature will show a continuous behaviour over a defined period as reaction to stressors. These periods end with sharp changes induced by internal dynamics or by exogenous events, at times large, at times small (Holling 1986:295). Nature resilient postulates not only multiple equilibria in a landscape. "The myth of resilience sees nature as nature naturing, i.e., nature actively altering and responding in various ways to predictable or unpredictable stresses. This means that not only must one account for the internal structure of a system and its potentialities, but also the external context of chance and unpredictable impacts must be incorporated. This is because the system is presumed capable of some sort of adaptive memory, i.e., learning trough historical time" (Timmermann 1986b:444). Nature Resilient – the hermit's myth of nature – is not easy to visualise by means of a ball in a landscape (the landscape *and* the ball are moving) and for this reason is not shown in Figure 3.3.

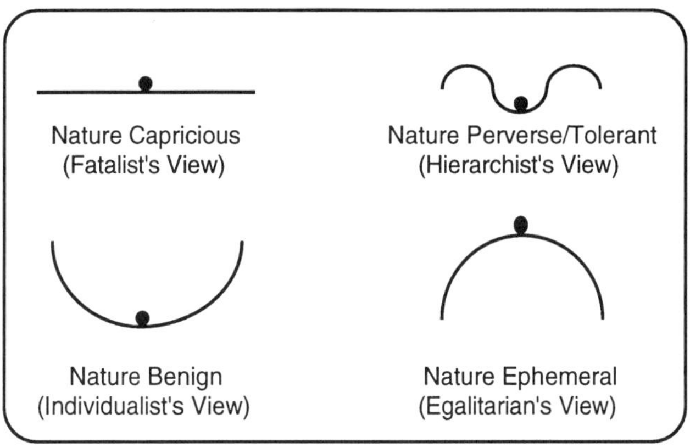

Fig. 3.3: The four primary myths of nature (derived from Thompson et al. (1990)). The rolling ball represents the state of nature which is shifted by human activities to the left or the right or up and down the curved shapes which represent the system's behaviour (metaphor of a sphere rolling in a landscape). The position of the ball indicated in the figure represents the state where human beings live in harmony with nature.

Thompson *et al.* (1990) themselves developed a visualisation of the fatalist's view that nature is unpredictable. They argue that "since fatalists seldom find themselves in charge of major national and international agencies, one of the five myths – Nature Capricious – was not fully elaborated by ecologists" (Thompson *et al.* 1990:37). They then linked these myths of nature with the five archetypes from Figure 3.2.

The myths of nature are in a first step interpreted as individuals' views on the behaviour of the natural system. The links between the archetypes and the views on the behaviour of the natural system presented in Figure 3.3 are the second step in the direction of linking CT with views about the ecosphere. The existence of this link can be questioned and proof of its existence awaits further work (see, e.g., Grendstad *et al.* 1997b)[11]. The most obvious message coming from this visualisation of the link is the hypothesis that individuals who subscribe to one of these myths of nature are increasingly less willing to accept a high dose of environmental measures as they move from the egalitarian via the hierarchist and individualist to the fatalist view. Nature Resilient may be understood as a sub-summation of all the other four myths. Each myth represents for a certain period in a given place the main characteristic of reality and alternate with one another. Holling (1986:307) postulated an ecosystem cycle starting with an exploitation phase (nature benign), followed by a phase of conservation (nature perverse/tolerant), of creative destruction (nature ephemeral), and of renewal (nature capricious).

For natural scientists it is obvious that each of these myths of nature can be true in some situations in some places for a defined period of time and yet fail to describe the situation adequately in other situations. This relation between myth of nature and archetype says only that a person belonging to an archetype has a bias to predominantly remember and impose interpretations on situations which support their own myth of nature, i.e., they have a biased perception. But when faced with a concrete situation defined in space and time and the knowledge about it, representatives of these archetypes may well accept a view of nature that is different from the one they generally hold and that is suggested by the links established in Figure 3.3.

CT has already been used to, e.g., explain and interpret societal changes, politics, attitudes towards technology, risk perception, and it has also been drawn upon to improve risk management. Thompson *et al.* (1990) includes a comprehensive bibliography up to 1990. Additional use has been made since then of CT for, e.g., the prediction and explanation of consumer behaviour (Thompson 199?, Jager *et al.* 1997), the understanding of mass belief systems (Coughlin *et al.* 1998), the routed modelling of uncertainty in integrated assessment (Rotmans *et al.* 1994, Rotmans 1995, van Asselt *et al.* 1995/1996a/b, Janssen *et al.* 1994/1995, Janssen 1996, Trisoglio *et al.* 1997, Rotmans *et al.* 1997), the different paths towards sustainable development (van der Wurff 1992, Roe 1996), and the valuation of environmental problems (Hofstetter 1996b, Mengel Jørgensen 1996, Chemla *et al.* 1997). The insights gained through these studies have been summarised in Table 3.1 which contains a large set of attributes for each of the four archetypes that have been retained in Figure 3.3.

To determine the attributes that are characteristic for the representatives of the fifth archetype, of autonomy, is more difficult. First and foremost, only a small group of individuals belongs to this archetype. Secondly, these individuals lack social interactions among themselves and common regulations of their behaviour; they are therefore largely uninfluenced by each other. And thirdly, it may well be that they adopt a meta-perspective that would cover simultaneously the positions of the other four archetypes together. However, this is no serious shortcoming as hermits play a

[11] It may well be that the first step is more problematic than the second one, i.e., to interpret myth as views of individuals to nature. This aspect is not addressed by cultural theorists.

very small role in our society in decision and policy making[12]. It is therefore safe to simply disregard them in the further course of our analysis.

Archetypes → *Predictions* ↓	**Hierarchist**	**Egalitarian**	**Individualist**	**Fatalist**
Ideal of Fairness	Equality before the law	Equality of result	Equality of opportunity	Not on this earth
Cultural bias	Ritualism and sacrifice	Fundamentalism/ millenarianism	Pragmatic materialism	Inconsistent eclecticism
Idea of nature (4)	Isomorphic nature	Accountable	Skill-controlled cornucopia	Not accountable
Myth of nature	N. is perverse/ tolerant	Nature is ephemeral	Nature is benign	Nature is capricious
Perception of time	Balanced distinction between short and long term	Long term dominates short term	Short term dominates long term	Involuntary myopia (short--sightedness)
Scope of knowledge	Almost complete and organised	Imperfect but holistic	Sufficient and timely	Irrelevant
Preferred economic theory	Bureaucratisation through increasing transaction costs (O. Williamson)	'Buddhist' and 'thermo-dynamic' economics (E.F. Schumacher and N. Georgescu-Roegen)	Neo-Austrian: competition without equilibrium (F. Hayek, A. Alchian)	Marginalisation through structural imbalance (neo-Marxist)
Benefit-risk dilemma(1)	Benefits versus risks	Risks	Benefits	Ad hoc
Temporal survival dilemma (1)	Present versus future outcomes	Future	Present	Ad hoc
Spatial survival dilemma (1)	Local versus global outcomes	Global	Local	Ad hoc
Social survival dilemma (1)	Individual versus collective outcomes	Collective	Individual	Individual
Sovereignty (2)	Institution	Collective	Consumer	-
Procedures applied(2)	Rules	Ethical standards	Skills	-
Criteria (2)	Evidence	Argument	Experience	-
Liability (2)	Redistributive taxation	Strictfault	Loss spreading	-
Trust (2)	Procedures	Participation	Successful individuals	-
Future generations (2)	Resilient	Fragile	Self-sufficient	-
Justification (3)	Contractualism	Rights-based	Consequentalist	No consistent justification
Goal (3)	System maintenance	New social order	Market success	Survival
View of resources	Scarce	Depleting	Abundant	Lottery
Ideal scale	Large	Small	Appropriate	-
Engineering aesthetic	High-tech virtuosity	Frugal and environmentally benign	Appropriate (as cheap and cheerful as possible)	-
Energy future	Middle of the road (technical fix)	Low growth (radical change now)	Business as usual	What you don't know...
Desired system properties	Controllability (through inherent orderliness)	Sustainability (through inherent fragility)	Exploitability (through inherent fluidity)	Copeability (through inherent chaos)
Preferred form of governance	Leviathan	Jeffersonian	*Laissez-faire*	It doesn't matter who you vote for
Information rejection style (5)	Paradigm protection	Expulsion	Networking	Risk absorption
Anomaly handling style (5)	Monster-adjustment	Monster-barring	Monster-accepting	-
Management style (4)	Control	Preventive	Adaptive	-
Attitude to nature (4)	Regulatory	Attentive	*Laissez-faire*	-
Attitude towards humans (4)	Restrict behaviour	Construct egalitarian society	Channel rather than change	-
Latent strategy	Secure internal structure of authority	Survival of the collectivity	Preservation of the individual. freedom to contract	Survival of individual
Leadership (5)	Pro-leadership	Anti-leadership but will accept charismatic leadership under certain conditions	Leadership minimisation (through self-organisation)	Leadership - enduring
Blame-pinning (5)	The victim	The system	The non-productive individual (or external distortions of the market)	"It is the poor that gets the blame"
Tragedy (5)	Technique triumphs over purpose	crabs in a barrel	Tragedy of the commons	(Inescapable ignorance)
Triumph (5)	sacrifice of parts to whole (*noblesse oblige* etc.)	Brotherhood of man	The hidden hand	Dignity

%

[12] Renn (1995) claims that autonomists may be the perfect mediators thanks to their independence.

Archetypes → *Predictions* ↓	**Hierarchist**	**Egalitarian**	**Individualist**	**Fatalist**
Consumption style (5)	Traditionalist: strong links to past and others	Naturalist: rejection of artificiality and excess	Cosmopolitan: neophiliac and wide-ranging	Isolated: traditionalist but with weak connections to past and to others
Impact on production system (5)	High product differentiation/ low product innovation	Low product differentiation/low (or negative) product innovation	High product differentiation/ high product innovation	Low product differentiation/ high product innovation
Advertising and history (5)	Advertising has to fit itself to a gradually accommodating history	Apocalyptic history rejects almost all advertising	Advertising an essential input to a rapidly accommodating history	Advertising rewrites a vestigial history
Style of cheating (5)	Wolves: cheat in hierarchical and exclusive teams, unequal redistribution of proceeds	Vultures: cooperative, but difficulties in equalising proceeds often leads to scism	Hawks: competitive back stabbing/shifting allegiances	Donkeys: sabotage and cheat, when possible, to excess (no group or network controls)
Evolutionarily stable strategy (and its power implications) (5)	Collectivist manipulation (power-wielding and power-deflecting)	Collectivist survival (power-deflecting)	Individualist manipulative (power-wielding and power deflecting)	Individualist survival (power absorbing)
Diagnosis of cause (6)	population	Profligacy	Pricing	-
Policy bias	Contractarian	Egalitarian	Libertarian	-
Distribution (6)	Proportionality	Parity	Priority	-
Intergeneration responsibility (6)	Present = future	Present < future	Present > Future	-
Discounting (6)	Technical standard	Zero/negative	Diverse/high	-
Commitments to institutions (5)	Correct procedures and discriminated status are supported for own sake	Collective moral fervour and affirmation of shared opposition to outside world	Only if profitable to the individual. If not, then exit	-
Nature of pollution (5)	Human defilement of social order through nature	Social transgression of natural order	Matter in wrong place at wrong time	Fecalmonism
Pollution solution (5)	Change nature to confirm to society	Change society to confirm to nature	Market incentives (transferable rights to pollute, etc.)	-
Audit criteria (5)	Legality of expenditures	Equalisation of differences	The bottom line: profit, cost-effectiveness, popularity	-
Search and change behaviour	High on search; low in (internal) change	High on search: high on (external) change	'Satisficing'; enough search for enough change	No search; fatalistic acceptance of change
Concept of human nature (4)	Sinful	Born good, malleable	Self-seeking	March of destiny
Learning Style	Anticipation	Trial without error	Trial and error	Luck
View of needs & resources (4)	Can manage resources but not needs	Can manage needs but not resources	Can manage needs and resources	Cannot manage needs or resources
Attitude to needs/ resources (4, 5)	Increase resources	Need-reducing strategy	Manage needs & resources upward limits of skills	Devise short term responses to cope with erratic mismatches of needs and resources
Rationality	Procedural	Critical	Substantive	Fatalistic
Model of consent	Hypothetical consent	Direct consent	Implicit consent	No consent
Salient risks	Loss of control (i.e., of public trust)	Catastrophic, irrev. and inequitable developments	Threats to the functioning of the market	-
Method for applying model of consent	Natural (or other ideal) standards	Expressed preferences	Revealed preferences	-
Attitude towards risk(4)	Risk-accepting	Risk-aversive	Risk-seeking	-
Risk handling style	Rejection and absorption	Rejection and deflection	Acceptance and deflection	Acceptance and absorption

Tab. 3.1: World views, attitudes, management styles and characteristics of the four archetypes (Schwarz *et al.* 1990:66f), (1) Jager *et al.* (1997), (2) Rayner (1991), (3) Rayner *et al.* (1987), (4) compiled by van Asselt *et al.* (1995) out of Thompson *et al.* (1990), (5) Thompson (1992), (6) Thompson *et al.* (1998).

The predictions presented in Table 3.1 for the four dominant ways of life can be used for several purposes, e.g.,

- to analyse the behaviour of certain groups, their attitudes towards societal problems, or societal change,
- to predict four extreme cases and to foresee their implications prior to making strategic decisions (e.g., which arguments should be used to win a vote), or to

use them for the generation of scenarios in support of decision making (e.g., energy planning, integrated assessment),

- to customise decision support systems for use by the adherents to one of the archetypes that have been identified here.

These are only some suggestions. In a more general vein, this information can be used to explain or model "situations" in which structural uncertainty and judgements play a relevant role (Schwarz *et al.* 1990). Its application to LCA is discussed in Section 3.4.

A detailed look at Table 3.1 makes clear what has been said before. The ways of life defined by CT are archetypes rather than concepts to one (and only one) of which each individual can be allocated. There may be only a few individuals which are fully committed adherents to any one of these extreme descriptions (see Subsection 3.2.4).

3.2.3 Will all the predictions be fulfilled? Surprise and change

It is a trivial observation that not *all* the predictions listed in Table 3.1 will be fulfilled at *the same time* in *reality*. What consequences result from this state of affairs for CT? First of all, the restriction suggested by the three terms printed in the first sentence in italic allow individuals to think that they perceive a real world that is compatible with their own world view to a large extent:

- Even if not *all* predictions show up in reality some of them will. Dissonance is prevented if the view is shaped primarily by the perception of just those events which confirm the predictions (Festinger 1957, Frey *et al.* 1993).
- Things change over *time*. If reality is only observed and perceived at those moments when predictions compatible with the archetype are fulfilled, then it is more likely and easier to overlook the many moments when they don't.
- *Reality* is a questionable construct in itself. What is the reality if it can be perceived in so many different ways? Many predictions in Table 3.1 are falsifiable only with respect to the perception from the perspective of other archetypes (relativism).

"But ways of life, like theories, cannot exclude reality altogether. As evidence builds up against theories, or as ways of life do not pay off for adherents, doubts build up, followed by defections" (Thompson *et al.* 1990:69). If the observation of the real world deviates from the convictions about how the world really is and if adherents of these convictions notice the "real" functioning of the world, one can speak of a surprise to the respective archetypes. A wide range of surprises can occur depending on exactly how the world is functioning and on whose perspective the observation is based. Table 3.2 presents a typology of these surprises. Only occurrences in the off-diagonal are surprises. The combinations of actual development and world view represented by the lightly shadowed boxes represent compatible and therefore expected combinations and thus make viable the way of life under the given circumstances.

The viability of a way of life is by no means an indicator that this way of life will remain stable during the whole life of a decision maker. Although individuals will tend to perceive only that part of reality which supports their own world view[13], they inevitably will sooner or later face surprises. They will sooner or later be confronted with the fact that the world does not necessarily develop in ways that are compatible with their own view and that they are often unable to bring about the world they desire (Table 3.2). Thompson *et al.* (1990:3f) formulate this idea as follows: "Change occurs when successive events intervene in such a manner as to prevent a way of life from delivering on the expectations it has generated, thereby prompting individuals to seek more promising alternatives." That means that a persistent pattern of surprise will in the end force individuals to look for an alternative to their way of life, probably making them adopt one or the other of the three remaining ways of life. Whether this reorientation happens slowly or abruptly depends on the way the individual is confronted with the incompatibilities between the actual world and his or her present way of life. As a given way of life is sustained by both cultural bias *and* social relations, abrupt changes are only possible if the social environment is changed abruptly too. Such abrupt changes are most likely if catastrophes, accidents, and a revolutionary reordering of social relations occur. Otherwise, change will be steady but slow.

Actual world → Way of life ↓	Capricious	Ephemeral (fragile)	Benign	Perverse/Tolerant
Fatalist	Survival, expected runs of good and bad luck	Expected windfalls don't happen	Unexpected runs of good luck	Unexpected runs of good and bad luck
Egalitarian	Caution does not work	New societal order, optimal balance with nature	Others prosper	Others prosper
Individualist	Skill is not rewarded	Total collapse	Market success, no collapse	Partial collapse
Hierarchist	Unpredictability	Total collapse	Competition	System maintenance

Tab. 3.2: A typology of surprises, adapted from Thompson *et al.* (1990:71)

A change is possible from any one archetype to any one of the others. This results in twelve possible change trajectories even if we limit the attainable alternatives to just the four archetypes that are characterised by intensive social relations. Classical theories which distinguish only between two archetypes, e.g., materialism and post-materialism (Inglehart 1977), can only observe two possible change trajectories and do normally focus on change in just one direction, i.e., the shift from materialism to postmaterialism. Thompson *et al.* (1990:75ff) show that each of the twelve trajectories that CT permits can be explained and justified and they find for some of them corresponding historical examples. We do not want to elaborate here on a theory of value changes (see, e.g., Inglehart 1979, Klages 1992, Klein 1995, Laszlo *et al.* 1996) because it is not essential to the topic of this book.

What is essential for CT is the suggestion that change is essential to the stability of a way of life. Individualism, for instance, in order to maintain itself, must push some individuals up-grid into the fatalist category. Stability without change is like

[13] Rosner (1995:109) remarks that mental models are usually taken for granted and that "we do not usually perform experiments to challenge them. Even if there is some evidence against an existing model, this results in pain and therefore first the evidence is questioned (cognitive dissonance), before the model – a proprietary knowledge – is given up." This is one of the causes that makes people so resistant in their beliefs and thus allows things to change only slowly.

trying to balance oneself on a bicycle without pedalling (Thompson *et al.* 1990:80). This positive view of change provokes some questions relevant to the theory's further application to LCA:

- If everything is changing, does it then make sense to use this heuristic in the less flexible context of LCA?
- Are these changes on the individual level slow processes or can individuals switch from one way of life to another within the same day?

The first question can be answered affirmatively. The changes are not de- but stabilising society and the heuristic with it. The archetypes as such will continue to conform to the predictions listed in Table 3.1 but the individuals adhering to them may change and the size of the adhering group may also change over time (see also Subsection 3.2.5).

The second question is not that easy to answer because cultural theorists themselves are of two opinions about the answer. The crucial point here is that most individuals spend their lives in more than one sphere, e.g., at home, at work, in leisure activities. Each sphere has its own social environment with its rules. The open question now is whether individuals arrange their lives in such a way that their cultural bias linked with their specific pattern of social relations is met by all spheres, or if they (have to) move frequently between institutions with different social organisations. In the former case, individuals will seek to attach themselves only to those institutions in the different spheres in which they move that have the same type of social organisation. In the latter case, individuals live during the same day and week in institutions that belong to different corners of the grid/group scheme and thus have to endure at least some of the time a contradiction between beliefs and behaviour.

Marris *et al.* (1996b) claim that Mary Douglas has been a proponent of the first view while Thompson *et al.* (1990) plead for the 'mobility' version. The existence of a frequently heard justification for NIMTOO, the acronym for "not in my term of office" (Kemp 1992 cited in Power 1993), suggests that the 'mobility' version better corresponds to modern conditions. NIMTOO is indirectly an admission that there are spheres of life in which this individual would react or decide differently. This suggests that at least this individual's preferences do change from one sphere to the next. Thompson *et al.* (1990:265) state that, because cultural bias depends on social context and *vice versa*, an "individual's bias will be consistent only to the extent that its social context is consistent. An individual may find himself in cutthroat competition with his business rivals, hierarchical relations in the military, egalitarian relations at home, while treating certain areas of life, say inability to carry a tune, with fatalistic resignation."

Although Thompson *et al.* (1990:263ff) believe that there are individuals living in the way described above, they relativise the 'mobility' version in three aspects:

- First, they claim that individuals living in such different contexts will in none of them be an extreme representative of a way of life. If they were activists in an egalitarian pressure group, they would have to change their other contexts in order to minimise personal dissonance.
- Second, they expect that individuals will make significant efforts to bring consistency to their social environments. With that they also make clear that – as in Goethe's Faust – there may be more than one soul dwelling within an indivi-

dual's heart, but that the competing allegiances are not equally divided among the possible ways. That is, one way of life dominates the others. Douglas may argue that these efforts will normally succeed in establishing a harmonised context.

- Thirdly, the compartmentalisation of biases may coexist peacefully for a long time only if they belong to different realms of life.

This short discussion suggests that the 'mobility' version with the mentioned relativising aspects is the one that is more congruent with everyday experience than the 'harmonising' one. The answer to the initial question is therefore: yes, individuals can switch from one way of life to another several times a day, but these contexts themselves are rather stable and change only slowly. (We disregard 'catastrophic' events for the moment.) The implications of this position can be summarised as follows:

- Empirical validation will be more difficult (see next subsection).
- Decision makers that have to choose 'their' LCA-model have to be aware of in or for which social context they intend to make the decision.
- Modelling the valuesphere by a small number of ways of life that are maintained by both cultural bias and social relation, i.e., by CT, may be the most meaningful procedure because even an atomised approach distinguishing between individuals would not suffice to describe consistent value patterns.

3.2.4 Empirical validation of Cultural Theory

One of the advantages of CT over other classifications of societal groups is that the formation of the ways of life is theoretically explained with their social relations, i.e., the grid-group dimensions. It is this characteristic that made possible the many predictions on world view and management style for the different ways of life just by analysing the grid and group dimensions, their consequences for social relations, and their further effects on the ways of life.

This advantage of CT becomes a disadvantage as soon as it has to be empirically validated. Such validation is not impossible in principle, but so far only a limited number of empirical studies have been undertaken (see, e.g., Rayner *et al.* 1987, Dake 1991/1992, Dake *et al.* 1993, Grendstad 1994, Sjöberg 1996/1997, Marris *et al.* 1996b, Grendstad *et al.* 1997a/b, Thompson 199?, Ellis *et al.* 1997, Coughlin *et al.* 1998).

A number of questionnaires are available to elicit the cultural bias of individuals. Most are based at least partly on the "British Edition" of "Dake's Cultural Biases Questionnaire" (Dake 1991). Its shortest version that can be found in the literature, developed and used by Grendstad *et al.* (1997b), is shown in Table 3.3.

Studies using qualitative methods such as participant observation and focus groups also have provided empirical support for CT (e.g., Rayner *et al.* 1987, Marris *et al.* 1996b). And quantitative studies have confirmed the predictions made, although the correlations found were not always statistically significant. Some problems of and insights from these empirical studies are:

- It can be assumed that individuals live in more than one social context and switch from one to another. (A point discussed in the previous subsection.)

Questionnaires, such as the one reprinted in Table 3.3, may elicit inconsistent answers from them. This effect can indeed be seen clearly when questionnaire results are used to categorise individuals according to the four archetypes. Only a very small share of individuals exhibit a dominant pattern that corresponds to one of the archetypes (see, e.g., Marris *et al.* 1996b, Boholm 1996). This problem should be solvable by using focus groups instead, or one should limit questionnaire surveys of individuals to persons with a coherent social context[14].

	strongly disagree	mildly disagree	both agree and disagree	mildly agree	strongly agree
Hierarchy					
One of the problems with people today is that they challenge authority too often.					
The best way to provide for future generations is to preserve our customs and heritage.					
Egalitarianism					
What this world needs is a fairness revolution to make the distribution of goods more equal.					
I support a tax shift so that the burden falls more heavily on corporations and people with large incomes.					
Individualism					
If people have the vision and ability to acquire property, they ought to be allowed to enjoy it.					
Everyone should have an equal chance to succeed and fail without government interference.					
Fatalism					
Co-operation with others rarely works.					
It seems that whatever party you vote for things go on pretty the same.					

Tab. 3.3: Example of a questionnaire to survey the views of individuals about society in order to derive a scale for cultural bias (Grendstad *et al.* 1997b). The question's wording was: "To what extent do you agree or disagree with each of these statements. Indicate the answers by writing an 'x' in one box for each of the following statements".

- Marris *et al.* (1996b:6) claim that Dake (1991/1992) has only shown that it is possible to identify the cultural bias described by CT, but they think it is necessary to also show that the four types of social relations can be identified and that the cultural biases correlate with the social relations as predicted by CT. CT cannot be validated without these second and third steps.
- Panellists have sometimes not understood that the archetypes with their extreme patterns of attributes and the illustrations of the myths of nature are just extreme flags but not concrete descriptions of reality. Grendstad *et al.* (1997b) showed that it was difficult to prove the correct attribution of cultural bias to the myths of nature[15]. One obviously has to be careful when confronting individuals with clearly exaggerated predictions.
- Several studies have revealed the existence of a strong correlation between hierarchy and individualism (e.g., Dake 1991, Marris *et al.* 1996b). It is therefore

[14] Olli (forthcoming) distinguishes between the coherent individual, the sequential individual, and the synthesised individual and finds that the last type, where only limited adherence to one perspective can be found, is also a frequently found individual. He suggests, therefore, not only to analysis support of a cultural perspective, but also its rejection. However, this additional separation enables a large number of additional combinations which enlarges the size of the necessary sample to arrive at statistically significant results.

[15] They showed that organised environmentalists believe 83% in the myth of nature as perverse/tolerant although 86% of them belong to the egalitarian way of life.

difficult to find statistically significant correlations between them and their predictions. The explanation here is that categorising the surveyed individuals into the four ways of life is possible to a limited extent only. Firstly, this is due to the rather extreme characteristics of the archetypes. Secondly, the questionnaires developed by or based on Dake have not been prepared for this purpose[16] and they are especially weak in separating hierarchists from individualists. Recent empirical studies working with different questionnaires and/or analysis methods solved most of these problems (Grendstad *et al.* 1997a, Ellis *et al.* 1997, Coughlin *et al.* 1998).

These problems should be kept in mind when empirical studies are planned and analysed. Yet it has to be said that the available studies all support at least some part of CT despite all the problems identified here and no study has rejected CT as such. Marris *et al.* (1996b) used the so-called 'psychometric paradigm' from Fischhoff *et al.* (1978) and Slovic *et al.* (1980/1983) (see Subsection 3.1.3) in comparison with CT to see which approach better explains the variation in risk perception (a set of 13 risk issues were used). The results of the survey with individuals showed that CT explains 12% while the psychometric paradigm explains 50% of the variation in risk perception. Nevertheless, Marris *et al.* (1996a/b) judge CT to be very useful because it is not just correlated closely with risk perception but it explains also why it is.

The criticism of CT that its empirical validation is limited can be answered on a more general level. The more encompassing a theory and its consequences are, the more difficult is the theory's empirical validation. Theories that concern just a small area of life are easier to validate, but they also have just a small reach.

3.2.5 The distribution of ways of life in European countries

Having introduced CT and the problems faced with its empirical validation, one can ask about the frequencies the five ways of life are distributed with within different countries. Grendstad (1994) has made a re-analysis of the survey undertaken by the *European Values System Study Group (EVSSG)* which included 9'839 individuals from eight European countries and reported roughly 330 variables for each individual (Harding *et al.* 1986). Eighteen of these variables were used in a factor analysis due to their good fit with the grid and group dimensions. The results were analysed in a second-order discriminant analysis using the country attribute as the grouping variable. Finally, Grendstad (1994) calculated the shares of four ways of life for all eight countries (Table 3.4). The autonomists' way of life could not be extracted from the available data set, but it can be assumed that its share is small in all eight countries.

It is interesting to see that the re-analysis of this survey reveals significant differences between the eight countries. Only France and Italy, and Belgium and Great Britain, respectively, show a similar pattern of the shares. All other countries have patterns of their own. The aggregation to a weighted average therefore does not make much sense given this wide variety. Nevertheless, it is interesting to note that the fatalists form the largest group overall with a share of 34%. The fatalists are an

[16] Dake used all four scores on each way of life for each individual to correlate them with predictions on, e.g., risk, rather than categorise these individuals into prototypes first and then calculate the correlations.

inherently necessary group when a country is dominated by a hierarchical system or by individualists.

Way of Life	West Germany	Nether-lands	France	Italy	Den-mark	Belgium	Great Britain	Ireland	*Weighted average*
Individualism	37.8	21.8	21.8	20.7	19.3	17.5	14.3	8.0	*23*
Egalitarianism	31.1	39.1	13.5	14.7	57.8	20.9	25.5	16.7	*23*
Hierarchy	11.2	17.9	19.5	18.7	17.3	25.4	29.3	46.7	*20*
Fatalism	19.9	21.2	45.2	45.9	5.6	36.2	30.9	28.6	*34*

Tab. 3.4: The relative size of cultures in eight European countries (Grendstad 1994) and the weighted average (population data from Stat. Jahrbuch (1996)) for the cluster of the eight countries.

The numbers given in Table 3.4 may provoke one to ask in which societal context these attributions are made. This question makes clear that it does not make much sense to derive such general averages.

If one knows the shares of the ways of life, one could construct a representative average attitude towards specific questions by constructing a weighted average of the attitudes specific to each way of life and its share in society. However, this procedure is unlikely to work in most cases because consensus processes favour the powerful representatives of a society and different groups will have this power for the different questions at hand.

3.2.6 Criticism towards and open questions in Cultural Theory

The criticism of CT is manifold yet modest (see, e.g., Nelkin 1982, Johnson 1987, Renn 1991/1995, Marris *et al.* 1996b, Boholm 1996, Sjöberg 1996, Grendstad *et al.* 1997b). The most serious point of criticism concerns the missing empirical evidence for many of the hypotheses of the theory. The number of empirical studies has increased after 1990, but many of them can be criticised for their design or do explain observed variations only to a limited extent (see, e.g., Marris *et al.* 1996b, Sjöberg 1996). Other recent studies even showed that certain assumptions do not hold up, e.g., the identification of archetypes with the symbolic graphical representation of nature (Grendstad *et al.* 1997b). The major conclusions from this limited empirical validations are (see also Subsection 3.2.4):

- It is not yet clear whether individuals or only groups of individuals should be used as the basic element in empirical studies.
- All three central assumptions of CT, i.e., the cultural bias, the social relations, and the viable correlation between them, have been demonstrated to exist as separate elements.
- The perspective is not falsifiable if the archetypes are all present at the same time within organisations.

Many empirical studies have confirmed most of the predictions that have been made despite these problems. In addition, Thompson *et al.* (1990:270) refer in support of CT to the many scientific applications of CT ranging from "the rules for keeping kosher, to why and what institutions forget, to the practices of different types of criminals, to how mathematicians deal with anomalous results". We could conclude that the empirical validity of the theory as such is limited, while the usefulness as a heuristic in different contexts has been demonstrated.

On the content level, one can insist that the myths of nature are too simple and they do not represent important ecological mechanisms such as persistence, i.e., the continued functioning of ecosystems away from the equilibrium point, and the continued development of new ecosystems (Kwa 1987). It has been suggested that at least two dimensions, e.g., stability and complexity, should be used to describe nature (van Asselt *et al.* 1996a).

Renn (1995:41) makes two additional critiques:

- The relationship between archetypes and organisational interests is unclear and problematic. If cultural affiliation precedes interest, then what determines to which archetype groups or organisations belong?
- The definition of the five archetypes as the only relevant cultural pattern in modern societies needs more evidence than the reference to tribal organisations or generic models of human interactions.

The first point becomes moot when one acknowledges that both cultural bias and social relations have the same relevance in supporting a way of life. Groups and organisations will then consist of an uneven mix of different archetypes that make, under most circumstances, the group or organisation belong to one or another of the archetypes. The second point is acknowledged by giving it the name of the 'impossibility theorem'. However, so far no proposals with comparable theoretical or empirical foundation for completing the set of archetypes have been forthcoming.

Johnson (1987) finds that CT does not explain all aspects of American environmentalism. He suggests complementing CT by taking into account social movement theories, because CT as such is so far too static an instrument. Johnson's critique is a modest one and he states (Johnson 1987:168): "Grid/group analysis[17] is a provocative and potentially powerful theory. Its critics have failed to disprove its contention that cosmology stems from the varying cultural negotiations of individuals within different social structures."

Renn (1995:42) concludes: "[Cultural Theory] should be treated as a hypothesis rather than the exclusive explanation. The emphasis on values and world views rather than interests and utilities is a major accomplishment of this theory."

Thompson *et al.* (1990:261) ask and answer some relevant questions arising from CT. One of them is: how do adherents to rival ways of life communicate with each other? Their answer is that anthropologists and travellers are able to do so, that a certain minimal agreement on the rules of logic (non-contradiction, for instance) provide a basis for communication, that the small number of ways of life limit the number of arguments and increase the chance that the same arguments are encountered over and over again by individuals. All these facts and others allow for communication between different archetypes, a necessary element for CT. An even more salient explanation is that only a few individuals are prototypical for the archetypes. Besides the characteristics of one way of life, most individuals also present characteristics belonging to other cultural biases. This can be because an

[17] Grid/group analysis has become generally identified as CT only after the publication of Thompson *et al.* (1990).

individual switches between more than one context or because an individual's adherence to just one way of life is not sacrosanct.

Another point addressed by Thompson *et al.* (1990), and also found frequently in discussions about CT, is that there are many situations in which individual self-interest overrides cultural bias. Thompson *et al.* (1990) acknowledge this, but claim that the determination of one's interest is often a difficult task in itself and again steered by cultural bias. In our case of applying CT to LCIA, we have already mentioned that we are not interested in modelling behaviour, but attitudes. Therefore, our application of CT is less sensible to the aspect of self-interest.

Finally, one can easily observe that people do not like to be put in a quadrant and labelled as corresponding to an archetype; they prefer to be perceived and acknowledged as individuals. This is a serious point of objection, because decision makers will be confronted with the need to select an appropriate quadrant, i.e., archetype. There are two possibilities to take this objection into account. Either, one applies CT the way it was done by Dake (1991), Grendstad *et al.* (1997b) and others, i.e., by measuring the degree to which an individual belongs to each one of the four cultural biases without placing individuals in the quadrant with the highest degree of concordance. Or, one explains exactly why such a grouping is made for the question at stake and probably should also show that society in daily life uses many other characteristics to group individuals, e.g., political parties, level of prosperity, race, religion, sex, hair colour. The answer Schwarz *et al.* (1990:72) give to this observation is that CT allows people to build the boxes of their choice while people rejecting these boxes are busy putting everyone else into just one box.

Although this last point seems to be merely a question of communication, one should always insist that people accept that the prescriptions of the ways of life are just valid for the extreme archetypes and that their presence may be extremely rare in the population.

3.2.7 Summary

In seeking to make sense of their lives, people inevitably organise themselves into patterns that enable them to do this. CT aims to explain these patterns and the processes by which they are sustained (Thompson *et al.* 1990:99). The introduction of CT in this section has provided only a small insight into the basics of sociocultural viability theory which can be summarised as follows (Thompson *et al.* 1990:84):

1. There are five, and just five, ways of life that are viable (impossibility theorem).
2. Each of these ways of life is viable only if all others are present (requisite variety condition).
3. These essential mutualities can be sorted out into two linked hypercycles: a primary hypercycle in which each of the four engaged ways of life does something vital for the others that they cannot do for themselves, and a secondary hypercycle in which the hermit is able to withdraw from all the intense transactional activity generated by the primary hypercycle.
4. Each way of life is dynamically stabilised, that is, the movement of individuals in and out is a necessary condition for its persistence through time.

5. These movements in and out can follow any of the twelve transitions that are logically possible (if we consider just the primary hypercycle).
6. It is the cumulative mismatches between promise and performance that, from time to time, dislodge an individual from his or her way of life.

The theory assumes that what matters most to people is how they would like to relate to other people and how they would like others to relate to them (Thompson *et al.* 1990:97). Most other theories in the social sciences focus on the degree of preference realisation and *how* people get what they want (see, e.g., Feldman 1980). CT tries to explain *why* people want what they want as well as how they get it, thus it focuses on preference *formation* as well.

The *validation* of the theory is still partly outstanding, i.e., not all predictions are empirically tested and some predictions are at least questioned by empirical studies. Empirical studies are difficult to design because it is not fully clear if surveys of individuals or only of social groups are capable to validate the theory.

CT is fully applicable thanks to a clear underlying theory and a long list of predictions concerning the world view and management styles of the single archetypes. Therefore, it is a useful heuristic to model the valuesphere.

The relation of CT to other theories and social science models and its application in LCA are discussed in the following sections.

3.3 Cultural Theory in relation to other typologies

If you are convinced that CT is a sensible choice for a heuristic to model the valuesphere, then you better skip this section. If you ask yourself if there are other typologies, if they are completely different, and why they were not chosen instead, then the following subsection, where a short bibliography of other typologies with comments concerning their relation to CT is given, will provide the answers. Although we offer no classification of the typologies[18], we nevertheless grouped the proposals in four subsections: the ones reviewed by Thompson *et al.* (1990), the ones which make an explicit statement about the view on nature, a selection of the ones which show interesting parallels to CT, and finally the ones which complete the picture of typologies.

3.3.1 Thompson *et al.* (1990) and the masters

The analysis and discussion of the masters of sociological theory (Montesquieu, Comte, Spencer, Durkheim, Marx, Weber, Malinowski, Radcliffe-Brown, Parsons, Merton, Stinchcombe, Elster) takes up more than 100 pages in Thompson *et al.* (1990). Further discussions of these theories would undoubtedly be of interest, but we refer the reader instead to Thompson *et al.* (1990) and the original literature cited there. Here, we present only the three main conclusions of this analysis by Thompson *et al.*:

- The archetypes of CT are superior to most of the ones suggested by the masters of sociological theory because they are derived from common social dimensions.
- Social forms closely resembling egalitarianism and fatalism are observed by the past masters but treated as anomalies or ignored.
- Functionalism works within CT although it is criticised by other approaches[19].

These conclusions should not mislead the reader. Many elements of CT are similar or the same as in the theories of the past masters. The types of social relations we distinguish in CT are for instance the same as those Montesquieu, Spencer, Marx, Durkheim, and Weber have identified. However, none of the past masters (maybe with the exception of Durkheim) formed a mutually exclusive and jointly exhaustive set of categories based on social dimensions. (In the case of CT they are the grid and group dimensions). From these dimensions one can not only deduce the frequently identified and discussed types of individualism and of hierarchy, but also the archetypes of egalitarianism and fatalism, both of which are missing in the preceding theories. These two archetypes strengthen the explanatory power of the typologies.

Functional explanation – as used in Thompson *et al.* (1990) – can be defined as an explanation "in which the consequences of some behaviour or social arrangement are essential elements of the causes of that behaviour" (Stinchcombe 1968:80). Egalitarians, for instance, blame "the system" and insist that new technologies have

[18] Such a classification could have used criteria such as, e.g., the discipline of origin, historical development, the distinguishing characteristics, i.e., whether subjective or/and objective factors are constituting factors, and the fields of application.

[19] This claim may be altered upon closer analysis (Grimen forthcoming).

inherently high risk potentials, or that other archetypes have incorrect views of nature etc. The functional argument behind that is that behaviour can be explained in terms of the contribution it makes to maintaining a way of life (Thompson *et al.* 1990:105). In response to one other objection to functional explanation, it has been shown that not only rational choice models, but also CT can generate a large number of explanations and predictions (see Table 3.1) from only a few theoretical assumptions.

In addition, it can be mentioned that Thompson *et al.* found no serious contradictions between the past masters and CT. This is not surprising as several of CT's elements had been already proposed by them.

3.3.2 Typologies which make reference to nature or environmental characteristics

The typologies which allow – like CT – correlating individuals or groups of individuals with views on nature are the most relevant alternatives to CT for our purpose. We found five approaches which might serve, to a certain degree, as alternative concepts:

- The concepts of anthropocentrism, eco- or biocentrism, and partnership were introduced as ethical concepts[20] which may stand for the individualist, egalitarian, and hierarchist myths of nature respectively, or which could be seen as an alternative set (van Asselt *et al.* 1996a). This set can be completed by pathocentrism and holism and used to justify the selection of safeguard subjects in LCA and which kind of interventions may be considered to do harm to them (Beltrani 1997). These concepts are widely used in ethical discussions, but little related to other spheres of life and few further characteristics are provided for them.
- The "new environmental paradigm" can be seen as an early attempt to characterise environmentalists and differentiate them from the general public. Many questionnaire items are close to the ones used for the egalitarian perspective in CT (Dunlap *et al.* 1978).
- In Table 3.4, a set of compatible characteristics for four archetypes are presented. Pearce (1993) intended with this compilation to position the two paths to sustainability he selected for his further analysis. It is not fully clear whether both weak and strong sustainability are considered as the only viable ways of development or if they are just the more probable ones. However, it is only a small step to label the 'cornucopian' as the individualist, the 'accommodating' as the hierarchist, and the 'communalist' as the egalitarian. 'Deep ecology' can be seen as an extreme form of egalitarianism which places a high demand on the hierarchic system. Pearce's system is already close to CT. What is missing are more predictions on the world view and management style and the sociological foundation.
- A motivation similar to Pearce's has led Fischer-Kowalski *et al.* (1994) to develop four paradigms: poison, natural balance, entropy, and conviviality. They claim that there exists a variety of conceptions to distinguish between what is

[20] For the respective empirical studies see Stern (1992), Stern *et al.* (1992/1993/1994/1995a/1995b).

good and bad for the environment. Scientific disciplines and political or ethical understandings of man-nature relationship can be correlated with the four paradigms. Fischer-Kowalski *et al.* (1994) used these paradigms to reason the need for different kinds of indicator sets to describe environmental damage caused by the socio-economic system[21]. In order to put these four paradigms into a structure, they postulate two so-called 'epistemological qualities'. One quality describes the dichotomy of "analytic - holistic" while the other dimension separates "well-being oriented" from "risk-oriented". These two dimensions are not further analysed by Fischer-Kowalski *et al.* (1994) and the concept is just used to justify the different nature of the indicator sets. The proposed scheme appears to be immature concerning its sociological foundation and the explicitness of statements, but some of the four paradigms might well be used to replace or to be combined with the myths of nature in order to take into account more complex images of nature.

Archetype→ Characteristics↓	TECHNOCENTRIC		ECOCENTRIC	
	Cornucopian	Accommodating	Communalist	Deep ecology
Green labels	resource exploitative, growth-oriented position	Resource conservationist and 'managerial' position	Resource preservationist position	Extreme preservationist position
Type of economy	Anti-green economy, unfettered free markets	Green economy, green markets guided by economic incentive instruments (EIs)	Deep green economy, steady-state economy regulated by macro-environmental standards and supplemented by EIs	Very deep green economy, heavily regulated to minimise 'resource-take'
Management strategies	Primary economic policy objective, maximise economic growth (GNP)	Modified economic growth (adjusted green accounting to measure GNP)	Zero economic growth, zero population growth	Reduced scale of economy and population
Sustainability labels	Very weak sustainability	**Weak sustainability**	**Strong sustainability**	very strong sustainability

Tab. 3.4: The different spectra of sustainability (Pearce 1993)

- Van der Wurff (1992) develops his own five ideal environmental perceptions based on an evaluation of nine classification systems of general environmental perception (including CT and Inglehart's theory) and labels these approaches as: 'back to nature', 'ecosocial', 'structural ecologisation', 'ecological modernisation', and 'effect-oriented'. The five perceptions are partly based on CT without referring, however, to the underlying dimensions of social relations. Therefore, they can partly be linked to archetypes. Although the typology is used to explain the national positions on environment and development in seven countries, there is little empirical experience available and the validity of the classification has not been demonstrated yet.

All these five approaches offer archetypes which have different views on nature. Some of them are embedded as well in some predictions on behaviour, world views

[21] They suggest indicators for emissions within the poison paradigm, economic-ecological system indicators (e.g., material balances, energy or material intensity, etc.) within the entropy paradigm, and purposive interventions in life processes (e.g., km roads, successfully applied pesticides) within the natural balance and conviviality paradigms. All of these indicators are far from predicting damage and can best be understood as proxy indicators. See Section 4.4 for a different application suggested in this book.

and management styles. However, these typologies offer little sociological foundation, almost no empirical validation, and are therefore not preferable to CT. At best, CT might profit from them by developing more appropriate views on nature than the myths of nature used so far.

3.3.3 Typologies with interesting analogies to Cultural Theory

Many typologies show parallels to CT in some respects and differences in others. A selection of four typologies which served in different context to classify attitude and/or behaviour is presented here:

- Inglehart's dichotomy of materialism-postmaterialism has attracted a large number of researchers, either working with the theory, or attempting to falsify it[22] (see, e.g., Inglehart 1977/1979, Klages 1992, Alheit *et al.* 1994, Klein 1995). The dichotomy has been considered as being made up somewhat of two dimensions, rather than just one. Klein (1995) supplements Inglehart's prototypes by a re-analysis of available empirical data with the 'realist' (value synthesis) versus the 'resignated' (value loss) dichotomy. The parallels with the archetypes in CT now become obvious. Materialists and individualists, postmaterialists and egalitarians, realists and hierarchists, and resignated and fatalists have a rather high degree of correspondence. However, neither Inglehart nor Klein suggest the grid-group dimensions and thus have no social relations as the underlying structure. The correlations produced by the two theories may therefore differ in some cases.
- Bourdieu's theory of the 'subtle distinctions' in society are based on empirical data (including many objective factors). Without going into the details of his theory and its validity (see, e.g., Bourdieu 1987a/b, Blasius *et al.* 1989), we see two parallels with CT: the social sphere is an important component of his theory and the identification of subtle distinctions may be seen as Bourdieu's requisite variety condition, as Thompson *et al.* (1990) would call it. Bourdieu (1987a) orders his milieus in such a way that there results a more hierarchic milieu (high power and capital volume), a more individualistic milieu (high economic capital, low cultural capital, and conventionality), a more fatalistic cluster of milieus (low economic capital, little influence), and a more egalitarian cluster of milieus (low economic capital, self control, high cultural capital). However, these characteristics do not really correspond to the attributes listed in Table 3.1 and Bourdieu's dimensions have a different origin than the ones used in CT.
- Bahro (1987) constructed a world scheme based on Galtung in order to explain the many political changes and instabilities we have been faced with so far. The four corners of his universe are characterised by:

[22] It is very interesting to note that Inglehart based his theory on Maslow's theory (need pyramid and predictions on need fulfilment) (Maslow 1954). Maslow is nowadays criticised as being too simplistic. Culture Theory would probably be more concrete by saying that Maslow's pyramid is valid for only one archetype. Other archetypes will have other needs and other priorities resulting in at least a different order of the needs within the pyramid but most probably also in a different pyramidal geometry. Maslow's theory may fit well for a certain group within society, e.g., western world people having experienced world war(s), but fail to describe other parts of society. A CT dependent Maslowian "building" of needs may be able to explain many effects observed in market research with respect to consumption patterns (Dake *et al.* 1993, Jager *et al.* 1997).

- First world, capital, market, co-operation, liberalism, capitalism
- Second world, state, plan, bureaucracy, Marxism, socialism
- Third world, locally, human beings in the centre, family, village, anarchism, Ghandism, Maoism
- Fourth world, state and capital, plan and market, bureaucracy and co-operation, Japanism

With the middle of the square thus defined, he localised socio-democratism. Nine of the possible changes are illustrated with historical examples. The four corners of Bahro's scheme do not completely match with the archetypes of CT and they are not built on an underlying theory or constitutive dimensions. However, the square seems to be a perfect heuristic to explain history and to make predictions and proposals for the future.

- A comprehensive analysis of cultures and organisations is provided by Hofstede (1991). He adapts the view of social anthropologists which state that all societies have the same basic problems, but approach them by different means. The three basic problems are: (1) the relation to authority; (2) the relation between individuals and society and the masculine and feminine views of individuals; and (3) the way to deal with conflicts, the way of controlling aggressions and expressing feelings. From these basic problems Hofstede (1991), distils four dimensions: power distance (from small to large), collectivism to individualism, masculinity to femininity, uncertainty avoidance (weak to strong). An additional fifth dimension of long/short-term orientation has been added based on an additional analysis focusing on China (Hofstede 1991). Seen from the perspective of CT, one could assign the grid-dimension to the power distance and the group-dimension to the collectivism-individualism distinction. Masculinity, uncertain-ty-prone, and short-term orientation would measure attributes of individualists, and femininity, uncertainty avoidance, and long-term orientation would measure attributes of the egalitarian way of life. From that comparison we can see that Hofstede (1991) considers the two dimensions of CT, but is more specific in differentiating between individualists and egalitarians by adding three dimensions. It is also clear that from Hofstede's data it is possible to derive the four archetypes of cultural perspective[23]. The scope of Hofstede's study did not include the environmental dimension. This is the main reason that only few environmentally related predictions of individual attitudes are possible. Therefore, his typology is more difficult to apply to other applications and it was therefore disregarded here for our purpose.

None of the presented typologies use the grid/group dimension, although Bourdieu and Hofstede both refer to social relations. Other theories (next to Bourdieu's), based on social distinctions, are discussed in Müller (1992). The lack of parallels between CT and the typologies presented here with respect to underlying social relations should not be taken as an indication that CT is unique in that respect. Luhmann (1995), for instance, confirms that individuals' values are largely dependent on their social relations, i.e., they are social constructs. Durkheim (1933/1951), too, explains world views by their social relations. By functional explanation, Durkheim believed, one could find the social sources of the thoughts and actions of individuals.

[23] Maybe such a re-analysis would be a good opportunity to get more empirical evidence for CT.

3.3.4 Further typologies

The label of 'lifestyle' covers many proposals for typologies. Most of them have been developed with the clear-cut aim of explaining or predicting behaviour in specific situations. The following books and reports may help to get a limited overview of this wide area:

- Reusswig (1994) provides a comprehensive overview of sociological lifestyle concepts (M.E. Sobel, M.J. Weiss, M. Zapf *et al.*, A. Mitchell, G. Schulze, P. Bourdieu, H. Lüdtke), of lifestyle concepts used in market and consumption research (SINUS, INFRATEST, Eurostyles), and of shorter references to many other classifications. Some of these concepts can easily be transformed into CT by assigning lifestyles to archetypes. Others allow only for the attribution of some lifestyles to archetypes and still others are a mixture of archetypes.
- Another comprehensive overview of different lifestyle concepts and their foundations is given by Lüdtke (1989) together with a general critique of empirical research.
- A book by Alheit *et al.* (1994) provides an overview of some well-known lifestyle studies. The relevant part is devoted to qualitative portraits of five individuals and the presentation of a pre-test for the operationalisation of a new set of lifestyles.
- Jungermann *et al.* (1993) use four personality prototypes characterised by the two dimensions 'values', ranging from ecological to economical, and 'knowledge', ranging from small to large, in order to structure the discussion on technology and risks. The prototypes with large knowledge are the 'utopistes' or 'alternative experts' and the 'technocrats' or 'traditional experts'. The prototypes with low knowledge are the 'green basis' and the 'broad public'. This mapping may have proved to be useful for the questions they have had. However, there is little empirical foundation for these dimensions which concern two very different aspects. No obvious parallel to CT can be made.
- Zwick (1996) developed a lifestyle typology distinguishing seven archetypes within the three dimensions of conformity, socio-economic status, and asceticism. This typology was developed to understand better people's attitude towards technology.
- A further analysis of attitudes towards the future that have been derived by cluster analysis can be found in Juchler (1995).
- A consumer-oriented classification called 'Eurostyles' has been developed for Europe by statistical analysis of a wide range of national surveys on consumers (Euro-Style 1991/1993). The resulting scheme offers 16 Eurostyles which can be ranked according to the two dimensions of 'materialism-postmaterialism' and 'modern, change - conservatism, persistence'. These prototypes are used by many national and international companies to strengthen and focus their marketing to meet the needs of single Eurostyles or groups of them.

Especially the market-oriented typologies are necessarily behaviour-oriented. They will not be analysed further as we are looking for attitude-oriented typologies (see Subsection 3.1.4).

3.3.5 Exclusivity *versus* transformability of Cultural Theory

The survey of other typologies in the previous subsections has shown that there exist many potential alternatives to CT. In order to support the choice of CT we make succinctly explicit once more what it is that makes CT so useful for our purpose:

- CT explains not just views on society or behaviour, but explicitly includes views on nature. CT therefore serves perfectly to model the interface between valuesphere, ecosphere, and technosphere.
- The theory is based on the two underlying dimensions of social relations, the grid and the group. This is the basis for its claim that all possible viable ways of life are covered.
- This foundation of CT makes it possible that functional explanations can be applied which in turn make possible the generation of many compatible predictions, thus increasing the coverage and the usefulness of CT as a tool.

The many fields of application, the increasing stock of empirical expertise, and the already large compilation of compatible predictions (see Table 3.1) make CT a widely applicable instrument. In addition, it is remarkable that the CT community is already co-operating with another instrument of environmental sciences, i.e., integrated assessment (Trisoglio *et al.* 1997). Although this is a very pragmatic argument, it is essential that social scientists support the adaptation to and application of their theories in environmental sciences.

However, some of the other typologies mentioned above also fulfil some of these criteria, are possibly better known within specific areas, have already proven their applicability to resolve certain questions, or are less criticised than CT. These are good reasons to chose such another typology! Therefore, it is argued, we should not insist on CT's exclusivity, but appreciate its transformability to/from other typologies. Modelling the valuesphere by applying elements of CT does not mean that the outcome is only useful to adherents of CT. On the contrary, the overview of other typologies has shown that many similarities exist between many of the archetypes used by them. The transformation of modelling outcomes to other typologies is therefore possible and desirable if, e.g., another typology is better understood by decision makers.

The use of CT to model the valuesphere is therefore best seen as the selection of a heuristic or of a tool rather than of an ideology. The transformability of CT is an additional support to our decision to exclusively use CT in our application!

3.4 Cultural Theory in LCA

After the introduction of CT and the identification of parallels with other typologies, it is time to ask and concretise the application of CT in LCA and to think about its implications. This consequence analysis of CT in LCA ends in the crucial question: "whose tool is LCA"? Further consequences of CT in LCA are discussed in Chapters 8 to 10 after the operationalisation and application of CT in LCIA (Chapters 4 to 7).

3.4.1 The intended use of Cultural Theory in LCA

In Section 3.1, an overview of the problem setting and the need for a modelling support had been given. The two main purposes of CT in LCA are:

- To model the valuesphere in order to define what are the ecosphere and technosphere and which of its characteristics are the relevant ones to be considered and modelled, i.e., to understand them as human constructs.
- To make sure that all choicess in LCA[24] are consistent in themselves and are compatible with one specific world view.

The intended use of CT in LCA is therefore to serve as an additional set of causal factors in the modelling of the valuesphere. Process engineering, environmental chemistry, environmental toxicity, ecology, and medicine are other disciplines which deliver insights into causality, rules, and laws.

The use of CT as a heuristic enables one to establish a link between the techno- and the ecosphere, on the one hand, both dominated by little questioned natural laws, and the 'soft' valuesphere, on the other hand. To make the soft valuesphere harder by postulating functionalism and by deriving rules and theorems may be judged as a too mechanistic approach to solve the problem. However, to do so will motivate decision makers to think about their own valuesphere (and the ones of other stakeholders), social scientists to improve LCA, and LCA methodology developers and analysts to make transparent their (often hidden) value judgements.

The ultimate goal is to provide for each decision situation a specific LCA where judgements are made compatible with the world view(s) of the decision maker(s) and concerned stakeholder(s). The goal in this book is more modest. The aim is for an archetype-independent basic structure that includes elements which are sometimes considered as relevant only by one or two archetypes. In addition, the application is limited to the impact assessment phase of LCA in which modelling of the ecosphere and of the valuesphere and of their interface is the dominant problem. Within this restriction, CT is used to model the choices compatible with the world views for each archetype separately wherever the analyst or methodology developer is confronted with value choices.

[24] Such values choices are necessary within all steps of a LCA and during methodology development as well.

Depending on the specific decision situation, a decision maker looks at just the outcome of his/her archetype[25], or looks at the outcome of the archetypes represented in the decision situation, or, finally, looks at the results for all archetypes to test the robustness of the outcomes. In principle, it would be possible to calculate a weighted average of the outcome if the shares of archetypes in society are known. However, as suggested in Subsection 3.2.5, such a weighted average should not be confused with a (democratic) consensus. It will provide almost no additional insight. It is therefore preferable to perform a robustness analysis instead of an aggregation in the case where all the archetypes are relevant.

In the case of integrated assessment, a similar procedure proved to be useful in order to find routes of scenarios which are based on compatible world views, i.e., it is mainly used to reduce structural uncertainty (Rotmans *et al.* 1994, van Asselt *et al.* 1995/1996a/b, Janssen 1996, Rotmans *et al.* 1997). The set of applications within integrated assessment is growing and so far it has been applied to, e.g., world population development and global warming (van Asselt *et al.* 1995/1996a/b, Janssen 1996, Trisoglio *et al.* 1997).

The valuation of the many attributes influencing the disutility assessment (Subsection 3.1.3) is an aspect going beyond the modelling of the structurally uncertain development of population or global warming. This aspect, introduced by Hofstetter (1996b), is new for environmental decision support tools. Chemla *et al.* (1997) and Finnveden (1997) both state that this line of further development may enhance the usefulness of LCA for decision support.

Van Asselt *et al.* (1996a) summarise their experience with the possibilities to apply CT to concrete choicess as follows:

- The translation of the structural uncertainty inherent in specific cases to the archetypes of CT needs an iterative effort involving modelers, experts from the different sciences, cultural theorists, and other experts of the social sciences.
- Given this precondition, it is possible in 80% of cases to arrive for a specific issue at unambiguous descriptions of the interpretations of the archetypes.

The first requirement could only be met in part by this book. The quality of the translations therefore may be less than predicted. However, the intention is still to empirically validate all the translations made here once the whole system of LCA is described and modelled in terms of CT. The translations made in Chapters 4 to 7 have to therefore be considered as suggestions *ad interim.*

[25] A vision in this direction could be that the archetypes are colour-coded and that, for instance, product ecolabels are labelled with a set of differently coloured bars. Decision makers, i.e., the consumers in this case, already know beforehand the colour which fits best with their world view. Therefore, they have the possibility to consistently base their consumer decisions on the, e.g., blue bar on products.

3.4.2 Are all archetypes relevant for LCA?

Having accepted that we model the valuesphere by CT, one then can ask whether we have to model all five of the archetypes. To answer this question we differentiate between two decision situations:

A) The decision maker decides in a way that is compatible with her/his world view.

B) The decision should represent a consensus in society.

In case A) all those archetypes which make decisions should be considered in the model. These are the active archetypes, the hierarchists, individualists, and egalitarians. Fatalists do not decide because it won't change anything anyhow[26]. Fatalists would not ask for an LCA at all. This is also true for the autonomist, i.e., the hermit. The extreme isolation and lack of interaction with the rest of the world limits the usefulness of LCA for his/her purpose.

In decision situation B), fatalists and autonomists should be represented as well as the active archetypes. However, fatalists will again claim that the active archetypes anyway will do what they want to anyway and that their own view will not change anything[27]. Autonomists will never participate in a consensus process and therefore find themselves excluded from any decision process, but their exclusion is of no consequence for the quality of the decision because of their low number.

Although the fatalists' share in society can be as high as 45 % or more (see, e.g., Table 3.4), they play a negligible role in decision making and therefore in LCA. Fatalists are, to some extent, the mass the active archetypes can manipulate and it is this which makes their decisions realisable.

3.4.3 Interest groups and their cultural bias

Based on Beentjes *et al.* (1995), Mengel Jørgensen (1996) asked herself if different stakeholder groups may prefer other kinds of LCA or, more specifically, other kinds of valuation criteria. For that purpose, she correlated stakeholder groups with their political culture, applying the typology of CT. Based on this correlation and the typical application of LCA in the fields of interest to the stakeholder groups, she made predictions on the stakeholder's attitude towards LCA and weighting, their valuation criteria, and their preferred weighing methods. A selection of her hypotheses are compiled in Table 3.6.

Although Table 3.6 presents only hypotheses which still have to be empirically validated, it is already possible to highlight some of the more important aspects:

---

[26] They do decide in daily life, of course. And no decision is also a decision. They just do not believe that they can change anything by making their decisions.

[27] This attitude makes fatalists refusing to voluntarily fill in questionnaires or participating in interview surveys. This bias of opinion polls is in principle known but often neglected. Martinez-Ebers (1997) presents a study approach where a better response rate was achieved by monetary incentives. However, one can question whether such a refined study design will lead to more meaningful predictions if fatalists will afterwards not join the public policy making process.

- Within most societal actors, one can identify interest groups which represent different archetypes, i.e., business is not just industry dominated by individualism, or environmentalists are not automatically egalitarians.
- Within all the main groups, there are interest groups which have a positive or even a very positive attitude towards LCA. LCA is therefore an instrument with a broad coverage of stakeholders and has the potential to become the instrument of choice in decision situations.
- However, there are interest groups which will not use LCA. It can therefore be assumed that they will refuse to become involved in a stakeholder panel interpreting LCA results[28].
- A wide range of weighting (valuation) methods would be preferred by the different interest groups. The types of preferences and of information used in these methods vary substantially. It is in fact one aim of this book to suggest a meta-method with which all interest groups interested in LCA would be comfortable (see Section 8.3).

Stakeholders/ Interest Groups	Cultural bias	Attitude towards LCA	Preferred weighing (valuation) methods
Environmentalists			
Grassroots	E	Negative	Panels which are citizen dominated or social veil of ignorance, Sustainability based DtT
Eco-establishment	I or H	Very positive	Monetarisation, Social panel which mirrors society
Business			
Hierarchic corporations	H	Little interest	Political DtT, Abatement-cost based monetarisation
Individualised corporations	I	Very positive	Monetarisation with WTP and cost-benefit analysis, Consumer panel
Egalitarian corporations	E	Very positive	Monetarisation with combined WTP, DtT with sustainability targets and social preferences
Politicians			
Conservatives	H	Neutral to neg.	DtT, cost-benefit analysis
Liberalists (Dutch)	I	Very positive	Monetarisation with WTP and cost-benefit analysis, Consumer or stakeholder panels
Socialists	egali- tarian H	Negative	Panels with worker and politicians, Politically based DtT
Greens	E	Very positive	Consensus stakeholder panel, Sustainability based DtT
Regulators	H	Very positive	DtT, Expert panel, Monetarisation with abatement costs
Scientists	H	Positive	Sustainability based DtT, Expert panel
Consumers			
Normal consumers	F or I	No interest	none
Potentially green consumers	I, pot.. E	Very positive	Sustainability based DtT, Expert/consumer panel combined with monetarisation
Green Consumers	E	Sceptical	Sustainability based DtT, Expert/stakeholder panels

Tab. 3.6: Selected hypotheses concerning the attitude towards the use of LCA and the preferred weighing methods (Mengel Jørgensen 1996)
(E = Egalitarian, H = Hierarchist, I = Individualist, DtT = distance to target, WTP = willingness to pay)

[28] A parallel to the grassroots opposition towards LCA has been described by Tal (1997) with his analysis of their attitudes toward risk assessment.

This very short summary on the positions of interest groups toward LCA confirms the statement from the previous subsection that only the three archetypes, the hicrarchists, individualists, and egalitarians, have to be considered in the modelling because they make decisions and will base them on LCA.

3.4.4 Cultural bias of LCA

In a last subsection, an obvious question is whether LCA as a tool already has intrinsically biased assumptions. If this would be the case, then only the corresponding archetype has to be considered within the modelling and other types of tools would be needed for the other archetypes.

Indeed, recalling Chapter 1 and comparing it with Table 3.1 reveals some egalitarian and hierarchical biases. The basic assumption that all environmental interventions along the life cycle of a product have to be considered as independent of country or of place has a strongly egalitarian bias. The same holds true for the practice in LCA *sensu stricto* of compressing the time scale in a way that all environmental interventions are considered as if they would occur today. However, the idea of a tool to support environmental management and the basic acceptance of environmental interventions and damages are elements that are more congruent with a hierarchical world view. The optimisation character of LCA on the micro-level and the voluntary nature of LCA are elements which attract individualists instead.

This first evaluation reveals that the tool's application and view of nature are basically hierarchic[29], while the way temporal and spatial equity is dealt with has a strongly egalitarian touch. This contradiction is well hidden so far and there is some chance that all three archetypes will accept LCA as their tool by perceiving only those elements that are in harmony with their own view.

But as indicated by Table 3.6 and suggested by Finnveden (1997), there is room for an archetype-specific orientation of the tool. This possibility to make LCIA more specifically adapted to different archetypes is one perspective worked out in this book[30] (see also Section 8.2 for other phases of LCA).

[29] As Table 3.6 postulates science is hierarchic as well.

[30] Thompson (1997) gives the CTist's view on the requirements for technological decision making.

3.5 Final remarks

The previous sections have suggested Cultural Theory with its three active archetypes, i.e., hierarchist, individualists and egalitarians, as the heuristic to model the valuesphere and its interface with the ecosphere.

Cultural Theory is considered to offer a typology of archetypes which hold extreme but consistent world views. CT is attractive for our purpose because of its theoretical foundation and its functional power of explanation. The many applications covering a wide range of different areas of life have helped in the formulation of a large number of attributes of and predictions about the world views and management styles of the archetypes. This large set of predictions support the LCA methodology developer and the analyst to make assumptions on the likely choicess made by the different archetypes.

However, we appreciate the charges that the scheme is too rigid, that only a few decision makers will fully identify themselves with one archetype alone, that there are other typologies which could equally well serve as a heuristic, and that it may even be necessary to refer to different kinds of classifications such as cultural bias, religion, or urbanity to explain the attitudes of individual attitudes towards all kind of questions[31].

Further, we appreciate that some people may disagree with the attempt to model a collective good, i.e., the ecosphere, by only considering the world view of a subgroup of society. Our answer to this objection is that if LCA is used as a voluntary tool in private decisions, then the tool should reflect the decision maker's view as precisely as possible.

Approaches from some scientific fields are completely overlooked, e.g., the big five taxonomy[32] used in psychology (John 1990, John *et al.* 1991), the personality attributes of differential psychology (Herrmann 1984), or the characterology developed by physiognomists (Kretschmer 1925). It is therefore obvious that others might model the valuesphere with completely different tools and means.

The three active archetypes of Cultural Theory will serve in the following chapters to differentiate between three different types of LCIA.

[31] This last remark is from a note of Dr. Thomas Baumgartner, CREATO, Thalwil (CH) from 26-4-1996 as a reaction to Hofstetter (1996b)

[32] This taxonomy includes the five dimensions extraversion/surgency, agreeableness, neuroticism *versus* emotional stability, and openness/intellect. They can be measured by questionnaire items (John *et al.* 1991) and are based on a long history of natural-language personality descriptions (John 1990).

4 Modelling the Ecosphere by the Structured Aggregation Procedure

While Chapter 3 described the model of the valuesphere, this one will discuss, explore, and finally describe how the ecosphere is to be modelled. After a specification of the problem setting, we propose to model the sphere by the three different aspects 'damage', 'unknown damage' and 'manageability' (Section 4.2). For each of them, a separate structure will be suggested which leads through aggregation to an index (Sections 4.3 to 4.5). As already argued in Section 2.1, the ecosphere can only be modelled by assuming an underlying valuesphere. Therefore, the relevance of the three indices depends on the cultural perspective adopted. The value choices within the single indices are suggested separately for each cultural perspective. An overview of the whole structured aggregation procedure is provided in Section 4.6. The prescriptions for the final rules of composition and aggregation have to be seen as preliminary at this stage of their development. Empirical work with decision makers may well alter the results of this last step.

4.1 Damage assessment and damage attributes

Section 2.1 introduced the top-down thinking in the modelling of safeguard subjects to represent the ecosphere's main properties. Here, we are able to partly extend the discussion and to make more applicable suggestions. A further aspect considered here is that a deterministic model linking environmental interventions to damages on safeguard subjects will fail to include all relevant consequences on the ecosphere. This observation is one motive for a further extension of the framework.

4.1.1 Environmental problems as a starting point

Early attempts to model the severity of environmental interventions which had been calculated in the inventory analysis, used a compartment-oriented aggregation, i.e., the *critical volume* of air and water[1], the mass of solid waste and primary energy use (Jansen *et al.* 1972, Basler&Hoffmann 1974, BUWAL 1984, BUWAL 1991). These

[1] The so-called critical volumes approach assumes the dilution of the emissions up to the respective air or water quality standard. The "used" volume per substance were added up to the so-called critical volume. Neither degradation nor partitioning was included and no attempt was made to combine the critical volume of water and air.

indices were occasionally further aggregated by making use of analogies and weighting (see, e.g., Suter *et al.* 1989, Hofstetter 1991, Schaltegger *et al.* 1992, Jolliet 1993a).

This line of development has been challenged by the introduction of impact categories representing the environmental problems singled out by Dutch environmental policy. A Dutch expert panel complemented these problems with a few additional categories and thus was born the so-called *policy themes* approach (Heijungs *et al.* 1992). The resultant list of 18 impact categories has been received well and served under the label 'CML Classification' as the basis for many LCA case studies. Goedkoop (1995) has developed this approach further. He retained most of the pollution-oriented impact categories and replaced the category of 'human toxicity' by the impacts on human health through winter smog, carcinogenics, and heavy metals. Pesticides are the only eco-toxic burden included in the list of impact categories in EcoIndicator'95 (see Table 4.1). This explicit definition of the toxicity categories was a necessary step in order to be able to define targets of acceptable damage.

Proposals from North American authors for impact categories make use of similar categories, although different category indicators are suggested in some of these approaches and toxicity is assessed in much more detail (Table 4.1). Their roots in risk assessment (RA) and environmental impact assessment (EIA) are clearly visible. Indeed, the CML classification is closer to national indicator systems and green accounting (see, e.g., Adriaanse 1993, Jesinghaus 1993, OECD 1994, Klaus *et al.* 1994) than to schemes used in EIA and RA.

Both the efforts of SETAC to define the state-of-the-art and of ISO to standardise LCA have included several attempts to define a so-called minimum or default list of impact categories. Udo de Haes (1996) provides the latest compilation of such a list designed to provide LCA practitioners with some sort of guidance. Two very pragmatic criteria have so far guided the compilation of such lists of impact categories:

- Each impact category should have a defined category indicator and a specified model of how to quantify the contribution to this indicator.
- The model for the impact indicator should either rely on a proposal from an international body or be well known and generally accepted.

The acceptability of the model (second criterion) was to be ensured or improved by the demand that only *one mechanism* should underlie each impact category, i.e., all the environmental interventions summarised by one and the same impact category should contribute to the same mechanism and be interchangeable with each other. Such a strict grouping (called common mechanism approach) would make it possible that the models were based largely on natural science. Especially the toxicity categories were considered to violate this criterion and therefore a frequent subject of criticism.

Looking back, it is now obvious that neither the *policy themes* nor the *common mechanism* approach have made it possible to produce a consensual list of impact categories which could serve to model the ecosphere. The original list from the policy themes approach had been already extended *ad hoc* by a Dutch expert panel and thus resulted even in a watered-down approach for use in the Netherlands. The approach of the common mechanisms, on the other hand, only offered a criterion for the definition of each impact category, but not of the *set* of environmental interventions to be considered here. (There are literally thousands of mechanisms.)

CML Classification (Heijungs *et al.* 1992)	**EcoIndicator'95** (Goedkoop 1995)	**Union Carbide - Classification** (Boguski *et al.* 1995)	**Battelle Classification** (Vigon *et al.* 1995)
Resource depletion			
Abiotic resources		Total Energy Requirement	*Fossil Fuel Depletion* *Mineral resource Depletion*
Drying out			*Decreased Water Availability*
Biotic resources			
Pollution			
Greenhouse effect	Greenhouse effect	Greenhouse Gas	Global Warming
Depletion of the ozone layer	Ozone Depletion	Ozone Depletion	Ozone Depletion
		Weather Alterations	
Human toxicity	Winter smog Carcinogenics Heavy Metals to Air and Water	Allergenicity/Sensitisation, *Behavioural Effects, Bone effects, Cardiovascular System Effects, Central Nervous System Effects, Human Carcinogen, Irritant/ Corrosive, Methoglobinemia, Odour, Renal Effects, Reproductive Effects, Respiratory Effects*	*Toxicity* *Respiratory Effects* *Human Carcinogens* Groundwater/Drinking Water Contamination
Ecotoxicity	Pesticides	*Aquatic Life* *Aquifer Contamination* *Air dispersion/Transport*	*Vegetation Stress from Air Contamination, Aquatic Biota Toxicity, Terrestrial Biota Toxicity, Increased Surface Water Turbidity Effect on Fish*
Photochemical oxidant formation	Summer smog	Photochemical Smog	*Photochemical Smog* *Decreased Visibility*
Acidification	Acidification	Acid rain, pH Alterations	*Acid precipitation* Altered Surface Water pH
Nutrification	Nutrification	Eutrophication Oxygen depletion	*Eutrophication*
Radiation			
Waste heat		Thermal Changes	
Noise			
Odour			
Working conditions			Worker Exposure Eye & Respiratory Irritant
		Solid Waste	*Plant Toxicity from Solid Waste* Decreased Landfill Space
Direct damage			
Physical damage to ecosystems		*Chem/Bio Content Alteration*	*Smothering of Spawning or Benthic Habitat* *Habitat loss*
Damage to the landscape		*Visibility Changes*	
Direct or indirect human victims			

Tab. 4.1: Applied or suggested classification systems in LCA for the most relevant environmental problems. Impact categories printed in italic have either not yet been operationalised or the authors of the classification systems suggest their further improvement.

The missing criterion so far has been the magnitude of harm done by an impact category to the representatives of the environment that was to be protected, i.e., to safeguard subjects. The safeguard subjects can be understood as the common endpoints (Udo de Haes 1998).

The value judgement, and with that the policy element, inherent in this *common endpoint approach* is the selection of the safeguard subjects. Once this societal choice is made, there is no need anymore to discuss standard lists of impact categories or interventions. If they contribute relevantly to the damage to safeguard subjects, then they have to be included, otherwise they can be disregarded[2].

This shift in the modelling framework undertaken in this book is the reason that we will not suggest a list of impact categories. The consequences that stem from this shift are the theme of the next subsections and of Sections 4.2 and 4.3.

4.1.2 Analysis at the level of safeguard subjects

Subsection 2.1.4 provided an overview of the proposals set forth so far in the literature for the determination of the sets of safeguard subjects. We concluded there that it is impossible to derive safeguard subjects in a unidirectional process from ethical principles or other principles of humanity. One could identify them on the basis of society's revealed preferences instead[3]. However, revealed preferences are purely descriptive and may even be nothing more than just surrogates for underlying characteristics. Hence, the safeguard subjects should not be derived, but be defined instead in a normative manner that complies with the world views that have been identified in Chapter 3. Ideally, they would be defined through a co-operative effort of representatives of the humanities, of adherents to the different world views, and of LCA experts, the latter pointing out the implications of the proposed set of safeguard systems and providing their operationalisation (Hirsch Hadorn 1997).

Müller-Wenk (1997:1) describes safeguard subjects as representative parts of nature which fulfil the following requirements:

1. the damage to safeguard subjects should be representative of the unknown damage to nature,
2. the damage can reasonably be described in practice, and
3. the number of safeguard subjects should be very small.

The first requirement is difficult to prove, but should be a guiding principle for the determination of safeguard subjects. We will present a solution to this problem in Section 4.2. The second criterion is very important for the operationalisation of the LCIA. Compromises with respect to this second requirement are impossible. The selection and the definition of safeguard subjects will therefore always be influenced by this criterion[4]. The third criterion is considered to be important because the

[2] A consolidated list of 56 environmental problems provided by the European Environmental Agency may be an inspiring starting point for such a test (Stanners *et al.* 1995:613).

[3] Contingent valuation would not adequately reflect the societal values because individuals and markets are not suited to do so (Holland 1997).

[4] This is one of the reasons why it is claimed that the determination of safeguard subjects is an interactive process between LCIA modellers, representatives from the humanities and adherents of different world views.

damages to safeguard subjects have to be combined or weighted before a final judgement can be made. This aggregation step at the level of safeguard subjects will always be subjective by nature and should therefore be kept tangible to decision makers (Principle of parsimony).

The question of the proper safeguard subjects has been debated intensively in the course of a joint Dutch-Swiss project (Müller-Wenk 1997, Goedkoop *et al.* 1997) on the redesign of 'EcoIndicator'95', the LCIA method proposed by Goedkoop (1995). Instead of following the interactive procedure suggested here, it was concluded there that 'human health' and 'ecological health' should be included among the safeguard subjects anyway in order to represent two relevant aspects of life. In addition, 'resources' was considered as a third safeguard subject. The inclusion of this latter choice has been mainly motivated by suggestions made in SETAC (1993b) and ISO (1997) and is not based on reasoned arguments, i.e., decision makers ask for this safeguard subject, but either do not offer reasons for the importance of resources or, if they do, provide very different justifications for the need to safeguard them.

The safeguard subject *'human health'* includes, in terms of LCIA, both pressures on and damages to human health, both of which are due to changes in environmental conditions. Chapter 5 will introduce 'disability adjusted life years' (DALYs) as a unit of measuring damages to human health. This metric is used by WHO and the World Bank (Murray *et al.* 1996a/b) and can be adapted for our purpose by adding only a few small refinements. The value choices inherent in this concept will be addressed in Section 5.4. The examples given in Chapters 6 and 7 will both concern human health. They are the basis for the claim that the operationability of at least this safeguard subject is given within this book.

Odum (1971:8) defines *'ecosystems'* as "..any unit that includes all of the organisms (i.e., the community) in a given area interacting with the physical environment so that a flow of energy leads to clearly defined trophic structure, biotic diversity, and material cycles (i.e., exchange of materials between living and non-living parts) within the ecosystems". This complex interaction of species, structure and function is far from being operational for the purpose of LCIA and this situation lets Müller-Wenk (1997:23) conclude that two principle directions can be pursued in future work:

- the known populations of *species* could be taken as a substitute for ecosystems, or
- instead of ecosystems, types of *habitats* could be taken as substitutes for the safeguard subject 'ecosystem health'.

Müller-Wenk (1997) has worked out a proposal based on the CORINE habitat concept (CEC 1991) for making operable the safeguard subject 'ecosystem health' and for quantifying damages due to land use, chemical or physical emissions, and the extraction of biotic resources.

Goedkoop *et al.* (1997) suggest – based on very recent developments at RIVM (Klepper *et al.* 1997a/b, Luttik *et ål.* 1997, Roghair *et al.* 1997) – following the 'species-approach' and using the 'potentially affected fraction' (PAF) of species as a surrogate for 'ecosystem health' (in this case, illness). PAFs were initially developed for the assessment of toxic effects due to chemical stressors, but this approach may well be expanded to include indirect effects on populations due to structural changes and physical damages as well (i.e., acidification and land use, respectively).

In order to reflect the aspects of biodiversity, structure, and function in Odum's definition, we will use the broader term of 'ecological health' instead of the terms 'ecosystems' or 'ecosystem health' used so far[5].

Damages to 'ecological health' will not be further addressed within this book. The reader is therefore referred to the literature cited here to gain further insights into these concepts and their pros and cons.

The safeguard subject *'resources'* is a problem child of LCIA. Although resources are mentioned in most LCIA methods, it is hardly argued why and which aspect of resources should be safeguarded (for reviews see, e.g., Finnveden 1994, Udo de Haes 1996, Scheringer *et al.* 1997:7, Heijungs *et al.* 1997). Therefore, many suggestions suffer from a certain arbitrariness. Müller-Wenk (1998) uses the notion of the *destructive* and the *dissipative* use of resources (if the concentration is increased, this may not be considered as damage at all). Fossil energy, for instance, is used in a destructive way while zinc is used in a dissipative manner. Müller-Wenk argues that these two kinds of use should be distinguished. The destructive use is considered to violate inter-generational equity. However, he argues that this is only a damage if the potential utilities of the remaining stocks are reduced, i.e., if the improvement in the efficiency of resource use is less than the used share of the resource. This view is not shared here because improvements in efficiency may well be necessary to satisfy, e.g., a possibly increasing world population. The smaller the stocks get and the more efficiently they are used, the lower the probability that the total utility potential of the resources can be stabilised in the future, because efficiency cannot exceed 100%. Future generations may blame us for having wasted too many resources in comparison to the small efficiency increase realised.

Even if the resource's concentration is increased in the anthroposphere, one can justifiably assume that it does not constitute a damage to the safeguard subject 'resources' because the mass does not only remain constant, but the resource quality in terms of an anthropocentric view is even increased (higher concentration). The dissipative use, in contrast, leads to a decrease in the concentration of ores and will compel future generations either to put more effort into resource extraction and beneficiation or to look for substitutes. Müller-Wenk (1998) quantifies this additional effort for extraction and beneficiation needed in the future and calculates their additional impacts, calling them 'virtual impacts'. Hence, the damage due to the dissipative use of resources is expressed in terms of damage to human health and to ecosystems and of the destructive use of resources, i.e., the dissipative use is not treated as a safeguard subject on its own. Müller-Wenk's calculations for some metals with a comparably small resource-to-use ratio and the use of several worst case assumptions, among others, on the technologies used and the decline in ore concentrations, show that the virtual damage is in most cases small compared to the damages resulting today from their production[6]. Based on these findings it may therefore be justified to focus for the time being on the destructive resource use only.

---

[5] The term 'ecosystem health' is widely used in North America (see, e.g., Constanza *et al.* 1992, Suter 1993, Calow 1993, Cairns *et al.* 1993).

[6] Metals showing a relevant surplus energy due to lower ore grades in the future are copper (60 MJ/kg), mercury (210 MJ/kg), tin (600 MJ/kg), tungsten (90 MJ/kg) and molybdenum (40 MJ/kg) (Müller-Wenk (1998:49). Most other metals and salts, gravel and stones show negligible surplus energy. These results suggest that there are only a few additional resources that will have to be analysed if they appear in the inventory table of specific case studies (Müller-Wenk 1998:50).

Figure 4.1 is a graphical representation of all that has been said so far. In this book we will provide a precise definition only for human health, and define a category indicator and provide models to quantify the indicator as well. The reader should look up Goedkoop *et al.* (1997) and Müller-Wenk (1997/1998) for first attempts at an operationalisation of 'ecological health' and 'resource use'. The impact profile is added here merely to illustrate the approach. The list of impact categories is not comprehensive and can be expanded if other mechanisms lead to damages to the safeguard subjects. The impact categories organise and structure the impact pathways, but have lost all meaning on their own.

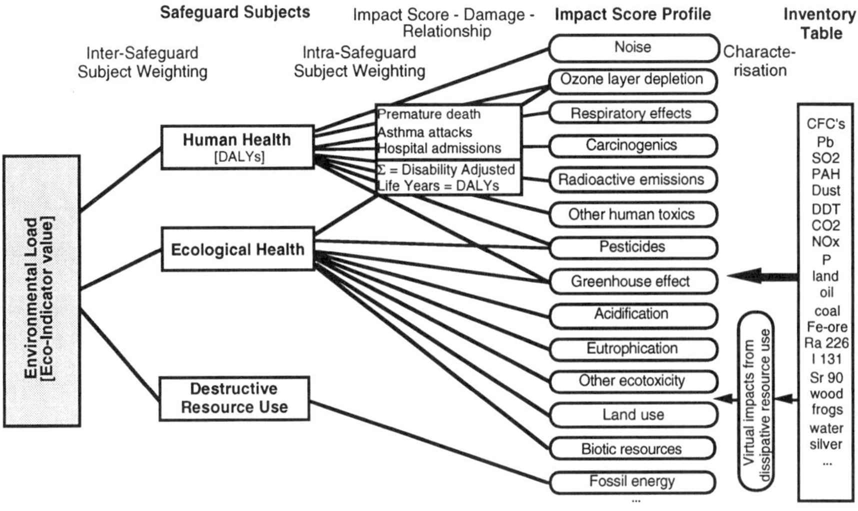

Fig. 4.1: Possible structure of an LCIA method following the 'common endpoint approach' by the prescription of safeguard subjects. The impact profile and its impact categories are only shown for illustrative reasons and are not constituting elements of the approach.

The structure presented in Figure 4.1 may be close to what will emerge from the ongoing operationalisation as part of the revision of EcoIndicator'95. However, the main messages that can be formulated already at this stage are:

- an LCIA method based on few safeguard subjects may be a realistically achievable goal,
- the safeguard subjects have to be clearly defined in order to be able to define and model a category indicator,
- the impact categories and their profile lose the importance they had so far and will serve for structuring and organising the data and the model rather than as a basis for valuation. (They will be organised according to common mechanisms rather than policy themes.),
- the number of quantitatively known impact damage relationships will determine the number of causal links to known environmental problems and the type of environmental interventions which have to be analysed in the inventory analysis, and

- the framework presented here will be operationalised in this book (only) for a set of impact pathways of human health.

More details on the modelling will be presented in Section 4.3 and Chapters 5 to 7.

4.1.3 Safeguard subjects revisited by Cultural Theory

The selection of safeguards subjects, their justification and the definition of what the damages to safeguard subjects are, all involve value choices. Chapter 3 and especially Section 3.4 have suggested that value choices can be modelled by Cultural Theory (CT).

It seems therefore obvious to ask what CT can contribute to support the selection and justification of the safeguard subjects and how much this selection depends on the cultural perspectives, i.e., the world views of the archetypes.

A first answer is disappointing: not that much. The reason for this hard and probably surprising statement is that LCA has a cultural bias in itself (Subsection 3.4.4). The idea that it is possible to account for the environmental impacts of a product system and to model the ecosphere based on a selection of representative elements of nature is in itself a reflection of the hierarchic view. The concept of accounting for the damages to safeguard subjects is therefore biased. One consequence is that only minor differences between the different perspectives can be identified:

- It may be argued that egalitarians will tend to prioritise ecological health and resource use and pay less attention to human health while individualists will focus on human health and claim that the scarcity of resources is already adequately reflected in market prices. Hierarchist, as mentioned before, pay attention to all safeguard subjects. However, egalitarians will, to some extent, also pay attention to the protection of human health as well because they acknowledge that more is known on causalities between environmental interventions and damage to human health (or to mice and rats) than on ecological health. They may therefore use human health as some kind of proxy for ecological health[7]. Individualists are, of course, quite aware that even an anthropocentric world view needs to take into account negative feedback from the environment to human health and welfare, i.e., they also pay some attention to damages to ecological health as far as they may be concerned from negative feedback.
- The way the safeguard subjects – once they have been selected – are defined may well differ between the perspectives. Section 5.4 will address this aspect of human health, where we will discuss if the question whether all humans, even though of different age, should be equitably treated, is a question that will or should be answered differently for the different cultural perspectives. The safeguard subject 'resource use', to take another example, may be judged to be relevant because resources have an intrinsic value (i.e., the egalitarian's reasoning), because resource quantities and qualities do decrease (i.e., the hierarchist's reasoning), or because of there are no substitutes for some of them (i.e., the individualist's reasoning).

---

[7] We do not suggest accounting for all causal damages to mice and rats by environmental interventions although such a model may represent best the available knowledge and serve as a proxy for (toxic) damage to life.

- As mentioned in Subsection 3.4.3, the concept that the ecosphere can be represented by safeguard subjects is a concept developed by scientists and they are hierarchists. Therefore, other attributes and aspects of the ecosphere may be more relevant to the other archetypes (see Subsection 4.1.5 and Section 4.2 to 4.6).

In short, the concept of representing the ecosphere by safeguard subjects is an inherently hierarchist concept and their selection may therefore well be based on the definition of human rights and their fixation on international treaties and declarations. CT plays a major role when the safeguard subjects are operationalised, both in terms of their reasoning and of the selection of the indicators and the values that are necessary to set up the sub-models. CT is relevant when the views from different perspectives are used to complement the hierarchists' damage assessment by egalitarian and individualist attributes that are relevant for the assessment (see Subsection 4.1.5 and Section 4.2 to 4.6).

These arguments provided here for the role of different perspectives for the selection and definition of safeguard subjects are not yet supported by empirical work. Research to test what should be properly called theses is currently underway (Brunner 1998).

4.1.4 Uni-directional view of the ecosphere in LCA

Whatever approach to LCIA is chosen – bottom-up or top-down – it always reflects a very unidirectional view of nature. The links from damages to emissions or from emissions to potential impacts are modelled as straight causal relationships. Nature's many feedback mechanisms, non-linearities, its dynamic and sometimes even chaotic behaviour all fail to be reflected in the model of the environmental system that is used in LCIA.

In Subsections 1.2.6 and 1.5.2, we have justified this simple model of the ecosphere with the argument that the product system under analysis will experience only very small changes and that this choice of the micro level precludes the application of dynamic world models.

In addition, LCIA explicitly intends to model not just changes in the environment, but adverse effects in terms of damages to all safeguard subjects. If human beings die prematurely due to environmental pollution, this is accounted for as a damage. The "benefit", in the form of avoided environmental pollution that is resulting from this prematurely ended life, however, is of no further interest in the course of LCA. This cynical example has been chosen to show that the selection of endpoints (safeguard subjects) is a value choice and that induced effects in the form of damages to these endpoints could be modelled in principle. However, LCIA stays with a simple uni-directional model of the ecosphere.

4.1.5 Damage attributes and the precautionary principle

Subsection 4.1.3 already suggested that the assessment of damages to a small selection of safeguard subjects may not be judged by all cultural perspectives as a sufficient basis for LCIA. The simplicity of the uni-directional view of the ecosphere underlying the damage assessment has been stressed in addition in the previous subsection. On top of that, it is clear that the knowledge on causal relationships is and will remain limited and that it will never be possible to analyse all existing mechanisms within an LCA case study. This means inevitably that the damage assessment will never be *comprehensive*.

This last point addresses a problem which is, in general, inherent to all information, but LCA is especially concerned by this 'comprehensiveness problem' because, both in the public's and the decision makers' perception, it is an all-encompassing environmental assessment tool. This myth originates in the enthusiasm of the late eighties and early nineties when LCA was considered to be the key to the analysis of and the solution to all kinds of problems. Of course, and Chapter 1 has made this clear, LCA is hedged in by a large number of assumptions which try to make reality less complex, more manageable, and thus easier to analyse. LCA considers known impacts on the safeguard subjects which represent the environment. The number of safeguard subjects that are considered is small and may be considered as a proxy for, rather than a picture of, the ecosphere. The knowledge about causal relationships between interventions and damages to safeguard subjects is very limited and the share of the relations that can be quantified is even smaller. Not all environmental interventions can be or are measured. All of these points should make the reader aware of the fact that by far not all the consequences for the environment of a product system are considered in LCA.

Knowledge on causation – the process that connects causes with their effects – is what we need to predict damage to safeguard subjects by environmental interventions. This is not the place to enter into a philosophical debate about the roots of causation (see, e.g., Ehring 1997). Some of the reasons for the limited knowledge on causalities within the ecosphere are therefore simply stated here:

- The ecosphere does not work like a uni-directional process for which one can identify inputs and outputs. It is best imagined as consisting of an unknown number of cycles which interfere with each other, which are partly closed, but also partly not (yet) closed, which change with time and allow for a rather stable, but evolving equilibrium.
- The ecosphere does not tell us about its causalities or, if it does, we do not yet understand its language. Hence, we are compelled to search for causalities with experiments and epidemiological studies. Experiments suffer from being closed off from the other interacting cycles and epidemiological studies suffer from confounding factors:
  - In the case of experiments, causality can be determined with accuracy, but the transfer of the findings to the real ecosphere with real system parameters may lead to questions about the accuracy of those causalities.
  - Epidemiological studies are strong in showing associations, but in most cases unable to prove causality. It is almost impossible to control for all confounding factors[8]. Therefore, the notion of evidence or the degree of evidence was introduced. The degree of evidence for the causality measures the strength of association and considers all other supporting factors such as known mechanisms, experimental data, and the results from other epidemiological studies.

[8] The knowledge on causation and its quantification for all confounding factors is a prerequisite to show more than just associations for the causing factor at study.

- Field tests and micro cosmos studies are often used as a step in between laboratory tests and epidemiological studies in order to have more realistic system parameters while still being able to show more than associations.

• One of the stabilising elements of the ecosphere may well be that it is able to invent mechanisms which interrupt the pathways of causation. Therefore, the same impact at two different places or at two different points in time may well lead to different effects.

After this short look at causality and evidence, it should not come as a surprise that "proofs" of causality are subjects of heated debates (see, e.g., Ozonoff 1994, Botti *et al.* 1996) and that science knows only of a comparably small number[9] of causalities that are supported by a high degree of evidence[10].

However, LCIA claims that the necessary simplifications and selections are made in a reasonable manner and allow to provide the intended decision support for, e.g., product improvements, product comparisons and assistance in eco-labelling. The part of the known reality that is analysed may even be considered as a proxy for the whole.

Subsection 3.1.3 introduced a set of criteria which were considered relevant by lay people for their perception of risks (Fischhoff *et al.* 1978). These criteria can be understood as damage attributes, i.e., aspects which have to be considered next to the damage assessment.

As a first try these attributes can be classified as follows:

1) Intrinsically given to environmental impacts considered in LCA: voluntariness of risk (always involuntary), chronic *versus* catastrophic risk (always chronic as large accidents are excluded from LCA so far), unfairness (unequal distribution of risks and benefits).
2) At least partly covered by the damage assessment integrating over time and place: immediacy of effect (delayed effect), knowledge about risk by science, severity of consequences, harm to future generations.
3) Contributing to uncertainty and unknown damage: immediacy of effect (delayed effect), harm to future generations, newness.

[9] In Chapters 6 and 7 we will use the information on about 1000 relationships between environmental interventions and damages to human endpoints. An optimistic guess is that there are, in total, maybe ten times more known causal relations. But there is little evidence for many of these 10'000 causal relationships. One can also start with an approximate estimate of 100'000 substances to which ecosystems and humans are exposed, each through three media. One assumes that there are about 100 endpoints in humans and about 100 for species and ecosystems. (There are of course thousands, but we are not (yet) able to define them.) A multiplication suggests that there are therefore about 60 million causal relationships which could theoretically occur. Thus, only 0.02% of these relationships are known and about a minuscule 0.002% are operationalised in Chapters 6 and 7.

[10] Carpenter (1995) identifies the problem of measurement as a major source of lacking knowledge. The following seven points are considered to be responsible for these difficulties:
• ignorance of how ecosystems behave and evolve at the regional scale,
• non-linearity in the response of ecosystems to stress,
• natural variability (signal-to-noise ratio),
• sampling and analytical errors under field conditions,
• inadequate monitoring and research over large areas and long time periods,
• deliberate falsification of data for sociocultural or political reasons, and
• inadequate research on the linkage of natural and managed ecosystems.

4) Individual factors: knowledge about risk by the persons who are exposed to those risks, common dread, control over risk.

Factors (3) and (4) are hardly addressed and poorly covered in environmental risk assessment when compared to the treatment of the well-established factors (1) and (2). The damage assessment in LCIA suggested here does likewise.

Adams (1995) and, based on him, Gaskell (1997) distinguish three different types of risk: (i) directly perceivable risks, (ii) risks perceived through science, and (iii) virtual risks which scientists do not know about or cannot agree upon. This last type of risk is not covered in damage assessment. Adams (1995) points out that the relevance of this third type of risk is perceived very differently by archetypes holding different world views and it should therefore be considered to depend on the cultural perspective held by decision makers.

Scholz (1996) argues that a risk evaluation procedure has not only to consider economic costs and environmental damages, but that it has to fulfil a third function in addition. The precautionary function should reflect the 'unknown' or the 'lacking knowledge' in the case of a substance that is ubiquitarily distributed in the ecosphere. He argues that a lack of knowledge is highly important, a judgement which is reflected by the investments our society makes in knowledge generation and the compilation of information.

That the attitudes toward risks depend very much on the world view of the archetypes, from risk seeking (individualists) up to risk averse (egalitarians), is a well-established fact (see Table 3.1 in Subsection 3.2.2). These archetypes consequently have their own preferred management style and these differ very much. Individualists are comfortable with an adaptive management style while egalitarians prefer a preventive management that reflects the precautionary principle.

Developers of LCIA realised some time ago that there is more than just one approach to damage assessment, i.e., that there are a number of quite different criteria which may be relevant. Table 4.2 lists the criteria mentioned in the literature and the shading indicates the degree to which they are already covered in damage assessment.

UBA's criteria set is the only one so far which has been operationalised to a certain extent and applied in a semi-quantitative way in a case study (UBA 1994). Lindeijer (1994) has put forward another proposal based on Kortman *et al.* (1994) (see Table 4.3). It differentiates clearly between the seriousness and the dynamics of a given harm. This aspect of damage assessment, complementing the static assessment with indicators that reflect the dynamic component of harm, has been overlooked so far. But the proposal has not been operationalised since it has been made.

The review of risk and causality presented here highlights the points that:

- the damage assessment will cover only a small number of causal relationships,
- the absolute proof under realistic conditions on causation is almost impossible to find. Therefore, the degree of evidence is an important additional information,
- there are risk and damage attributes which are not covered by the damage assessment, but are perceived as relevant by society, and
- the damage assessment relies in most cases on a static analysis, yet the dynamics of damages may influence the perception of their importance.

Used by **UBA** (1994) for LCA	Proposed by **Müller-Wenk** in Udo de Haes *et al.* (1994) and Müller-Wenk (1997)	Used in **8 LCA weighting methods** reviewed by Volkwein *et al.* (1996b)	Implicitly used by **experts** for weighting (Kortman *et al.* 1994)
Ecological threat potential	Substitutability	Ecological threat potential	Relative harmfulness of expected effects
Irreversibility	Reversibility (hysteresis)	Reversibility	Probability of occurrence
Scale of effect (global-local)	Geographical extension of damage	Extension	Expected effort to return to an acceptable level
Preferences of population		Environmental preferences of the population	Extent to which Dutch population is threatened
Distance to target	Ecological scarcity (distance to target)	Distance to target	Extent to which ecosystems are threatened
	Uncertainty	Uncertainty	Uncertainty
	Transient response (overshoot of damage)	Time lag between emission and impact	Endangering human health
		Willingness to pay	Contribution of the Netherlands
		Others	Nature of the effects
			Possibility for administrative solutions
			Others

Tab. 4.2: Weighting criteria used or proposed within LCIA. Boxes shaded dark grey indicate criteria which are fully considered in damage assessment; light grey shades indicate that these criteria are only partly covered in damage assessment and boxes left white identify those criteria which are missing in the damage assessment.

Criterion		Unit
Seriousness of harm		
• Extent of exceeding reference level		[-]
• Reversibility		
for irreversible harms:	• Risk of extinction	[% of total pop. endangered]
	• Extent of damage	[% disfunction]
	• Importance to life on earth	[score scaled 1-100]
for reversible harms:	• Extent of stress	[% disruption]
	• Time-extent of stress	[score scaled 1-100]
	• Geogr. scale of stress	[score scaled 1-100]
	• Importance of system	[score scaled 1-100]
Dynamics of harm		
• Trend in future seriousness of harm		[score scaled 0-2]
• Complexity of the causal chain		[score scaled 1-100]
• Administrative, technical, economic effort to reduce harm		[score scaled 1-100]
• Time span required to reduce harm		[score scaled 1-100]

Tab. 4.3: Weighting criteria proposed by Lindeijer 1994 for LCIA.

In summary, the damage assessment has to be complemented by additional damage attributes and it has to acquire a more preventive orientation in order to be able to consider the 'virtual risks' as well and represent characteristics of precaution. This holds especially true if one looks from the egalitarian perspective.

Based on that observation, the next section introduces the modelling framework for the ecosphere.

4.2 The model framework: Damage, unknown damage, and manageability

Based on Section 4.1 and especially Subsection 4.1.5, it is a small step to claim that:

The model of the ecosphere shall consist of a submodel to account for the causal damage known to science, a submodel representing unknown damage and causality, and a submodel for the dynamic aspects of the damage.

Figure 4.2 graphically represents this new modelling framework. The light grey oval symbolises the damage to safeguard subjects which can be predicted by knowledge on causal relationships between environmental interventions and damages. The dark grey fuzzy area symbolises the entire unknown damage due to the environmental interventions. This fuzzy area is composed of a share where the damage can be observed but no causal relationships are known, and a share where the damage is not (yet) known at all. The black arrows symbolise the need and effort to reduce the known damage to an acceptable one (the striped circle), i.e., the dynamic aspect of the damage which is called from now on *manageability*.

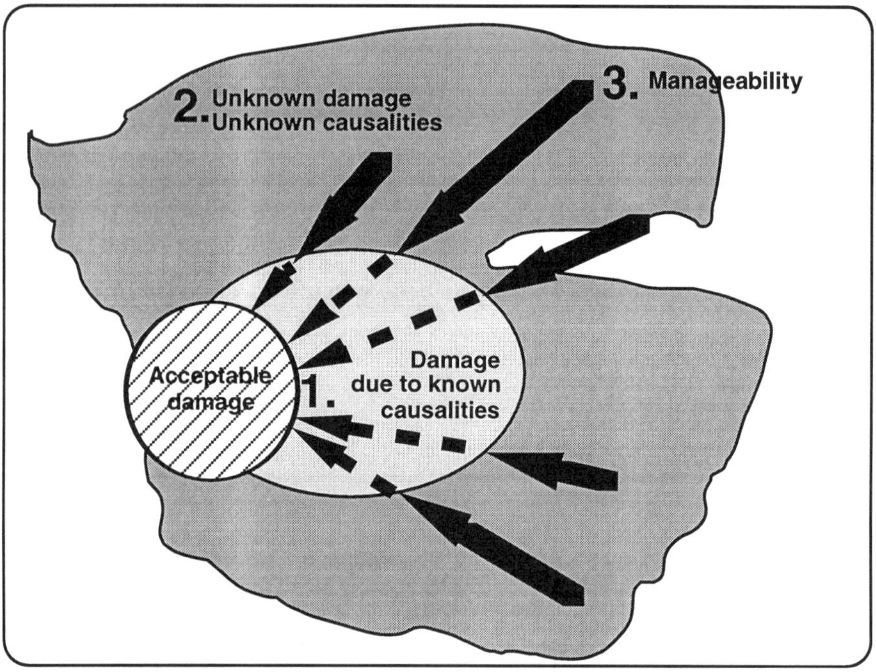

Fig. 4.2: The modelling framework for the ecosphere (the arrows – the third modelling level of 'manageability' – symbolise the dynamic aspects of a damage reduction towards an acceptable damage).

The damage symbolised by the oval area can be modelled by a 'traditional' *damage assessment* that includes a fate, exposure, effect, and a damage analysis. The causalities of dose-response relations can only be proven to a certain degree of evidence as stated earlier. Degree of evidence is, apart from its definition, a subjective element. The question of which degree of evidence still needs to be considered in order to represent a causal relationship is a value choice. The model of the valuesphere from Chapter 3 provides the tool for distinguishing between value choices and supporting more than one of them. In fact, Chapters 6 and 7 will provide for each of the three archetypes a different "oval" which represents their interpretation of the degree of evidence which still indicates a causal relationship. Subsection 4.1.3 already mentioned that the safeguard subjects may well be defined and operationalised differently for each cultural perspective. Together with the different degree of evidence necessary to accept a damage as a causal one, one can predict that the "oval" will have a different shape *and* a different size dependent on the cultural perspective adopted. Section 4.3 will provide guidance for this part of the damage assessment.

The fuzzy area representing the *unknown damage* and the unknown causalities cannot be determined, otherwise we would know them and thus be able to model them like the known damage. Section 4.4 will therefore propose a proxy indicator with a high predictive power that can serve as an indicator representing the precautionary principle. This proxy indicator will be operationalised independent of the cultural perspectives. Nevertheless, individualists will pay less attention than egalitarians to this indicator. This way of approaching the problem ensures that the same indicator will stand as a proxy for two different "areas" representing the two perspectives.

The indicator for *manageability,* measuring the power of the "arrows", i.e., the dynamics of the damage, will be based on the review that has already been undertaken in Subsection 4.1.5 and especially on the attributes mentioned in Table 4.3. Its operationalisation in Section 4.5 will show that the index is dependent on management style and world view, i.e., the need and effort to reduce harm are not natural constants but depend on the kind of measures that are supported and on the effort with which they are supported.

In order to keep the overview on the submodels and its indices[11] introduced in this section and worked out in the next section, Table 4.4 summarises some properties and gives a preview on the characteristics to be introduced in Section 4.3 to 4.5.

This new framework that explicitly includes indicators for unknown damage and for the dynamics of damage as complements to the damage assessment is the answer to the growing awareness that these aspects play a decisive role in risk perception and decision making. The aim is to have a framework that can serve as an umbrella over the many different approaches which address, most often, just one of the three submodels. This will make LCIA inclusive instead of exclusive and prevent it from being seen as an (over)deterministic tool, a fate that risk assessment has suffered at the hands of the environmentalists (Tal 1997).

[11] In this book we use the term 'index' as the result from a submodel. The 'index' is in most cases calculated based on 'indicators'. In order to determine the 'indicators' 'parameters' and measured 'data' are used.

Submodel	Abre-viation of its index	Main parameters	Modelling dependent from cultural perspectives	Aggregation levels	Further information
Known damage	D	Fate and exposure factors, Effect factors, Damage factors	Yes	Environmental inter-entions, Environmental problems (mechanisms), Safeguard subjects	§4.3, §5, §6, §7
Unknown damage	U	Bioconcentration, Anthropogenic and geogenic emissions	No	Environmental interventions	§4.4
Managea-bility	M	Ease of damage reduction, Excess of long-term policy targets, Success of regulation	Yes	Environmental problems (mechanisms), Safeguard subjects	§4.5, §6.6, §7.6

Tab. 4.4: Preview on characteristics of the three submodels of the ecosphere

In Sections 4.3 to 4.5, this framework will be operationalised and in Section 4.6 first conclusions will be drawn. Further implications of the new model for the ecosphere will be elaborated upon in Section 8.3 where we postulate a meta model that is based on the three submodels.

4.3 Damage assessment by Impact - Pathway - Analysis

4.3.1 Introduction

The use of cause-damage-analysis[12] in the field of LCIA requires the *development of damage functions which link the environmental interventions from the inventory table with the damage to the different safeguard subjects.*

Most elements of the damage assessment that are used here have been introduced into the field of LCIA by Steen *et al.* (1992). They used this approach to describe the damage to five safeguard subjects[13]. Goedkoop (1995) proposed an approach using physical damage functions that were based on the assumption of a simplified linear damage function. The slope was determined with the help of the distance-to-target approach, i.e., the ratio between the unit damage at target flow and the target flow itself was considered to be the best available surrogate for the slope of the damage function. In the meantime both Braunschweig *et al.* (1996) and Müller-Wenk (1997) developed further elements of the damage function approach. A joint Dutch-Swiss project team is currently in the process of operationalising these concepts and hopes to develop a full set of consistent damage functions to be used in LCIA (Goedkoop *et al.* 1997).

LCA is not the only field where such damage functions are needed and developed:

- The calculation of external costs - the so-called externalities - is based on similar work and is still going on at the present time. ExternE (1995) coined the term "impact-pathway-analysis" to describe the methodology they use for the calculation of external costs. In fact, the damage cost approach, which differentiates between single interventions, uses a damage-cause-analysis and the damages are expressed in monetary units[14] in the end (e.g., ExternE 1995, ESEERCO 1995).
- The same methodology has also been used within "green accounting" recently. In this case, the single damages can be averaged to national damage functions of a more generic kind (Metroeconomica *et al.* 1996). These results are easier to adapt to LCIA than the ones from, e.g., ExternE (1995), because the single damage functions can easily be averaged over a country's area, i.e., they can be made less site-specific.
- In another vein, RIVM (NL) has recently started a kind of risk mapping. The first reports already presented a wide range of damage functions to health (radiation, carcinogenic substances, noise, particles, and some other risk factors) (Pruppers *et al.* 1996, Pruppers 1996, Pruppers *et al.* 1997). These functions included the geographic distribution of risks within the Netherlands and differentiated between Dutch and country-external sources of risk. These cause-damage functions, that

[12] The terms "cause-damage analysis" and "impact pathway analysis" are used interchangeably.

[13] Several reasons may explain the little recognition that EPS (the name of the method) has found outside of Scandinavia: there is not much documentation available; the format of presentation did not fit the SETAC (1993b) structure; the monetarisation of the five safeguard subjects may be judged as premature; or the high relevance of metallic resource depletion has been judged as suspicious (Braunschweig *et al.* 1994).

[14] However, the physical damage is an intermediate result within the damage cost approach.

link potential damage (human health risks) to the sources of risk (emissions, economic activities), have been developed with the purpose of the project in mind, which is risk mapping. They are therefore not fully appropriate for the purposes of LCIA. The analysis is at present restricted to airborne risks.

- Chemical or environmental risk assessment is the traditional impact pathway analysis. Typically, risk assessment consists of four steps: hazard identification, exposure assessment, toxicity assessment, and risk characterisation. Its strength lies in the exposure assessment of single substances which considers all impact pathways. Due to its purpose, it is site-independent only during the initial screening, but includes a lot of site-specific information in the detailed analysis. Additionally, the tool was primarily designed to predict whether effect levels will be surpassed. Therefore, the aggregation of effects or the damage analysis are little developed within risk assessment (see, e.g., Paustenbach 1989, Ozonoff 1994, Kolluru *et al.* 1996).
- Last but not least, another area exists where functions similar to damage functions have to be built: the setting of threshold or target values by regulators. The need of regulators for such functions increases if safe concentrations are exceeded or if threshold behaviour cannot be expected (Lühr *et al.* 1991, LAI 1992).

Data from and knowledge in all these fields will be necessary to construct as many relevant damage functions as possible within LCIA in order to model the area of known damages as accurately as possible.

4.3.2 The safeguard subjects as a prerequisite for the damage assessment

The concept of safeguard subjects in LCIA has been introduced and reviewed in Subsection 2.1.4 and further elaborated in Subsections 4.1.2 and 4.1.3. Chapter 5 will define the safeguard subject "human health" and explain the choice for and the modelling assumptions behind an index for human health.

Here, we check the claim implied in the title that the definition of safeguard subjects is a prerequisite for the damage assessment. If this is so, we should also be able to identify the use of such subjects in the applications mentioned in the previous subsection:

- Studies calculating external costs of, e.g., energy systems (ExternE 1995) or national economies (Metroeconomica *et al.* 1996) select all those goods where the market already assigns values (revealed preferences) or for which individuals can express values, e.g., through contingent valuation methods. Human health, buildings, agricultural yields, aesthetic values, and biodiversity are typically considered as safeguard subjects in damage cost assessments.
- The risk mapping by RIVM uses, for the time being, the mortality risk as an indicator and considers at present to extend it to human health including diseases (Pruppers *et al.* 1996). The safeguard subject therefore is human health.
- Quantitative risk assessment is used in many different areas. Kolluru (1996) separates safety risks from health risks, ecological/environmental, public welfare/goodwill, and from financial risks. Health risks and ecological/environmental risks are relevant to LCA. Health risks are assessed in terms of damages to single

endpoints such as, e.g., the risks of developing cancer. Endpoints for the environmental risk assessment are ecosystem or habitat impacts on the one hand, e.g., population abundance and the diversity of species, and global impacts on the other hand (Kolluru 1996). As mentioned above, the main aim of risk assessment is to predict whether effect levels or thresholds will be surpassed. It is therefore rather a no-damage than a damage assessment.

- Regulators tend to set targets and thresholds in such a way that politically acceptable damages by direct and indirect effects to the safeguard subjects are not surpassed. The safeguard subjects are normally defined in the constitution or in the respective laws. In Switzerland, not only human beings but fauna and flora too belong to the safeguard subjects. Other countries protect the fauna and flora only to the extent that they would, if damaged, indirectly damage human health or welfare.

This very concise review of a few specific applications that make use of damage functions is an indication for the relevance of safeguard subjects in damage assessment.

4.3.3 From damages to causes – an illustration

Figure 4.3 illustrates the analytical path that leads from observed damages to human health and on to its causes. From a damage-oriented point of view, the analysis can be described as follows:

The analysis starts with a normative determination of what is the safeguard subject and which damages represent an impairment of the safeguard subject. This step rests here upon the assumption that disease and mortality of humans can be conceptualised as damages to the safeguard subject of *human health* (see also Chapter 5). The next step in the analysis is the observation of patterns of diseases and of cases of mortality. With help from medical sciences, it is possible through diagnosis to identify the effects which have caused disease and mortality, i.e., the internal organ that is damaged and the mechanism causing the harm are identified.

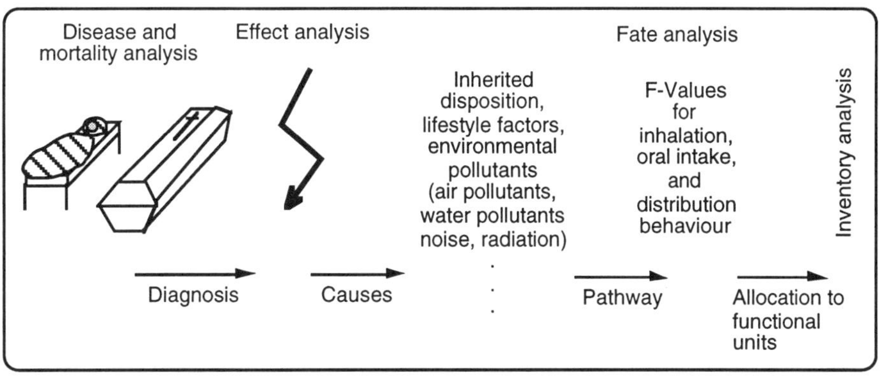

Fig. 4.3: The top-down procedure links damages to causes by using know-how from several disciplines in a multistep approach.

In a next step the causes for this harm have to be identified by using epidemiological studies, for instance. In order to identify the causal risk factors it is necessary to have a reliable exposure assessment. If the exposure to certain substances is identified as the cause, the causes of the exposure have to be identified. Through a pathway analysis, it is possible to identify the amount of emissions causing the exposure situation. Sometimes even the emission source can be identified. One logical step further removed from this source identification is the attribution of the emissions to functional units.

This description of the damage-cause analysis implies that it focuses very much on the descriptive part of the disciplines (medicine, toxicology, environmental chemistry, and engineering).

A cause-damage relationship can also be found by calculating the emissions due to the provision of one functional unit. The exposure that is caused by this provision can be modelled through multimedia fate modelling. On this basis, an effect analysis can be performed with help of dose-response relationships that have already been established by toxicologists. Such an effect will cause disease and mortality events with a certain probability. In a last step, the cases of disease and of mortality will be judged according to the extent that they damage safeguard subjects. This second procedure to describe the relationship between causes and damages makes use of the same disciplines as the first procedure, but the knowledge they have to provide is prescriptive instead.

These illustrations of a descriptive "top-down" procedure and its prescriptive reverse address the dichotomy that exists between a top-down and a bottom-up analysis[15]. These two procedures have to be combined (in a form that will become clear in the next subsection, in Subsection 4.3.6, and in the Chapters 6 and 7) in order to:

- use all the available and accurate information to describe as many causal relationships as possible. (There is never enough information available to understand the existing network of influencing factors.)
- use the descriptive models as a reliability check to improve the quality of the prescriptive (model-based) techniques.

The long chain from the industrial metabolism to damages makes LCA a truly interdisciplinary field of research. Together with the intermediate steps of analysing the environmental behaviour of substance flows and of decay processes, and of studying the toxicokinetics and toxicodynamics, this requires not only the cooperation of different sciences, but also a linking of their models and a combination of their different methods.

[15] The following paired terms have a similar meaning in different disciplines:
- damage-oriented versus cause-oriented perspectives
- epidemiological versus inductive perspectives
- descriptive versus prescriptive perspectives

4.3.4 The general set-up of the impact pathway analysis

The damage functions are based on three distinguishable steps of analysis. This procedure is called the impact pathway analysis (see, e.g., ExternE (1995), Rabl *et al.* (1995)). Figure 4.4 graphically presents a general set-up which is applicable to most impact pathways. Some examples for models or model families are mentioned to the right of the labels that identify the level of analysis. The upper arrows lead to examples for prescriptive models. The lower arrows indicate models that are primarily of a descriptive nature.

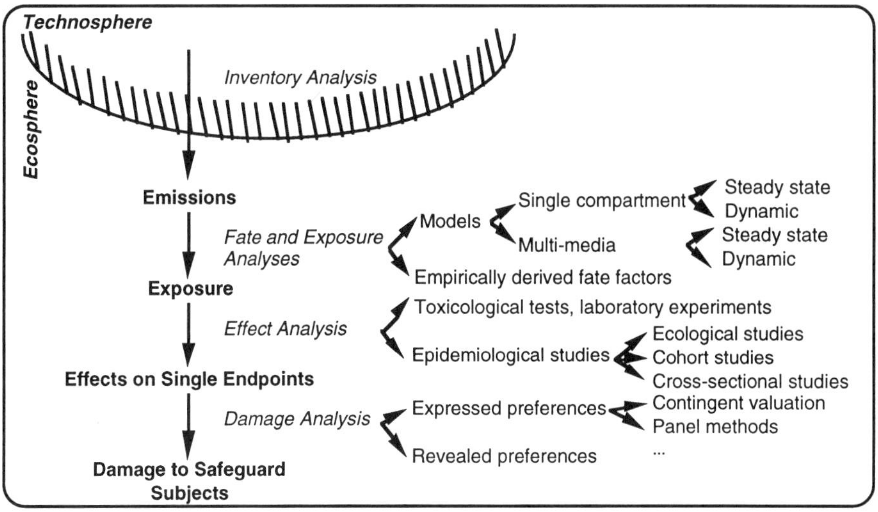

Fig. 4.4: General set-up of the impact pathway analysis within the ecosphere. The upper arrows for each level of analysis give examples for the cause-oriented modelling and the lower arrows specify the descriptive modelling

The different steps can be described as follows:

The *fate and exposure analyses* model the relationship between emissions to air, surface water or soil and the exposure of humans, animals, or plants to a contamination due to "inhaled" air, dermal absorbed air or water, water, and food. The exposure is quantified in either one of two ways depending on the effect analysis. It makes use of the concentration of pollutants in the compartments mentioned (e.g., if epidemiological studies are used) or of the part of pollutants which enter the organism. Secondary formation and metabolites have to be considered here as well (see Subsection 7.2.3).

The *effect analysis* uses dose-response relationships to quantify the effects that can be expected due to the exposure. The endpoints affected are elements of the safeguard subject, e.g., cough or lung cancer. LCA includes the effects that occur all over the world without limitations to time or place. The different sensibilities of receptors are reflected in the use of an average pattern, e.g., a given percentage of human beings are asthmatics or a certain percentage of all species are vertebrates.

The *damage analysis* finally links the effects on single endpoints to an index for the damage to human health. The additional information used here may be the relevance of the endpoint or the duration of the effect. The element of relevance, e.g., one day of coughing is half as harmful as one day of suffering from an asthma attack, or, the class of vertebrates is equally important as the class of invertebrates, is an element which is based explicitly on value judgements. Its choice therefore should be based on models of the valuesphere.

The damage function linking emissions with the damage caused by the emission can be approximated by the slope of the damage function under the assumption that all the steps in Figure 4.4 can be modelled with linear functions passing through the origin (i.e., no threshold or sigmoid behaviour) This slope is called the *damage factor.*

The combination of these steps are formalised in Equation (4.1):

$$D_c = \sum_{ijkm}\{I_{ij} \cdot F_{ijk} \cdot E_{ikm,c} \cdot DALYs_{m,c}\} \qquad \text{[DALYs,...]} \qquad (4.1)$$

where D outcome of the damage assessment for human or ecological health measured in the respective damage units (here DALYs for human health) [a]

$DALYs$ Disability Adjusted Life Years, used as metric for the damage to human health [a]

E effect factor [see Sections 6.3 & 7.3]

F fate factor [see Sections 6.2 & 7.2]

I environmental intervention per functional unit [e.g., kg]

c index for the three cultural perspectives (individualists, egalitarians and hierarchists)

i index for substance

j index for compartment

k index for exposure path

m index for endpoint

The next section will address those cases where the prerequisites to this simplest of the cases are not fulfilled.

4.3.5 The cases of non-proportional damage functions

This subsection addresses a series of questions which will arise when one starts to operationalise the impact pathway analysis. These merely technical answers will therefore attract readers working with the impact pathway analysis.

a) The shape of the functions

As mentioned above, the impact pathway analysis combines three levels of analysis, the fate, effect, and damage analysis. Each of them can be described as a blackbox and the output can be described as a function of the input. Figure 4.5 takes the effect analysis as an the example and suggests four different shapes for this function:

- The *proportional function* describes an effect without threshold characteristics. Each increment in the dose causes the same increment in response quite independent of the intensity of the dose. It is impossible to prove that the dose-response function is really is such a straight line through the origin. This form is in most cases the result of an extrapolation to low doses from knowledge about higher doses. Or, it reflects a population effect, i.e., it results from the superposition of individuals with different sensitivities to the agent at hand. This function can be described by just one slope. It represents the simplest case and can be easily handled within LCIA.
- The *linear function with threshold behaviour* is the second possibility of a linear function. Threshold behaviours occur if a natural repair mechanism can counteract damages up to a certain burden. In such cases, it is important to know whether the emitted substance will cause or contribute to the thresholds being surpassed or not (see Paragraph (b)).

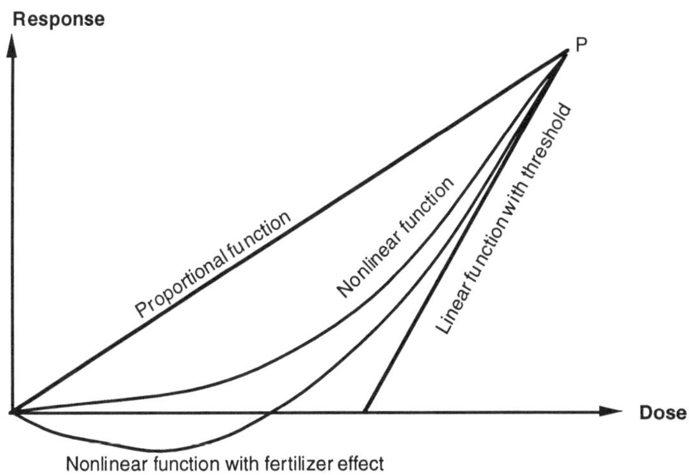

Fig. 4.5: A variety of possible forms for dose-response functions (adapted from ExternE (1995))

- The *non-linear function with a fertiliser effect* is relevant in cases where the pollutant can act as an essential element necessary for, e.g., growth. ExternE (1995) accounts for such a behaviour in the link between the combination of NOx and $SO2$ emissions and crop yield. In such a case, it is important to know either the exact background dose or the frequency distribution of all doses.

- The *non-linear function* (lying between the two linear functions in Fig. 4.5) may be the most realistic curve, although it cannot be determined for a large number of substances. It reflects best the situation in which repair mechanisms are available, but do not work in all individuals with the same efficiency. Taken at the population level, this leads to the shape of the function presented in Fig. 4.5. In this case too, it is important to know either the exact background dose or the frequency distribution of all doses.

We have used the example of the effect analysis in this case, but there exist also nonlinearities in the fate analysis. Two such cases will be described in Section 7.2. The photochemical formation of ozone in Europe is a strongly non-linear process that depends on the combination of specific meteorological conditions and the emission of the precursors VOC and NOx. The ozone formation process depends additionally on the absolute mixture of the precursors. At present European background concentrations for NOx and VOC, the marginal increase in the formation of ozone for a unit increase in precursor concentrations is already very small. Hence, we already seem to be above the saturation level. A similar saturation effect occurs in the process of the formation of ammonium-nitrate as secondary particles due to NOx emissions. This process is strongly dependent on the availability of ammonia as IER (1997) has shown.

The damage analysis assumes a simple additive characteristic of proportional linear functions. This assumption is obviously a simplification. It may well be that one and the same person or specie suffers from different effects at the same time and that this superposition may lead to a non-proportional increase in "pain" or prolongation of the disease time.

In Subsection 1.2.6, it had been decided to model the change-oriented approach, i.e., to apply a *marginal analysis*. Therefore, the shape of the damage functions at the present background concentrations and doses are relevant for the analysis in all cases where the functions are not proportional.

The next paragraph (b) will re-evaluate the need and the possibilities to consider more information on time and place and, with that, on the actual background load. In paragraph (c) we will suggest a feasible procedure to overcome the problem raised.

b) Place and time – the neglected children in LCA

LCA *sensu stricto* is very poor in modelling place and time, a point that has already been made in Subsections 1.2.5 and 1.2.6. Usually one assumes that all environmental interventions linked with the product system are added up independently of the point in time when they have occurred or will occur, of the time duration during which they occur, and of the place where they occur or where they lead to exposure.

We do therefore not know the background concentrations at the points of release and of exposure. We do not know the increase in concentrations due to the product system at hand, and we know nothing about the sensitivity of the areas (including their population density) so exposed.

A simplified modelling neglecting site- and time-specific variations is fully justified if:

- the same environmental effect that has occurred in the past, occurs today, and will occur in future is valued as being of identical importance, i.e., no *time preference* exists and the discount rate is set to zero, and
- no information on the place of release can be given because the analysed good is the product of a *homogenous market* (e.g., electricity), or
- no information on the *place of release* can be given because the places of production are still undetermined or changing in time, or
- the environmental interventions will be *ubiquitous* in the environment (e.g., CO_2).

Additionally, there is the pragmatic argument that we have to be satisfied, at present anyway, to just get the necessary information about processes for the inventory even without specifications of time and place. The present way of modelling in LCA which neglects information on place and time, leads to the notion that only potential impacts or damages can be assessed (White *et al.* 1995, Udo de Haes 1996, Barnthouse *et al.* 1997). This limitation may be relevant if large shares of impacts are predicted to occur from sources which will actually cause only very little damages, e.g., emissions from ships on oceans, damages to human health in very sparsely populated areas, or damages due to summer smog by emissions released in winter time. Of course, the opposite also may occur, i.e., the high importance of fossil waters in dry areas, or of emissions in mega-cities or in especially vulnerable places may be underestimated.

If the conditions justifying site-independent analysis at the beginning of this paragraph are fulfilled there is still the possibility to improve the model by the consideration of:

- A *source factor*. Potting *et al.* (1997) suggest differentiating, for instance, according to stack height or temperature and source strength of the released exhaust gas. Thanks to such release parameters, it is possible to make more reliable assumptions about the dilution volume and with that of the potential exposure of target species (see also Plewnia *et al.* 1983, Spadaro (forthcoming)).
- *Branch-specific* particularities in siting plants. Raw material extraction is partly performed in only a few places on earth which strongly deviate from the world average background concentrations and sensitivities. Therefore, it may be possible to define some typical branch-specific standard environments, including one for ocean shipping.
- *Season-dependent* characteristics. The contribution of hydrocarbons and NOx emitted during the winter period to the formation of smog in summer time is very limited. Emissions from installations which are running only during cold winter days could therefore be neglected when effects of summer smog are calculated.

If the conditions justifying site-independent analysis, that have been listed at the beginning of this paragraph, are not fulfilled one can:

- Increase the effort in *gathering data* on the process, the geographical and meteorological conditions, and the sensitivity (and density) of the receptors at the places of exposure (Ahrens *et al.* 1981, Tolle 1997). The modelling may be supported by *geographical information systems* (GIS) which are already being applied to risk mapping (Fedra 1997, Pruppers *et al.* 1996) and cover partly single compartments such as rivers (Feijtel *et al.* 1997). First attempts to combine LCA and GIS have been made by Bengtsson *et al.* (1997).

- *Divide the product system* into a foreground system with high geographical and time resolution and a background system with unit world assumptions. This division can be made, pragmatically based, on the available information. Or, it can be the result of a dominance analysis after a first round assessment of all environmental interventions with the unit world model and where information for the most relevant processes and substances are added afterwards[16].

Place and time are very important dimensions for the adequate modelling of the ecosphere. The steps mentioned here to improve the temporal and geographical resolution of LCA can form an indispensable requirement depending on the case at hand.

However, this book focuses on the LCIA for a background system, i.e., no site-specific information is used and a unit world representing the average situations in Europe is assumed as the modelling area. In Chapters 6 and 7 we will indicate which of the factors considered may have to be assessed in a more site-specific manner if the foreground system is analysed. Besides this type of flags we will – for pragmatic reasons – make no further attempts to improve the spatial and temporal resolution of LCIA.

c) What to do if background concentrations and doses matter?

One consequence of the limited temporal and spatial information in LCA *sensu stricto* is that one is compelled to make assumptions about the exposure characteristics, the receptor sensitivity and density, and the background concentration.

The consensus for the exposure assessment is to define unit worlds with average receptor sensitivity and density and average assumptions, but the opinions diverge on the question of how many different unit worlds are needed and how the background concentrations should be considered. As introduced in Subsection 1.2.5, the term 'only above threshold approach' is used when only exposure to substances is considered which surpass thresholds. In this case it is necessary to add more information in order to be able to make a judgement on the surpassing of a threshold (Hogan *et al.* 1996). Another approach assumes that either the threshold is already surpassed, or that it will probably be surpassed in the future, and that the product system at hand contributes therefore to "filling up" the reserves. This approach is called 'less is better' (see for a further discussion White *et al.* (1995) and Udo de Haes (1996)).

However, there is a way in between which allows for a more generic and less data intensive assessment. One can calculate the share of a pollutant (with today's emission pattern) which will surpass the threshold in a steady-state multi-media

[16] The use of the terms foreground and background here is not consistent with the definition in Subsection 1.2.5. If the terms will already be used to differentiate the product system in accordance with the criterion of decision makers' control, then new terms have to be used or invented.

model. This share can then be used to correct the slope of the dose-response factor above the threshold.

This procedure allows one to consider that there are pollutants where – if at all – only a certain share will surpass thresholds even if a steady-state situation is assumed. In this way, one can consider the accumulating behaviour of persistent and accumulating substances. This way of proceeding needs only an extra effort in the development of the LCIA method, but not in the LCA case studies.

For substances with a short half-life, this procedure suggests to consider the present pattern of concentrations. In the case of photochemical ozone formation (Subsection 7.2.3), it suggests that the present background concentrations are compared with the concentrations that would result in the case of the two scenarios under which all European emissions of VOC and NOx are to be cut by 30% respectively. These average declines could then be considered as a reasonable linearisation of the fate function in the relevant sector. It could therefore be taken as a representation of the marginal exposure per mass unit of precursor emissions.

If the loss in crop yield would have to be assessed instead, one would have to look at the change in the number of days during which the threshold concentrations are surpassed in the case of the two emission scenarios.

These procedures for averaging allow the production of more accurate estimates of the changes in effects than in the case of assuming fully proportional damage functions, but without increasing the need for detailed information in the inventory phase of LCA studies.

d) On/off mechanisms and LCIA

There are also mechanisms which show an on/off characteristic. This means that either an agent is there to cause allergies or it is not present. The quantity of the agent is in these cases irrelevant for the size of the effect.

Such a characteristic does not fit well with the assumptions made within LCIA. It violates the second axiom of the epistemological foundation (Subsection 1.2.2). If such allergies prove to be relevant, and the development in allergic problems suggests that they are, then LCIA may still aim for modelling the marginal increase of the area in which people are affected due to the additional emission (and with that of the area where damages occur). In this case, the fact is included that the probability that receptors within the polluted area are indeed exposed will increase with higher concentrations.

This aspect will not be further developed in this book.

4.3.6 The case studies chosen

a) The reasons leading to the selection

The framework presented in Section 4.2 and the model of the valuesphere discussed in Section 3.2 have to be made operable. For this purpose two case studies will be presented in Chapters 6 and 7. Case studies in this case does not mean LCA cases where products are analysed or compared, but subsets of endpoints which are harmed by common mechanisms.

For pragmatic reasons only mechanisms that damage the same safeguard subject will be included. Our choice fell on the safeguard subject "human health". Boguski *et al.* (1996:30) suggested to distinguishing between the following mechanism damaging human health:

- Carcinogenesis
- Irritant, corrosive effects
- Respiratory effects
- Central nervous system effects
- Allergenicity, sensitisation
- Methemoglobinemia, blood diseases
- Effects of odours
- Cardiovascular system effects
- Reproductive system effects
- Behavioural effects
- Bone or renal effects

From this list we have selected the carcinogenic and respiratory effects. A number of quantitative studies are available to show that, under actual environmental conditions, these two effect categories are responsible for large shares of health damages[17]. These studies cover a range of approaches: studies on health effects due to environmental pollution (World Bank 1993, WHO 1994a), studies calculating external costs (ExternE 1995, ESEERCO 1995) and a study making use of qualitative priority setting (Victorin *et al.* 1997). The responsibility of environmental conditions for the production of respiratory and carcinogenic effects becomes especially obvious when looking at death causes. Otherwise, one could also, e.g., consider noise as another environmental problem relevant to the damage to human health. Section 9.2 will summarise our own results and allow for a quantitative estimate of the importance of the chosen mechanisms.

Müller-Wenk (1997) has already published a preliminary damage function for increased ultraviolet radiation due to ozone depletion leading to cancer (see also Slaper

[17] Both themes have recently been the theme of expert workshops in Switzerland. This underlines their importance for future policy-making and has also facilitated the reception of up-to-date information (Waeber *et al.* 1997).

et al. 1997). Braunschweig (1997) and Frischknecht (1998) have operationalised the damage functions for ionising radiation due to the release of radionuclides leading to cancer. The case studies here, therefore, look only at chemical carcinogenesis as the third relevant source of damages due to cancer from environmental interventions[18]. Detailed introductions to the effects and their definitions will be provided in Sections 6.1 and 7.1.

The choice of these two mechanisms leading to damages to human health is the reason why we look more closely at the safeguard subject of human health and will proceed to define a damage index (see Chapter 5).

The following paragraphs (b) and (c) will explore points which have already been addressed in subsections 4.3.3 and 4.3.4, i.e., the combination of descriptive and prescriptive models.

b) Chemical carcinogenity caused by environmental pollutants

In order to illustrate the principal thoughts on the links between and the combination of models, we use here the case of chemical carcinogenity (to be discussed in detail in Chapter 6).

Table 4.5 distinguishes between the four substeps in the assessment of cause-damage-chains and the two perspectives that can be used to perform this assessment. Each cell lists the types of models or techniques which will be used in Chapter 6 to "construct" the damage function for human health for the case of carcinogenic chemicals. The last two steps of the more prescriptive or cause-oriented procedure (i.e., the fate and effect analyses) could be partitioned into many more steps (Lühr *et al.* 1991). But as we will see in Chapter 6, all the models actually used for transmission analysis, external exposure, internal exposure, and the determination of toxicokinetic and of toxicodynamic effects, combine the five substeps into just the two distinct steps identified in Table 4.5.

The definition of the damage categories, as described in Chapter 5, will mainly be based on health sciences. The concept of DALYs (disability adjusted life years) which is used, and its value choices, will be based on a panel of health experts. The information on the share of people which die due to tumour incidence and the life years lost due to premature deaths will mainly be taken from health statistics. The data for the effect analysis will come from epidemiological studies using small groups of people subject to high exposure and from toxicity data from animal testing which is extrapolated to human beings. The fate analysis will be performed with an inductive-stochastic model in a unit world. However, some of the results will be checked against and improved by comparisons with empirically derived fate factors. The different importance of the contributions from the descriptive and from the cause-oriented paths are indicated in Table 4.5 with the use of a scale of shades. The darker the shading is, the greater the importance of the particular technique for the analysis.

[18] The effects of fibres such as asbestos have also been excluded from the case studies as they fall within a separate family of mechanisms.

Chosen techniques / Steps in the procedure		Descriptive, damage oriented (empirical track within disciplines, "top-down -oriented")	Prescriptive, cause-oriented (modelling track within disciplines, analytical functional, "bottom-up -oriented")	
Definition of the damage categories	↓	Willingness-to-pay, contingent valuation (CVM)	Equivalency system from health economy (QALY, DALY) or insurance statistics	↑
Damage analysis	↓	Cancer registers and statistics, epidemiological cohort studies for patients with tumours	Information on latency time, tumour growth etc.	↑
Effect analysis (dose-response relationship)	↓	Epidemiological studies (case-control and cohort studies for highly exposed groups)	Toxicological studies, extrapolation from animal experiments and knowledge on mechanisms	↑
Fate and exposure analyses	↓	Empirical relationship between measured concentrations and emissions	Multimedia fate models to predict concentrations caused by emissions, risk assessment	↑

Tab. 4.5: The main models and information bases for the damage analysis of the carcinogenic effects of chemical emissions. The degree of importance of the chosen models for each step in the procedure is indicated by the increasing shading of the cells.

For reasons of practicability, the analysis will be restricted to 55 carcinogenic substances that lead to damages to human health, but data and information sources to calculate additional damage factors will be provided.

c) Respiratory effects

A short look at both Tables 4.5 and 4.6 immediately reveals differences in the shading of the cells. The damage categories for the respiratory effects will still be defined based on Chapter 5, but the damage analysis will be based more on clinical data and expert judgement[19] than is the case for the analysis of chemical carcinogenity. The effect analysis will be based on a large number of epidemiological studies. The fate analysis will be based, to a large extent, on empirical relationships between measured concentrations and emissions. However, concentration calculations by sophisticated atmospheric distribution models will also be used.

The main analysis will consider only seven substances to which human beings are exposed. However, for particles, we will distinguish between three different size classes. For the formation of ozone, we will include about 120 precursor substances in the analysis. This results, therefore, in more than 120 damage factors for pollutants emitted by anthropogenic activities (Chapter 7).

[19] As will be shown, non-expert judgement – unfortunately – will also be necessary.

Chosen techniques / Steps in the procedure		Descriptive, damage oriented (empirical track within disciplines, "top-down -oriented")	Prescriptive, cause-oriented (modelling track within disciplines, analytical functional, "bottom-up -oriented")	
Definition of the damage categories	↓	Willingness-to-pay, contingent valuation (CVM)	Equivalency system from health economy (QALY, DALY) or insurance statistics	↑
Damage analysis	↓	Health statistics, epidemiological cohort studies	Information from clinical disease history	↑
Effect analysis (dose-response relationship)	↓	Epidemiological studies (case-control, cohort, and cross-sectional studies)	Toxicological studies, extrapolation from animal experiments and knowledge on mechanisms	↑
Fate and exposure analyses	↓	Empirical relationship between measured concentrations and emissions	Multimedia fate models to predict concentrations caused by emissions, risk assessment	↑

Tab. 4.6: The main models and information bases for the damage analysis of the respiratory effects of emissions. The degree of importance of the chosen models for each step in the procedure is indicated by the increasing shading of the cells.

4.3.7 The role of cultural perspectives

Damage assessment is the one submodel for the ecosphere which is, as stated in Section 4.2, judged to be relevant by all cultural perspectives. However, the value choices within the damage assessment will be made in a manner which is compatible, as much as possible, with the three cultural perspectives. The following value choices can be identified:

- In the *fate analysis,* one has to choose a time horizon for the steady state modelling of persistent substances, otherwise the concentrations increase infinitely. Egalitarians can be expected to adopt a very long time horizon and consider low immobilisation rates. Individualists will consider those time horizons that are mentioned in the laws that set legal liability. Hierarchists will take an in-between position because it is the individuals or the public that will have to take responsibility for damages when the companies' liability has already come to an end. But the fate model used in Section 6.2 is of limited suitability for the highly persistent heavy metals and the cultural dependence could therefore not be considered in this specific case.
- In the *exposure analysis* and in the *damage analysis,* one could consider a range of measures which could be taken in the future to prevent damages due to environmental interventions. Such measures would depend on the adopted management style. They can be considered either in a culturally dependent damage assessment or in the index of manageability. We chose in this book to follow the second option.
- The acceptance of a degree of evidence as sufficient for declaring a given dose-response "association" as causal is a decisive value judgement in the *effect analysis.* Individualists will accept only associations which are understood and where causality is proven, hierarchists will rely on expert judgement and egalitarians may tend to include all associations that have been identified, even if the underlying mechanisms are not (yet) understood (see Subsections 6.3.2 and 7.3.4 for details).

- The explicit definition of the index for damages to human health opens up two questions: should future health damages be weighted equal to health damages occurring today or less (discounting), and should a year of life lost at the ages of 5, 30, and 80 be judged of equal importance or not (age-weighting) (see Subsection 5.4.7 for the cultural interpretation).

Additional value choices have to be made if other than those damages to human health that are analysed in this book and if damages to ecological health and to resource stocks are assessed. Table 3.1 will provide support for making predictions in these cases for each archetype.

The cultural dependence of the value choices in the damage assessment are not only the reason that the magnitude of damage per kg emitted substance will be different for the different perspectives, but also that some substances will, e.g., be considered in the first place by egalitarians, but disregarded by individualists.

4.3.8 Final remarks

It is evident that this section has been too short to provide a detailed introduction to damage assessment. It is recommended that readers who would like to learn more about this topic look at the comprehensive treatments available in the different fields of application (Paustenbach 1989, ESEERCO 1995, ExternE 1995, Kolluru *et al.* 1996).

This section's aim was to introduce the conceptual elements of damage assessment and to address some problems which arise when it is applied to LCIA. The main settings for the damage assessment are that (1) marginal analysis will be applied to derive damage factors and (2) the analysis is made for background processes without specification of time and place, i.e., averages are taken wherever possible[20]. The detailed description of the adaptation and the use of the models for the different substeps will be directly given in Chapters 6 and 7 where the adaptations can be demonstrated on the cases at issue.

The splitting of the damage function into the three levels of analysis makes it possible to include all the information available from environmental chemistry, the environmental sciences, and the health sciences. However, this way of proceeding also increases the number of elements and parameters which have to be quantified, but for which there is not just one right number due to uncertainty and variability. A (simple) uncertainty assessment will therefore be performed for all substeps and finally for the whole damage function in order to provide more than only a best estimate.

[20] In this case, the conditions found in Europe are taken as reference for purely pragmatic reasons.

4.4 Proxy for unknown damage

As introduced in Section 4.2, the ecosphere will be modelled by three submodels: the damage assessment (Section 4.3), the unknown damage assessment (this section), and the manageability of the damage (Section 4.5). The combination of these three submodels will be discussed in Section 4.6.

4.4.1 Overview

This section is dedicated to the small difference between *damage assessment* and *assessment of known damage*. *Damage* is composed of two parts, of *known, attributable, and causally linked damage* and of *unknown damage*. The first has been extensively discussed in Section 4.3 and will be further discussed in Chapters 5 to 7. The second is the subject of the discussion in this section. For an overview on its place within the model of the ecosphere, the reader is referred to Section 4.2 and especially to Figure 4.2.

Subsection 4.4.2 opens the discussion and lists the principle arguments justifying proxy indicators. Subsection 4.4.3 discusses the position of different cultural perspectives when aspects beyond known damages are addressed. Subsection 4.4.4 includes:

- an initial discussion of the paradox of measuring unknown damage
- the specification of the formal requirements for the indicator
- the discussion of a set of existing proxy indicators
- the limitation to represent emissions only
- a proposal to solve the problem of the dominance of high volume substances in proxy indicators
- the justification of a final choice of the characteristic to serve as a proxy
- the introduction of bioaccumulation, and, finally,
- the calculation of a set of equivalency factors.

The operationalisation is restricted to unknown damage due to emissions. Resources and land use are not (yet) included. A final discussion (Subsection 4.4.5) summarises the arguments for, and limitations of, the chosen proxy indicator for unknown damage.

4.4.2 Discussion to clarify the meaning of unknown damage

A significant number of researchers in environmental sciences, biology, chemistry, medicine, physics, and many other disciplines are working on the identification of causal relationships between interventions or causes and damages or effects. A large part of this research is concerned with the assessment of causal damage to safeguard subjects due to environmental interventions. However, human beings will never be able to explain the full web of interactions (not only physical!) on earth as it is composed of an almost infinite number of interacting systems. If finally one interaction or causality identified, at least two other unsolved questions will arise.

Nevertheless, if safeguard subjects can be clearly described and if they are observable, such as, e.g., human health, and if damages to such safeguard subjects can be measured or observed, then causal damage assessment can contribute significantly to the understanding of the relevant elements of the system concerned and, finally, to the design of specific interventions. It is desirable that the safeguard subjects are clearly defined and that, thanks to new analytical possibilities and observational means (e.g., satellites), damages can be measured and observed. This will increase the probability that a growing number of systems and their interactions can be understood. Still, there are good reasons why this approach will fail to provide a sufficient basis for assessment:

- Scientists are still far from describing ecological health in terms of a safeguard subject. Essential functions of ecosystems are still to be discovered. Ecology teaches us that ecosystems are not in equilibrium (see, e.g., Holling 1973, Ryder 1990:619); at best they are at a steady state non-equilibrium, a so-called flowing equilibrium. Such a situation makes it difficult to differentiate between a natural change and a change representing damage. This is an unsatisfactory starting point for the observation and the measurement of damage to ecological health. (The same also holds true for other safeguard subjects, see e.g., the case of resources in Subsection 4.1.2 and Müller-Wenk (1997), Scheringer *et al.* (1997).)
- Observation of effects implies that they have already occurred and that they occur at places where human beings look for them. Many effects may only reveal themselves in the distant future after accumulation processes have taken place and have altered biological or geological systems. These effects just cannot be observed today. Other effects occur at places where people do not stay or where they would not think to look for them (Scheringer 1996:23f).
- More and more substances are ubiquitous; they can be found all over the world. The so-called "global distillation" process transports persistent semi-volatile compounds from warmer emitting (i.e., evaporating) regions to higher latitudes where the substances are condensed and deposited (Anonymous 1997). Persistent substances are globally spread within the downwind zone and exchanged with upper levels of the atmosphere. Globalisation of trade sees to it that the same kind of products and substances are used and emitted all over the world (Ballschmiter 1992). These are undesired conditions when one wants to assess causalities. Our common large scale field experiment does not fulfil the basic principles for a scientific experiment such as providing us with a unexposed control group and test groups with exposure to single substances.
- A consequence of the state described in the previous point is that a large number of substances are used and emitted in comparably small quantities which lead to very low concentrations in the environment. The causal attribution of damages to such a cocktail of low-concentrated substances by means of epidemiological studies is impossible. Toxicity tests, on the other hand, suffer from the lack of realistic long-term conditions and the inability to consider antagonistic and synergistic effects.

These are some of the reasons why knowledge on causalities in damage assessment is insufficient and will remain so. They provide a first indication for what type of proxy of unknown damage should stand for:

- ill-defined safeguard subjects and damages to safeguard subjects

- persistent and accumulating substances
- non-perceived damages due to missing "eyes" (sensors) at the right places
- low volume substances and substance mixtures.

It may be helpful after this concretisation of the meaning of unknown damage to try to define where to draw the line between known and unknown damages. Known damage is not a defined and given range of subjects for which the causalities are known. The decision whether causalities are sufficiently known due to measurements or model calculations is a subjective one. Some researchers and politicians consider the relationships between the emission of greenhouse gases and global change, between emissions of chlorofluorcarbons and increased UV-radiation, or the emission of fine suspended particles and respiratory diseases as causally proven while others do not. For each causal hypothesis, there exists a certain degree of consensus which varies over time. In the next subsection, this aspect will be discussed in more detail. For the time being, it is important to retain that the border between known causal damage and unknown damage has to be fixed and that it is therefore somewhat arbitrary or subjective.

How should this borderline be drawn? Subsection 4.4.4 will show that a proxy should be used which is not located on the damage, but on the exposure level. Figure 4.6 illustrates this distinction by differentiating between four levels of the impact path. Starting with the production of a chemical substance, we have on the first level, the amount of production and the amount stored in the technosphere. A more or less small share of this substance production will be emitted into the environment (second level). After emission, the substance will dilute, probably decay, and nature and humans will be exposed to it (third level). The fourth level is an optional one. The exposure to the substance may or may not lead to effects in human beings and in nature. Knowledge on the last level is scant and many of the links from exposure to damage are unknown.

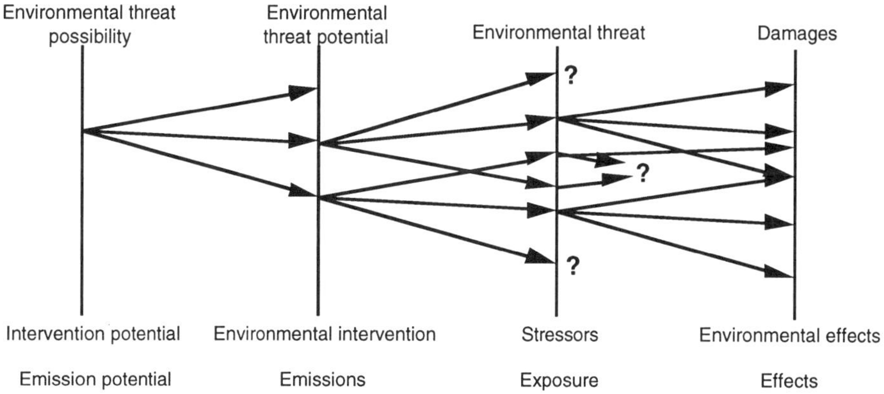

Fig. 4.6: The different levels from possibility of an emission to effect and its normative parallels from threat possibilities to damages[21] (after Scheringer (1996), Berg *et al.* (1994))

[21] The terms used here diverge partly from what is currently used as LCA terminology in Udo de Haes (1996) or proposed in ISO (1997). For most terms, the LCA community would add a 'potential'. This potential serves as a flag indicating that all steps are modelled in LCA by ignoring time, space, and

Choosing a proxy for unknown damage means that all the information to be gained from an insufficiently broad consensus on cause-effect relationships and from the discussion about these relationships is lost. This is an argument for not drawing the borderline between the known and the unknown damages too close around the small number of cause-effect relationships that everyone agrees with, and instead, to also include less validated knowledge together with appropriate tools to deal with the inherent uncertainty.

This means, in other words, that the damage assessment should cover causal chains leading to possible or known effects. For either situation, the probability of occurrence is known (leading to risk) or unknown (leading to uncertainty). The proxy for unknown damage should primarily cover the case where neither the effect at all nor the probability of occurrence is known (indeterminacy) (see, e.g., Wynne 1992, Dürrenberger 1994).

4.4.3 The role of cultural perspectives

There are two subjective aspects to this borderline between known and unknown damages which should be discussed from the vantage point of Cultural Theory: What is *known* and what is *unknown*, and how far can unknown aspects influence decision making? The question of what constitutes a damage is not re-addressed here (see Subsections 4.1.2 and 4.1.5).

The first question has already been addressed in the previous subsection with the discussion of the borderline problem. However, it is obvious that the proposed division (if possible effects with known or unknown probability are known, they should be covered by the damage assessment; if effects are not known, a proxy for unknown effects should be used) still requires a decision whether effects are known or not.

Here the discussion can profit from the archetypes of decision makers which have been introduced under the heading of cultural perspectives (Section 3.2).

Individualists are risk-seeking and use an adaptive management style. These characteristics, compounded with their belief in the benign behaviour of nature, let individualists make their decisions based on experience rather than on evidence or arguments (Rayner 1991). Only undisputed epidemiological results for cause-effect relationships which concern obviously damaging effects will be accepted by them as the relevant basis for decisions. 'Known' means to individualists that damages really occur, are observed and measured and do directly or indirectly harm human beings. In addition, no established researcher is supposed to have doubts on the causal factors. Under the individualists' perspective, only a small number of environmental problems will be covered in the damage assessment.

Egalitarians hold the opposite view in this special case. Their world-view is based on the concept of an ephemeral (fragile) nature. This implies that there are many factors which can damage it. This requires a preventive management style that not only considers observable and proven damage, but predicted and modelled damage based on arguments as well. However, egalitarians do not just tend to act on the

background conditions and that the respective modelling results cannot be compared with observed concentrations or effects.

basis of worst case scenarios. They simply pay attention not just to known cause-effect relationships, but to lesser understood problems. The inherently higher degree of uncertainty is dealt with in an uncertainty assessment.

Hierarchists show a high belief in expert judgements and the existence of evidence is their main criterion for deciding if they will include an environmental problem in the damage assessment or not. Hierarchists will also pay a great deal of attention to the procedural aspects. Results from established scientific communities with a high reputation are given a high relevance while new findings from unorganised research groups may be considered to be of lesser relevance.

This short discussion leads to the conclusion that the borderline between known and unknown damages depends on the cultural perspective held by decision makers in a number of different ways. The examples that will be given in Subsections 6.3.2 and 7.3.4 of carcinogenesis and respiratory effects will also confirm that the borderline depends on the degree of evidence necessary to consider that an association between causes and damages can be accepted as causal. The indices for known damage (one for each perspective) are based for these two examples on different sizes of the analysed systems of cause-effect relationships due to the differences in the evidence used in their support (Subsections 6.3.2 and 7.3.4). However, the proxy indicator will remain unchanged even if other numbers of causal relationships are considered in the damage assessment, i.e., the proxy for unknown damage is independent of the damage assessment.

The second question about the relevance of a proxy for unknown damage for decision making does not deal with the practical question of how it is possible to find a sensible proxy for something we do not know (see next subsection). Rather, it is a question of the significance that the different perspectives give to such a proxy in their decision making than of its modelling assumptions. Only the modelling aspects will be further discussed in this section.

From the discussion above, it is clear that individualists will pay little or no attention to such a proxy indicator. Hierarchists and Egalitarians may be more in favour of using such indicators. Hierarchists would claim though that such indicators have to be developed by established experts. They recognise that there are good reasons to base decisions on such indicators in situations where the subject is overcomplex[22]. Egalitarians, finally, see in proxy indicators the only way to deal with a lack of information on, and understanding of, the overcomplex system.

A further discussion of the importance of the different indicators for manageability, known damage, and unknown damage based on cultural theory can be found in Section 4.6.

[22] This term is used by Schmidt-Bleek (1993) and Berg *et al.* (1994) to stress that "ecosystems can neither be described sufficiently nor they can be defined clearly" and the evolution with time of ecosystems is unpredictable and irregular.

4.4.4 Operationalising unknown damage

The paradox of measuring unknown damage

The idea of deriving an indicator for something which is not known may look like an absurd way of proceeding. This contradiction deserves some comment before we begin with the operationalisation of the proxy for unknown damage.

There is no doubt that people tend to include not only a set of known aspects and causalities in decisions, but a more holistic view on the whole problem area as well. They consider aspects which are not made explicit or develop a "feeling" for unknown interactions that might be relevant for solving the problem. It is much too reductionistic to assume that decisions are made only based on known and explicitly stated aspects.

However, the argumentation in favour of the relevance of unknown damage, in the case of the assessment of environmental damage, does not automatically justify the conclusion that this unknown damage can be measured in the form of an indicator. Nevertheless, there are three reasons why a proxy indicator is quantified here:

- Firstly, as already stated in Section 1.2, it can be assumed that decision makers prefer, in general, a small number of indices as decision support instead of a long list of qualitative statements. This preference for quantified information is increased by the circumstance that in most decision situations an indicator for the economic dimension and expressed in money terms will be available. This indicator will attract all the attention as long as no comparably powerful indicators for the other dimensions of relevance in decision making are available.
- Secondly, LCA is a highly quantitative tool with the LCI delivering a comprehensive list of environmental interventions. It would seem to be completely inappropriate to add a purely qualitative and holistic step to this quantification of aspects that are of very different relevance after all (orders of magnitude).
- Thirdly, the pressure to quantify an index for unknown damage is a motivation to think about more basic mechanisms of environmental threat and it opens up the mind for a more comprehensive and future oriented view of the ecosphere and its mechanisms (see also Berg *et al.* 1994). It makes it possible, in addition, to bring in supplementary information and knowledge from other than the damage level.

We will be searching for an indicator for unknown damage based on these arguments in this section. We will use the term proxy indicator[23] from now on and with this choice of terminology acknowledge the paradoxical situation that one will never find an identical indicator[24] for unknown damage.

[23] Which has the characteristics of a non-identical indicator (see next footnote).

[24] Systems analysis distinguishes between identical, partly-identical and non-identical indicators. The descriptive character of the indicators decreases in this order and the tendency to act as a proxy increases accordingly.

Specification of the proxy indicator

There are some questions which should be answered before we make a proposal for the operationalisation of the proxy for unknown damage:

A Should we aim for one proxy indicator, or is it possible to include several indicators which will later be aggregated to a proxy index?

B If there are indicators to be aggregated to a proxy index, will they be linked additively or multiplicatively?

C Should the index (or the indicators) be based on the level of environmental interventions, of stressors, or of damage?

D Which type of scale has to be used to measure the index (or the indicators)?

There is more than one indicator suitable to reflect the aspects of system behaviour that we are interested in. In principle, all of them should be part of the proxy index. However, thinking one step ahead to the aggregation of indicators to an index, suggests that we may better stay with one indicator (question A). A proposal from Scheringer et al. (1994a) that makes use of two indicators is presented below in some detail and it will become clear how difficult it is to aggregate proxy indicators for unknown damage to an index.

Question B is meaningless once we have made the decision to stay with one proxy indicator. If one decides otherwise (as we will later on), the choice between an additive or a multiplicative aggregation depends on the kind of characteristics that are always relevant when faced with this choice. In the course of the development in this subsection, we will see that a multiplicative linkage fits best (for a test procedure see Appendix (4)). On the level of the main criteria 'known damage', 'unknown damage', and 'manageability', the proxy indicator for unknown damage should be designed as an additive indicator because unknown damage is not a correction factor for one of the other criteria.

The question C is linked to the discussion of a point illustrated by Figure 4.6. From this discussion, it is clear that the effect level – or, more normatively, the damage level – is inappropriate for a proxy for unknown damage[25]. Which of the other levels is most appropriate will be discussed below.

From the argumentation above in favour of one proxy indicator, it is clear that we aim at a quantitative indicator which is based somehow on the inventory table. A cardinal scale seems to be the most obvious scale if the inventory table is presented in the form of ratio scales and the equivalency factors have to be linked to the table (question D).

---

[25] It was argued in Subsection 4.4.2 that the proxy for unknown damage should stand for situations where neither the effect nor the probability of occurrence is known, i.e., in the case of indeterminacy. It is therefore clear that we cannot base it on the effect or damage level.

Overview of existing proxy indicators

Subsection 1.3.2 already contains an overview of proxy indicators. We will discuss here some of the proposals made there in light of the intended use as a proxy indicator for unknown damage.

Probably the first proxy indicator, and the indicator with the largest dissemination today, is the *market price*. This indicator measures the time and place-specific valuation of the use of natural and human resources, i.e., market adjusted costs. In terms of Figure 4.6, it is an indicator on the level of intervention potential, i.e., very early in the impact path. The prices – but even more the costs – reflect indeed to a certain extent the use of and the intensity of processing natural resources. Due to its early place in the impact path, no understanding on ecosphere behaviour is added, however. I.e., the indicator reflects mainly the mechanisms of the anthroposphere. Therefore, market price is not proposed as a 'brother' to the index for known damage.

The *cumulative* (direct and indirect) *energy demand* had been introduced as an indicator when the mining of increasingly large volumes of coal required large amounts of wood for the pits in the 19th century. The methods were improved during the 1960's and 1970's and applied to optimise, e.g., energy systems (IFIAS 1974). The indicator is still used today and some even claim it to be a proxy for environmental relevance (VDI 1995). The indicator fits in terms of Figure 4.6 partly on the level of intervention potential and partly on the level of intervention. Resource use can be treated within LCA as a safeguard subject, which means that energy use will be treated as environmental intervention and assessed within a given valuation framework. Therefore, only energy use on the level of intervention potential may have relevance as a proxy for unknown damage[26]. However, the same arguments as above apply. While energy demand could stand as a proxy for the system characterisation as such, it does not seem fit to be a 'brother' to the index for known damage.

The *mass intensity per service unit (MIPS)* is the latest representative of indicators on the level of intervention potential (Schmidt-Bleek 1992/1994). Although no significant differences between MIPS and the market price and cumulative energy demand can be identified, it is worthwhile to note that it is the only one of these indicators explicitly developed for the purpose of being a measure of environmental threat or even damage. However, little justification is given for the claim that it is a more meaningful proxy than the other two already mentioned above. The objections against using this indicator as a proxy for unknown damage are the same as those made above for the other two proposals.

Scheringer *et al.* (1994a) have chosen a different level for the construction of a proxy measure. They developed two indicators, one for the *spatial range* and one for *persistency* (the time range), to characterise the environmental threat from chemicals. Scheringer (1996) starts out with a fundamental discussion of the problems of damage assessment, the normative implications of the valuation of environmental problems, of equity considerations, and of the best ways to deal with

[26] Frischknecht *et al.* (forthcoming) critically discuss this statement and the implications for the aggregation rules.

overcomplexity. He calculates the persistency for a large number of substances and determines the percentage of the earth's circumference which would be exposed by a point source of emission (indicator for the spatial range). Both indicators are calculated by means of a multi-media model adapted for these purposes. The indicators, or proxies as they are called by their developers, cover aspects of the exposure, i.e., they are on the level of environmental threat (Figure 4.6). The two indicators cover the time and spatial aspects of exposure, certainly two very important dimensions. These are features which could make this approach to be a prime candidate for the role of proxy for unknown damage. However, there are also some disadvantages:

- There are two indicators which, as was already indicated, poses a problem as there are no suggestions for the aggregation. Indeed, the developers of the indicators themselves refrain from a further aggregation of them.
- The spatial range is largely influenced by the environmental life time in air. Because of that the two indicators are not fully independent of each other (van Pul *et al.* 1997).
- The approach gives a great deal of weight to non-degradable substances. It does not differentiate between them being inert or not and does not ask whether they are available to living organisms. In this way, the approach reflects more the exposure of the abiotic sphere than of the biota.

Nevertheless, if the two indicators could be aggregated to one proxy, and if, in addition, their bias against biological availability of the substance in the different compartments could be corrected, they would fit for our purpose.

The ratio between present concentrations and *geogenic concentrations* or between present emission flows and *geogenic flows* is sometimes used in material flow analysis (e.g., Baccini *et al.* 1991) and has been adapted for LCA (Hofstetter 1991). The idea behind this proxy is that geogenic loads are what nature knows how to deal with. The larger the anthropogenic induced change in concentration or flow is, the more serious an intervention has to be judged. According to this way of thinking, xenobiotic compounds are the most serious environmental burden (a division by geogenic concentrations leads to an infinite ratio!). Major drawbacks of this proxy are the difficulty to include xenobiotic substances, the large variations of geogenic concentrations and flows, and the need to choose between geogenic concentrations and flows. E.g., anthropogenic emissions of CO_2 are very small compared to geogenic flows, but the concentration increase in the atmosphere is predicted to equalise the geogenic concentration in the next century.

A last class of proxy indicators which have been developed is close to the effect level. Christoffel *et al.* (1996) examined in a student thesis the criteria of reversibility and of spatial range on the level of impact categories. Reversibility was based on the environmental lifetime of substances and regeneration time of ecosystems. It was assumed that the environmental intervention will be stopped completely from now on. (This is, of course, no realistic phase-out scenario.) For the spatial range, the authors undertook a detailed world-wide analysis of damaged areas and of areas sensitive to further burden by environmental interventions. The latter areas are where the loads are already high and the conditions to cause damage are given, but the damages not (yet) observed. Their estimates are reproduced in

Table 4.7. They should be seen as first estimates rather than as the results of extensive modelling.

From the results in Table 4.7, it is clear that both criteria discriminate in a relevant manner. The least and the most relevant impact categories differ by orders of magnitude. In the light of the proposed framework in this study, it is clear that reversibility and damaged areas are, in principle, already considered in the index of the damage assessment. The additional indication of sensitive areas may add information for a proxy of unknown damage. However, as mentioned earlier, the proxy indicator for unknown damage should not imply that the set of environmental problems is known as it is done here. Information of the type given by Christoffel *et al.* (1996) is very useful in order to get a better understanding of the meaning, on a global scale, of environmental problems identified, for instance, in Europe.

indicators for	Reversibility	Damaged areas	Sensitive areas	Damaged plus sensitive areas
Impact categories	years	1000 km^2	1000 km^2	1000 km^2
Depletion of abiotic resources	Irreversible	n.d.	n.d.	n.d.
Victims	Irreversible	n.d.	n.d.	n.d.
Damage to ecosystems and landscapes	50 - 9'520	19'700	n.d.	>19'700
Ecotoxicity	3'000	2'000	1'300	3'300
Depletion of biotic resources (here only forests considered)	200	60'000	57'000	117'000
Enhancement of the greenhouse effect	108	n.d.	1'600	1'600
Depletion of the ozone layer	70	n.d.	53'100	53'100
Acidification	10	13'000	20'000	33'000
Nutrification	4.5	1'200	960	2'160
Photochemical oxidant formation	0.6	2'600	n.d.	>2'600
Human toxicity	0.022	2'800	10'300	13'100
Waste heat	0.01	44	n.d.	>44
Odour	0.008	n.d.	n.d.	n.d.
Noise	0	180	n.d.	>180

Tab. 4.7: Reversibility and spatial range of environmental problems (Christoffel *et al.* 1996), n.d.: not determined

The limitation on a proxy for emissions

At this stage, the proposal starts to become concrete in order to operationalise a proxy indicator for unknown damage. As mentioned before, only emissions will be considered to contribute to unknown damage. All aspects of resource use and direct physical impacts on land and waters are not reflected in the proxy indicator developed here.

The paragraphs below will suggest that the accumulating characteristic is important for emissions. Maybe the decumulating aspects in resource and land use could serve as a proxy for these interventions. However, no proxy for input oriented interventions will be presented in the course of this book[27].

[27] This choice was made in order to limit the scope of the development work and of this book.

The dominance of high volume emissions in proxy indicators

If we agree to look for a proxy indicator on the level of environmental threat and to define a kind of equivalency factor to weight and aggregate single environmental interventions in the form of:

$$U = \Sigma_i \, (p_i \cdot I_i) \qquad [-] \qquad (4.2)$$

where U proxy indicator for unknown damage
p_i proxy equivalency factor for substance i
I_i emission of substance i per functional unit

then we will end up in many cases with indicators dominated by high volume emissions. If this indicator, for instance, would be based on spatial range or on persistency, it would, in both cases, largely be dominated by the emission of CO_2, a globally distributed and relatively persistent gas (about 120 years). The same would be true in case of the MIPS approach or, as will be discussed later, the one focusing on bioaccumulation.

Should high volume substances dominate this indicator? This is a tricky question since it is very hard to discuss and argue about *unknown* damage. In addition, it is rather unscientific to construct an index and then to reject it simply because one does not like the outcome, i.e., in this case its dominance by high volume substances. There is no easy way out of this quandary. However, we can go back to the subject of Subsection 4.4.2 and ask which substances do we not know enough about? This is the case when, for instance, substances with high persistency and accumulation potential will lead to effects only in the future that can then be seen to occur. Substances with high emission rates have already today generated concentrations that are high enough to have been noticed and measured. Indeed, policy towards chemical substances has, in the past, very much concentrated on high volume substances. It might therefore be more important to look at the characteristics of low volume and, therefore, probably less understood substances.

To overcome this problem of the dominance by one high volume substance, it is proposed to normalise the environmental intervention by a flow representing the present background, i.e., the sum of the anthropogenic and geogenic yearly emission flows. Adding the geogenic flows is relevant because there exists much more experience[28] with substances with high geogenic background flows than with xenobiotic substances where there is no geogenic background flow.

$$U = \Sigma_i \left(p_i \cdot \frac{I_i}{B_i} \right) \qquad [a] \qquad (4.3)$$

where B_i world-wide anthropogenic emissions of substance i plus world-wide geogenic flow which leads to concentration available to the biota [kg/a]

This normalisation represents an important weighting step, although it is usually labelled as a scaling or a normalisation step. It gives a lot of weight to substances with small anthropogenic emissions and or little or no geogenic background. In other words, it is supposed that substances with high geogenic and/or high

[28] This refers above all to humans, but is also true for the whole biota.

anthropogenic emissions are better understood than substances with low emissions and/or flows. This supposition is given if one is convinced that the damage assessment already delivers reliable assessments for such high volume substances.

The importance of a substance, measured in terms of the contribution to the proxy indicator for unknown damage, is high on the world level (*Ii* is set equal with world-wide anthropogenic emissions) if the equivalency factor pi is high and the geogenic emissions low.

Choice of the proxy indicator

There is a lively discussion ongoing within the chemical industry on the evaluation of new and existing substances used in or produced by the industry that turns, among other things, around the right criteria to be used for such evaluations. Klöpffer (1994) mentions the following criteria:

- emitted volume per year
- mobility (tendency to be distributed)
- persistency (long life time, no available sinks)
- accumulation (in organisms, soil and sediments)
- adverse effects (toxicity)

Klöpffer (1989/1994) thinks that in the absence of sufficient knowledge on substance behaviour and toxicity, the main criterion for environmental valuation should be persistency and that it should serve as a proxy for ecotoxicity. He argues that only persistent substances can accumulate (depending on their volume emitted, their mobility, and their potential to accumulate). In addition, he makes a strong argument concerning the attitude to adopt towards substances about which we lack knowledge. It should be possible to eliminate adverse environmental effects, once detected, simply by stopping further emissions to the environment. This condition is fulfilled only if the substance has a short environmental lifetime.

The opinion that toxicity, especially ecotoxicity, is so far not sufficiently understood is not just one held by scientists, but also by the Swedish Chemicals Policy Committee (Anonymous 1997). It proposes to drop toxicity as a criterion from existing evaluation schemes for chemicals and to stick to the two criteria persistency and bioaccumulation. They should be used to identify those chemicals that are of concern. The Committee proposes – in absence of available test methods – that not readily degradable substances (in internationally recognised tests for ready or inherent biodegradability) should be considered as persistent. For the bioconcentration factor, a threshold of 10 and for the octanol-water partition coefficient a threshold of 100, are proposed.

In Subsection 4.4.2, we listed what a proxy index for unknown damage should stand for: persistency, accumulation, mobility (to places where damages are not perceived), and synergistic behaviour of a large number of low-concentrated substances. Persistency and accumulation stand for the tendency that it is the dose that makes the poison (according to Paracelsus). Persistency and mobility stand for the impossibility to 'clean' up the environment after unexpected effects have shown up (precautionary principle and equity considerations, see also Scheringer (1996)). And the problem of a cocktail of low volume substances addresses the problem of synergistic behaviour and cases where it is not the concentration that makes the effects, e.g., allergies.

In the beginning of this subsection it was argued that the equivalency factor *pi* (see Equation 4.2) should consist of only one indicator because aggregating indicators to one index would be not only a subjective, but also a largely arbitrary task. Without this limitation, a multiple of indicators for mobility, persistency, and accumulation would have been proposed instead. The importance of low volume substances is already assured through the introduction of the normalisation step (in Equation 4.3).

The following argumentation leads to the choice for bioaccumulation as a proxy indicator:

- The criterion of mobility has lost some of its relevance due to the globalisation of trade and the industrialisation of so-called less developed continents. Less mobile substances that are used and emitted all over the globe lead to similar problems as highly mobile substances do.
- Persistency is certainly relevant for the distribution and accumulation of substances in the environment. It is therefore an interesting candidate for a proxy indicator. However, persistency does not indicate the share of the substance that is available and will result in infinite values for many substances (e.g., metals). Non reactive, elemental environmental interventions will show little or no decay. The law of mass preservation leads therefore to high environmental lifetimes for such substances.
- Bioaccumulation as a proxy is closest to the biota. It directly indicates internal exposure and is therefore closer to potential effects than the other indicators mentioned above.

A critical discussion and operationalisation of bioaccumulation will be given below. One could argue that this choice of indicator is subjective and arbitrary as well and means in fact that the other characteristics are weighted by zero. This criticism is acknowledged and the choice of bioaccumulation as the proxy should be considered as preliminary only.

Characteristics of bioaccumulation

Living organisms tend to accumulate substances that are available in their food and in their surrounding compartments. Biomagnification stands for the increase in the concentration of substances along the food chain and is seen as one potential risk path to animals on a higher trophic level. Bioaccumulation is a function of the uptake of a substance determined by the concentrations in the exposure paths and its internal absorption, and of the elimination processes determined by passive (simple diffusion processes) or active elimination (enzymatic detoxification systems biotransform substances to metabolites).

Bioaccumulation in water organisms is known best. Bioaccumulation and bioconcentration factors were originally developed as parameters to characterise the accumulation of substances. The following definitions are used (ECETOC 1995):

- *Bioaccumulation Factor (BAF)*: The ratio of the steady-state concentration of a substance in an organism due to *all routes of exposure* in relation to the concentration of thc substance in water.
- *Bioconcentration Factor (BCF)*: The ratio of the steady-state concentration of a substance in an organism due to *water-borne exposure* in relation to the concentration of the substance in water.

Relying on organisms in water and relating the parameters to the concentration in water have not only historical reasons. Aquatic organisms find themselves in intensive interaction with the medium water and, in most cases, the uptake of a substance through the water is much more relevant than the uptake through food. This means that aquatic organisms are normally in a steady state equilibrium with respect to the substance's concentration in water. Therefore, it is easy to measure the BCF and BAF for aquatic organisms, something which is much more difficult for terrestrial animals.

Many experimental BCFs are available for plankton, algae, and fish (Rippen 1996, Nagel *et al.* 1991, Connell 1990). Therefore, it would be pragmatic to rely on this data. Such a choice provokes two questions to be answered: can we rely only on aquatic organisms and are the test organisms usually used appropriate for our purpose?

The question with respect to the compartment to be considered can be answered by referring to explanations given above. The choice of aquatic organisms has the advantage in these animals are in equilibrium with the concentrations of the substances in water. The choice of organisms living in water will therefore reveal the highest bioaccumulation observable. This may fail to catch those specific terrestrial species (including birds) which show a higher accumulation due to the composition of their organism or to the enzymes their organism produce.

The best answer to the question with respect to the usually used test organisms is that it is a question of choice. Plankton and microorganisms show generally higher BCFs than fish. Each specific species of fish or of plankton shows an individual behaviour. Arguments in favour of microorganisms or plankton are that they are very low in the food chain, they have little specific elimination mechanisms and show therefore a larger range for the BCFs (which supports the discriminatory power of the indicator), and they would make unnecessary the use of animal tests. In favour of data from fish, one can mention the better representation of other animals and the broader use for chemical assessments (ECETOC 1995). It is this last reason which makes us prefer to work in this study with BCF of fish. This is a preliminary choice and is not really relevant for the presentation of the principle behind proxy equivalency factors.

Some critical aspects connected with the choice of BCF should be mentioned before the data are derived and the calculations are made (Lillelund *et al.* 1987):

- The BCF is dependent on the concentration in water. The BCF is generally higher at low rather than high concentrations due to saturation effects, maximum levels of stock capacity, etc.
- The BCFs vary quite a bit from one organism to the next. Biomagnification does not normally occur in aquatic organisms even though it is sometimes assumed. Organisms of higher trophic levels often show lower BCFs than those of lower

trophic levels due to their increased capacities for biotransformation. Still, they do accumulate more pollutants than organisms of lower trophic levels due to their larger size. Terrestrial organisms may show biomagnification due to the fact that many organisms are not in a steady state equilibrium with the surrounding compartments. The uptake by food becomes therefore the important intake path and leads to the accumulation in the food chain.

- Comparisons of BCF tests performed with laboratory and with field organisms revealed significant differences. One has to assume that different kinds of diet and of living conditions make field animals accumulate less pollutants.
- The retention behaviour of the different organisms varies widely. Some excrete or break down substances as fast as they accumulate them; others are slow in their elimination, but finally approximate the zero load level. Some organisms have a minimum stock below which they will not manage to get, and some show no decontamination at all. These differences in retention behaviour are not reflected in the BCFs.

These additional aspects are met with the use of comparable test conditions for all substances. These requirements are largely fulfilled given their wide use in chemistry and the description as a standard test procedure on an international level (OECD 1981). In addition, we stay with aquatic animals where biomagnification is less important. For aquatic organisms, the BCF and BAF are normally very close due to the dominating intake path by water.

Empirical data and QSARs for Bioconcentration Factors (BCFs)

Empirical BCFs can be found in literature and databases. Large collections of BCFs for organic substances can be found, e.g., in Rippen (1996) and Nagel *et al.* (1991). BCFs for metals and other substances can be found, e.g., in Connell (1990) and Jørgensen *et al.* (1993).

However, BCF's are not available or easily accessible for all substances inventoried in LCA. For those substances for which BCF's are not available, methods have been developed that make it possible to calculate them from easily obtainable physical and chemical parameters. Such Quantitative Structure-Activity Relationships (QSARs) are derived from the relationship between measured BCFs and the physical and chemical parameters. Such QSARs are available for different substance classes, organisms, and different input parameters (Connell 1990, ECETOC 1995, Nagel *et al.* 1991). For simplicity reasons, we present in Table 4.8 only two frequently used equations based on the octanol-water partition coefficient Kow that are valid for various substance classes (but only lipophilic chemicals) and that are used to calculate BCFs for fish.

QSAR	Valid for K_{ow}	QSAR based on	Regression coefficient r	Source
$\log BCF = \log K_{ow} - 1.32$	0.03 - 4.7	44 Substances	0.97	Mackay (1982)
$\log BCF = 0.79 \log K_{ow} - 0.4$	1.0 - 6.9	122 Substances	0.93	Veith *et al.* (1983)

Tab. 4.8: Regression equations for estimating BCF in fish from octanol-water coefficient (log Kow), most frequently used QSARs for various lipophilic substances (according to ECETOC (1995))

It is possible, with this empirical basis and the possibility of calculating missing BCFs, to calculate the proxy equivalency factor *pi*. However, it should be emphasised that the databases and calculation models mentioned are mostly based on lipophilic substances. Especially substances with no solubility in a polar media and high Henry constants, i.e., substances which primarily stay in the atmosphere or are bound to soil, are poorly reflected in the operationalisation here[29].

Equivalency factors for the calculation of the proxy indicator

We have to rewrite Equation (4.2) in order to give a first list of equivalency factors:

$$U = \Sigma_i \left(Ii \cdot \frac{BCFi}{Bi} \right) = \Sigma_i \left(Ii \cdot EFi \right) \quad \text{[a]} \qquad (4.4)$$

where U proxy indicator for unknown damage
$BCFi$ bioconcentration factor in fish for substance *i*
Ii environmental intervention *i* per functional unit
Bi world-wide anthropogenic emissions of substance i plus world-wide geogenic flow which leads to concentration available to the biota [kg/a]
EFi $BCFi/Bi$ = equivalency factor

According to Equation (4.4), the BCFs in fish and the world-wide emissions have to be known in order to calculate the equivalency factor for each substance. The results given in Table 4.9 are based on the average of the empirical data given for BCFs in fish by Rippen (1996). We used the calculated BCFs given by Rippen (1996) when no empirical data was available. As a third alternative, we used the equation of Mackay (see Table 4.8) to make our own calculations in case neither of the two previously mentioned types of data, nor test data were available.

The world-wide emissions were taken from Rippen (1996), which in most cases are nothing more than just rough estimates. They do *not* include the geogenic flows. This data was used nonetheless in order to be able to present examples for the operationalisation of the proposed proxy indicator. Additional normalisation data is given, e.g., in Guinée (1993), Goedkoop (1995), Schmucki (1996), Axenfeld *et al.* (1992/1994), UBA/TNO (1997) and Nriagu *et al.* (1988). To quantify more precisely the equivalency factors presented here would require a more detailed analysis of the literature than has been possible to undertake for this study.

[29] Several gases will show no or only little accumulation due to immediate decay or very little absorption. In such cases, one could start to calculate with a default value of, e.g., BCF = 1, and put more effort into the analysis of accumulation behaviour if the substance shows to be relevant in the calculation of the proxy for unknown damage.

Substance-Name	CAS-Number	log Kow	BCF Microorganisms	BCF fish	Calculated	Totally emitted world-wide	BCF fish for calculation	World-wide emission *B* for calculation	Equivalency factors *EF* = *(BCF/B)*
		Rippen (1996)					Choice from given data		Own calcul.
		-	-	-	-	1000t/a	-	1000t/a	a/kg
1,3-Dichlorobenzene	541-73-1	3.47		90-700		0.01	400	0.01	4.0E-02
p,p'-Dichlorodiphenyl dichloroethane	72-54-8	5.86	9100	64000		<5	64000	3	2.1E-02
Hexachlorobenzene	118-74-1	5.8	290000	2300-20000		0.1-10	10000	1	1.0E-02
1,2,4-Trichlorobenzene	120-82-1	4.06	3300	490-2300		0.3-0.6	1000	0.4	2.5E-03
Benzo[a]pyrene (BaP)	50-32-8	6.04	140000	200-2700	20000	5 (1969)	1000	5	2.0E-04
Butyl-benzyl-phthalate	85-68-7	4.76		510-770		7	600	7	8.6E-05
Diethyl-phthalate	84-66-2	2.39	210	117		1.5	117	1.5	7.8E-05
m-Dinitrobenzene	99-65-0	1.49		4.7		0.01-0.1	4.7	0.1	4.7E-05
1,2-Dichlorobenzene	95-50-1	3.4	730	90-560		10	300	10	3.0E-05
Dichlorvos	62-73-7	1.65			79	3	79	3	2.6E-05
beta-Hexachloro-cyclohexane	319-85-7	3.85	1500	290		15	290	15	1.9E-05
alpha-Hexachloro-cyclohexane	319-84-6	3.77	1500	1600		100	1600	100	1.6E-05
gamma-Hexachloro-cyclohexane	58-89-9	3.66	1 500-2300	230-1250		38	500	38	1.3E-05
1,1-Dichloroethane	75-34-3	1.79			1.2	<1	1.2	0.2	6.0E-06
Di(2-ethylhexyl)phthalate	117-81-7	7.48	230000000	150-890		10-150	500	100	5.0E-06
Naphthalene	91-20-3	3.33	420	30-300		20	100	20	5.0E-06
Perchloroethylene	127-18-4	2.87	250	900-4800		630	2000	630	3.2E-06
1,1-Dichlorethylene	75-35-4	2		2		2	2	2	1.0E-06
Aniline	62-53-3	0.95		5		10	5	10	5.0E-07
Carbon-tetrachloride	56-23-5	2.77	220	18-30		50	25	50	5.0E-07
Ethylene-diamine	107-15-3		740	<10		15	5	15	3.3E-07
Nitrobenzene	98-95-3	1.85	24	30		70-120	30	100	3.0E-07
1,1,2-Trichloroethane	79-00-5	2.34		<10		20	5	20	2.5E-07
Allylchloride	107-05-1	1.53				8	*1.62*	8	2.0E-07
Epichlorhydrin	106-89-8	0.3			4.6	23	4.6	23	2.0E-07
1,3-Dichloropropene	542-75-6	1.41			2.9	16	2.9	16	1.8E-07
Trichlorethylene	79-01-6	3.03	97	17-90		600	50	600	8.3E-08
Ethylbenzene	100-41-4	3.2	470	15		200	15	200	7.5E-08
Vinyl chloride	75-01-4	1.27	5.7	<10		200	5	200	2.5E-08
Chloroform	67-66-3	1.95	26	6		100-300	6	300	2.0E-08
Toluene	108-88-3	2.66	148	90		6000-8000	90	7000	1.3E-08
1,1,1-Trichloroethane	71-55-6	2.49	81	9		750	9	750	1.2E-08
Benzene	71-43-2	2.12	19	10		500-1000	10	1000	1.0E-08
1,2-Dichloroethane	107-06-2	1.46	9	2		400	2	400	5.0E-09
Dichloromethane	75-09-2	1.31	6	2.3	0.91	500	2.3	500	4.6E-09
Acetaldehyde	75-07-0	0.5			1.2	100-500	1.2	300	4.0E-09

Tab. 4.9: Octanol-water partition coefficient (logKow), experimental BCF for different microorganisms, experimental BCF for different fish, calculated BCF, and world-wide emissions (all from Rippen 1996), best estimate of BCF fish (BCF for allylchloride is an own calculation), best estimate of world-wide emissions, and the equivalency factors to calculate the proxy indicator (sorted in ascending order)

For this reason we will refrain from calculating individual confidence intervals for each equivalency factor. It is assumed that both the BCFs and the emissions are distributed in a lognormal way and that the two distributions are independent of each other. The square of the geometric standard deviation (σg^2) (describing the 95%-confidence interval) is estimated for all BCFs together to be a factor[30] 10, and for the emissions, a factor[31] 30. Both of these ranges could be narrowed down by an additional analysis of the available data. The σg^2 for the equivalency factor *EF* can be calculated by using the equations given in Appendix 6.8. Doing this gives a σg^2 = 60. This means that the value for *EF* lies with 95% probability in an interval [*EF*/60, *EF*·60].

A first analysis of these rough estimates reveals some interesting characteristics:

- Seven orders of magnitude between the lowest and the highest *EF* show a good discrimination between the substances.
- Most substances with a high *EF* have a high BCF and low world-wide emissions and *vice versa* for the substances with a small *EF*.
- There are some substances with rather high emissions world-wide that still have a rather high *EF* due to high BCFs (but about 1000 times smaller than the highest *EF's*). These are substances such as α-hexachlorocyclohexane, γ-hexachlorocyclohexane, di(2-ethylhexyl)phthalate, and perchloroethylene. All these substances are known to cause serious environmental problems. The proposed proxy indicator would already have flagged them when they were emitted in low volumes. I.e., the proxy indicator would have proven its effectiveness as an early warning device.
- On the other hand, there are substances with a low BCF and a high *EF* due to low emissions. These are, for instance, m-dinitrobenzene and 1,1-dichloroethylene. They receive only high *specific EF* per kg, but their resulting relevance is nil on the world level.

A further interpretation of the results is insofar dangerous since using the proxy to discuss unknown damage provides it with a very virtual touch, without bringing more insights, however.

4.4.5 Summary and concluding remarks

'Bioaccumulation' has been chosen from a large array of candidates as the one characteristic to reflect best unknown damage due to emissions and to be easily operationalised as a proxy indicator. Bioaccumulation is a characteristic very close to the biota and measures how low environmental concentrations accumulate to high internal exposures.

The chosen Equation (4.4) leads to a high relevance of low volume substances without geogenic background concentrations, but with high bioconcentration factors. This takes into account that we are more knowledgeable about high volume sub-

---

[30] This factor is larger than what is suggested by the ranges for the bioaccumulation factors given for fish. However, this value seems appropriate when one bears in mind that this factor should reflect the additional uncertainty introduced when fish are chosen as reference organism as well.

[31] The ranges given in Table 4.8 suggest a factor 10. However, some estimates are very old and geogenic emissions are missing for most of the estimates. For substances with geogenic background the deviation may be even larger than the estimated standard deviation.

stances and have less experience with xenobiotic substances, i.e., substances with a geogenic level of zero. Some aspects of persistency are included in bioaccumulation as well. We therefore can conclude that many of those aspects mentioned as important for the constitution of a proxy indicator are covered by the one chosen.

The requirement defined for a good proxy was that the proxy for unknown damage should consist of only one indicator so as to avoid aggregation that is hardly possible based on argumentation or plausibility alone. This requirement could not be satisfied. The bioconcentration factor and normalisation by the anthropogenic plus the geogenic flows can be considered as constituting two indicators which are multiplicatively linked to the proxy indicator. However, most other proposals for proxy indices would prioritise high volume substances without such a normalisation.

One should be aware of the following limitations of the approach chosen here:

- The empirical validation of proxy indices for unknown damage will never be possible.
- Whether bioaccumulation or, e.g., persistency is the better proxy indicator is finally a question of choice rather than reasoning. A combination may even be considered if data for both are available.
- The way the normalisation has been introduced and the choice of an equal weighting for BCFs and world-wide emissions are elements that have been chosen on a subjective and partly implicit basis[32].
- The BCF chosen as an indicator for bioaccumulation is water-oriented. Substances which are not dissolved in water but remain airborne, for instance, have no measured BCF. Their accumulation behaviour has to be assessed based on terrestrial biota. This leads to certain incompatibilities between different accumulation factors.
- The BCFs vary for the same substance from organism to organism. The BCFs should therefore be derived from just one organism wherever possible.
- The BCFs measured in laboratory animals or in field animals, or those calculated from physico-chemical parameters based on QSARs, show relevant differences. The estimation procedure should therefore be uniform for all substances.
- A major limitation of the proxy indicator is its focus on emissions. Input oriented and use parameters, such as, e.g., resource depletion and depreciation, land use and soil degradation, are neglected so far and no proposal is made here for their inclusion.

Despite these limitations, we can conclude that the proposal for a proxy indicator for unknown damage presented here is:

- reflecting the tendency of accumulation and persistence of the substances, i.e., two main criteria for the discussion of unknown damage (future damage),
- considering that we know more about high than low volume substances due to the practice of the regulation of chemical substances,

[32] E.g., it could be argued as well that the BCFs should be entered with a power factor 2 into Equation (4.3).

- considering that xenobiotic substances show a larger potential for unknown damage than substances abundantly available in nature, and
- operational in the sense that BCFs are available for most substances or can be calculated by making use of QSARs (normalisation factors are more difficult to find).

The data given in Table 4.9 are the preliminary results of a first analysis. They have to be improved and complemented by a further analysis of available data and the use of more accurate estimates for the global emissions (anthropogenic *and* geogenic origins). The substances included in the example given in Table 4.9 contribute all to a certain degree of evidence to carcinogenic effects. However, it is not clear that this is the main effect for all substances. Therefore, the proxy index includes all substances disregarding its treatment in the damage assessment.

Readers who disagree with the appraisal made, i.e., if they can think of effects due to emissions which will not (adequately) be reflected by the suggested proxy index, are invited to introduce their knowledge into the damage assessment, rather than complain about its poor consideration in the proxy for unknown damage.

Whether or not this proxy indicator can have an important position in decision making will be discussed in Section 4.6, from the vantage point of cultural perspectives.

4.5 Index for manageability

As introduced in Section 4.2, the ecosphere will be modelled by three submodels: the damage assessment (Section 4.3), the unknown damage (Section 4.4), and the manageability of the damage (this section). The composition of these three submodels is discussed in Section 4.6.

4.5.1 The relevance of manageability

Subsection 4.1.5 revealed that damage assessment covers not all dimensions of risk relevant for risk perception (see attributes of Fischhoff *et al.* (1978)). In addition, the need to represent the dynamics of the damages was identified. Arguments for the relevance of the criterion of manageability are:

(1) Known and understood damages that occur in the future can only be assessed on the basis of a baseline emission scenario. Its design requires predicting the measures society will take to prevent damages due to stressors.

(2) Decision makers will give higher priority to an environmental problem if the damage caused by it is difficult to correct and undo.

(3) Decision makers may tend to give environmental problems higher priority if they exhibit a significant tendency towards excess sustainable damage levels. A large 'target damage excess factor' implies a high demand for changes in behaviour, technique and legislation.

(4) The reverse effect may lead decision makers to give lower priority to environmental problems for which legislation already exists and if long-term policy targets seem to be within reach thanks to foreseeable reductions in pollution. They will concentrate their attention instead on problems which, so far, have not been addressed by legislation, where no long-term policy targets have been set, or where it is unlikely that such targets will be met in the foreseeable future.

The first argument (1) describes a well-known problem in damage assessment. Even for modelling and estimating marginal damages it is often necessary to know the background concentrations and the effectiveness of measures that could be used to prevent damages. Nevertheless, it is better not to treat argument (1) as part of the 'manageability' issue. The design of emission and damage prevention scenarios, where relevant, is better accomplished as a part of damage assessment. The contents of these scenarios depend very much on the assumptions one makes about the world view of decision makers and their management styles. They therefore can be based on cultural perspectives. The direct consequences of measures on the magnitude of damage is reflected in a more sensible way by this integration with damage assessment.

The other arguments (2-4) can be clarified further by a discussion of the following decision situation: imagine the situation where two different environmental problems cause the same magnitudes of damage (caused, e.g., by the emissions during one year on a global level). What are the reasons to evaluate these environmental problems differently?

Argument (2) says that if the *reduction of damage* is much more difficult for one of the environmental problems than for the other, one should give more importance and pay higher attention to the environmental problem whose damage is less easily reduced[33].

Argument (3) says that if one of the environmental problems has a higher *target damage excess factor* than the other problem, its damage should be given higher priority because its correction requires more stringent reduction measures and because achieving this reduction potentially requires more time.

The last argument (4) says that if one of the environmental problems:

- is known and understood
- is under control through some environmental policy
- has already seen its size reduced significantly thanks to these regulatory policies, and
- can be assumed to cause negligible damage up to, e.g., 2025 because the policy measures will by then have shown their effect,

then its damage can be considered less important than the same damage from a lesser or *not yet regulated problem* where no long-term policy targets have been set or where their attainment is uncertain.

Argument (2) is close to the philosophy of end-of-pipe management, i.e., the emission level is taken as given and solutions are only sought through the reduction of damages. The aim of arguments (3) and (4) is to anticipate future situations (dynamic behaviour) and to already influence the current allocation of resources.

4.5.2 The role of cultural perspectives

Before we turn to the operationalisation of the index for manageability, we ask in this subsection which one of these arguments about the relevance of the criterion of manageability is used by the different cultural perspectives. The use of a particular criterion of manageability is, to a large extent, a question of management style rather than of the world view held. But management styles are culturally dependent (Section 3.2). The different management styles will be used when the arguments in the previous sections are taken up again and looked at from a cultural perspective.

- For *individualists* the criterion of manageability is of little relevance. They are interested most in an estimate of the damage which is as accurate as possible, and they believe that market forces will lead to a reduction of damages. If they favour policy intervention, they will choose to reduce the environmental interventions of those processes that have the lowest abatement costs. Arguments for weighting the same magnitude of damage higher because a large excess of target damage will occur, or because there is no regulation in force to produce a relevant reduction, are irrelevant in their view. Legislation will simply be changed if it turns out that existing regulations do not succeed in controlling an environmental problem and all market players will again have the same conditions for competition. Argument (2) is nevertheless accepted because weighting lower the damage that is easier to

[33] This argument does not address the question of how easy it is to control the environmental problem through a reduction in environmental interventions. The argument starts on the damage level only, i.e., on a given emission level.

reduce than damage reductions that are difficult to achieve means that one can wait to deal with the more easily reducible damage until the time when the damage really proves to be serious.

- *Egalitarians* subscribe to a preventive management style that favours need-reducing strategies. Already when assessing damages they presume that all measures that will reduce them should also be taken (argument (2)). The arguments with respect to the target damage excess factor and to the anticipation of future environmental problems fit in well with the precautionary principle to which they subscribe. Egalitarians will assign some relevance to the criterion of manageability because such an index helps to anticipate coming problems and places more weight on the damages they cause. However, they do not believe that recognising the manageability of environmental problems is a significant step towards their solution.
- *Hierarchists* strongly believe in the possibilities of managing through control and regulation. Environmental problems which are not yet under control (4) and which have a tendency to exceed the target damage (3) will therefore be valued as more important than problems which are already regulated. The possibility to reduce damages at given emission levels (argument (2)) by, e.g., allocating additional resources, is attractive to them. It induces them to assign a lower weight to such predictable damages (end of pipe philosophy).

This short discussion from the perspective of cultural theory of the use that can be made of these arguments shows that each one of the arguments (2) to (4) is used by at least one of the perspectives. This is reason enough to work towards the operationalisation of all three arguments for use in the index for manageability.

4.5.3 Operationalising indicators for manageability

The operationalisation starts from scratch as there does not seem to exist any operationalised proposal for an index of manageability in life cycle impact assessment. The most advanced proposal for the consideration of dynamic aspects of harm can be found in a text by Lindeijer in Udo de Haes *et al.* (1994). This contribution (see Table 4.3) lists some criteria which were considered of importance after an expert panel on the weighting of environmental problems had concluded its work (Kortman *et al.* 1994). But so far there have been no attempts to operationalise these criteria.

A number of preliminary issues should be dealt with first before we make a proposal for the first operationalisation of the index for manageability:

A Should we aim for one or for several indicators which subsequently would be aggregated to one index?

B If there are indicators to be aggregated to an index, will they be linked additively or multiplicatively?

C Should the index (or the indicators) be based on the level of environmental interventions, of stressors, or of damages?

D Which type of scale should be used to measure the index (or the indicators)?

Question A can be answered easily. There is no reason why the criterion of manageability should be measured by one index alone. A set of indicators, to be aggregated to an index, is quite a possibility.

We need to go back to the arguments in Subsection 4.5.1 for answers to questions B and C. The relevant arguments (2-4) are all made on the damage level for each environmental problem. The aim of the proposed impact assessment is to assign potential damages caused by the environmental interventions from the analysed product system. The ease of reducing the environmental interventions is therefore not a question to be answered in the impact assessment, but rather in the improvement analysis. Resource extraction and emissions are therefore given entities which are not questioned in the index of manageability. Within the scope of manageability are all management interventions in the impact pathway between the emission and damage level. All facts that may give higher or lower priority to calculated potential damage are at the core of the index of manageability. As we already have a central estimate of the potential damage (the index 'magnitude of damage'), it is most elegant to relate the attributes of manageability directly to the damage level. The index should therefore be based on the magnitude of damage caused by each environmental problem considered (answer to question C).

The index itself has the form of a sum of weighted magnitude of various damages. The combination of the indicators to such a weighting factor m is not clear beforehand. This will be addressed in Subsection 4.5.4 and guidance will be given by Appendix (4) (answer to question B). It is obvious from this last answer that only ratio scales will be flexible enough for all kind of combinations and finally result in a quantitative manageability factor m.

There are no decision makers available for this study that could state their motivation for including a criterion of manageability in the structured aggregation procedure. We propose instead to develop indicators which operationalise the three arguments (2-4) formulated in Subsection 4.5.1 and discussed within the context of different archetypical decision makers in Subsection 4.5.2.

Therefore, the index for manageability $M_{p,c}$ for the environmental problem p *and* cultural perspective c can be written as

$$M_{p,c} = f(R_{p,c}, X_{p,c}, S_{p,c}) \cdot D_{p,c} = m_{p,c} \cdot D_{p,c} \qquad (4.5)$$

with $R_{p,c}$ indicator for the ease of damage reduction [-]
$X_{p,c}$ indicator for the excess of long-term policy targets [-]
$S_{p,c}$ indicator for the success of regulation [-]
$D_{p,c}$ outcome of the damage assessment for human or ecological health measured in the respective damage units
$m_{p,c}$ manageability factor [-]

The operationalisation of the three indicators are the objective of this section. $M_{p,c}$ can be further aggregated to M_c by a simple addition of the manageability-corrected damages per environmental problem for all environmental problems p damaging the same safeguard subject.

$$M_c = \Sigma_p M_{p,c} \qquad (4.6)$$

The final composition of the index will be presented in Subsection 4.5.4.

Indicator for damage reduction

As mentioned in Subsection 4.5.1, the indicator to operationalise argument (2) should start at a given emission level, i.e., lowering the emissions is not addressed by this indicator.

Efforts to reduce damage can take the form of financial expenditures, technical measures or new legislation. Technical measures can be expressed in financial terms if one excludes inventions that would be necessary to reduce the magnitude of damage[34]. One can imagine a decreasing magnitude of damage for each environmental problem if financial expenditures and the number of legislation is increased (Figure 4.7) (Clift 1995).

Figure 4.7 shows fictitious graphs for three different, but typical, developments of the magnitude of damage as a function of additional effort for damage reduction. The graph that shows small but steady reductions may be representative of those environmental problems where only little success can be expected, whatever the efforts that are undertaken. Global warming could be such a problem. Global change cannot be combated by means of single measures on a damage level such as constructing higher dikes or starting to irrigate when drought threatens. The development of a new vaccine is an example of the second graph where one major measure results in a significant decrease in damage. Another example is the reduction in damages to humans due to increased UV-radiation from stratospheric ozone depletion subsequent to the adoption of laws which require the textile industry to produce clothes with low UV transmission rates and that restrict sunbathing. The third graph shows decreasing marginal utility for each subsequent measure taken. This may hold true for most environmental problems when a whole set of measures is taken. Some of them are very efficient and others less so. Following the recommendation to stay indoors and to refrain from sport activities between 11.00 and 15.00 may reduce the damage to humans from summer smog more efficiently than an improvement in the medical treatment of asthma.

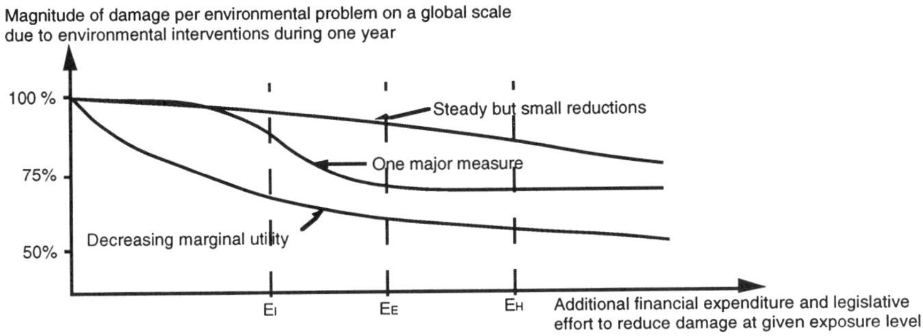

Fig 4.7: Three typical graphs for the reduction of the magnitude of damage at given environmental interventions as a function of the spent expenditure in financial and legislative terms

[34] They have been excluded because they cannot be commanded. One therefore cannot count on them for manageability purposes.

The concept and activity of damage reduction is of course a human concept. Using financial resources and passing laws for the purpose of reducing damages are activities that only humans undertake. The indicator as such is designed in principal to work for damages to all the safeguard subjects. However, damage reduction through human interventions with their anthropocentric and 'end-of-pipe' orientations may bias the indicator towards the reduction of damages to human health. The measures which are known and capable of protecting human beings from damage are more numerous than those which protect ecosystems. Human beings can change place and behaviour to reduce a damage; but change of place and behaviour of ecosystems is, by definition, considered to be damaging in itself (see Subsection 4.4.2). Examples of human measures to reduce damage to ecosystems are the spreading of lime in acidified forests or the artificial oxygenation of eutrophic lakes. This indicator for damage reduction will therefore generally change little concerning the relevance of damages to ecosystems.

The concretisation of the graphs requires the definition of the units for the abscissa and the axis of ordinates, and of the way damage reduction is to be measured. On the axis of ordinates, the world-wide magnitude of damage to human or ecological health during one year due to the environmental interventions is set equal to 100%. Damages are measured according to the proposals made in Section 4.3 and in Chapter 5.

The abscissa represents effort. Effort consists of financial expenditures (measured in $) for damage-reducing measures and legislative activity to establish new laws and decrees. The latter can be seen as an indicator of the society's willingness (at least in direct democracies) to change its behaviour. Such efforts would have to be undertaken together in all the countries concerned. The unit of financial expenditures can therefore be normalised for one inhabitant ($ per inhabitant) and the number of laws and decrees can be measured in absolute terms based on individuals' views, i.e., how many new laws and decrees are necessary at the different political levels (country, state, county, or commune).

Measuring damage reductions requires finding a common way to measure the damage reduction for all different types of graphs which can occur. The slope of these graphs, i.e., the efficiency or the ease of damage reduction varies with the amount of effort undertaken. A pragmatic proposal is to fix a unit effort E_c and to determine the damage reduction which is possible through such an effort (Figure 4.7). The choice of this unit effort E_c is somewhat arbitrary and the resulting linearisation of the damage-reduction as a function of the effort between $E = 0$ and E_c is a simplification. However, the alternative is to work with the slopes of the graphs. The slopes are very dependent on the value of the abscissa and would completely neglect high or low slopes at lower efforts, i.e., the outcome would be even more arbitrary.

The measure of damage reduction is so far defined as a percentage of the potential global damage (due to the environmental interventions of one year) at a given effort E_c. The choices that had to be made so far are all based on a constructivistic view. The determination of the magnitude of E_c and of the equivalence between financial expenditures and legislative effort are subjective, however, and the choices made are therefore dependent on cultural perspectives (Table 4.10).

The relevance for the different cultural perspectives of the indicator 'damage reduction' can be determined on the basis of the discussion in Subsection 4.5.2. A consideration factor *f* is defined for this purpose, set according to whether or not the damage assessment is already based on cultural dependent management styles. For the moment, it is assumed that the different perspectives do not pay any attention to the criterion of ease of reduction ($f = 0$) if the damage assessment has been performed on the basis of cultural dependent damage management scenarios. If, however, no special attempt has been made to consider cultural dependent management styles in the damage assessment, the indicator of damage reduction is considered to be of relevance by the adherents of the different management styles ($f = 1$).

Default values were set for the financial resources. It is assumed that individualists and egalitarians will allocate less resources than hierarchists do. Individualists believe that only small interventions are sufficient. Egalitarians agree to invest financial resources, but would strive to reduce needs at the same time, thus obviating the need for heavy interventions. The amounts are determined from the perspective of an individual living in a developed market economy. The lower amount is set at 0.5% of the GNP per capita in view of the fact that individuals may have to spend additional money themselves to prevent damages caused by a total of about 20 environmental problems. The higher default value for the hierarchists is set at double this percentage (1%)[35].

No difference is made between laws and decrees when setting the default value for legislative effort; this makes it unnecessary to consider the different political systems. Hierarchists and egalitarians tend to operate through legislation while individualists are chary of using even more regulation. All three perspectives consider the change of laws and decrees, but egalitarians and hierarchists include changes in the constitution as well. Changing the constitution is considered to represent an effort comparable to the financial resources requested. It is necessary to get many interested parties to agree on such changes and several years are necessary until a proposal for a new decree can be translated into structures that make possible its application.

The equivalence suggested here between financial resources (to be spent yearly) and one-off changes in regulations is of course highly contentious (Table 4.10). It should be taken here as just an indication of the magnitudes involved. Trade-offs between financial resources and legislative efforts are possible. Each of the three management types would accept a somewhat greater legislative effort (if this could be had in a cost-neutral way) in exchange for a smaller increase in financial expenditures and *vice versa*.

---

[35] Leipert (1989) estimated the external costs for West Germany in 1988 at 6% of the GNP. This amount includes both the external costs due to damage costs to the environment and actual prevention costs for reducing pollution and cure health damages. Ellwanger (1997) estimates that the external costs of traffic in the EU are equal to 4.6% of GDP. Maibach *et al.* (1996) estimated the external costs in Switzerland to at around 5% of GNP (for a review see Perkins 1998). We therefore assume that external costs in established market economies are today about 5% of GNP. A monetarisation of all effects might double this percentage amount. This 10% can be interpreted as an upper level for all expenditures to prevent environmental damages (based on the assumption that prevention costs should be smaller than or at most equal to damage costs).
These lower and upper bounds translate approximately into about 50 $ and 100 $ per capita. They add up to 25 to 50 billion $ per year for Europe (with its 500 million inhabitants). The sums are about 5 billion $ per year for each of the larger countries (Germany, UK, or France). Such budgets are sufficient to finance relevant measures such as, e.g., an improved health screening program.

Cultural perspective	Individualists	Egalitarians	Hierarchists
Consideration factor f=	0 (#) or 1(‡)	0 (#) or 1(‡)	0 (#) or 1(‡)
E_c in terms of financial resources	50 $/individual and year	50 $/individual and year	100 $/individual and year
E_c in terms of legislative effort	1 New law or decree	1 Change in the constitution and 2 new laws or decrees	1 Change in the constitution and 2 new laws or decrees

Tab. 4.10: Default values for the cultural-dependent choice of the unit effort Ec at which the damage reduction should be determined.
(#) this indicator of damage reduction is of no relevance if a strongly cultural dependent management scenario is used in the damage assessment.
(‡) this indicator is considered to be relevant if no assumptions on cultural dependent management styles are made in the damage assessment.

The indicator for damage reduction R is a triple due to the different cultural perspectives and is equal to the remaining relative damage after the reduction due to the additional unit effort E_c and is multiplied by the consideration factor f.

$$R_{p,c} = 1 - (\text{relative reduction of damage } p \text{ at } E_c) \cdot f \qquad [-] \qquad (4.7)$$

Indicator for excess of policy targets

The *target damage excess factor* is defined as the ratio between the magnitude of damage caused by the current environmental interventions of a specific environmental problem and the negotiated long-term policy target or an estimation of the sustainable level of damage. Graphs for three environmental problems with target damage excess factors of 1.2, 2.6 and 4.5 are given in Figure 4.8.

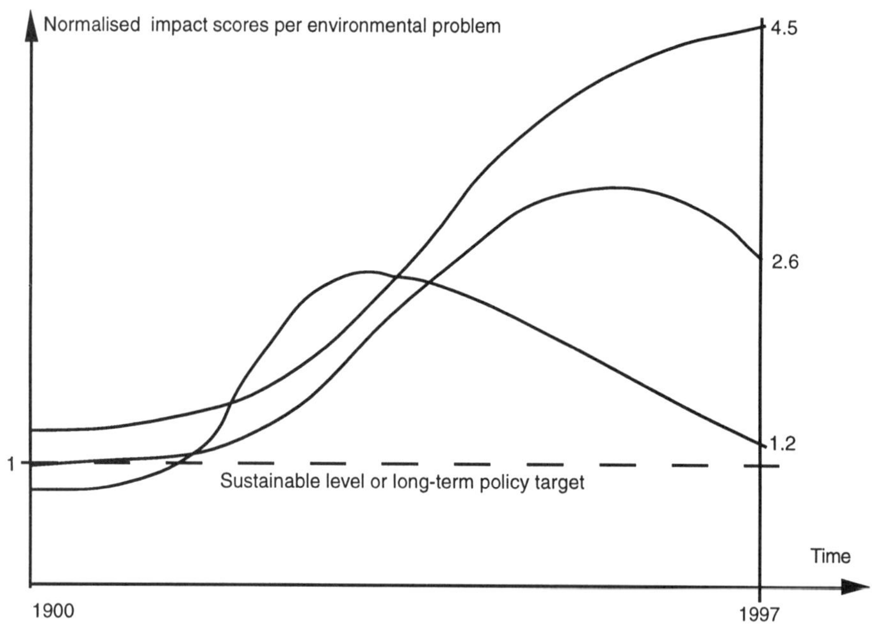

Fig. 4.8: Present excess compared to sustainable level or long-term policy target.

The indicator for the target damage excess factor is an indication of the need for changes in behaviour, technologies used, and legislation. The same damage is weighted more heavily if this need is large than if there is little need for change.

The target damage excess factor had already been introduced and widely used as weighting criterion in the so-called distance-to-target methods (e.g., Müller-Wenk 1978/1980, Braunschweig 1988, Ahbe *et al.* 1990, Braunschweig *et al.* 1993, Kalisvaart *et al.* 1994, Kortman *et al.* 1994, Goedkoop 1995). They used the distance-to-target approach as a proxy for the importance of environmental problems in general. They calculated the distance-to-target either on an emission level or on the level of impact scores. Here, it is just an indicator that suggests the need for change and thus serves as a help for better anticipating political actions. It is based on the magnitude of damage at present and target situation. The indicator for the target damage excess factor X can be written as follows:

$$X_{p,c} = \frac{N_p}{T_p} \qquad [-] \qquad (4.8)$$

where N_p is the magnitude of damage caused by the current environmental interventions contributing to the specific environmental problem p and where T_p is the long-term policy target or the estimated sustainable level for the environmental problem p. Both values have to be determined for the same region.

It has to be mentioned here that this indicator may have to be adjusted due to its discriminating nature. If X equals 100 for one problem and 10 for an other problem then, although the indicator is ten times higher, it may still be that the need for management measure is less than 10 times higher, i.e., there may be no linear relationship between X and its intended meaning. This question will be addressed when the index is composed in Subsection 4.5.4.

The discussion in Subsection 4.5.2 has suggested that individualists give little relevance to this indicator while egalitarians and hierarchists give more weight to it. What constitutes the *adequate* relevance is again a highly subjective matter. Subsection 4.5.4 will discuss the cultural dependency and suggests weighting factors.

Indicator for regulatory success

This third indicator, reflecting the success of regulation, addresses an aspect which again can be visualised by Figure 4.8. The lower two graphs represent environmental problems where the load is already falling below their historical highs (e.g., acidification in Europe), while the upper graph reflects an environmental problem where measures have not yet been taken or where the measures' effectiveness are compensated by population and/or economic growth (e.g., global warming).

Criteria for the definition of such an indicator have already been given in Subsection 4.5.1. To attribute a lower weight to a damage, the environmental problem causing it:

- should be a problem that is well known and understood,
- should be regulated by environmental policy,
- should already be declining in absolute terms thanks to these regulations, and

- can be assumed to be within its long-term policy target before 2025 because the policy measures already taken will by then have been effective.

If none of the three first criteria is fulfilled, there is no reason to assume that the regulations will show success by the target date. In this case, the value for the indicator for regulatory success *S* is set equal to 1. If the first three criteria are fulfilled, there is reason to acknowledge a certain success by attributing a value of between 0 and 1 to factor s_1. If the fourth criterion is met as well, then a value of between 0 and 1, but smaller than s_1 can be attributed to another factor s_2 (see Figure 4.9 for the decision tree).

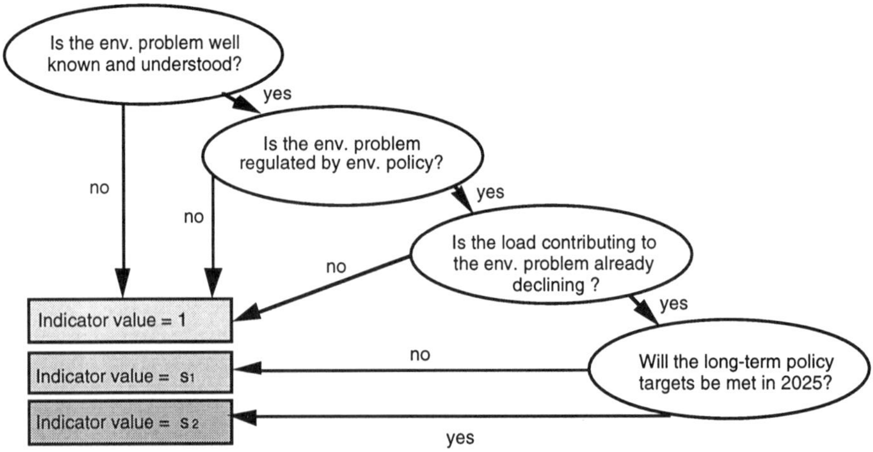

Fig. 4.9: Decision tree to define a indicator value for regulation success per environmental problem.

The exact values for the parameters s_1 and s_2 have to be fixed in a next step. This choice is again a highly subjective one. For this reason, different default values for the parameters are suggested for each cultural perspective (Table 4.11). The discussion in Subsection 4.5.2 has suggested that individualists see little relevance in such an anticipatory indicator. The parameter for the change in trend $s1$ is of some relevance, but the parameter reflecting compliance with policy targets is unimportant. Egalitarians give more importance to a change in trend. Hierarchists consider both the change in trend (first sign of the regulations) and the meeting of the policy targets to be very important.

Cultural perspective	Individualists	Egalitarians	Hierarchists
Parameter s_1 (reduction but still a problem)	0.9	0.8	0.8
Parameter s_2 (long-term policy target met up to 2025)	0.9	0.7	0.6

Tab. 4.11: Default values for the cultural-dependent choice of the parameters $s1$ and $s2$

The indicator for regulation success $S_{p,c}$ can be written as:

$$S_{p,c} = \{1 \text{ or } s1_c \text{ or } s2_c\} \qquad [-] \qquad (4.9)$$

4.5.4 Composition of the indicators to an index

The composition of the manageability factor per environmental problem was left open in the first paragraph of the previous subsection. The structure was set there as follows:

$$M_{p,c} = f(R_{p,c}, X_{p,c}, S_{p,c}) \cdot D_{p,c} = m_{p,c} \cdot D_{p,c} \tag{4.5}$$

with $R_{p,c}$ indicator for the ease of damage reduction [-]

$X_{p,c}$ indicator for the excess of long-term policy targets [-]

$S_{p,c}$ indicator for the success of regulation [-]

$D_{p,c}$ outcome of the damage assessment for human or ecological health measured in the respective damage units

$m_{p,c}$ manageability factor [-]

The determination of the structure of function f and with that of the manageability factor m is not purely a technical one. It has to be defined normatively which values of R, X, and S will result in a certain weighting factor m. For a detailed description of a procedure to derive the function f refer to Appendix (4). As it is a subjective step, there is need for a panel. In Appendix (4) we have concluded that in its absence the structure fitting best is:

$$m_{p,c} = R_{p,c} \cdot X_{p,c}{}^{gc} \cdot S_{p,c} \qquad [\text{-}] \tag{4.10}$$

The value of the exponent g_c should reflect two considerations. It first makes sure that Xi,c will be appropriately relevant when combined with the two other indicators for manageability. Secondly, it reflects the importance given to this indicator by the different cultural perspectives. The discussion in Subsection 4.5.2 has suggested that individualists give little relevance to this indicator while egalitarians and hierarchists give more weight to it. An upper value of $gc = 0.2$ for hierarchists and egalitarians seems advisable. Individualists give much less importance to this indicator. This could be reflected in $g_c = 0.1$ which would alter the final damages by less than factor 1.4. These values for g_c are just preliminary proposals. If the feasibility test proposed in Sections 6.6/7.6 shows that the index of manageability is applicable and supports intuitive judgements, then the sensitive parts of the proposal, like, e.g., g_c or the long-term target T, have to be determined by panels of representatives of the three cultural perspectives.

4.5.5 Summary and concluding remarks

In the absence of real decision makers, three indices of manageability were constructed compatible with the three cultural perspectives identified in Chapter 3. These three indices are based in turn on three indicators for each perspective which are used to adapt the outcome of the damage assessment. The combination of Equations (4.5) to (4.10) leads to

$$Mc = \sum_p [R_{p,c} \cdot X_{p,c}^{\ gc}\ S_{p,c} \cdot D_{p,c}] = \tag{4.11}$$

$$Mc = \sum_p \left[\left(1 - rel.\ red.\ of\ D_p\ at\ E_c \cdot f\right) \cdot \left(\frac{N_p}{T_p}\right)^{gc} \cdot \{1\ or\ s1_c\ or\ s2_c\} \cdot D_{p,c}\right] \tag{4.12}$$

with	
Mc	index of manageability
$R_{p,c}$	indicator for the ease of damage reduction [-]
$X_{p,c}$	indicator for the excess of long-term policy targets [-]
$S_{p,c}$	indicator for the success of regulation [-]
$D_{p,c}$	outcome of the damage assessment for human or ecological health measured in the respective damage units
E_c	additional unit effort in financial and legislative terms
f	consideration factor dependent on the modelling assumptions in the damage assessment
N_p	impact due to present environmental interventions contributing to environmental problem p
T_p	target level for the environmental problem p
g_c	cultural perspective dependent exponent
$s1_c$, $s2_c$	parameters for the regulatory success factor
p	index for environmental problem
c	index for the three cultural perspectives (individualists, egalitarians and hierarchists)

The default values which have been proposed for the parameters introduced here are summarised in Table 4.12.

The proposal presented here for an index to measure the manageability of environmental problems has the status of a hypothesis. The arguments and reasons, the structure of the equation, and the default values for the parameters may all provide an input into empirical work with decision makers and representatives from the three cultural perspectives. The *verification* or *falsification* of these assumptions and the steps required for their improvements are not part of this study (a procedure is suggested in Appendix (4)).

However, the proposal is applicable apart from this critical validation. First attempts at an application will be made in Sections 6.6 and 7.6. In a kind of preview it can be said that this application will reveal a need for considerable amounts of additional information before the index can be accurately calculated. This is not an argument to withdraw the proposal. The required information has to be collected only once at the time the method is made operational; it is not necessary to collect it anew for each case. And this additional demand of information from other fields of science only shows that additional aspects are added by the index to the decision support system.

Cultural perspective	Individualists	Egalitarians	Hierarchists
Consideration factor *f*	0 (#) or 1(‡)	0 (#) or 1(‡)	0 (#) or 1(‡)
E_c in terms of financial resources	50 $/individual and year	50 $/individual. and year	100 $/individual and year
E_c in terms of legislative effort	1 New law or decree	1 Change in the constitution and 2 new laws or decrees	1 Change in the constitution and 2 new laws or decrees
Exponent g_c	0.1	0.2	0.2
Parameter s_1 (reduction but still a problem)	0.9	0.8	0.8
Parameter s_2 (long-term policy target met up to 2025)	0.9	0.7	0.6

Tab. 4.12: Default values (to be confirmed by empirical studies) for the operationalisation of the index of manageability M (for explanations see Subsection 4.5.3)
(#) this indicator of damage reduction is of no relevance if a strongly cultural dependent management scenario is used in the damage assessment
(‡) this indicator is considered to be relevant if no assumptions on cultural dependent management styles are made in the damage assessment

As claimed in Subsections 4.1.5 and 4.5.1, the index for manageability covers aspects such as need and effort to reduce, dread from, control over, and dynamic behaviour of, the damage. Aspects concerning the *spatial characteristics* of damage may be judged to be missing. On the one hand, this is not really true because the ease of reduction (*R*) and the success of regulation (*S*) are both indirectly influenced by the geographic pattern of the damages and the spatial behaviour of the substances. On the other hand, we can repeat the argument given in Subsection 4.4.2 that global trade and the industrialisation of emerging countries may be more relevant for the spatial patterns than the distribution behaviour of the damages.

Although the reasoning behind the index for manageability was based on damages caused by emissions, the index can in principal be used as well for input-oriented damage categories. In the case of resources, one may address, within the indicator 'ease of reduction', the aspects of substitutability or measure to prevent the dissipation of, e.g., highly concentrated metals. The calculation of indicators for target damage excess (*X*) and for success of regulation (*S*) are merely a question of targets and long-term policy goals and not of the nature of the damage category.

The manageability will be higher for the environmental problems causing damages to the safeguard subjects human health and resource use (i.e., lower index for manageability) than to ecological health. That is because there are only about 5.5 billion human beings while the ecological health is much richer in species and population and slower in movement processes.

This proposal for an index of manageability is labelled *preliminary* because no verification for, validation on, and application to, a large number of environmental problems have been or will be made here.

4.6 The structured aggregation procedure

Section 4.2 is suggested to model the ecosphere with three submodels for the known damage, the unknown damage, and the manageability, respectively. Sections 4.3 to 4.5 justified the choice of these submodels, and described the model suggested and its implications.

This section will address the embedding of these submodels in the whole framework and reveal why we speak of the structured aggregation procedure. In Subsection 4.6.1, the three submodels are summarised. Subsection 4.6.2 shows how the indices of the submodels can be composed and linked to the model of the technosphere. Finally, we will highlight the role played within this procedure by Cultural Theory and present hypotheses about its influence on the weighting scheme. Concrete proposals for the preparation of the structured aggregation procedure for decision support will be made in Section 8.1 after its operationalisation in Chapters 5 to 7.

4.6.1 The outcome of the three submodels

The main equations for the three submodels are put together in this subsection. For the known damage, unknown damage, and for manageability Equations (4.1), (4.4) and (4.11) can respectively be taken to represent the relevant submodels. Each factor or indicator is supported in turn by a model or calculation procedure of its own. The three submodels and their units are described here for emissions and both D_C and M_C are specified for human health.

$$D_c = \Sigma_{ijkm}\{I_{ij} \cdot F_{ijk} \cdot E_{ikm,c} \cdot DALYs_{m,c}\} \qquad \text{[DALYs,...]} \qquad (4.1)$$

$$U = \Sigma_i \{I_i \cdot \frac{BCF_i}{B_i}\} \qquad \text{[a]} \qquad (4.4)$$

$$M_c = \Sigma_p \{R_{p,c} \cdot X_{p,c}{}^{gc} \cdot S_{p,c} \cdot D_{p,c}\} \qquad \text{[DALYs,...]} \qquad (4.11)$$

where B world-wide anthropogenic emission plus world-wide geogenic flow which leads to the concentration available to the biota [e.g., kg/a]

- BCF bioconcentration factor in fish [-]
- D outcome of the damage assessment for human or ecological health measured in the respective damage units (here DALYs for human health) [a]
- $DALYs$ disability adjusted life years, used as metric for the damage to human health [a]
- E effect factor [see Sections 6.3 & 7.3]
- F fate factor [see Sections 6.2 & 7.2]
- I environmental intervention per functional unit [e.g., kg]
- M index of manageability [a]
- R indicator for the ease of damage reduction [-]
- S indicator for the success of regulation [-]

U	proxy indicator for unknown damage [a]
X	indicator for the excess of long-term policy targets [-]
g_c	exponent dependent on cultural perspective [-]
c	index for the three cultural perspectives
i	index for substance
p	index for environmental problem
j	index for compartment
k	index for exposure path
m	index for endpoint

Three properties of the submodels should be considered before one proceeds with their further composition and aggregation:

- The manageability index is based on the damage index by weighting it with a manageability factor.
- To calculate the manageability index, it is necessary to provide not only a damage assessment per substance and per safeguard subject, but also per environmental problem. This is necessary because the manageability factor will be modelled for each environmental problem.
- The indices for damage and manageability will depend on the cultural perspective while the unknown damage is culturally independent.

One should also be aware that it is possible to give upper estimates for the total damage and for the total manageability adjusted damage, but not for unknown damage[36].

The next subsection will suggest a composition procedure.

4.6.2 A proposal for the composition of the spheres and their indices

LCAs should serve as a decision support system by providing information on environmental impacts due to the use of products that are defined in terms of a functional unit. We suggest constructing this link between environmental impacts and the functional unit based on a highly structured multi-step analysis. Figure 4.10 on the next page summarises this structured aggregation procedure. Although the procedure has been developed in a top-down manner, i.e., starting with the definitions of safeguard subjects, we will provide a description couched in terms of a bottom-up application.

The environmental interventions for a set of alternatives that provide the same functional unit will be determined through the analysis of the technosphere and by allocating sub-elements to the product systems at hand. In LCA language this is called 'inventory analysis' and the result is the inventory table containing a list of quantified environmental interventions.

[36] If a small amount (e.g., 1 kg/a) of a new xenobiotic substance with high accumulation potential is released, this will contribute to a large increase in the world-wide unknown damage.

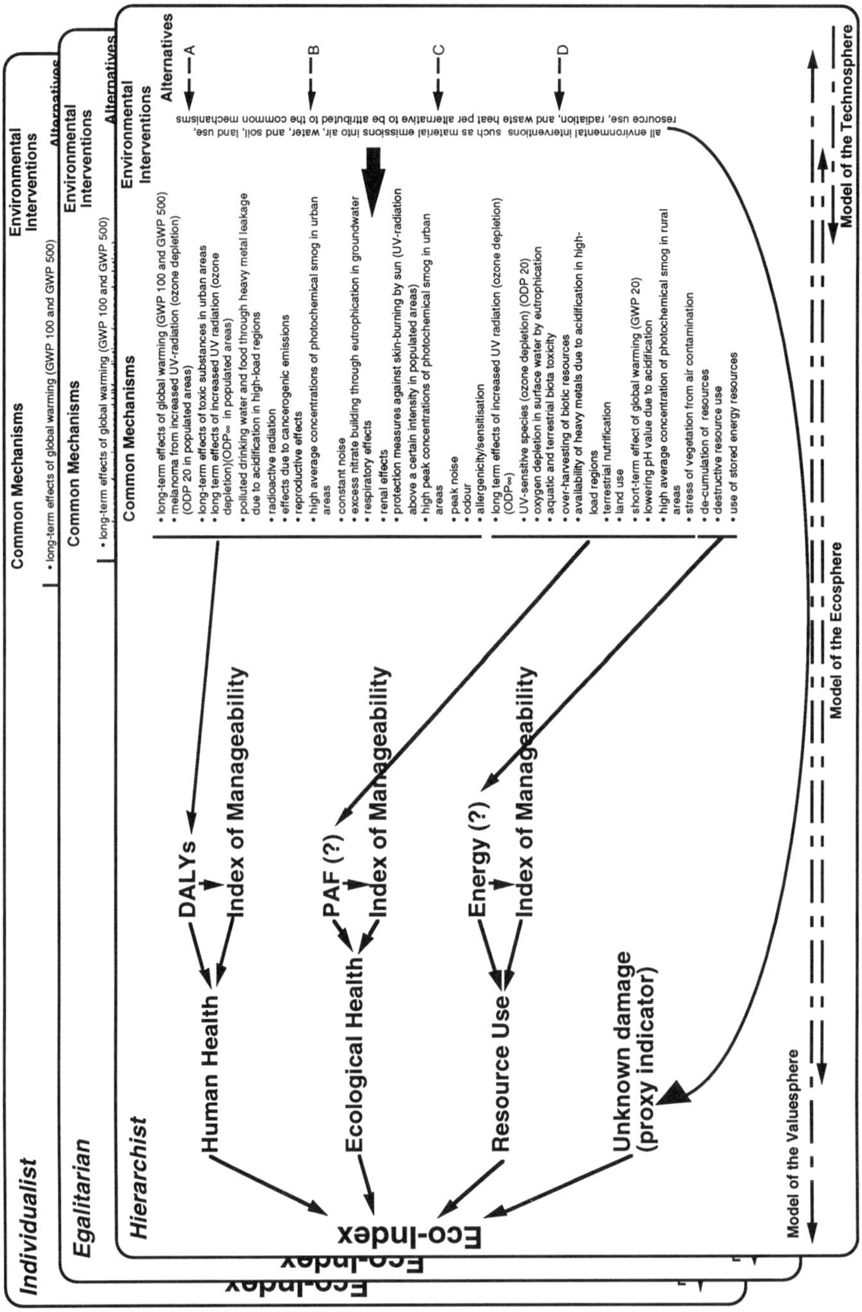

Fig. 4.10: The structured aggregation procedure for the three spheres and the three models of the ecosphere (the list of common mechanisms is just an example)

The inventory table alone tells us little about environmental impacts without further analysis. It can be used alone only in one specific case as decision support. This is the case if one of the alternatives scores higher (i.e., is more polluting) for all interventions. It will remain dominated by the other alternatives even after additional assessment steps. This is assured by the principles stated in Subsection 1.2.2.

The next step links the environmental interventions with the damages to the safeguard subjects and to the unknown damage. While the link to unknown damage can be performed directly by applying the model introduced in Section 4.4, the link to the safeguard subjects is less straightforward. In principle the structure presented in Figure 4.4 applies for this link. However, here Figure 4.10 introduces the additional structural element of the common mechanisms. The main reasons for this additional level are:

- Scientific communities, research groups, and models are also organised according to common mechanisms. To facilitate communication with these groups it is essential to subdivide the tasks accordingly.
- Results on this intermediate level may offer additional insight as this is often the level of public and political debate. To present results on that level may increase the usefulness of the whole assessment system.

The common mechanisms are just a means to organise the damage assessment. Its constituent elements are the steps of fate, exposure, effect, and damage analyses which are, however, not shown separately here. In fact, it is these steps that make possible the final aggregation on the level of indices for the known damage.

So far we have just repeated what has been suggested earlier in this chapter. Figure 4.10 goes one step further by suggesting a further composition and aggregation of the results obtained from the three submodels of the ecosphere. In a first step, it is suggested that a weighted average of the indices for damage and for manageability be calculated for each safeguard subject. These two indices have the same unit. The aggregation can therefore be done by the simple attribution of a weight between 0 and 1 for both indices; the sum of the two weights has to be equal to one[37].

This first weighting step leads to the aggregation of six indices and a proxy into three indices and a proxy. In the next subsection we will discuss their meaning and in Section 8.1, we will introduce an attractive procedure to present the results.

The resulting three indices for the manageability adjusted damage (MAD) to safeguard subject plus the proxy for unknown damage will either form the most aggregated input to the decision making process from the LCA or be further enriched with information by:

1) calculating the specific contribution of a product alternative to the total *MADs* in a certain region for a certain period of time, i.e., the normalisation step (as mentioned earlier, this is extremely difficult to do for unknown damage, because one will never be sure that the most important contributors are included in the assessment.),

[37] The determination of this weighting factor is not demonstrated in this book. In Figure 4.12 a first guess is presented for the archetype-dependent weighting. The weighting factor has to correspond with the perception by the decision maker(s) of the indices' relevance. Either they are asked directly to assign weights or, e.g., focus groups are used to derive archetype-specific weights.

2) providing the combinations of weighting factors where the ranking of alternatives will change (this will be explored in Section 8.1.), and

3) attributing weights to the four indices and aggregating them to a final Eco-Index.

In case (1) this leads to the following outcome for the three indices for the safeguard subject:

$$NoMADs_c = \frac{MADs_c}{\Sigma\{MADs_c \text{ in area } A \text{ during 1 year}\}} =$$

$$\frac{w \cdot D_c + (1-w) \cdot M_c}{\Sigma\{w \cdot D_c + (1-w) \cdot M_c \text{ in area } A \text{ during 1 year}\}} \quad \text{[a]} \quad (4.13)$$

and for the unknown damage:

$$NoUDs = \frac{U_c}{\Sigma\{U_c \text{ in area } A \text{ during 1 year}\}} \quad \text{[a]} \quad (4.14)$$

where:
- D outcome of the damage assessment [a]
- M index of manageability [a]
- U proxy indicator for unknown damage [a]
- $MADs$ manageability adjusted damages
- $NoMADs$ normalised manageability adjusted damages
- $NoUDs$ normalised unknown damages
- A area of the normalisation basis, e.g., country, continent or world
- w weighting factor for the share of the index for damage in the $MADs$ [0...1]
- c index for the three cultural perspectives

The *NoMADs* and *NoUDs* are measured on a scale from 0 to 1 and the units given in the Equations (4.13) and (4.14) are of no further relevance.

Case (2) will be explored and worked out for a simple example in Section 8.1.

Case (3) requires the set-up of a panel that is relevant for the questions at hand. The way to proceed in this case is suggested in Brunner (1998) who also explores its implications. However, Section 8.1 will show that, thanks to the way of case (2) is presented, the very difficult derivation of reasonable weights can often be avoided.

It is assumed that the structured aggregation procedure is followed separately for each cultural perspective. This aspect will be addressed in the next subsection.

4.6.3 The submodels revisited by Cultural Theory

Section 4.2 introduced the three submodels for known damage, unknown damage, and manageability as representations of the ecosphere. The necessity for these three submodels was partly explained by the different importance they have for the specific archetypes.

The operationalisation of the submodels in Sections 4.3 to 4.5 makes it now possible to come back to two questions:

- What are the main influences of the world view on the submodels?
- How important are the submodels for the archetype's model of the ecosphere?

The question on the cultural shape of the submodels can be answered as follows:

- *Known damage* has a different meaning to different archetypes. Individualists will stick to proven causalities, hierarchists will ask scientific bodies to draw the borderline between causal and non-causal associations, and egalitarians will tend to include associations even if the causal mechanisms are not yet understood. This suggests that the indices for known damage will score highest for egalitarians and lowest for individualists. Other value choices and judgements concerning ideals of fairness, perception of time, preferred procedures, trust, and the model of consent (see Table 3.1) will also depend on the cultural perspective adopted and influence the damage assessment too. Therefore, not only the size but also the shape of the submodel will depend on the archetypes.
- In Section 4.4 we suggested to model the proxy for *unknown damage* independently from the archetypes' world views. However, their relevance for decision making is itself strongly dependent on the cultural perspective applied.
- The quantification of the third submodel depends on the adopted world view and management style. It includes aspects such as ease of reduction, target damage excess, and regulatory success. These are summarised in the *index for manageability*. Hierarchists will tend to minimise damages by regulatory means and by prescribing costly measures to reduce damages. Individualists will prefer to use economic instruments to reduce damages, which will lead to smaller decreases in damages than in the hierarchist's approach. They will give little relevance to a high excess of target damages or to non-conformance with long-term policy targets. Egalitarians and hierarchists, on the other hand, will judge both these factors to be important because they represent uncertainty and non-control, respectively.
- The *acceptable damage* has been disregarded so far. It is meant to be set through the political consent about long-term targets. This definition makes clear that it represents the consensus of the politically active part of society and will therefore be different from the consensual targets for each cultural perspective taken separately. The definition of the acceptable damage is only used within the quantification of manageability.

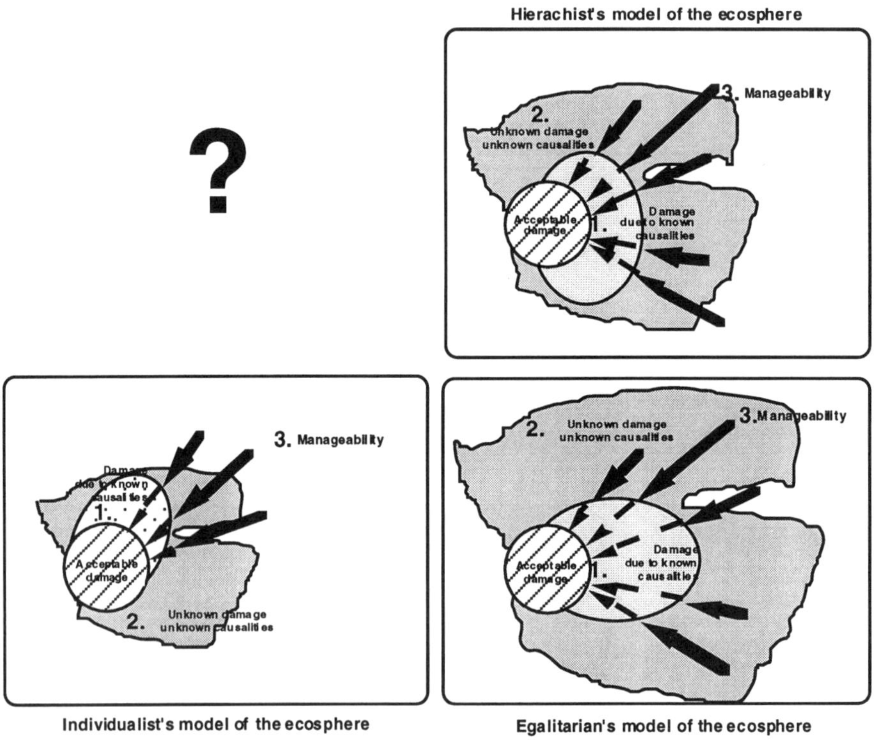

Fig. 4.11: The relevance of the three submodels for the ecosphere judged from the viewpoint of the three active perspectives. The question mark indicates that fatalists need not to be considered here because they are no active decision makers.

With these answers to the first question, the answer to the second question on the relevance of the three submodels for the modelling of the ecosphere is almost given. Figure 4.11 uses the size of the areas and the number and dimension of the arrows to illustrate the importance of the submodels:

- *Hierarchists* will aim for a balanced consideration of the three submodels, but give some priority to the known damage and to manageability.
- *Individualists* will give most priority to the known damage. Unknown damage will get little attention or will be disregarded completely. Manageability will be considered, but the individualist's shape or version of the index will give little importance to it because the manageability factor will be close to one.
- *Egalitarians* will give high priority to the unknown damage because they show little confidence in today's scientific findings or distrust the damage assessment to reasonably represent the ecosphere at all (holistic world view). At the same time, the index for the known damage is higher than for the other perspectives because more of the unproven causalities are included in the modelling. Although egalitarians dislike the technocratic touch of reducing damage, they give some importance to the index of manageability because it also stands for certainty and control.

The fatalist's model of the ecosphere is not drawn in Figure 4.11 because, as argued earlier in Subsection 3.4.2, their perspective is not relevant in decision making.

We have reviewed here our models of the ecosphere from the perspective given by Cultural Theory. One can of course also try to go in the opposite direction. Figure 4.11 can be seen as a potential candidate to replace the much-criticised Figure 3.3 in which the myths of nature were plotted and attributed to single archetypes. Of course, Figure 4.11 is graphically less appealing and the meaning of the areas and arrows is less self-explanatory. Nevertheless, empirical work should be done (but cannot not done here) to show which of the two figures explains more of the variance in world views.

Figure 4.12 summarises the hypotheses stated above and suggested in Figure 4.11. The areas shown indicate the weighting triples[38] which appear to be the most probable one for each cultural perspective. These hypotheses have to be verified by empirical studies which are yet to undertaken.

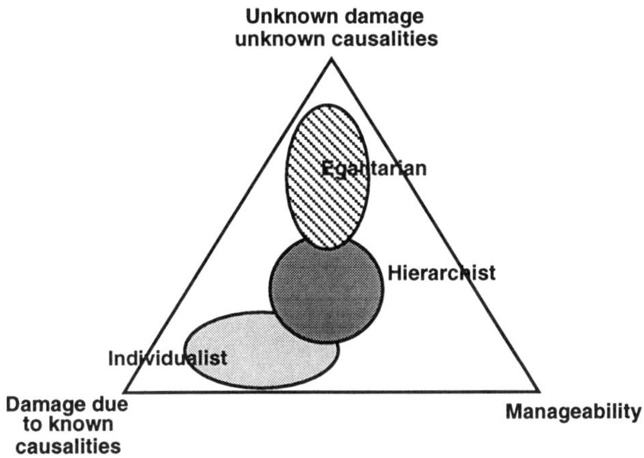

Fig. 4.12: Hypotheses on the preferred weighting triples for the three submodels by the three active cultural perspectives. (to be read like a mixing triangle: the closer a point is to one attribute (corner) the higher is the attribute's weight)

[38] The triangle has the nature of a mixing triangle, i.e., each point within the triangle represents a weighted triple of the three corners. The closer a point is to one of the corners, the higher is its weight (see also Section 8.1).

4.7 Concluding remarks

This chapter is the backbone of this book because it:

- describes the *modelling of the ecosphere* with the help of the three submodels for known damage, unknown damage, and manageability,
- links the ecosphere not only to the analysis of the *technosphere,* but also with the *valuesphere,*
- can be seen as a meta-framework that fits very different world views, and
- suggests a *structured aggregation procedure* to bring together all elements judged to be relevant for the decision support.

The submodels of the ecosphere are worked out to such an extent that they can be operationalised. In the absence of an authoritative panel, Cultural Theory has been chosen as the basis for modelling the valuesphere and to support value choices compatible with each archetype.

However, one has to keep in mind that:

- this chapter contains a number of (as yet unverified) hypotheses, and
- only feasibility tests for them will be made in Chapters 5 to 7.

A further appraisal will be made in Chapters 9 and 10 in order to reconsider the experience that will be gained in the following chapters.

5 DALYs – An Index for Human Health Assessment

5.1 Overview

The structured aggregation procedure presented in Chapter 4 has been designed to measure the importance of environmental problems by three main criteria: the magnitude of damage they generate, the manageability of these damages, and the unknown damage. Suggestions for how these criteria could be operationalised and concepts for doing so have already been given in Sections 4.3 to 4.5. This chapter is limited to a further elaboration of the way the magnitude of damage to human health can be measured. It focuses exclusively on the problem of aggregating different health outcomes and introduces a health index for this purpose. This limited focus allows for going into details and looking at the problems likely to occur when the damage assessment introduced in Section 4.3 is put into practice. The same level of detail is likely to be needed when one would want to look at the criterion of manageability or develop an index for damage to ecosystem health in greater detail than has been done so far in Section 4.3. An important difference between the areas of human and ecosystem health is that, in the former, there is extensive literature available from medical science and health policy which goes back many decades, while the literature on environmental health is less comprehensive because of a more recent origin and the coverage of only a limited range of issues.

This chapter starts with some facts about and figures from global health statistics and discusses the position of environmental risk factors in such statistics. The purpose of this discussion is to motivate others to further elaborate on the treatment of human health in LCA. The manifold methodological problems that occur when measuring and aggregating damage to human health are addressed in Section 5.3. Two approaches are described in more detail: the economic accounting and the concept of Disability Adjusted Life Years (DALYs), which is the one that is finally chosen for further consideration. These sections have a broad overlap with health economics but, do not intend to review and reflect the whole discussion in that field.

5.2 Some facts and figures about human health

5.2.1 Health statistics

The premise on which this discussion of health statistics rests is that the assessment of the impacts of environmental interventions and problems on human health can make use of epidemiological data and information. It is therefore appropriate to start the discussion of damages to human health by looking at how national and international bodies report such damages.

Health statistics are the instrument to report mortality and sometimes even morbidity during a given year according to their causes which can be quite specific or remain unspecified. The term *cause* is used in health statistics in a very specific way. It always refers to the type of disease that has caused the death or sickness and not to the reason for the disease. The reasons for diseases are called *risk factors*. The statistics normally differentiate between the sex and the age group to which the reported cases belong. Health statistics have a very long history, but the first systematic classification systems for the reporting of diseases was introduced only in the 18th century in Australia. The introduction of health statistics in Europe began in 1837 when the General Register Office of England and Wales started its reporting of health statistics (WHO 1993). A first statistical congress, held in Brussels in 1853, started the preparation of a list of diseases which was adopted in 1855. In 1898, the American Health Association recommended that the list should be revised for the beginning of each decade in order to reflect the intervening progress in medical science. From this moment on, the list began to be adopted widely and was updated every 10 years (Alderson 1988). Nowadays, WHO is standardising the classification of diseases world-wide. The tenth revision (WHO 1993) has now been adopted by most countries.

The classification system has become very detailed over the years. International reporting makes use of a list of about 100 broadly defined disease classes (WHO 1995b). A more detailed classification is used only in national or regional (continental) statistics that have a special focus, e.g., on carcinogenesis (e.g., SC 1995, IARC 1995). These more specific classifications may be important for the assessment of environmentally caused diseases if the diseases of interest belong to very specific subgroups (see Chapter 6.4).

Most national and international statistics only report mortality. The reporting of morbidity is becoming more frequent, however, because this information is of increasing relevance to health management (WHO 1993, Murray *et al.* 1996a/b). The wider availability of statistical data on morbidity will increase the possibilities of conducting epidemiological studies on environmentally caused diseases.

The completeness and validity of the data in health statistics varies from country to country and for the different causes of disease. The need for diagnosis and the diagnostic capabilities have changed over the last decades for the different countries and their governments. The data for certain countries and causes, however, is still of limited quality. Alderson (1988) presents an extensive survey of existing health statistics, their methodologies, and their validity.

Murray *et al.* (1996a/b) have published a very comprehensive and consistent health statistic covering the eight world regions which includes information on mortality, years of life lost due to premature death (YLL), and years lived disabled (YLD). (See Section 5.4 for an explanation of this concept.) One aspect that differentiates this report from other statistical sources is that it strives to cover all countries and to allocate the unknown or unregistered cases to meaningful causes. This interpretation of the raw statistical data provides it with an increased internal consistency. Some of the data from this statistic are shown below and will be used to address a number of issues relevant to the assessment of the environmental causes of disease.

There are significant differences in the leading causes of disease in developing and developed regions of the world. Table 5.1 shows that the 10 leading causes of death that together are responsible for more than 50% of all deaths are different for the two regions. Heart and circulatory diseases, and several types of cancer and respiratory ailments are dominating the causes of death in developed countries (53.8%). The same causes are responsible for less than 30% of all deaths in developing countries. No single cancer site belongs to the ten leading causes of death in developing regions. Here the list is dominated by communicable diseases.

Developed Regions	Deaths ('000s)	Cumulative %	Developing Regions	Deaths ('000s)	Cumulative %
All Causes	10 912		All Causes	39 554	
1 Ischaemic heart disease	2 695	24.7	1 Lower respiratory infections	3 915	9.9
2 Cerebrovascular disease	1 427	37.8	2 Ischaemic heart disease	3 565	18.9
3 Trachea, bronchus and lung cancer	523	42.6	3 Cerebrovascular disease	2 954	26.4
4 Lower respiratory infections	385	46.1	4 Diarrhoeal diseases	2 940	33.8
5 Chronic obstructive pulmonary disease	324	49.1	5 Conditions arising during the perinatal period	2 361	38.7
6 Colon and rectum cancers	277	51.6	6 Tuberculosis	1 922	43.4
7 Stomach cancer	241	53.8	7 Chronic obstructive pulmonary disease	1 887	46.1
8 Road traffic accidents	222	55.8	8 Measles	1 058	48.7
9 Self-inflicted injuries	193	57.6	9 Malaria	856	50.9
10 Diabetes mellitus	176	59.2	10 Road traffic accidents	777	52.8

Tab. 5.1: The ten leading causes of death world-wide, 1990 (Murray et al. 1996c)

In Figure 5.1 the age and regional specificities of death from the three main groups of communicable (group I) and noncommunicable (group II) diseases and from injuries (group III) are shown. For the purpose of this study, it is important to note that:

- Each region shows a specific pattern of causes at different ages. It is therefore essential to think about the global applicability of damage assessment based on conditions found in established market economies.
- For most LCAs, noncommunicable diseases are the most relevant causes of death. (Global warming could change this picture by favouring the emergence of new communicable diseases.) The share of noncommunicable diseases in the cause of death of children is very small. For adults the shares are similar for all regions. The probability of dying die from a noncommunicable disease (Group II) is

distributed therefore more uniformly across regions than for the other two cause groups.

- Life expectancy varies widely between the regions due to the different probabilities of death and is influenced mainly by the mortality of children.

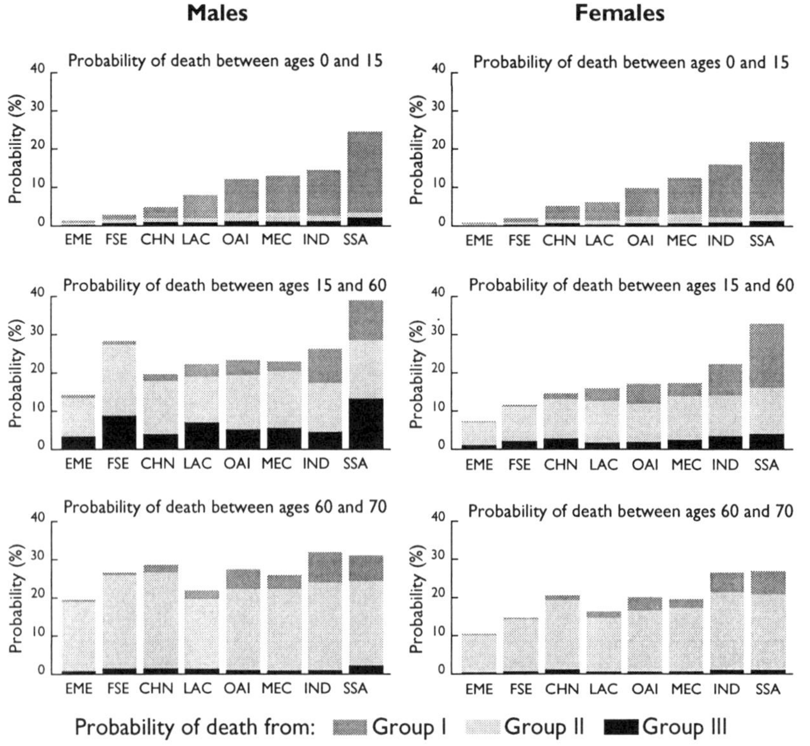

Fig. 5.1: Risk of death from each broad cause Group, by region, 1990 (Murray *et al.* 1996c)Group I = communicable diseases, Group II = noncommunicable diseases, Group III = injuries EME = Established market economies, FSE = Formerly socialist economies of Europe, IND = India, CHN = China, OAI = Other Asia and islands, SSA = Sub-Saharan Africa, LAC = Latin America and the Caribbean, MES = Middle Eastern crescent

The information from Figure 5.1 makes it clear that the number of deaths reported in Table 5.1 for the main causes of death do not all occur at the same age for the different causes. The years of life lost (YLL) due to premature death are therefore not proportional to the death rates. Figure 5.2 shows, for the world averages of deaths, that the diseases occurring early in life (mostly communicable diseases) acquire a greater weight when the YLLs are used to measure them. For health assessment in LCA, it is therefore important to take into account for each disease the corresponding average YLL.

Morbidity statistics are becoming more important in the field of health policy as has already been mentioned. Morbidity due to environmental risk factors becomes relevant for the assessment of health in LCA if its magnitude, weighted by a factor of severity, is significantly out of line with mortality. Table 5.2 lists the ten leading causes of disability in the world. It is notable that five out of the ten causes are psychiatric conditions (if alcohol use is counted as one of them). Only one of them, chronic obstructive pulmonary disease, is also among the ten leading causes of death listed in Table 5.1. The use of a measure of disability instead of the simple number of deaths (mortality) is therefore likely to influence the ranking of the most important environmental risk factors to human health.

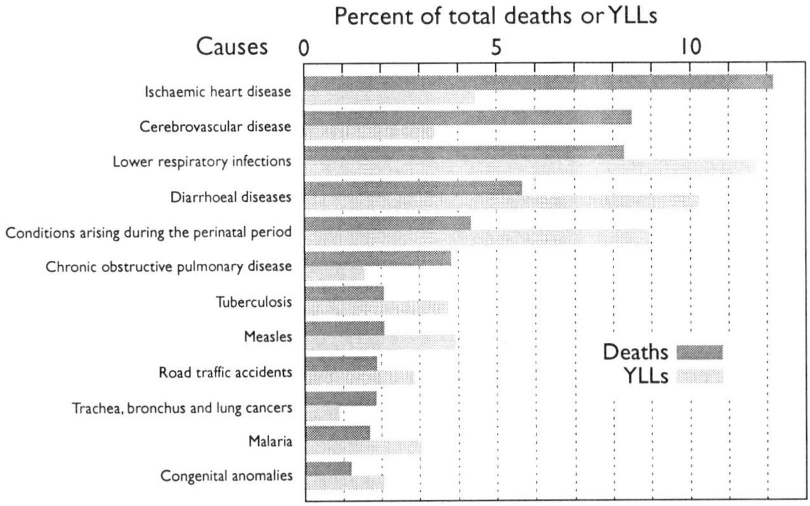

Fig. 5.2: The leading causes of death and of premature death, i.e., years life lost (YLLs), world-wide, 1990 (Murray *et al.* 1996c)

		Total (millions)	**Per cent of total**
	All Causes	472.7	
1	Unipolar major depression	50.8	10.7
2	Iron-deficiency anaemia	22.0	4.7
3	Falls	22.0	4.6
4	Alcohol use	15.8	3.3
5	Chronic obstructive pulmonary disease	14.7	3.1
6	Bipolar disorder	14.1	3.0
7	Congenital anomalies	13.5	2.9
8	Osteoarthritis	13.3	2.8
9	Schizophrenia	12.1	2.6
10	Obsessive-compulsive disorders	10.2	2.2

Tab. 5.2: The leading causes of disability, world-wide, 1990 (Murray *et al.* 1996c)

This limited exploration of the state of health statistics and their interpretation in general provides the basis from which to look in Subsection 5.2.2 more closely at the risk factor *environment*.

5.2.2 Environmental risk factors

A certain share of the global burden of disease can be attributed to environmental risk factors. The term *environment* has to be used carefully within the context of health assessment. In this Subsection, only the effects from environmental interventions and problems in the strict meaning of LCA are of interest. Thus, effects from poor sanitation, personal and domestic hygiene and water supply[1] are excluded. The same also holds true for health effects of environmental tobacco smoke (passive smoking) and occupations.[2]

The share of health effects caused by environmental risk factors can be estimated either top-down (World Bank 1993) by attributing certain diseases fully or partly to environmental factors or they can be calculated bottom-up with information from other sources (Murray *et al.* 1996a, WHO 1994a). The estimates will be highly uncertain in both cases because many health effects cannot be attributed causally to *a* risk factor. If such factors can be identified at all, it is likely that more than one risk factor is involved. Human health assessment indeed would become rather easy if all health outcomes caused by environmental risk factors could be attributed fully.

There are other sources with relevant information on health and environment than those mentioned so far. But they provide a more qualitative discussion and are therefore not reviewed here (WHO 1992a, WHO 1995a, WHO 1996c, WHO 1996d).

At present the problem with the determination of environmental causalities is that many of them are not (yet?) known or do not exist as independent variables. The numbers in the two following Tables 5.3 and 5.4 can only represent rough lower estimates of the unknown real shares. Damage oriented impact assessment methods for LCA or green accounting - such as the one proposed and developed in this study - will undoubtedly produce more accurate estimates of these shares in the future. This optimism is grounded in the large number of damage factors for single interventions and environmental problems which are now being developed here and by others. Their presentation in a site-independent form or as averages that are at least valid for large areas is a beginning on which more differentiated functions can be built.

The World Bank has been the first organisation to estimate the number of disability adjusted life years (DALYs) lost due to selected environmental threats (World Bank 1993). (Section 5.4 will elaborate on this concept of DALYs.) Table 5.3 reproduces these estimates. They include occupational factors and road transport injuries although usually they are left out of LCA as explained earlier in Subsection 1.2.6.

Type of environmental disease	Burden from this disease in Mio. DALYs per year	% of total burden
Respiratory infections due to urban air	123	9.0
Chronic respiratory effects due to urban air	47	3.5
Occupational risk factors (including cancers, neuropsychiatric, chronic respiratory, musculoskeletal, and unintentional injury)	318	23
Motor vehicle injuries	32	2.3
Total	*473(a)*	*35*

Tab. 5.3: Estimated global burden of disease from selected environmental threats, 1990 (World Bank 1993)
(a): Adjusted for double counting

Murray *et al.* (1996a) estimate human health effects from world-wide particulate and sulphur emissions using a bottom-up approach and an updated aggregation method

[1] Poor water supply here refers to biologically infected and not to chemically poisoned water.
[2] The exclusion of these two causes of bad health holds true only if one agrees with the limitations of LCA *sensu stricto* as described in Subsection 1.2.6.

to calculate DALYs. This updated method does not affect the distribution of the burden of the different diseases reported in Table 5.3. But Murray and his co-authors end up with much lower absolute numbers (by a factor of 20) than the World Bank does for air pollution (Table 5.4). The conservative lower estimate for occupational factors is also much lower than the number given by the World Bank (1993). Given the difficulties in attributing risks to health effects that have been mentioned above, it is indeed not surprising that Murray *et al.* (1996a) attribute less than 40% of the total DALYs to the ten risk factors they have selected and which are presented in Table 5.4. It is therefore quite possible that further analyses and investigations will substantially alter the results given in Table 5.4.

Risk factor	Deaths (thousands)	As % of total deaths	YLLs (thousands)	As % of total YLLs	YLDs (thousands)	As % of total YLDs	DALYs (thousands)	As % of total DALYs
Malnutrition	5 881	11.7	199 486	22.0	20 089	4.2	219 575	15.9
Poor water supply sanitation and personal and domestic hygiene	2 668	5.3	85 520	9.4	7 872	1.7	93 392	6.8
Unsafe sex	1 095	2.2	27 602	3.0	21 100	4.5	48 702	3.5
Tobacco	3 038	6.0	26 217	2.9	9 965	2.1	36 182	2.6
Alcohol	774	1.5	19 287	2.1	28 400	6.0	47 687	3.5
Occupation	1 129	2.2	22 493	2.5	15 394	3.3	37 887	2.7
Hypertension	2 918	5.8	17 665	1.9	1 411	0.3	19 076	1.4
Physical inactivity	1 991	3.9	11 353	1.3	2 300	0.5	13 653	1.0
Illicit drugs	100	0.2	2 634	0.3	5 834	1.2	8 467	0.6
Air pollution	568	1.1	5 625	0.6	1 630	0.3	7 254	0.5

Tab. 5.4: Global burden of disease and injury attributable to selected risk factors, world 1990 (Murray *et al.* 1996c)

From Table 5.4 we can see that the average incidence of death occurs at a high age. Only about 10 YLLs are reported per death and the years lived disabled (YLDs) contribute more than 22% of the DALYs. The conclusion is that YLDs can therefore not be neglected in the determination of human health effects.

As a last example, we present in Table 5.5 some of the results of a semi-quantitative estimate for several environmental interventions undertaken by WHO (1994a). The percentage of people exposed in Europe to levels of concentration that are defined as constituting a health concern rises from around a low 1% to 10% in most cases, but for some factors, up to 25% of the European population are concerned. It is clear from this analysis that SO2 and particles, both of which are included by Murray *et al.* (1996a) in their analysis, are not the only relevant environmental risk factors.

The main conclusions from this incomplete survey are:

- The estimates given for environmental risk factors are rather vague and the uncertainty behind the numbers is large. The knowledge on causalities seems too limited to allow for the calculation of reliable numbers.
- The contribution of environmental factors (exclusive of injuries and occupational factors) to the burden of disease (expressed in DALYs) amounts to between 0.5% and, possibly, 20%. In established market economies, this is a relevant share of risk factors that are independent of lifestyle. It follows that an investigation of

human health impairments due to environmental risk factors seems to be fully justified.

- Risk factors such as traffic injuries, occupational hazards, and indoor air pollution are relevant risk factors even though all of them are rarely addressed in LCA. It follows that injuries and indoor air pollution should be included in LCA where they can be attributed to a product or service. The assessment of occupational health, due to its uniqueness and relevance, could be treated as a separate life-cycle tool.
- At least two statistics (Murray *et al.* 1996a/b, World Bank 1993) use a single index to measure premature death and differences in health states. Such single indices are a powerful instrument to discuss risk factors and health consequences.

From the points in this conclusion, the first is taken into account by drafting an assessment framework in this study and using it for the concrete examples of carcinogenity and respiratory effects. The fourth point made above is the main interest of Sections 5.3 and 5.4.

Environmental factor	**Potential health effects**	Europeans exposed at level of concern in Mio.
Air pollution (ambient)		
SO_2 - short term exposure	Transient respiratory disorders, aggravation of chronic respiratory diseases potentially precipitating death	200
SO_2 - long-term exposure	4-7% Decrease in average level of pulmonary function	6
TSP - short term exposure	Transient respiratory disorders, aggravation of chronic respiratory diseases potentially precipitating death	29
TSP - long-term exposure	5% Decrease in pulmonary function, increased incidence of chronic airways disease	5
NO_2 - short term exposure	Lower respiratory illness in children, throat and eye irritation in adults	31
O_3 - short term exposure	Cough and eye irritation, small transient changes in pulmonary function in children	85
Lead	Impaired mental development of children	0.5
Air pollution (indoor)		
Mother smoking at home	Lower respiratory illness in children	2
Being married to smoker	Lung cancer	85
NO_2 from gas stove	Lower respiratory illness in schoolchildren	15
Water and food		
Microbiological contamination	Mild gastrointestinal disturbance to severe gastroenteritis	130
Housing		
Lack of piped water	Waterborne infections	110
Dampness	Allergies, including asthma and respiratory infections	170-250
Ionising radiation from Radon	Lung cancer	43
Noise	Annoyance and sleep disturbances	180

Tab. 5.5: Estimated exposure of the general population to selected environmental risk factors and their potential health effects for the population of 852 Mio. Europeans (WHO 1994a)

5.3 Indices to measure human health

5.3.1 What is human health?

The World Health Organisation defined already 50 years ago: *"Health is not only the absence of infirmity and disease but also a state of physical, mental and social well-being"* (WHO 1947). In the *European Charter on Environment and Health* environmental health is defined to *"...include both the direct pathological effects of chemicals, radiation and some biological agents, and the effects (often indirect) on health and well-being of the broad physical, psychological, social and aesthetic environment, which includes housing, urban development, land use and transport"* (WHO 1994a:2).

This second definition of health quoted here is very broad and includes indirect effects. These are normally excluded from LCA (see Subsection 1.2.6 and Müller-Wenk 1997). The focus in this chapter is not on the risk factors, but on the assessment of different health states and of premature death. In this context it is important to realise that health is not just constituted by the absence of disease, but that physical, mental and social well-being all are components of health. It follows that handicaps, headaches, psychiatric conditions (e.g., depressions), impaired mental development (e.g., due to lead ingestion), and reduced fertility all are relevant elements which make up the health states and which therefore have to be considered in health accounting.

5.3.2 Requirements for a human health index

The index has to measure damage to the safeguard subject's *human health*. From the subsection above, it follows that such damage can be constituted by infirmity, disease and the absence of physical, mental and social well-being. In addition, it seems justified to include premature death as damage to human health (total absence of physical capabilities). As we want to measure primarily direct and partly indirect effects from environmental interventions (in LCA terms) on human health, we can restrict ourselves to include only the physical, mental and social consequences on well-being caused by physical and chemical effects.

Therefore, the index has to measure and aggregate different health states including premature death. From these initial requirements and definitions some additional requirements can be derived (partly from Murray 1994, Murray *et al.* 1996a, Busch Spycher 1997):

a The value choices in the construction of health indices should be made explicit and consistent with each other. This applies to elements such as the estimate of the duration of life lost due to death at each age, the comparison of time lived with a non-fatal health outcome with time lost due to premature mortality, discounting future health, age-weighting, and incorporating considerations of equity (Murray *et al.* 1996a).

b The health state should, in principle, be measured on the level of damages and in a manner as objective as possible. In the health sector one differentiates between impairments (defined on the level of organs), disabilities (defined in terms of impact on an individual's performance) and handicaps (defined in the context of the overall consequences for the individual's ability to function, which in turn depends on the individual's social environment). Although handicaps would be best because the concept comes closest to damage, their degree appears to be predominantly influenced by the socio-economic environment. The next level closest to damage is disability, which could be a good measure[3] (Murray *et al.* 1996a).

c The index should be able to encompass a large range of disabilities and not focus only on one kind of disability.

d At least a nominal or ordinal scale is required in order to measure the different health states, but in order to allow for a straightforward aggregation, we need a cardinal scale for all health outcomes including death.

e The index should be valid, i.e., it should reflect the properties which it is supposed to measure.

f The index has to be sensitive, i.e., small changes in the health state should be shown up through a change in the value of the index.

g The index should be reliable and reproducible, i.e., changes in the index should only be caused by differences in the health state.

A more pragmatic and strategic argument for using a certain health index in LCA would be that there already exists already an international consensus on the appropriate method and/or that there exists already operationalised data ready for use in such an index. An evaluation of existing approaches to health indices will be undertaken in the next section and the seven requirements set out above will be used to select a subset of these approaches for a more detailed analysis.

5.3.3 Existing approaches

Health indicators and indices already have a long history and a great deal of literature exists on them. Busch Spycher (1997) cites as references Rosser (1983), Brooks (1986), Pedroni *et al.* (1990), Ganz (1990), and Till (1991) who have all presented overviews and reviews of existing methods. Murray (1994) and Murray *et al.* (1996a) discuss existing methods to position their own DALYs approach (see Section 5.4). Murray *et al.* (1996a) cite Spilker *et al.* (1996) who had published a survey of about 300 different instruments for the comparison of different health states. They remark in this context that only a few individuals have actually read the vast literature on these instruments.

Both Busch Spycher (1997) and Murray *et al.* (1996a) make a main distinction between *time-based* and *time-point related* methods. Both methods can be further separated into disease-specific and disease-unspecific instruments. Disease-specific instruments are unsuited to the comprehensive human health assessment which is desired within LCA. All time-point related methods are irrelevant for our purpose because one of the requirements defined above was that different health outcomes should lead to a change in value of the health index. This means that if one person

[3] The assumed handicaps resulting from disabilities will, of course, influence the attributed weights in the weighting of different disabilities.

suffers from a sickness during one year and another one from the same sickness, but for 10 years, the difference should be reflected in the value of the index, but isn't when using time-point related methods. This therefore leaves us only with disease-unspecific time-based instruments.

Time-based instruments which cover broadly different diseases and preferably treat both YLDs and YLLs due to premature death in an equivalent manner, best fit our purpose. Busch Spycher (1997) describes three instruments belonging to this category which assess both the quality and the quantity of disease in one common index. The best known of them is called *Quality-Adjusted Life Years* (QALY) and is used by health economists. The *Health Years Equivalent* (HYE) was developed in response to criticism of the QALY concept. The *Quality of Well-Being Scale* (QWB) is another comprehensive and complex measure of health, but it is not widely applied. Another index in this category, but not described by Busch Spycher, is the *Disability-Adjusted Life-Years* (DALYs). It is a young index that has been jointly developed for the *World Development Report 1993* (World Bank 1993) by the World Health Organisation, the World Bank, and the Harvard Centre for Population and Development. This method has been widely disseminated through Murray (1994) and Murray *et al.* (1994). It has been extensively discussed and revised already in the meantime. It has been used to calculate the global burden of disease (Murray *et al.* 1996a/b). These sources also provide all the background data required for its calculation.

Common to all time-based instruments is the need to find or somehow measure weights that can be attributed to the different health states and that reflect both the duration of a disability and the loss of quality of life associated with such a state of disability. It is rather tedious to describe in detail a number of the instruments that have already been developed for this purpose. It is more interesting to analyse directly the different weighting principles that are made use of by these instruments. One can identify six main methods to measure personal preferences for different health states (Murray *et al.* (1996a:71), Busch Spycher (1997:38ff), who make use of a number of other references):

- *Rating Scale/Visual Analogue:* A typical rating scale consists of a line with clearly defined endpoints. The most preferred health state is placed at one end of the line and the least preferred at the other. The remaining states are placed between the two endpoints so that the intervals between the placements correspond to the differences in preferences as perceived by the subject that is asked to determine the weights.
- *Magnitude Estimation:* Subjects are asked to provide the ratio of undesirability for pairs of health states. For instance, State A is felt, for example, to be two times worse than State B. A series of questions allows the subjects to locate all the health states on one scale of undesirability (similar to the procedure used in the Analytical Hierarchical Process (AHP) (Saaty 1980)).
- *Standard Gamble:* A subject is offered a choice between two alternatives. Alternative 1 is a treatment with two possible outcomes: probability p of being restored to normal health and living another t years, and probability $(1-p)$ of dying immediately. Alternative 2 is the certain outcome of living in a given health state i for t years. The probability p is varied until the respondent is indifferent between

the two alternatives. The probability p at the point of indifference is the preference weight for health state i.

- *Time Trade-Off:* A subject is offered two alternatives. Alternative 1 is health state i for t years followed by death and alternative 2 is normal health for x years. x is varied until the respondent is indifferent to the choice between the two alternatives at which point the preference weight for state i is x/t.
- *Person Trade-Off:* A subject is offered two alternatives. Alternative 1 is to extend life for x individuals in normal health and alternative 2 is to extend life for y individuals in health state i. y is varied until the respondent is indifferent to the choice between the two alternatives, at which point the preference for state i is x/y. Other forms of person trade-offs can be structured where subjects are asked to trade-off restoring health to x individuals in health state i versus restoring health to y individuals in health state j.
- *Monetary Valuation:* Subjects can be asked in at least four different ways to estimate their own willingness-to-pay or willingness-to-accept certain health states. One can then measure which amount individuals would accept to pay (1) for reaching a better health state, or (2) to prevent a worse health state from occurring. Or one can determine the payment they would accept to receive in order (3) to give up the opportunity for achieving an improvement in their health, or (4) to accept a further decline in their health state. (For more details see Subsection 5.3.4, Jones-Lee *et al.* (1997), and Wenstøp *et al.* (1996).)

These different methods all pursue the same aim of deriving personal preferences, but use different ways to get there. All of them have advantages and shortcomings (Dolan *et al.* 1996a). The Standard Gamble is a very sophisticated method. It suffers though from people's inability to deal with probabilities. Other methods have a bias due to the respondents' tendency to discount time. The monetary valuation approach is presented in more detail in Subsection 5.4.3 because it allows a direct comparison of human health impacts and economic factors. The concept of DALYs, which makes use of the person trade-off method and compares the result with the one from the visual analogue method, is described fully in Section 5.4 .

Another area of heated debate concerns the problem of whose values should be measured in the first place (see, e.g., Murray *et al.* 1996a). In principle, one can distinguish between people experiencing a given health state, family members of individuals experiencing a given health state, the general public, and health care providers. We will not discuss all possible combinations of panel type and health state weighting methods. It is more useful to state instead a number of recommendations. The panel chosen for the determination of weights should be relevant for the question at stake.[4] Panel members should be able to understand the different health states that are to be weighted.[5] Finally, if a time-intensive method is chosen, the respondents should be able to participate in the exercise until its end

[4] The individual whose health state is under discussion and members of his or her family may be more relevant than members of the public at large or health care providers if there exists a specific decision situation where one has to choose between different therapies. In LCA, the individuals concerned are unknown and it is society as a whole that has to state its preferences. In this case, a panel drawn from the general public seems to be the better choice (Dolan 1996, Dolan *et al.* 1996b).

[5] All health states due to environmental interventions have to be weighted consistently for LCA purposes. Health care providers might be the only group which has the broad knowledge about the different diseases that is required for such an exercise.

(i.e., people in bad health might not live until the end). De Haes *et al.* (1985) presented a large number of instruments to measure the quality of life of cancer patients. Some of the instruments they reviewed were used to compare the quality of life of cancer patients with that of healthy persons. Most studies showed that the quality of life that cancer patients gave to their own health state was not below the quality of life assigned to the same health states by healthy persons. The authors argued that human beings tend to compare their present well-being with the one during previous episodes of sickness and that these may well have been dominated in the case of cancer patients by severe disabilities. Other explanations justify this result with changes in personal relationships, increased solidarity within the family, and a more conscious views of life on the part of the patients. Important here is the insight that these results demonstrate the ambiguity of the result if patients themselves determine the weights.

The methods discussed so far are all dependent on sophisticated models to describe, measure, and aggregate different health states *and* disease histories and projections. None of them has so far acquired widespread authoritative power although the QALYs are well known and the concept of DALYs has already been used by international bodies. This suggests that, for LCA purposes, it might be preferable to base the choice of values on societal values. It is even more obvious to use them if these values have already been expressed in the form of authoritative legislation for the same purpose, i.e., for the health issue at stake.

Along these lines, Müller-Wenk (1997) discusses the use of integrity tables developed in Switzerland as part of a national decree on accident insurance. SUVA (1996) differentiates between 18 types of damages to personal integrity. Most of them reflect health states after accidents; only a few of them are applicable to health states resulting from disease. The weights are defined as percentages of insured income, i.e., the time weighting is restricted to the time before retirement. They are therefore unsuitable for diseases which occur typically later on in life. This system would require major adaptations if it is to be adopted for LCA purpose although some of the required principles such as the consideration of physical, mental and social consequences is already met by it.

In the case of the Swiss *Störfallverordnung* (decree on large accidents), value choices between different safeguard subjects[6] had to be made in order to classify potential events in terms of their severity. In this context, it was decided to equate 1 death with 10 injured persons. The general categorisation as 'injured persons', without providing more information on the level of injury and the resultant length of time of disability, makes this approach unsuitable for the intra-safeguard subject weighting of human health. Nevertheless, these value choices on inter-safeguard subject weighting may well be considered for adoption in LCA.

[6] In fact, not only human health, but also the volumes and areas of contaminated surface waters, the volume of contaminated ground water, the surface with reduced biological productivity, and economic damage not covered by insurance are compared with each other.

5.3.4 Economic accounting

Damage assessment, i.e., the use of damage functions for environmental interventions, has been progressing for many years in the shape of the calculation of external costs (ExternE 1995), as already mentioned in Subsection 4.3.1, and has been adapted to LCA quite early in its development (e.g., Steen *et al.* 1992). The measuring of damages in monetary terms has the obvious advantage that all damages are expressed in one single unit and that in addition it uses at least[7] the same unit as the criteria used in the economic dimension (Figure 1.3). These two properties are the main reasons for the large research effort undertaken in this area and the wide application this way of assessing damages has found, but they are also a source of criticism. Some of the critics' arguments are:

- Ecological health cannot be measured adequately in monetary terms because of intrinsic values and because of our insufficient understanding of the factors that are responsible for the health of an ecosystem.
- Mortality and/or pain should not be measured in monetary terms. Ethical considerations forbid such an accounting and the trade-off with other monetarily measured utilities that is implied by this type of assessment.

An additional major problem is the general use of discount rates in the monetary evaluation of damages. This problem is of central relevance for environmental safeguard subjects with long lasting changes. Proponents of monetarisation argue that the trade-off between health and the provision of other utility is done in the daily life and therefore not immoral[8]. In a detailed discussion in Subsection 5.4.4 we will show that the problem of time preference and, with that, of discount rates is not unique in monetarisation.

The application of monetarisation to environmental damages has generated a wide range of methodological developments in order to handle the specific problems that have emerged in the course of this work. There exists a wide literature on methodology and its application to energy planning, waste incineration, transport and green accounting (see, e.g., Metroeconomica *et al.* 1996, GVF 1996, VDI 1996, Rabl *et al.* 1996a/b, Holland *et al.* 1996, ESEERCO 1995, ExternE 1995, Bickel *et al.* 1995, Pearce *et al.* 1994, Ott *et al.* 1994, Pearce 1993, Prognos 1992, Hohmeyer 1992, Teufel *et al.* 1991, Friedrich *et al.* 1989/1990, Frey *et al.* 1985). This literature, and the other literature on which these studies build, attempt to calculate damage functions for a wide range of environmental problems and to monetarise the specific damages concerned by each of them. Since in this chapter we are only interested in the indices to measure human health, we will not consider further the fact that the measure for the index is expressed in monetary terms and could be

[7] We make here this reservation because the same unit does not yet mean that one unit of each has the same meaning, i.e., in the case of damage costs that are uncertain and occur over a very long time they can be judged as lower estimates while the internal costs (economic dimension) are (daily) negotiated actual costs.

[8] In order to be more precise on this point, one has to distinguish between the *ex ante* and the *ex post* valuation. Society and individuals take measures and spend money to minimise health risks. This is done *ex ante* in order to save statistical lives. However, if an individual is affected by a health risk, everything will be done to save its life. The value of a statistical life is irrelevant in this *ex post* situation and will not constrain the effort exerted.

compared to other indices measured in this way, i.e., we disregard the probably most important argument used in favour of monetarisation.

We cannot present here the full theory of monetarisation of human health. We will just look at some widely used approaches (ExternE 1995, ESEERCO 1995). The value of a statistical life (VSL) can be measured by:

- Willingness-to-pay (WTP) or willingness-to-accept (WTA) methods (see also Subsection 5.3.3). These methods are called *contingent valuation methods* (CVM) and apply mostly questionnaire or interview techniques asking individuals about their WTP and WTA towards changes in the risk of death.
- Actual voluntary expenditures on items that reduce the risk of death. This approach can be called the *market* approach and can be interpreted as WTP. A frequently used example is the air bag for car drivers.
- *Wage-risks*, i.e., the increased compensation individuals demand, other things being equal, to work in occupations where the risk of death at work is higher than what is deemed normal (see, e.g., Viscusi 1993). This approach provides an estimate of the WTA.

All of these methods have serious shortcomings which are summarised in, e.g., ExternE (1995):

- In most cases, the willingness-to-pay (WTP) or the willingness-to-accept compensation (WTA) for a change in risk of death is measured. The VSL is calculated based on this information by dividing the WTP or WTA by the change in risk. This transformation is only possible if a set of assumptions such as the linearity between risk and payment is accepted.
- The contingent valuation methods tend to overestimate the VSL because of the choices are just hypothetical.
- Wage-risk methods tend to underestimate it due to limited freedom of job-choice in an economy with unemployment.[9]
- The market approach is dependent on the actually existing allocation between risks of injury and illness and of death risk that are revealed in the willingness to pay for certain safety measures but not others. This allocation is to some extent arbitrary.
- All of these approaches assume that people are rational and able to deal with measures of risk.

These assumptions are weakly grounded empirically and the resulting VSL have to be regarded as rough approximations only. The VSL calculated on the basis of these approaches range from 0.3 to 16 millions ECU (1990). A further analysis of the results and some averaging reduced the range to 2.0 to 4.4 millions ECU (1990) (ExternE 1995).

It is generally accepted that measuring the VSL just with the costs of treating sick and injured persons and with the loss of production due to premature death is a poor substitute measure for the VSL[10]. However, estimates for morbidity effects which

[9] The freedom to chose a job is also curtailed if dual labour markets exist in the economy.

[10] Immaterial damages would have to be added at a minimum. See, e.g., GVF (1996).

cause relevant costs in the health sector sometimes take the costs of illness (COI) as the starting point for an extrapolation to external costs.

The WTP for an illness is composed of the following elements (ExternE 1995):

- the value of the time lost because of the illness,
- the value of the utility lost due to pain and suffering, and
- the sum of all expenditures for averting and/or mitigating the effects of the illness.

Both ExternE (1995) and ESEERCO (1995) calculate COI for illnesses which require admission to hospital or other relevant treatment and multiply them by a generic WTP/COI-factor. In ESEERCO (1995) this factor was set as a default to 2, i.e., the study's authors assumed that the WTP to prevent an illness amounts to twice the health costs. Morbidity classes where pain and suffering dominate were in this study monetarised by pure WTP approaches.

This short review of the literature leads to the general observation that many different methods are proposed and often used in combination. The methods also focus much more on the determination of absolute values and less on the relative values for different morbidity classes. The information available from the QALY approach is hardly made use of nor do the studies make references to this approach.

Measuring the methods against the evaluation criteria listed in Subsection 5.3.2, we see that criteria c), d), and f) are most likely fulfilled. Criteria a)[11], b)[12], and e)[13], are mostly unfulfilled or not addressed in an explicit way. It has to be repeated here that the main reason for these obvious shortcomings may be rooted in the goal of getting *absolute* values that are as realistic as possible. In most cases, only one or two categories of morbidity and mortality are responsible for almost the whole total of external costs due to the impairment of human health and to premature death. The *relative* weighting within morbidity is thus much less important for the externality studies referenced above than for the assessment of human health in LCA.

We do not want to get into a discussion of the bases for, the backgrounds to and the assumptions behind the values given in Table 5.6, but a few remarks relevant for the subsequent arguments have to be made here nonetheless:

- The values given by the two studies are very similar if we disregard the values for chronic illness where the reference endpoints are defined differently by the studies.
- The comparison is insofar biased as both studies use the same data and extrapolation methods. The good agreement is therefore to some extent an artefact.
- The endpoints are very often defined according to the causal factors (illness) and the risk factors (pollutant). The values listed therefore sometimes cover the full episode of a given illness and thus depend on the assumptions about the duration and the severity of the illnesses which vary according to the different risk factors.

[11] Most cases so far have valued premature death only as an event (and morbidity during a defined time period). The ExternE-team is now changing this perspective to account for years life lost (YLL), i.e., they switch to a time-based accounting (ExternE 1997).

[12] Monetarisation measures on the level of handicap rather than disability.

[13] Presently, costs of illness or the acceptance of air bag costs are extrapolated to value health states, i.e., the properties to be valuated are not directly measured.

- Translating the value of a statistical life into the value of one premature death day results in about 200 ECU/day. All other values in Table 5.6, if expressed on a per day basis, are lower than these 200 ECU/day. This is according to expectation. Other endpoints, such as hospital admission for COPD symptoms, where the average duration of morbidity is 9.5 days (ESEERCO 1995), lead to much higher daily values. The technical explanation for this difference is that not only the severity of the morbidity is considered, but that medical costs are also included in the value of a statistical life and that *both* are multiplied by a WTP/COI factor (ESEERCO 1995). As the aim of this procedure is to quantify externalities, it makes sense that a morbidity day causes higher externalities than a premature death day.

Endpoint	ExternE (1995) 1990 ECU	ESEERCO (1995) 1992 US$
Hospital admission for respiratory and pulmonary (COPD) symptoms	6'600	14'000
Emergency Room Visit (ERV)	186	530
Restricted Activity Days (RADs)	62	70
Minor RADs (MRADs)	62	24
Chronic illness	1'000'000	210'000
Symptoms of chronic bronchitis	138	
Symptoms of chronic cough	138	
Hospital visits for childhood croup	186	
Asthma attacks	31	34
Minor symptoms of asthma	31	
Symptoms days	6.3	10
Non-fatal cancer	250'000	204'000
Severe hereditary effect	2'600	
Value of statistical life	2'600'000	3'300'000

Tab. 5.6: Summary of values recently used to monetarise damages to human health (1.25$ ≈ 1 ECU (ExternE 1995))

This last remark should be kept in mind when the disability weights rather than the externalities are discussed in the next section. The second of the above remarks is only relevant if one would want to assess the quality of the values given in Table 5.6 based on the two data sets that are available. The third remark will become important when the values are applied to other risk factors.

We have identified in this subsection some characteristics of the monetarisation methods currently being used to assess different states of human health and evaluated them with the criteria listed in Subsection 5.3.2. The result of this review is that it is still premature to include the operationalised approaches of externality studies in human health damage assessment. Both ExternE (1995) and ESEERCO (1995) list many shortcomings and themselves promise future improvements in the WTP estimates and predict a change from the VSL approach used at present to a time-based years life lost approach.

However, it has to be stated here that many shortcomings are not inherent to the monetarisation as such and can be solved by the ongoing research. Other shortcomings such as the problem of discounting are inherent to the question at hand and show up in most other systems. As soon as the promised improvements are available it should be evaluated again using the criteria given in Subsection 5.3.2.

5.4 The DALYs concept

In this section we will give a comprehensive introduction to the concept of Disability Adjusted Life Years (DALYs) and discuss the adaptations required when one wants to apply it to LCA. All information on the DALYs is taken from Murray (1996) who gives, in 100 pages, a very detailed, clear and self-critical description of this concept and of the assumptions on which it rests. The description of the concept presented here has profited greatly from this open discussion by the concept's creators.

5.4.1 Objectives, normative background and basic assumptions

The concept of DALYs was developed as part of the Global Burden of Disease Study (GBD) started in 1992. The objective of the study was the quantification of the burden of disease and of injury on human populations. First results have been published in World Bank (1993) and the methodology in Murray (1994) and Murray *et al.* (1994). The publication, wide dissemination and subsequent use of DALYs have initiated considerable discussion in international forums and literature. These discussions have forced its authors to take up some of the critiques and rethink and modify the concept for its latest publication in Murray *et al.* (1996a/b). They may also have been the motivation behind the careful description of the concept of DALYs in Murray (1996).

In order to understand the rationale behind the concept and the limitations of its use in LCA, one has to keep in mind the three major objectives behind the initiation of the GBD:

1. Non-fatal health outcomes should be included in debates on international health policy.
2. The epidemiological assessment should be decoupled from advocacy in order to produce objective, independent and demographically plausible assessments of the burdens of particular conditions and diseases.
3. The measure should permit the determination of the cost-effectiveness of alternative health policies in terms of the costs per unit of disease burden averted.

This third objective was the direct reason to develop the concept of DALYs, but it is the realisation of the first objective which ensures the international compatibility and applicability of DALYs in health policy-making. Satisfaction of the second objective is the basis on which to establish a large consensus. All three of them ensure that the concept is imbued with characteristics that are very relevant for its use in LCA.

Murray (1996:2) starts the discussion of the concept with what are the relevant questions from the perspective of LCA: "*Should DALYs be designed as a positive or a normative measure?*[14] *And what is the parent intellectual tradition for DALYs –*

[14] These are terms used, e.g., by economists. A positive analysis is one where no value choices are incorporated, i.e., the statements are capable of verification with reference facts.

welfare, human rights, capabilities, or "justice as fairness"?" The discussion of the first question leads him to conclude that: *"...the distinction between the positive nature of a health indicator and the normative use of health indicators to influence resource allocation may be difficult to maintain".* To support this view Murray (1996:3) states: *"...an indicator that is widely used will soon become normative through its use".* Accepting (and supporting) this position means making the foundation of the normative aspects the centre of interest, a position which is also highly relevant for indices for environmental burdens in LCA. Murray (1996:4) defines three normative perspectives and suggests the likely consequences each one of them might have for the construction of a health index:

- *"A welfarist might choose to design an indicator of burden based on assigning a value to each health event according to its contribution to welfare loss.*
- *An advocate of human rights might believe that the right to live has lexicographic dominance over a right to a better quality of life and propose the crude death rate as the best measure of burden.*
- *Someone inspired by Rawls*[15] *would argue for a measure that emphasises the health condition of those who have the worst health."*

Murray himself notes that the consequence of considering normative aspects is that several possibilities to draft internally consistent approaches exist by first defining the perspective that is to inform the construction of a health index. Murray's approach presented so far would conceptually fit well with the approach presented in Section 4.3 and the Cultural Theory discussed in Chapter 3. The normative archetypes defined by Murray are very radical, though, and do not fit as such into the cultural perspective. That, at least, goes for the perspective of the 'advocate of human rights'.

Murray appreciates the internal consistency and the intellectual elegance of a perspective-based construction of a health index, but he believes that such a construction would be going against the primary aim of constructing a health index in the first place, namely that it reflect a consensus between the different perspectives. Only in doing this can the index become the base for an international health policy. The danger for an index reflecting just one specific perspective is that all those who disagree with the perspective which happens to have been chosen would refuse to use it. Murray (1996:5) evades the problem though when he advocates – after an excursus on common values – *"...a principle of 'filtered consensus' which borrows from the common values and 'laundering preferences' approaches".* Murray's argumentation could be accepted if he were able to show that makers of health policy for whole nations or even for the whole world can only cope with one single number. But the decision-maker that would be using the three LCA results, each one based on one of the three different cultural perspectives, as parts of one unified decision support system, might well consider this three-dimensional information useful and not question the quality of the decision support as such (see Chapters 3 and 4). Thus, Murray might as well develop a multiple of internally consistent

---

[15] Rawls published 'A Theory of Justice' in 1971. One aspect of this theory is the notion that individuals, ignorant of their position in society and shrouded in a "veil of ignorance", would choose to maximise the position of the worst off.

numbers, each one of them reflecting a different cultural perspective on a given health situation.

It is important at this point of the discussion that the reader is aware that the original concept of DALYs does not conform to the statements made in the previous chapters in which the structured aggregation procedure has been developed. We will therefore first describe the original approach and then, in Subsection 5.4.7, propose an adaptation of it in light of Cultural Theory.

Murray (1996:6) starts his presentation of DALYs with two propositions in order to facilitate the argumentation and to make the principle of filtered consensus more transparent:

I *"The burden calculated for like health outcomes should be the same ("like as like" proposition)."*

II *"The non-health characteristics of the individual affected by a health outcome that should be considered in calculating the associated burden of disease should be restricted to age and sex."*

The first proposition is in agreement with the requirements for a sound health indicator listed in Subsection 5.3.2, but this proposition, standing on its own, is weak, as Murray himself correctly notes. Each health outcome can be made unique only if the number of attributes used to describe a health outcome is set sufficiently large (and, anyway, no human being is identical to another).

The second proposition dramatically restricts the range of possible solutions and ways to go in the construction of a health index. Few may disagree with the exclusion of information on race, religion, beauty, and other individual characteristics that one may personally care about. There is likely to be more disagreement on the observation or exclusion of socio-economic information. Some welfarists argue that the index should give a greater weight to the disabilities of high income persons compared to those of poor ones, but those subscribing to Rawls' position might argue for the opposite accounting principle.

Murray (1996:7) suggests that: *"The combination of Propositions I and II gives DALYs a strongly egalitarian flavor"*. We will look at this suggestion in more detail in Subsection 5.4.7 by making use of Cultural Theory.

A last introductory note concerns the question of whether either an incidence or a prevalence perspective should be chosen when setting up morbidity health statistics. There are three reasons given by Murray (1996:9) in favour of the incidence perspective, which is the one used by the GBD:

- *"...the method of calculating time lived with disability is more consistent with the methods for calculating time lost due to premature mortality...*
- *...an incidence perspective is more sensitive to current epidemiological trends...* [and]...
- *...measuring incidence or deriving it from prevalence data and information on case-fatality and remission rates imposes a level of internal consistency..."*

Calculating DALYs on the basis of this incidence perspective requires the making of four important value choices:

- estimating the duration of life lost due to a death at each age level,
- comparing time lived with a non-fatal health outcome with time lost due to premature mortality,
- discounting future health, and
- age-weighting.

They will be discussed in the following subsection.

The incorporation of equity considerations as a design feature for a health index has already been discussed earlier in this subsection. It also constitutes an important value choice, the fifth one, but the distribution of benefits across individuals and the distribution according to socio-economic status are both irrelevant for LCA. Murray, too, does not incorporate them in the design of his concept of DALYs. This value choice will therefore not be discussed any further.

In order to be able to follow the line of argument in the next sections, one has to be aware that the DALYs are composed of two terms that are summed up to form the index value proper: The years of life lost (YLLs) due to premature death and the years lived disabled (YLDs) due to different diseases. Subsection 5.4.2 deals only with YLLs. Subsection 5.4.3 begins with a discussion of YLDs first and then looks at their relationship to YLLs. The discussion in the two Subsections 5.4.4 and 5.4.5 are relevant for both of these terms .

5.4.2 Life Expectation and standard life tables

How long "would" people have lived if they had not been affected by disease and injury? For the construction of DALYs, we need to know the number of life years lost due to the premature deaths of persons at any given age. The actual years of life lost (YLL) for a dead individual can never be known. One therefore has to assume that the individual conforms to an ideal or reference population.

Murray discusses both the choice of the reference population and the choice of the calculation method for the YLL. He distinguishes four families of methods:

- Potential Years of Life Lost (PYLL): An arbitrarily chosen limit of life is set as reference and the difference between it and the actual age at death is the potential years life lost. The disadvantage of this approach is that the extension of a life beyond this arbitrary limit of life does not count as a benefit.
- Period Expected Years of Life Lost (PEYLL): Here, the period life expectancy for each age is chosen as a reference instead of a fixed limit of life. The period life expectancy does vary across countries and over time.
- Cohort Expected Years of Life Lost (CEYLL): This is an attempt to improve on the PEYLL. It is assumed that a child born today will be at each age subject in the future to the currently observed age-specific mortality rates. This results in a significantly higher life expectancy and might vary less over time. National differences continue to exist.
- Standard Expected Years of Life Lost (SEYLL): Here, a standard life expectancy for each age is chosen instead of using individual PEYLLs for each country.

The approach which makes use of PYLL has obvious shortcomings. One of them has been mentioned above. The PEYLL and CEYLL can be rejected because both of these choices conflict with the proposition of "like as like". This leaves the SEYLL for use. Murray chose as the standard life table for women the 'Coale and Demeny West Level 26'- model life table. It is close to the present life table for Japanese women (with an average life expectancy of more than 82 years), but some peculiarities of Japanese age-specific mortality have been eliminated from it (Table 5.7). This model life table has been widely published by the United Nations Population Division which also distributes the corresponding software. It is thus easily available.

The average difference in life expectancy for the sexes is at present equal to 7.4 years in developed regions. A detailed analysis of Canadian mortality statistics by socio-economic status, using special models which correct for the higher risk factors of men, leads Murray to the conclusion that the genetic difference in life expectancy between men and women might lie by about 2.5 years to the disadvantage of men. The UN does not have a schedule for a population of men that have an average life expectancy of 80 years. Murray therefore chose to use the 'Coale and Demeny West Level 25'- model for men even though it had been initially developed for women only (Table 5.7).

Age	0	5	10	15	20	25	30	35	40	45	50
Females	82.5	77.95	72.99	68.02	63.08	58.17	53.27	48.38	43.53	38.72	33.99
Males	80.0	75.38	70.40	65.41	60.44	55.47	50.51	45.56	40.64	35.77	30.99
Age	**55**	**60**	**65**	**70**	**75**	**80**	**85**	**90**	**95**	**100**	
Females	29.37	24.83	20.44	16.20	12.28	8.90	6.22	4.25	2.89	2.00	
Males	26.32	21.81	17.50	13.58	10.17	7.45	5.24	3.54	2.31	1.46	

Tab. 5.7: Standard life expectancies at each age measured in years (Murray *et al.* 1996a)

It is at this place that the differentiation between the sexes enters the DALYs concept. So far, it is not known whether such a difference in average life expectancy is justified genetically or not. If the assumed difference of 2.5 years would turn out to be unjustified, we could assume that the difference will, in most cases, lead to minor deviations only, especially if the disease concerned is sex-independent. For the sake of simplicity, it would then be possible to use only one death table for both sexes.

5.4.3 Weighting different health states and premature death

The subject of this Subsection is the determination of the degree of disability that comes with a disease or injury. Murray *et al.* (1996c:10) state that *"All non-fatal health outcomes of disease are different from each other in their cause, nature, and their impact on the individual, and the impact on the individual is in turn mediated by the way the surrounding community responds"*. This is obviously too complex for statistical treatment and a much simpler framework for analysis is needed with all the simplification of reality that this involves.

The levels at which health outcomes can be measured range from disease via pathology, manifestation, impairment and disability to handicap. This last level of handicap may be the most suitable one if we take reduction of complexity and the weighting perspective as the main choice criteria. Murray (1994) proceeded in this way and was correctly criticised for his choice because this model poorly accounts for disabilities in children and light disabilities in general[16]. Furthermore, the severity of a handicap is not an objective result of an impairment, but depends very much on the social environment within which the handicapped person has to function. It is context dependent. Murray has accepted these points and, in the latest version of his model, has switched to a disability perspective .

Murray chose to use, from among all the methods presented in Subsection 5.3.3, the Person Trade-Off (PTO) method to weight different health states. Murray (1996) reproduces and discusses the concretely used protocol, the questions asked, and the 22 weighted indicator conditions. The most relevant aspects of these elements are mentioned here:

- A *zero* weight represents perfect health and a *unit* weight represents death.
- The panel procedure incorporated the individual weighting of handicaps with PTO, ranking exercises, and group discussions. Panellists were forced to reconsider their initial valuations by presenting them with differently formulated settings.
- The weights for 22 so-called indicator conditions had to be determined in a one-day meeting. The indicator conditions chosen included physical manifestations (e.g., blindness), neuro-psychiatric conditions (e.g., Down Syndrome), vitiglio and its consequences for group interaction, pain (e.g., angina), and sexual/reproductive dysfunction (e.g., infertility). All other disabilities resulting from the diseases reported in the GBD were weighted later by the same panel by making use of a short-cut method.
- Murray (1996:35) applies two forms of the PTO method: *"In the first form, participants are asked to trade-off life extension of healthy individuals and life extension of individuals in a given health state. For example, would you as a decision-maker prefer to purchase, through a given health intervention, one year of life for 1000 perfectly healthy individuals or 2000 blind individuals? In a second form of the PTO, participants trade-off between raising the quality of life to those in health state i to perfect health for 1 year versus extending life for healthy individuals for one year.* The panellists were forced to remove eventual inconsistencies between the outcomes of their two trade-offs so as to end up with only one disability weight for each indicator condition.
- Murray tested the same protocol with nine different panels of health care providers in order to gain some experience. The groups were internationally well balanced. Health care providers were chosen as panellists because of their knowledge about indicator conditions. Extensive coaching would have been otherwise necessary before one could have started with the trade-off exercises. But only the results of a meeting convened at the World Health Organisation in Geneva, 14-19 August 1995, have actually been used. The comparison of the disability weights in Figure 5.3. shows good agreement between the weights that issued from the meeting in Geneva and those formed by the average of all nine meetings.

[16] Two more criticisms were mentioned in Murray (1996). There was no formalised protocol on the weighting process available and the members of the panel of public health practitioners were at that time unaware of the policy implications of their valuations.

The protocol prepared beforehand proved useful and it did indeed force panellists to reconsider their weightings and to rationalise their valuations. One drawback of this procedure is that the interactive set-up of the panel could make it possible that so-called opinion leaders and group effects influence the outcome. It is therefore surprising that the correlation coefficients between the weights that have been determined independently from each other by each of the nine groups are very high while one would have expected that they are highest within the groups. The conclusion is that the weights are not contaminated by opinion leader effects.

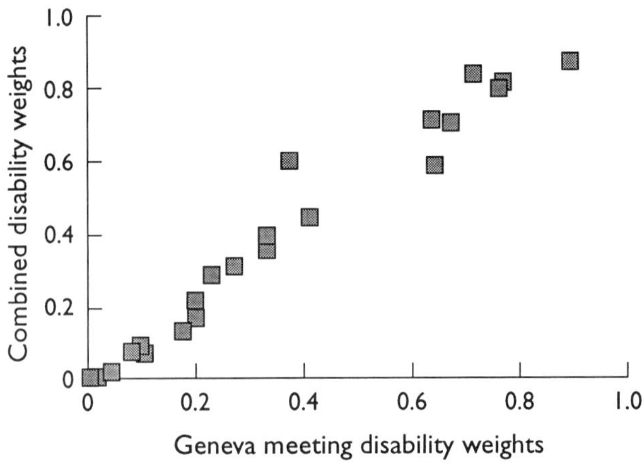

Fig. 5.3: Weight set for 22 indicator conditions based on the combined results of nine exercises using the same protocol, compared with the results of the Geneva meeting (Murray *et al.* 1996c)

Disability class	Severity weights	Indicator conditions
1	0.00–0.02	Vitiligo on face, weight-for-height less than 2 standard deviations
2	0.02–0.12	Watery diarrhoea, severe sore throat, severe anaemia
3	0.12–0.24	Radius fracture in a stiff cast, infertility, erectile dysfunction, rheumatoid arthritis, angina
4	0.24–0.36	Below-the-knee amputation, deafness
5	0.36–0.50	Rectovaginal fistula, mild mental retardation, Down syndrome
6	0.50–0.70	Unipolar major depression, blindness, paraplegia
7	0.70–1.00	Active psychosis, dementia, severe migraine, quadriplegia

Note: These weights were established using the person trade-off method with an international group of health workers who met at WHO in Geneva in August 1995. Each condition is actually a detailed case. For example, angina in this exercise is defined as reproducible chest pain, when walking 50 meters or more, that the individual would rate as a 5 on a subjective pain scale from 0 to 10.

Tab. 5.8: Disability classes for the Global Burden of Disease Study based on the results of the PTO protocol used at the Geneva meeting on disability weights (Murray *et al.* 1996c)

The results of the Geneva meeting were used to define seven disability classes (Table 5.8). This classification is useful if the weights for health states that are not specifically named have to be determined although much knowledge on health care is still required to be able to do so.

The Geneva meeting also provided weights for the approximately 250 diseases included in the health statistic provided by Murray *et al.* (1996a). The participating experts differentiated between the treated and untreated forms of each disease. They gave different weights, where necessary, to each age group and considered the many different disabilities caused by the same disease. The weights that issued from this exercise are given in Table 5.9 for those diseases that later will be assessed in Chapters 6 and 7. Using the estimated weights from the Geneva meeting compiled by Murray is one possibility among others. A large number of other lists are available which report the quality of life of cancer patients. An older review of these lists (de Haes *et al.* 1985) pointed out that their consistency is often poor and the number of patients surveyed had been insufficient in most cases. For these reasons we prefer to work here with the weights derived by Murray (1996).

	Untreated Form	Treated Form	Share with treatment in Europe	Average disability weights
Cancers Preterminal				
Mouth and oropharynx	0.145	0.09	0.9	0.096
Oesophagus	0.217	0.217	0.9	0.217
Stomach	0.217	0.217	0.9	0.217
Colon and rectum	0.217	0.217	0.9	0.217
Liver	0.239	0.239	0.9	0.239
Pancreas	0.301	0.237	0.9	0.243
Trachea, bronchus and lung	0.146	0.146	0.9	0.146
Melanoma and other skin	0.045	0.045	0.9	0.045
Bladder	0.085	0.087	0.9	0.087
Lymphomas and multiple myeloma	0.089	0.057	0.9	0.060
Leukaemia	0.098-0.112	0.083-0.097	0.9	0.085-0.099
Cancers terminal	0.809	0.809		0.809
Lower respiratory infections				
Episodes	0.280	0.280		0.280
Chronic sequelae	0.099	0.099		0.099
Upper respiratory infections (Pharyngitis)	0.070	0.070		0.070
COPD	0.428	0.388	0.9	0.392
Asthma	0.099	0.059	0.95	0.061

Tab. 5.9: Disability weights for untreated and treated forms of diseases, the column indicating the share with treatment indicates the share of tumour patients which are treated by the medical services (the untreated state may result from missing access to or supply of medical service or missing willingness to be treated); selection for the use in Chapters 6 and 7 (Annex Table 3, Murray *et al.* 1996a)

The disability weights presented in Table 5.9 should be seen as indicative of the current state of knowledge. Revisions are to be expected in the future when the protocol used by Murray will have become more refined and more representative groups will have been involved in the weighting exercises. From the view of Cultural Theory, it would be desirable that weighting sets for different cultural perspectives will be determined in the future. Such a refinement is not urgent for the moment as the correlation coefficient for the results of the small groups (8-10 participants) is high, even though one cannot assume that the groups were characterised by an equal distribution of different cultural perspectives[17]. We suggest that the differentiation

[17] On the other hand, it is also possible to argue that the international experts and health care providers who participated in the meetings are already a positive selection from society and one could expect that the hierarchist's perspective has been dominant among them.

by cultural perspective is explicitly planned for in future panels as one could expect that especially the weighting between physical manifestations, neuro-psychiatric conditions, consequences for group interaction, pain, and sexual/reproductive dysfunction will be informed by the cultural perspective of participant experts. The explicit consideration of this aspect within the present study lies outside of its scope.

5.4.4 Time preference and discounting

Health economists are confronted with the discounting of health expenditures that occur in the future. They tend to discount health benefits as well[18]. In this Subsection we take up some of the arguments given by Murray (1996) on the reasons for discounting from an individual and a societal perspective.

As a beginning, it is necessary to clearly define the terms (Murray 1996:44):

- *"Time preference refers to a preference for utility or well-being sooner rather than later, chosen simply because it is sooner and not because of other changes that might be correlated with time.*
- *Discounting refers to the practice of valuing the same thing in the future as less (or more) valuable than the present. Reasons for that may be, e.g., uncertainty increases with time or the likelihood that we will be better off in the future."*

The definitions given above are obviously ambiguous. Time preference as defined cannot be determined independent from personal experiences of uncertainty and feelings of optimism with respect to the future. In discussing this problem, we will focus here only on the special case of discounting health outcomes as the time aspects in general and the problem of discounting in LCA have been addressed already in Hofstetter (1996a:114f).

Individual Discount Rates

A number of explanations are usually given in order to explain why individuals use positive discount rates:

- The concept of opportunity costs implies that individuals prefer to receive a dollar today rather than tomorrow as this enables them to invest this dollar and earn money on this investment in the mean time. I.e., they do not prefer the dollar today *per se*. This is a circular argument, but it might reflect the present behavioural situation very well. Nobody assumes that all of a sudden everybody will become indifferent to the common practice concerning time preference and, e.g., refuse to pay more in the future for a service than they would have to pay for today.
- From an individual point of view, there is a risk of death within the next year. This risk increases with growing age. It is therefore rational to discount the future by this likelihood to die in the next year.

[18] It is worthwhile to note here that the questions of time preference and of discounting appear in a different light from an LCA perspective (Subsection 1.2.6) than from the perspective of economics. There is, of course, no need for a discussion of time preference if we agree that there is no time information in the inventory table. This subsection serves two purposes. It explains the treatment of discounting health benefits in the original concept of DALYs. And it summarises a number of arguments that can be used to decide to include or exclude the time dimension from LCA.

- If someone assumes that she will get richer in the future than she is today, the marginal utility of this additional income is below the one for the present income. (The paradoxical implication is that a pessimistic view, i.e., that income will fall in the future, would consequently lead to the use of a negative discount rate.)

There exists a large debate on the relevance of these arguments for discounting health and environmental impacts. Some just accept that an indirect measure of the discount rate is given by the real interest rate.

Philosophers and some (non-mainstream) economists think of pure time preference as a defect in human judgement. The three arguments listed above do not conflict with such a judgement. The second and third argument above can be related to uncertainty and to being better-off in the future. They are therefore related to the practice of discounting and are not a matter of time preference. The first argument is just the rational consequence for someone who accepts that the market works on the basis of discounting. Negative discount rates could occur if the growth rate of consumption exceeds the individual's rate of pure time preference (Murray 1996). Murray cites a survey which revealed that 10% of the responding individuals had a negative, 62.1% a zero, and 15.7% a discount rate greater than 10%. The average discount rate of the sample was 3.3%.

Social Discount Rate

The social discount rate may reflect the risk for the extinction of the whole society rather than the average individual's risk to die. The risk that the collective is extinguished is much lower than the one that an individual is going to die, i.e., it is close to zero. Murray (1996:47) cites two other arguments that support the choice of a social discount rate which is lower than the (average) discount rate used by individuals:

- People tend to be more concerned about the fate of future generations when they act in their political or public roles than when they take decisions during their daily market activities.
- The isolation argument suggest that individuals join in a collective contract of more savings by all even though they are unwilling to save more in isolation for themselves (prisoner dilemma!).

This short summary of Murray's arguments suggests that individuals may use discount rates which are different from the social discount rate, and, what is important in the light of cultural perspectives (Chapter 3), individuals having a strong group binding might tend to discount the future differently than non-group-bounded individuals.

Consequentalist Arguments

Under this header, Murray summarises arguments which assume that there is no time preferences, but which look instead at the paradoxical consequences of the failure to discount:

- The *opportunity cost* argument has already been introduced. If health benefits only occur in the distant future, but have to be paid today, their nominal costs at the time of benefit seem to be very large if one adds to them the financial charges (interest), i.e., does not use discounting.

- The *time paradox* results from an attitude which argues that it is always better to wait with health interventions and instead multiply the future health budget by spending money now on investments that provide a high return in the coming years. This attitude would lead to no health interventions at all if a zero discount rate for future life-years is used.
- The *disease eradication and health research paradox* looks at strategies such as the one that would finance a disease eradication program now which would lower the future rate of disease forever, or the one that would finance new research results now which would generate infinite efficiency gains in the future. In the absence of discounting, the requests for spending on research and disease eradication would explode. The consequence would be an excessive sacrifice of resources by society today in favour of the sole health sector.

All these arguments are discussed in Murray (1996) and solutions to avoid these paradoxical consequences without a recourse to discounting are also presented.

Consequences for the original formulation of DALYs

The consequences from all the arguments presented here led Murray (1996:53) to waver in his choice between two alternative procedures for discounting when calculating the DALYs:

A) "to use a low positive discount rate to capture the fact that uncertainty increases with time and, more importantly, to reduce the problems of excessive sacrifice"; or

B) "to use a zero discount rate, ignoring the cumulative small effects of uncertainty [i.e., for example the extinction of society], and to capture the problems of excessive sacrifice through other means, such as an arbitrary division of the health resources into separate budgets for the health of present generations and the health of future generations".

Murray chose case A) as a baseline solution, using an arbitrarily chosen discount rate of 3%, but some results in the GBD are given on the basis of a zero discount rate as well. Instead, in Subsection 5.4.7, we will discuss a choice for a discount rate which is more compatible with either the framework of Cultural Theory or LCA.

5.4.5 Should there be age-weighting?

A case can be constructed where two individuals with meningitis arrive simultaneously at the emergency room, but the available supply of antibiotics is only sufficient for one course of treatment. The prognoses for a successful treatment is identical for both patients. Their only difference is their age (2 and 22 years, respectively). The question is which one of the two should be treated? Murray (1996) cites several surveys which suggest that *in the average* the respondents would prefer to treat the young adult instead of the young child. It is worth noting, though, that in each survey there are respondents which were indifferent between the two cases or which chose treatment for the young child instead.

Murray gives three main explanation for this observed preference:

- Individuals assign greater importance to the good health of infants and of adults at an age where they do raise children than of children up to the age of five and of adults after the age of 60.
- People basing their judgement on the human capital approach assign greater weight to the age at which people are productive than when they are unproductive. Individuals at the age of 20 are the most important ones in this view because they have already been educated and are now able to contribute for the greatest length of time utility to society. Taking the position of society's willingness-to-pay leads to the same result.
- Another function of individuals in society is to care for other persons (children, elderly people, handicapped or otherwise disadvantaged individuals). Young and middle-aged adults (women?) are again assumed to contribute most to these activities.

All these arguments speak in favour of using age-weighting with a maximum weight assigned to young adults. Many of the arguments above can be questioned or they can be used to justify using weights for other factors than age, such as the degree of altruism in or the level of income of individuals, but the use of such attributes conflicts with Propositions I and II (see Subsection 5.4.1).

Two critical questions can be asked about the results of all those surveys which show this weighting according to age:

- How can respondents abstract from their own age when they determine age-related weights? People in general do tend to perceive the duration of time in function of the time they have already lived, i.e., a year at a higher age is perceived to be shorter than a year lived.
- How can respondents judge the weight to be given to *one* additional year of life when they know that life expectancy is falling with increasing age? Does this not lead them to weight twice the patients' life expectancy?

These two questions do not have to be answered here. It is obvious that people subscribe to the human capital approach will prefer weighting according to age. This is also the procedure used in the original concept of DALYs.

Murray chose to use a continuous function for the determination of the age-dependent weights that was easy to define mathematically. Its form is:

$$W(a) = C \cdot a \cdot e^{-\beta \cdot a} \qquad [-] \qquad (5.1)$$

where $W(a)$ is the weighting factor in function of the age a. β determines the shape of the function and the survey results suggest that it should lie between 0.03 and 0.05 with a best estimate of 0.04. C is a correction factor to make sure that the average weight for all ages is equal to one. C is equal to 0.1658 for the disease pattern calculated in Murray *et al.* (1996a/b). The resulting age-weighting curve is reproduced in Figure 5.4.

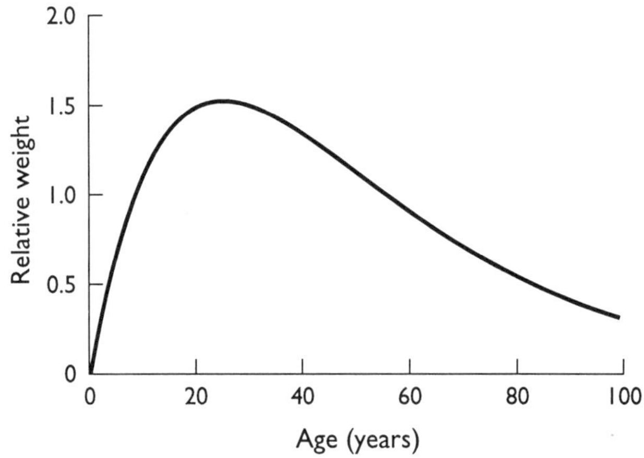

Fig. 5.4: Relative value of a year of life lived at different ages incorporated into DALYs (β = 0.04, C = 0.1658) (Murray *et al.* 1996c)

5.4.6 The original concept of DALYs

In this subsection, we link the elements discussed in Subsection 5.4.1 with those in Subsection 5.4.5 in order to arrive at a closed mathematical description of the DALYs' approach. We will add some reflections on some of the assumptions made in order to gain some more insight into the original concept of DALYs.

DALYs are the sum of the years of life lost (YLL) and the years lived with disability (YLD).

$$DALYm = YLLm + YLDm \qquad [a] \qquad (5.2)$$

where m is the type of disease. The YLLs lost are calculated with the standard expected years of life lost (SEYLL, abbreviated with L). A continuously falling discounting function of the form of e^{-rt} is used, where r is the discount rate (set to 0.03) and t the time. Age-weighting is done by the expression $C{\cdot}a{\cdot}e^{-\beta{\cdot}a}$ where C and β are constants and set equal to 0.1658 and 0.04 respectively. An additional factor K is introduced to allow for an equal age-weighting. The factor a is the age of death and depends on the cause m. Thus, the general formula for the YLL from cause m is:

$$YLLm(a,r,K) = \frac{KCe^{ram}}{(r+\beta)^2}\{e^{-(r+\beta)(L+am)}[-(r+\beta)(L+am)-1] - e^{-(r+\beta)am}[-(r+\beta)am-1]\}+ \frac{1-K}{r}(1-e^{-rL}) \qquad [a] \qquad (5.3)$$

If the discount rate is set to zero, the formula is reduced to:

$$YLLm(a,0,K) = \frac{KCe^{-\beta am}}{\beta^2}\{e^{-\beta L}[-\beta)(L+am)-1] + \beta am + 1]\}+ (1-K)\,L \qquad [a] \qquad (5.4)$$

and if age-weighting is deleted, i.e., K = O, then:

$$YLLm(a,0,0) = L \qquad [a] \qquad (5.5)$$

The same procedure can be followed for YLD. *am* is now the age at the onset of the disability *m* and *Lm* is the duration of the disability. *Dm* is the disability weight as given in Table 5.9. All other notions are unchanged from Equation (5.3). The YLD from a single disabling event can be written as follows[19]:

$$YLDm(a,r,K) = Dm \left\{ \frac{KCe^{ram}}{(r+\beta)^2} \{e^{-(r+\beta)(Lm+am)} [-(r+\beta)(Lm+am)-1] - e^{-(r+\beta)am} [-(r+\beta)am - 1]\} + \frac{1-K}{r} (1-e^{-rLm}) \right\} \qquad [a] \qquad (5.6)$$

If the discount rate is set to zero, the formula is reduced to:

$$YLDm(a,0,K) = Dm \left\{ \frac{KCe^{-\beta am}}{\beta^2} \{e^{-\beta Lm} [-\beta(Lm+am)-1] + \beta am + 1\} + (1-K)\, Lm \right\} \qquad [a] \qquad (5.7)$$

and if age-weighting is deleted, i.e., $K = O$, then:

$$YLDm(a,0,0) = DmLm \qquad [a] \qquad (5.8)$$

With this set of formulas, we are able to calculate the DALYs not only for the parameters preferred by Murray ($r = 0.03$ and $K = 1$) (Table 5.10), but also for other combinations of them.

Age	0	5	10	15	20	25	30	35	40	45	50
Females	33.12	35.85	36.86	36.23	34.52	32.12	29.31	26.31	23.26	20.24	17.33
Males	33.01	35.72	36.71	36.06	34.31	31.87	29.02	25.97	22.85	19.76	16.77
Age	**55**	**60**	**65**	**70**	**75**	**80**	**85**	**90**	**95**	**100**	
Females	14.57	11.97	9.55	7.33	5.35	3.68	2.45	1.53	0.94	0.57	
Males	13.92	11.24	8.76	6.55	4.68	3.20	2.12	1.30	0.76	0.42	

Tab. 5.10: YLL (a, r=0.03, K=1), i.e., standard expected life years lost at a given age a with a discount rate of 0.03 and age-weighting, measured in years (Murray et al. 1996a)

Three questions can be asked with respect to this algorithm which allows us to calculate all possible combinations of discount rates and age-weightings:

A Is the interpretation of different health outcomes sensitive to variations in the discount rate and age-weightings?

B Is the crude death rate a good indicator for DALYs, i.e., do we need the DALYs concept at all?

C How important are the other value choices (standard life table, equity principle, and disability weights)?

Murray *et al.* (1996a) compared the DALYs with and without age-weighting and discounting for a set of diseases. Figure 5.5 shows the changes in rank order of the diseases he analysed. The main changes in rank order occur for psychiatric condi-

[19] The DALYs concept assumes that the YLDs increase linearly with the time spent in a disabled state. Dolan (1996) showed in a large panel study based on the general public that a non-linear valuation can be observed. However, the simplified linearised approach used here is sufficient given the comparably small non-linearity.

tions. These conditions occur especially in young adults, which is exactly the group where the discount rate significantly alters the result. For most other conditions the rank order is quite robust. Nevertheless, in absolute terms, the world-wide DALYs (0,0) add up to about 160 million DALYs while the DALYs (0.03,1) add up to less than 100 million DALYs. The answer to Question A) therefore is that the relative ranking of diseases will be altered only minimally by using age-weighting and discounting for health outcomes caused by environmental risk factors, but the size of the absolute change is sufficiently large to merit further consideration.

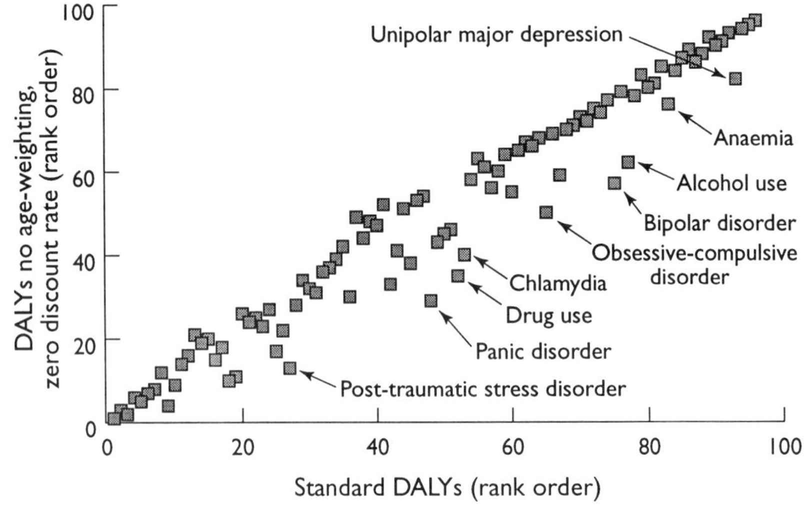

Fig. 5.5: Relationship between the rank order of causes of global burden using DALYs calculated without age-weighting and discounting and standard DALYs calculated with age-weighting and a 3% discount rate, data from whole world 1990 (Murray *et al.* 1996c).

After having developed a sophisticated system, it is always worthwhile to check whether much simpler systems lead to the same interpretation. This is the sense of the second question (B) above if the crude death rate could be a sensible indicator in support of decision making. Figure 5.6 demonstrates that the correlation between the DALYs and the crude death rate is quite poor. We obviously do need the DALYs' concept with its differentiation between YLL (not just death rate) and YLD. This finding had already been suggested by the different proportions between YLL and YLD for the different causes of death in Figure 5.2.

The third question (C) formulated above cannot be answered easily by making a comparison. Other weighting systems would have to be used or even developed first. Nevertheless, some remarks can be made in this context:

- The assumptions behind the standard life table are appropriate ones for LCA purposes because we look for a site-independent assessment. Most information on dose-effect relationships for environmental risks originate anyway in the industrialised world where some countries have national life tables which arc close to the standard life table. We can expect the standard life table to be a better representative of reality than actual national life tables as we want to assess to a certain extent the future damage to human health.

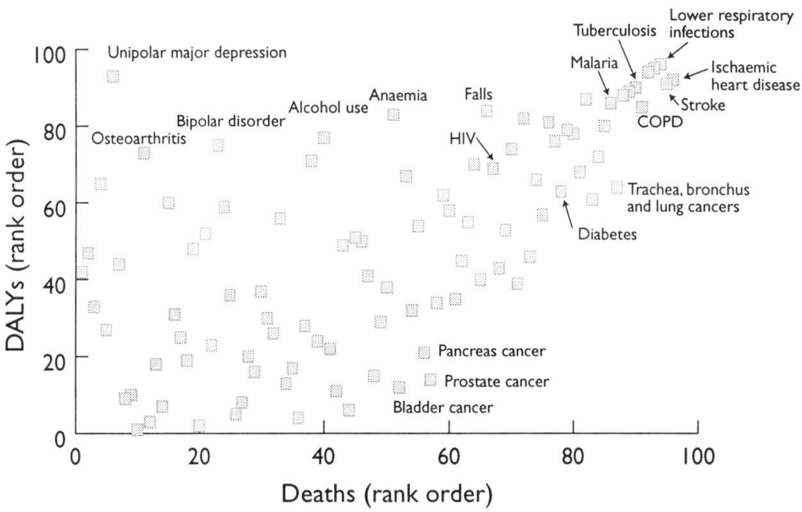

Fig. 5.6: The relationship between the two rank orders for causes of global ill-health, measured either by death alone or by total disease burden (DALYs) (for the reference year of 1990) (Murray *et al.* 1996c)

- The equity principle (i.e., making no distinction between socio-economic groups, religious beliefs, and races) is irrelevant for the purpose of LCA because it does not differentiate between nationalities nor rich or poor districts within a country anyway. LCA does not even report the information which would enable us to make such a differentiation.
- The change in disability weights which would result from the use of panellists other than health providers could significantly alter the YLDs and the DALYs. Especially patients who find themselves in the health states for which they have to determine the weights may judge their disability in a very different manner than has been done by the health providers (de Haes *et al.* 1985). The influence of such a change of weights on DALYs has not yet been tested, but is also rather irrelevant. Earlier, we listed good arguments in favour of using a survey of health care providers for the determination of the weights and the outcome is surprisingly stable after all. An exercise with disability weights on a visual analogue scale resulted in increased relative weights for mild disabilities (classes I and II, as defined in Table 5.8). The influence on the ranking of diseases is very small (Murray *et al.* 1996a:283), but the share of YLDs compared to total DALYs is increased from 30% to 39%. Thus, the total DALYs are changed by only about 10% due to this change of scale (with the application of an extreme transformation).

This discussion should demonstrate the relevance of certain arguments and will facilitate a more focused discussion in the subsequent sections.

5.4.7 DALYs revisited by Cultural Theory

This subsection will look at the concept of DALYs through the glasses of Cultural Theory (see Chapter 3). In the introduction to this section, it was mentioned that Murray (1996:5) tried to apply *"...a principle of 'filtered consensus' which borrows from the common values and 'laundering preferences' approaches..."*. At the same time Murray (1996:7) granted that the propositions for the DALYs-concept have *"...a strongly egalitarian flavor..."*.

We take here a different path. We imagine that all the decision makers who belong to one cultural perspective, i.e., the individualists, the hierarchists, and the egalitarians, are to be asked to develop the concept of DALYs which would best fit in with their perspective of how to measure human health outcomes in LCA. At the end of this exercise, we will then discuss how far the "strongly egalitarian" Propositions I and II led to an egalitarian flavour of the original concept of the DALYs.

In order to provide focus to this thought experiment, we restrict the argumentation to the value choices involved in determining age-weights and in discounting future health states. In the previous subsection, we already mentioned that the choice of the life table and the disregarding of differences in religion, race, and socio-economic status are implied by the concept of LCA[20], i.e., although this represents a value choice it is one that is made when the instrument is chosen (see Subsection 1.2.6). The determination of disability weights is based on value judgements and it is this that could be made more explicit by Cultural Theory. For this purpose, additional empirical work on the relation between cultural perspectives and the determination of disability weights would be necessary. It can be assumed that the relative weights that had been given by the panellists to the different consequences of disease (physical, neuro-psychiatric, social, reproductive, and pain) have been shaped by the cultural perspective proper to each one of them. But without further investigation, it is impossible to estimate the implications this has for the weights determined by panels with members who have different cultural perspectives. We therefore adopt *nolens volens* – as a fallback position – the view that disability weights are independent from cultural perspectives.

Discounting and Cultural Theory

The discussion on discounting in Subsection 5.4.4 showed that arguments can be made for large, small, zero, and even negative discount rates. In none of the surveys used in support of this point does a relevant share of respondents state that they do prefer the use of a positive discount rate. In fact, fully 72.1% of respondents argue for a non-positive one. Nevertheless, all the surveys cited do show that the average of the discount rate suggested by the respondents is positive. Cultural Theory can provide the arguments in support for using a multiple of discount rates, one for each perspective (Subsection 3.2.2 and Janssen *et al.* 1995):

[20] This has implications for the cultural perspective that lies hidden behind the instrument as such. For this discussion see Subsection 3.4.4.

- Egalitarians consider all past and future human beings equal and have a "compressed" time horizon (Rayner 1991). Egalitarians apply therefore a zero discount rate.
- Individualists have a short-term perspective influenced by market behaviour. Each of them individually applies a positive, but different discount rate. Rates up to 10% are cited by Murray (1996). Janssen *et al.* (1995) proposed a discount rate of 5% for individualists.
- Hierarchists have a longer time horizon and look at the problem from a group perspective, i.e., they apply a social discount rate. This social discount rate is close to zero and Janssen *et al.* (1995) propose to set it equal to 2%.

This set of discount rates, reflecting different cultural perspectives, could now be applied in the calculation of DALYs with the help of Formulas (5.3) and (5.6) above. Instead of proceeding in this manner, we come back to the argument made in the footnote to Subsection 5.4.4. Why should we include the time preference and discount future health states when calculating DALYs when LCA itself is based on a compressed time horizon? In Subsection 1.2.6 we stated that LCA *sensu stricto* does not differentiate between emissions in the past, present, and future. As a consequence, we do not know:

- when an environmental intervention occurs,
- when an exposure of humans occur,
- when an exposure will lead to health effects, and
- when there is the onset of a certain disability.

With all this relevant information on time remaining unknown, it makes little sense to include the individualists preference that, if someone dies at the unknown time point t_0 due to an environmental risk factor, the life year from the year t_0 to t_1 is valued more than the life year lost from t_{10} to t_{11}. The lack of time information in LCA *sensu stricto* compels us to refrain from discounting future health states. The consequence is that we are unable to design a human health assessment system that would be compatible with the individualist's view and can do so only to a limited extent for hierarchist's view.

Age-Weighting and Cultural Theory

The arguments in favour of age-weighting (Subsection 5.4.5) can now be looked at again from the concept of Cultural Theory:

- Individuals assign greater importance to being healthy at younger years. This argument might be more relevant for individualists than for the group-bounded hierarchists and egalitarians.
- The human capital approach is, in principle, a very strong argument for individualists because it is a market-oriented argument. Nevertheless, we have to keep in mind that the whole society might profit from this approach and this is in the interest of hierarchists and of egalitarians as well, at least as far as taxes and social assurance contributions are concerned. Egalitarians, however, would not like to have to differentiate according to the degrees to which the different members of society contribute to the GNP. Although both, hierarchists and egalitarians, would prefer to have access to a high GNP, they would not consider the human capital

approach as important. Individualists would prefer this approach to the extent they see an advantage in it for the operation of the market.

- The function of caring for other persons is supposed to be performed mainly by young and middle-aged adults. Individualists would consider this argument as irrelevant. Hierarchists might indeed tend to agree with this argument. There are laws that establish the duty for adults to care for their children and oblige them to support their parents. Egalitarians would argue that both children and aged adults fulfil important societal roles which is overlooked when one is focusing only on care-giving.

This short discussion demonstrates sufficiently well that the aspect of age-weighting is much more controversial than the issue of discounting when discussed from the perspective of Cultural Theory. The position of the three cultural perspectives on age-weighting can thus be summarised as follows:

- Individualists consider the human capital approach to be important and probably judge that the importance of their own health changes with their own age. This variability is insofar relativised as they value their health relatively high during their whole life.
- Egalitarians struggle with two contradicting facts: They support the *credo* of equity which includes a position of equality at all levels of age; and they put the group's well-being above that of the individuals that form it. The second position may lead them to assign unequal importance to the different individuals. Nevertheless, as mentioned above, egalitarians would reject the generalisation that children and older adults are generally of lesser importance to society than those in the prime of their life.
- Hierarchists believe that it is the group that is the important entity. In addition, they tend to obey the law. The laws postulate in general the equality of human beings. There are exceptions to this rule as mentioned above, e.g., concerning taking care of other people, in assuming certain duties, and in what one can do before and after the age of majority. In the example given in Subsection 5.4.4 with the two individuals that had contracted meningitis, the hierarchist would probably choose to save the life of the two-year old patient because more potential life years can be saved in this way and he would at the same time put much effort into increasing the treatment capacity in the future. The reasoning behind this choice, however, is not one concerned with age-weighting but one based on the consideration of *life years lost.*

The upshot of this discussion is that the age-weighting factor K in the Formulas (5.3-5.7) should be set equal to one for individualists and equal to zero for egalitarians. Hierarchists might choose a value of zero as well or plump at most for a moderate age-weighting. We think that the arguments for a $K = 0$ predominate and will work with this hypothesis as of now.

Conclusions

We have derived here parameters for a reformulation of the concept of DALYs from the vantage point of cultural perspectives, using admittedly some rather vague hypotheses (Table 5.11). The hypotheses on different discounting rates formulated here are of little relevance because LCA *sensu stricto* does not include information on time and thus does not provide the information required for discounting anyway.

The proposal for age-weighting is just preliminary and should be tested through future empirical studies.

	Individualist	Egalitarian	Hierarchist
Discount rate derived from Cultural Theory	5%	0%	2%
Discount rate due to LCA *sensu stricto* restrictions	0%	0%	0%
Age-weighting derived from Cultural Theory	yes	no	no

Tab. 5.11: Discounting and age-weighting in the DALYs-concept per cultural perspective

We now have the basis from which we can investigate whether Propositions I and II, with their strongly egalitarian flavour that underlie the concept of the DALYs, have indeed led to an egalitarian's tool. The original concept of the DALYs makes use of age-weighting and applies a discount rate of 3%. Comparing this with the information in Table 5.11 shows that the original concept neither reflects the egalitarian's, nor the individualist's or the hierarchist's concept. Murray's "laundering of preferences" and "filtering of consensus" led indeed to a tool that lies in between all three developed here.

5.4.8 Compliance with requirements and uncertainty

The requirements for a human health index have been defined in Subsection 5.3.2. Here, we discuss the extent to which the concept of the DALYs is in accordance with them. The value choices (a) are made explicit and are transparent. The adaptation suggested in the preceding subsection increases the consistency of the DALYs and the compatibility of the concept with the reference value patterns. Morbidity is measured on the level of disability; this is in agreement with (b). The concept of the DALYs measures a large number of different health outcomes (c&d) on a cardinal scale. The index is valid (e) and small changes in the duration or the severity of a disability influence the indicator value (f). The reliability and reproducibility are assured in most instances, although additional experience has to be gained before a definite judgement can be made. The concept is embedded in large international organisations such as the World Health Organisation and the World Bank. Considerable effort to identify a consensus between interested parties has already been undertaken and a lot of information on disease weights and many health statistics are available.

A number of factors of uncertainty still exist, though. The use of age-weighting alters the YLLs by up to 30% (compare Table 5.7 with Table 5.12). The difference is smaller than this because we assume compatibility with the underlying cultural perspective. For the estimates of YLLs we assume a geometric standard deviation σ_g^2 of 10% (see Appendix 6.8). The disability weights are estimated to show a variation smaller than a factor of 2 (for a 95% confidence interval) for classes I and II (see Table 5.8) based on a comparison with the visual analogue scale (Murray *et al.* 1996a). Smaller factors (< 1.5) apply for the classes III to VII which comprise the more severe disabilities. These factors are chosen for the geometric standard deviation σ_g^2 of YLD.

5.4.9 Summary

One major adaptation of DALYs is required before they can be used in today's LCA *sensu stricto*. The discount rate has to be set to zero because the inventory analysis provides insufficient time information[21]. If the concept of DALYs is modified to reflect Cultural Theory (Chapter 3, Subsection 5.4.7), we can calculate DALYs without the use of discounting and with no age-weighting. This is compatible with the view of egalitarians and hierarchists. The YLLs for this case are given in Table 5.7. The individualists apply age-weighting. The computation with Formula (5.4) yields the YLLs given in Table 5.12.

YLL	0	5	10	15	20	25	30	35	40	45	50
Females	87.19	85.60	81.06	74.82	67.67	60.14	52.61	45.33	38.47	32.13	26.37
Males	85.88	84.27	79.72	73.47	66.31	58.75	51.20	43.89	37.00	30.63	24.86
YLL	55	60	65	70	75	80	85	90	95	100	
Females	21.23	16.67	12.70	9.28	6.46	4.26	2.68	1.63	0.98	0.59	
Males	19.70	15.18	11.27	8.05	5.50	3.64	2.29	1.37	0.79	0.43	

Tab. 5.12: Individualist's *YLL (a, r=0, K=1)*, i.e., SEYLLs at a given age *a* with a discount rate of 0 and age-weighting measured in years calculated by Formula (4)

With the Formulas (5.4) and (5.5) for YLLs and the Formulas (5.7) and (5.8) for YLDs, it is possible to calculate the DALYs for different health outcomes and for each of the cultural perspectives. Examples will be given in Chapters 6 and 7.

This modified DALYs concept provides us with a powerful tool for aggregation which is promoted for use in health policy on both global and national levels. Timely updates of health statistics and disability weights can be expected. This concept of DALYs fulfils therefore many of the requirements that are important for LCA and is at the same time the concept of choice of the health experts.

5.4.10 Critical reflection

These major advantages have at least one serious consequence for the nature of the concept: we have chosen a concept that is embedded in the field of health and medical science and have to accept therefore science's narrow view on human health. The broad definition of health used by WHO and described in Subsection 5.3.1 is reduced to a mechanistic medical view of disease. Only that mental and social well-being is adequately reflected in the weighting procedure which is caused directly by diseases as defined by medical science. Allergies, which do reduce dietary choice, do limit the choice of the place of living or of the clothes to wear, have (yet?) no place in this aggregation scheme. Nor do degraded aesthetic surroundings which can affect well-being (depression) and heighten the sensitivity to other risk factors that often come together with such surroundings. This reflection should make the reader aware that the choice of unit in the form of single damages, and even more the use of the

[21] Individualists and hierarchists may well conclude that it is not the discount rate that should be set to zero, but other LCA concepts next to LCA *sensu stricto* have to be developed. However, this is not the purpose of this study.

aggregation principle, which strongly influences the choice of the former, introduces a bias towards a mechanistic way of understanding human health.

Kleinman *et al.* (1996) discuss the concept of DALYs and criticise it for its strong medical view and its culture-independent weighting of, for instance, 'female reproductive system disorder' or 'mental health problems'. The journal issue in which Kleinman *et al.* (1996) have published their paper deals with the theme of 'Social Suffering'. This is a condition at the border between social and health problems and was defined by Kleinman (1995) in the following way:

> *"What difference does it make–for theory, for research, for policy, and for societal ethics–to change the border between a social and a health problem. Now pulling the edge towards the social side, later on pushing it toward the medical margin–does that disclose a comparative advantage for 'medicalization' of human misery under certain conditions, or for 'socialization' under others? The moral, the political, and the medical are culturally interrelated, but how do we best interpret that relationship and its implications?"*

The consequences from this reflection have to be relativised by looking to the framework for LCA we proposed in Section 4.2. The concept of DALYs proposed here in Chapter 5 is the aggregation procedure that corresponds to the track "known causalities", *the* damage assessment. The social dimension and its influence on human well-being is excluded from LCA (see Section 1.5) and has to be assessed separately.

6 Damage to Human Health from Environmental Chemicals that Cause Cancer

The objective of this chapter is to demonstrate the quantitative feasibility of the framework introduced in Chapters 3 to 5, evidenced by the example of environmental chemicals causing cancer in humans. The damage to human health will be assessed by the modelling of an impact pathway starting with the fate or exposure analysis following an emission, the effect analysis following an exposure of human beings, and an analysis of the resulting diseases due to tumours. The causal relationship between emissions to air or water and damage to human health will be presented in terms of disability adjusted life years (DALYs) per kg substance emission. Further, the index for manageability will be assessed following the proposal in Section 4.5. Both, the resulting index for the magnitude of damage and the index for manageability will be derived in dependence of the cultural perspective applied, i.e., they look differently for the individualists, egalitarians, or hierarchists perspective.

6.1 Introduction

6.1.1 Mechanisms of chemical carcinogenesis

John Hill reported already in 1759 that tobacco snuff caused oral cavity cancer. Later on, soot, aromatic amines, benzene and tobacco smoke were also linked to different cancer types (DeVita *et al.* 1993). Tomatis *et al.* (1993) mention 1942 as the year when, for the first time, experimental evidence was produced in support of the thesis that urban air pollutants (dust) are carcinogenic. But the mechanism of carcinogenesis is even today not yet fully understood and is still a topic of research. There is general agreement in the relevant literature that carcinogenesis is a multistage process consisting of at least the three stages of initiation, promotion, and progression (e.g., Mehlman 1990, LAI 1992, DeVita *et al.* 1993, Philp 1995, Lutz 1997).

The current understanding of *chemical* carcinogenesis is represented in Figure 6.1 as a simplified multistep procedure that builds on these three stages. It can be described, based on Philp (1995:30-31), as follows:

Initiation: The initial step is believed to be the induction of a mutation by an electrophilic chemical or its metabolite (a genotoxic carcinogen) that binds to DNA.

Promotion: Promoters are agents that increase the number of tumours, increase their growth rate, or decrease the latency period. They do not themselves generally cause tumours, although there exists evidence that some promoters are merely weak carcinogens that act synergistically with other carcinogens[1].

Progression: The phase of malignant growth is the last stage within the natural history of the disease.

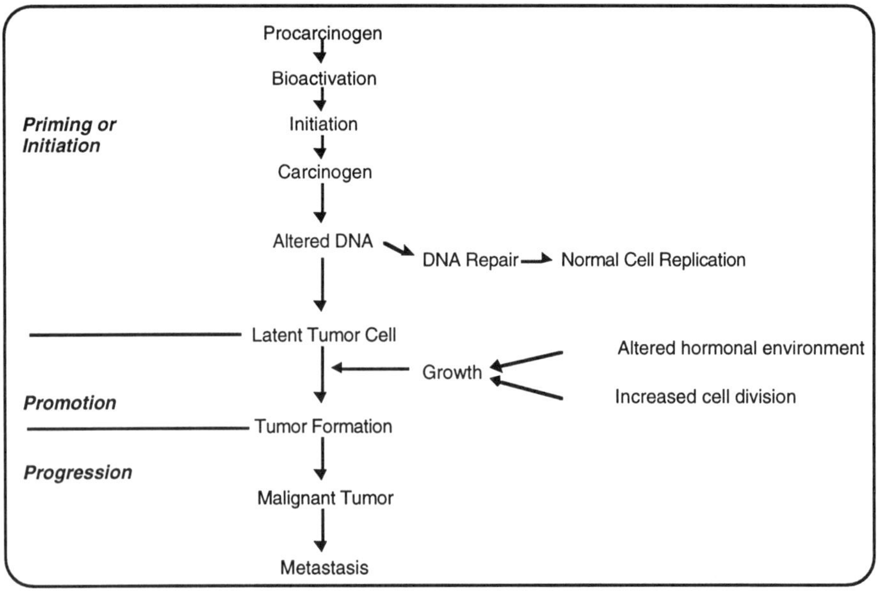

Fig. 6.1 The stages and their steps in the progression of chemical carcinogenesis (after Philp 1995:31)

It can be assumed that genotoxic agents which act as initiators or progressors exhibit no threshold characteristics (stochastic behaviour), but it also has been assumed that promoters do have a threshold. However in most cases, it is hard, in practice, to identify pure initiators and pure promoters. Nevertheless, WHO sometimes lists thresholds in its guidelines on promoters (WHO 1987/1996a). Barrett (1993) considers both the three-stage model shown in Figure 6.1 and that is behind the separation of agents into either initiators or progressors to be an oversimplification. He states that, in humans, three to ten genetic events are involved in the emergence of common adult malignancies. He also argues that, in addition, most promoter substances (if applied alone) have turned out to also be initiators. DeVita *et al.* (1993) mention that physical perturbation of the normal micro-environment (including wounding and radiation) and microbial agents (viruses)[2] may lead to selective clonal expansion of initiated cells. This suggests that the model presented

[1] The categorisation of agents as either initiators or promoters may be largely artificial as nearly all promoters have been shown to be carcinogenic in animal studies.

[2] The viral hypothesis was formulated about 20 years ago and its relevance has only recently been supported by epidemiological investigations (DeVita *et al.* 1993). Up to 15% of all cancer cases worldwide can be attributed to viruses, bacteria and parasites as risk factors. In industrialised countries, this share is much lower and can be estimated at about 5% (Trichopoulos *et al.* 1996).

in Figure 6.1 can be made much more complex. Such a detailed description of carcinogenesis is given in Figure 6.2.

The operationalisation of carcinogenesis in life-cycle impact assessment cannot (and does not need to) reflect this complexity. For this purpose, it is necessary to disregard the possibility that cancer may be caused by different modes of action and result from the combined effects of a mixture of substances (or of physical factors and of viral influences). Subsection 6.3 will show the possibility of treating the many stages of chemical carcinogenesis as one step like a blackbox.

6.1.2 Selecting pathways for analysis

Not all the known and suspected pathways can and will be analysed in this chapter. The chapter's focus is on human carcinogenesis. There are pragmatic reasons for this important limitation, but it also reflects a prioritising of content. One pragmatic reason is that human carcinogenesis is much better understood than carcinogenesis in animals and plants. A large amount of quantitative information is by now available on this topic. A second reason is that the analysis of the damage functions for human health is already a comprehensive task all by itself.

However, there are also substantive reasons for prioritising work on damage functions for human carcinogenity. It is assumed that most species do not live long enough to show damages due to carcinogenesis (latency time!). Additionally, the safeguard subject 'ecological health' is defined in such a way that the damage to individuals within a specie is not considered as a damage to the safeguard subject itself (see reasoning in Subsection 4.1.2). Most standards and guideline documents (WHO 1987, LAI 1992) assume that human beings are the most sensitive specie. The conclusion is that if humans are protected, i.e., if the lifetime risk to them is deemed acceptable, then all other species are also protected at the same time[3]. Mix (1986:1f) reviewed available studies on aquatic animals and concludes: *"Although environmental pollutants have been suggested as the cause of neoplasm in fish and shellfish in at least some cases, the evidence does not permit a firm conclusion. In contrast to fish, there is little evidence that neoplasm of clams, oysters and mussels are associated in any significant way with environmental pollution."* This statement, and the fact that toxicity tests to evaluate the carcinogenic risk to humans is mostly done on animals (rodents), leads to the conclusion that, in some cases, damage to individuals of non-human species can be attributed to environmental pollutants. The need to evaluate damages to ecological health by carcinogenic substances therefore depends on the definition of the safeguard subject and on the information available in the literature (which is not reviewed here).

Figure 6.2 reproduces the view of Arcos *et al.* (1995) of the presently known network of the causal effects operative in human carcinogenesis. In this chapter we are only concerned with the causal factors located in the upper left corner of Figure 6.2 (genotoxic chemical carcinogens) and partly with the substances taken up through food (diet composition). For their assessment, we assume that all the many other risk factors (doubly framed cells) in this model remain constant (*ceteris paribus*) and

[3] This conclusion holds only true if the exposure is comparable. Fish in polluted water are subject to a higher exposure than humans who just drink this water. Animals with a special diet may be exposed much more than humans (e.g., radioactivity in mushrooms).

assume an average value for them, i.e., the *marginal* damage is assessed based on the average constitution of the population.

Only a few cancer risk assessments of chemicals look simultaneously at all the possible intake paths[4]. Sagunski *et al.* (1991) considered inhalation of indoor and of outdoor air, intake by food, by drinking water, and by eating of soil by young children. The results show that all paths are relevant and that the path of intake by food is especially important. The authors identify one shortcoming in the data though: the dose-response data for oral intake are of a lower quality than the other effect data because they are mostly based on animal tests. Subsections 6.2.6 and 6.5.2 will demonstrate the importance of non-inhalative pathways for certain substances. The development of damage functions for human carcinogenity, therefore, must include oral intake. Soil intake by young children, though, is excluded due to its high site-specificity and low relevance in comparison with intake by food. Indoor air pollution is approximated for the time being by outdoor air quality. The literature fails to mention dermal transfer (i.e., through the skin) of carcinogenic chemicals as a relevant exposure path and it is therefore not considered in this case study.

In Subsection 6.2.3 a selection of chemical substances that are carcinogenic will be made based on relevance and data availability. The 55 substances finally retained are only a small share of all the chemicals that act as initiators or progressors. A further limitation of this operationalisation of carcinogenesis is the exclusion of the physical factors that are relevant in LCA[5]:

- Radon and other ionising radiation are therefore not considered, although Frischknecht (1998) made an attempt to build damage functions for them.
- Long-living halogenated substances are also not considered. The resultant ozone depletion has the secondary effect of increasing UV-radiation which, in turn, leads to additional cancer cases. Müller-Wenk (1997) has made a first attempt to assess this damage function. He confirms that an increase in UV-radiation indeed results in significant damages to human health.
- Asbestos will be excluded here because it is of little relevance today in European industrial production. But this substance has to be assessed as soon as an LCA for different asbestos remediation techniques is undertaken. Other fibres, such as rock wool and glass wool, have been excluded as well.

On the effect side, all tumour types for whom environmental pollutants act as causal agents will be considered and all the resultant damages in terms of mortality and morbidity will be included.

In summary, this chapter considers mortality and morbidity of humans that are due to tumours caused by chemical environmental pollutants.

[4] This situation reflects the organisation of legislation and of research.

[5] These physical factors would be grouped together in the impact categories "radioactive radiation", "ozone depletion", and – maybe – "fibres" if one were to use the concept of grouping substances into categories according to the mechanism through which they promote a cancer.

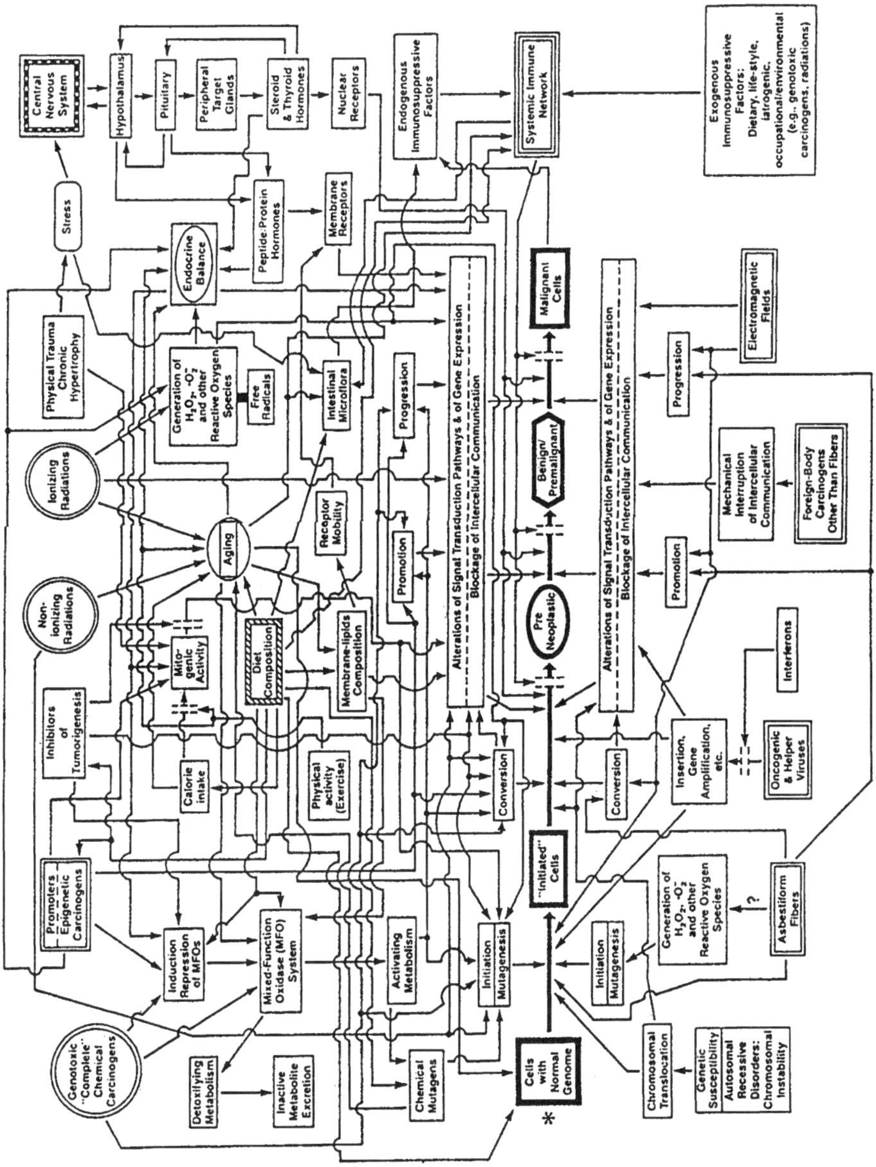

Fig. 6.2: Multifactor interaction network in carcinogenesis based on some of the major relationships identified (dashed double lines that break an arrow symbolise inhibition or blockage of the path) (Arcos *et al.* 1995)

6.1.3 Overview of the calculation of the damage factors

As argued in Section 4.3, the damage-cause analysis is a top-down way of thinking which benefits from the combination of top-down and of bottom-up elements. We begin this introduction to the construction of the damage functions with the formalisation of the emissions and will end it with the one for the damages[6] (see Figure 6.3).

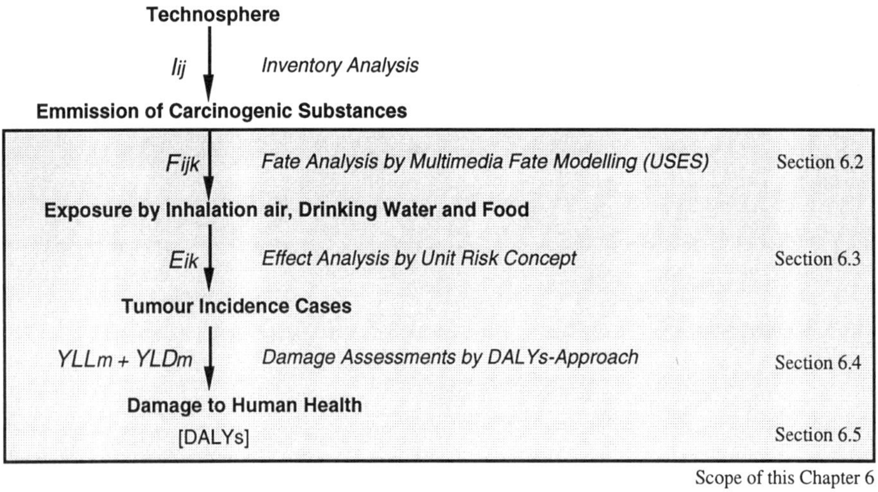

Fig. 6.3: View of the steps making up the impact pathway from emission to damage that have been modelled in Equation (6.2)

- For the emission *Iij* of substance *i* to be assessed, we make the assumptions that it can be measured in kg and that it is emitted to compartment *j*, being either air or surface water (e.g., after sewage treatment). Emissions to other compartments, e.g., direct emissions to soil, are not considered, but would fit into the methodology.
- The fate analysis (Section 6.2) models the fate factors *Fijk* for substance *i* in order to estimate the resulting concentrations in the exposure path *k* (air for breathing, drinking water, or food) due to the emission into compartment *j* (air or surface water). The fate factors transform emissions into external exposures.
- The effect factors *Eik* for substance *i* are estimated as absolute numbers, based on their dose-response relationships and on the potentially exposed population (Section 6.3).

The product of the fate and of the effect factors result in the tumour incidence factors *Tijk*:

[6] This might be considered to be inconsistent with what has been said before. Nevertheless, it turns out that most elements used present themselves as bottom-up rather than top-down procedures. Damage functions themselves are automatically understood as the function that describes the answer (damage) due to a cause (emission). As the LCA-procedure is a bottom-up element as well, we consider this

$$Tijk = Fijk \cdot Eik \qquad \text{[tumour cases/kg]} \qquad (6.1)$$

- The survival rates and morbidity periods will be derived from available data for different tumour types. Years of life lost (*YLLm*) and years lived disabled (*YLDm*) per tumour site *m* will then be established (Section 6.4).
- In a final step (Section 6.5), all elements in the cause-damage function are linked and the different damage categories are aggregated into the indicator for the damage to human health. It is expressed in DALYs, i.e., disability adjusted life years, per kg substance emission (see Section 5.4).

$$\frac{DALYs\ ij}{Iij} = \sum_k \{Tijk \cdot (YLLm + YLDm)\} = \sum_k \{Fijk \cdot Eik \cdot (YLLm + YLDm)\} \qquad \text{[a/kg]} \qquad (6.2)$$

This construction of the indicator, strictly speaking, establishes for each substance just the slope of the relationship between the emission [kg] and the damage [DALYs] at one single emission intensity. A universal damage function would consist of many different slopes, each one for another emission intensity. But due to the assumed linearity and the threshold-less behaviour of chemical carcinogenesis, this single slope (for each substance) represents the slope of a line that passes through the origin and which forms the damage function (for the range of concentrations found in the environment).

Figure 6.3 identifies the substeps modelled in Equation (6.2) and thus makes explicit the approach underlying the assessment using impact pathways.

6.1.4 Manageability of human carcinogenesis

The calculation of an index for the magnitude of damage is one thing. Another is to ask whether this damage can be reduced through additional efforts and whether additional importance should be given to a damage for which one anticipates the need for future management. The calculation of the index for manageability presented here follows the preliminary proposal made in Section 4.5 and uses the default values proposed there. Section 6.6 can be considered a feasibility test for such an index and, as such, does not conform to the scientific foundation of the other sections.

The derivation of the index presupposes the availability of an index for assessed damages and builds on its outcome, i.e., a kind of weighting factor composed of three indicators is multiplied with the magnitude of damage that is calculated in Section 6.5.

---

inconsistency as an acceptable pragmatism, i.e., the construction from a top-down perspective is possible but artificial and would require the adaptation of most available elements if done that way.

6.2 Fate analysis (from emissions to external exposure)

6.2.1 Introduction

The aim of this section is to model the environmental fate of 55 carcinogenic substances and to determinate their fate factors *Fijk* which will then make it possible to calculate the concentrations (times time) for different exposure paths *k* for an emission of 1 kg of the substance *i* emitted to compartment *j*. The substances will be selected later in Subsection 6.2.3. In order to reach this aim, it is necessary to apply and adapt a number of different models. These are introduced in the subsections that follow.

Before proceeding with the selection of the type of models to be used, it is appropriate to recall the different purposes for which they might be used:

I If we want to protect the most vulnerable and most heavily exposed persons (or ecosystems), we have to work with scenarios that use maximum values for all parameters (weather conditions such as inversions, behaviour of persons at their living and working places and their choice of diets, individual absorption characteristics, etc.). Such a scenario could also be deemed to be a reasonable worst case scenario, mostly executed by inductive stochastic bottom-up modelling.

II If we want to measure today's total risks due to the general background situation as accurately as possible, risks have to be assessed directly based on measurements of the background concentrations for some selected indicator substances. Many epidemiological studies limit their scope, e.g., to the identification of damages due to air pollution and fail to specify all the substances involved, i.e., they correct mainly for non-environmental risk factors.

III A third type of question asks for the additional exposure (and damage) caused by the emission of an additional mass unit of substance *i* to compartment *j* in a current, average background situation. This is the marginal approach and looks for the average exposure increase.

The purpose described in (III) is, in principal, adequate for LCA. 'In principle' is written here to remind the reader that today's LCA *sensu stricto* assumes a linear system (Subsection 1.2.6). The marginal approach therefore results in the same relation as the average approach. As a consequence, it is possible to profit from elements developed in (II) as long as they can be attributed to single environmental interventions.

A number of ways to model the average exposure situation for the average population exist. Three approaches can be distinguished (Boström *et al.* 1994):

A) The concentration of carcinogenic substances in the ambient air in different environments can be recorded or modelled together with movements of individuals or population groups between these environments.

B) Personal samplers[7] can be used.

C) The target dose[8] in individuals can be determined, e.g., in blood.

Personal samplers (B) are not feasible because most carcinogenic substances cannot be measured with small-scale methods. The target dose approach (C) is of little relevance for our purpose because we need a causal relationship from emissions to external exposure (the effect analysis (Section 6.3) starts with inhalation and intake data). These two approaches are especially appropriate for answering parts of questions (I) and (II).

This leaves the approach (A). It can be simplified at a number of levels, but has to be linked to the emission data for LCA purposes. We distinguish between two[9] ways of modelling the transformation from *emissions to concentration*: 1) multi-media fate modelling (Mackay 1979/1991, USES 1994, Guinée *et al.* 1996), and 2) statistical methods with empirical data (Hofstetter 1991, Jolliet 1994, Jolliet *et al.* 1997b).

These two ways of modelling fate can be seen in analogy to the effect analysis. The multimedia fate modelling (Subsection 6.2.2/6.2.3) stands for an inductive stochastic perspective where the most relevant paths are modelled to compare the exposure behaviour of different chemicals. The statistical method (Subsection 6.2.4) is close to an epidemiological perspective because it is not the mechanisms and single flows that are measured, but the resulting concentrations. Here, we use both approaches together (Subsection 6.2.5) to improve the fate factors.

Under real-life conditions, the fate factors depend on meteorological factors, the environment and the physical and chemical conditions of the release. In combination with the different emission patterns, this leads to varying background concentrations. Exposure, therefore, varies considerably depending on where and when people breathe air, drink water and get their food and from where it comes.

Boström *et al.* (1994) proposed a solution to this problem. They started with an in-depth analysis of NO_x-concentrations in different environments and the time-activity patterns of human beings in the Western world (about 22 hours indoor, 0.5 hours outdoor and more than one hour for all types of travelling). On this basis, they were able to calculate an overall average for the weighted exposure concentration in ambient air for the Swedish population (23 $\mu g/m^3$, including travels to the large cities). Assuming that most concentration patterns for air pollutants are similar to the one for NO_x (i.e., traffic dominated), they could then calculate weighted averages for other substances even if only limited concentration measurements were available to them. (But information on NO_x-concentrations has to be available for these sites.)

This approach suggested by Boström *et al.* could be adopted if one were to use method 2), i.e., statistical methods, for the fate analysis. As it will be shown later, we use method 2) only to adapt the dilution height of the unit world, to check the reliability of the multimedia modelling results (method 1), and for particles. The

[7] An analytical technique which permits a continuous or a cumulative measurement of individuals' exposure. The measurement device is normally attached to the individual or placed in a suitcase that the individual has to carry around.

[8] I.e., the dose that is relevant for internal exposure.

[9] There are, of course, more ways of modelling environmental fate. An especially large number of models considering only one compartment (e.g., troposphere, or surface water) is available. Such models will be used in Subsections 7.2.3 and 7.2.5.

method proposed by Boström *et al.* (1994) is an elegant way to estimate exposures caused by traffic. A large share of the total cancer risk is caused by traffic-related emissions, but only a limited amount of substances (diesel soot particles, benzene and many PAH) determine this risk. Most other carcinogenic substances are process specific and are mostly emitted by industrial processes. In this case, the proposed approach fails. In addition, the approach is only appropriate for the inhalation path.

LCA is comprehensive in the sense that it includes all environmental interventions in and by way of all compartments, disregarding time and place of release. It is this comprehensiveness that lies at the heart of the need for a multi-media model capable of dealing with a wide range of substances. At the same time, the model should not depend on the availability of information on time and place, i.e., a calculation with reasonable assumptions on average environmental conditions (unit world) is required (Guinée *et al.* 1996, Meier 1997).

We describe a multimedia fate model that fulfils these requirements (Subsection 6.2.2) and the input data that is used (Subsection 6.2.3). Subsection 6.2.4 shows the use of statistical methods and, as a side-result, it is shown there how to estimate the substance specific dilution height in the atmosphere. On the basis of this additional information, the available multimedia fate model can be developed further. The initial calculations of the fate factors with the multi-media model are compared with the ones that result from the statistical method (Subsection 6.2.5). The final results are discussed in Subsection 6.2.6. An estimate of the geometric standard deviation for the calculated fate factors is also presented there.

6.2.2 Introduction to multimedia fate modelling

Multimedia fate models were developed as a prerequisite for the assessment of the risks of new and existing chemicals. The need for chemical risk assessment was an important reason for environmental chemists and physicists to develop multimedia models, i.e., models which are able to predict concentrations in more than one compartment (in most cases more than four) due to substance flows from the technosphere to the ecosphere. Within this subsection we give just a short introduction to the model family developed by Donald Mackay and his co-workers (Mackay 1979/1991, Mackay *et al.* 1993/1996b) and to the software tool developed by RIVM (USES 1994) for this purpose and modified for LCA applications by Guinée *et al.* (1996). Readers who may want a broader overview and additional references to other models should turn to, e.g., Mackay (1991), SETAC (1995), Rippen (1996), EEC (1996), Mackay *et al.* (1996a), and Power *et al.* (1998).

Focus on the generic fate modelling

Comprehensive tools for risk assessment include multimedia fate models taking into account the production, use and discharge of chemicals, background concentrations, and meteorological and geographic information. Mackay *et al.* (1996a), e.g., propose a five-stage strategy: chemical classification, acquisition of discharge data, evaluative assessment of chemical fate, regional or far-field evaluation, local or near-field evaluation.

For LCA purposes one is looking for generic fate data, at least as long as there is no specification in the inventory table of the way the substances are emitted and where the emission occurs. For LCA purposes it is sufficient to focus on stages 1 and 3 of the five-stage strategy proposed by Mackay *et al.* (1996a):

- *Chemical classification: Classify the substance as to its chemical type and collect physical, chemical, and reactivity data for that substance in a manner that is appropriate for its classification. Then select an appropriate model.*
- *Evaluative assessment of chemical fate: Deduce the general features of chemical behaviour from running the chosen model in a generic environment.*

This selection of just two elements from the five-stage strategy proposed by Mackay *et al.* is one aspect that differentiates LCA fate analysis from risk assessment for new substances. The two main differences between risk assessment and fate analysis in LCA are:

- Risk assessment includes the estimate of the emission flow scenario for the full region in order to calculate absolute concentrations in the different compartments and to compare them with predicted no effect concentrations (PNEC) and acceptable daily intakes (ADI). In LCA we are instead just modelling the concentration increase due to a known emission pulse.
- Risk assessment uses, in its first tier[10], conservative default values where data or knowledge is missing because its aim is to check whether effect concentrations are surpassed. Conservative means here that the actual concentration might be smaller than estimated. LCA, on the other hand, is not interested in a reasonable worst-case estimate, but in as accurate a modelling as possible given the limited information on time and space that is available in LCA. It is especially important in this case that the systematic errors that are inevitable have the same size for all the substances so as to increase the quality of their relative rating.

The consequences of these differences is that the model has to be re-interpreted so as to model concentration increases by emission pulses (see below) and that both the model and the substance data have to be adapted for LCA purposes by replacing conservative default values with measured data (see, e.g., Subsection 6.2.3)[11].

Nonequilibrium steady state model

Four modelling levels can be distinguished within the family of multimedia models. They are ordered by the increasing power to model reality. This implies also an increased need for input data characterising the substances and the environments (Table 6.1).

The discussion in the recent past on the choice of the appropriate model level for LCA purpose has been lively (Guinée *et al.* 1993, Assies 1994, Heijungs *et al.* 1994a,b, Guineé *et al.* 1996). It focused mostly on the possibility to accurately model the fate of substances with an unknown pattern of emission pulses with models designed for emission fluxes (the so-called 'flux-pulse problem'). The reader should recall here that the inventory table normally shows the aggregated mass loading per substance without any information on time and space (Subsection 1.2.6, Hofstetter 1996a). Level I and II models are not appropriate for LCA purpose

[10] A risk assessment is normally performed in a tiered approach. The multi-media fate model used here is especially designed for the first screening-like tier.

[11] The same procedure would be necessary if one turns from the first tier in risk assessment to a higher order tier.

because the emission compartment is known in LCA and the transport to other media is needed information.. Level III and IV models are both able to deliver this information, but level III models need less input information and computing effort.

Model level	Evaluated conditions	Obtained fate information
Level I	Equilibrium partitioning under steady state	The primary compartments to which the substance will partition and the approximate relative concentration in the compartments, including tendency to bioaccumulate
Level II	As in level I plus losses by advective transport and degrading reactions	The approximate residence time or persistence in the environment, dominant mechanisms of loss by reaction and advection, or tendency for transport out of the generic environment in either air or water
Level III	Nonequilibrium because includes intermedia transport processes, steady state	How fate is affected by the media of discharge, which intermedia transport processes are most important, and which processes account for contamination in media other than that receiving the discharge; persistence
Level IV	Same as level III, but unsteady state	Time necessary to build up to or recover from a given concentration; this can be approximated from a level III model as the residence time, persistence, or amount in system divided by discharge rate

Tab. 6.1: Levels of multimedia fate models (Mackay 1979, Mackay *et al.* 1996)

In Heijungs *et al.* (1994b), it was mathematically proven that level III models are able to calculate the fate factors of substance emission in LCA and appropriate for this task. Here we give a verbal summary of this proof:

1 Most conventional environmental models assume a proportional behaviour of all processes, i.e., the fugacity is constant for each phase and independent from the concentration. This is equivalent to assuming that partition coefficients are constant. This assumption is usually valid at environmental concentrations, but not at concentrations when surfaces or sorption sites become saturated (Mackay *et al.* 1996a). This important assumption is responsible for the fact that a doubling of an emission to any compartment leads to a doubling of the concentrations in all compartments (under the assumption that no other emissions occur).

2 In LCA we assume that the additional production of one functional unit will lead only to a marginal increase in the background concentration. The violation of threshold values is therefore not directly caused by the functional unit. We are mostly interested in the concentration increase during a certain time in a certain area due to an emission into a certain compartment. If the emission is doubled we get either:

- double the concentration during the same time and in the same area, or
- the same concentration during twice the time in the same area, or
- the same concentration during the same time in twice the area, or
- a mixture of all that and where the multiplication of the concentration increase with time and with area results in the same number $[m^2 \cdot a \cdot g/m^3]$.

For LCA it is therefore sufficient to multiply the concentration increase with time and with area.

3 Level III models assume a constant emission flow from the technosphere to a compartment of the ecosphere and calculate the steady state answer to this inflow. Due to the proportionality of the model, it is possible to interpret the steady state answer as an answer during the same time as an inflow time, e.g., both can be set to equal one year. The relation between total inflow per year and

concentration increase during one year in the model area results in the fate factor. With the relation described above, it is possible to drop the condition of constant emission flows and apply the fate factor to the mass loading independent of the pattern of emission.

4 If the life cycle inventory is not able to deliver information on time and space, it does not make sense to choose a fate model which is able to deal with the time dimension. Both the input data and the computing effort required would be increased without improving the model output. Therefore, the level III model seems to be the optimum modelling level as long as the inventory table does not deliver detailed information on time and space and as long we assume that the functional unit that is analysed only leads to incremental concentration increases.

This choice holds for carcinogenesis, i.e., carcinogenic substances increase the risk that tumours are formed proportionally with their emissions. For global warming or the formation of tropospheric ozone, more accurate models were developed to take non-proportionality and non-linearity into account (see also Subsection 7.2.3). For the modelling of the increase of the radiative forcing per kg of the emitted greenhouse gas, models are used which take non-proportional behaviour, and therefore background concentration, into account. Emission scenarios are used in addition. These examples show that the decision to use a level III model here does not exclude choosing another model for selected classes of substances or mechanisms where necessary.

Chemical classification

The approach developed by Mackay (1991) and embedded in the software USES (1994) used here for the calculations is not applicable to all kinds of substances. The selection of subcompartments and the description of the substance behaviour itself is oriented to lipophil (non-polar) and non-dissociating/associating compounds. Many environmental pollutants fall into this group, but the models are weak or do not work for most metals, inorganic air pollutants, and polar chemicals. Mackay *et al.* (1996b) suggest a classification of chemicals into five different types (Table 6.2).

With the support of Table 6.2, the appropriate type for the chemical can be chosen and the fugacity capacity Z can be calculated by a different formula for each type according to Mackay *et al.* (1996b) (only for type 1 to 3). Type 4 and 5 substances can only be modelled with the same model if the input data is adequately manipulated, based on an in-depth knowledge of their environmental behaviours (Guinée *et al.* 1996)[12].

[12] It should be noted that sometimes the limitations are not only due to the different characteristics of the substances, but also due to different ways of emission, i.e., there exist better models than USES to model the fate of pesticides after application. One of them is, e.g., PESTRAS (Freijer *et al.* 1996). An overview of 16 different models used and/or developed at RIVM is given in Vermeire *et al.* (1997). Relevant for LCA purposes are, for instance, the models for radioactive substances and radiation (MiniBIOS, NUCRED, PC COSYMA, REM2, RISKA) and for UV-radiation increase due to the emission of ozone-depleting substances (UV-KETENMODEL).

Chemical category	*Partitioning data required*	*Examples*	*Range of properties*	*Equilibrium criterion*
Type 1	Water and fat or lipid solubility, vapour pressure, Henry's law constant, and octanol-water partition coefficient	Most organic chemicals, e.g., chlorobenzene, hexachlorobenzene, PCBs, etc.	$V_P>10^{-7}$Pa $S_W>10^{-6}$g/m^3	Fugacity
Type 2	Partition coefficients to solid surfaces and to organic carbon, solubility in water and fat	Cations, anions, and involatile organic chemicals (e.g., lead, LAS)	$V_P<10^{-7}$Pa $S_W>10^{-6}$g/m^3	Aquivalence
Type 3	Partition coefficient to solids from air or from pure phase	Very hydrophobic compounds, e.g., long-chain hydrocarbons, silicons, and polymers (e.g., eicosane)	$V_P>10^{-7}$Pa $S_W<10^{-6}$g/m^3	Fugacity
Type 4	Sorptive properties from a pure phase to various solids	Large molecular weight substances, polymers, many elemental metals, and inorganic substances such as minerals (e.g., Polyethylene)	$V_P<10^{-7}$Pa $S_W<10^{-6}$g/m^3	Models may not be useful
Type 5	Partitioning data for all species	Organo-metals, phenols of low pK_a (e.g., mercury, pentachlorphenol)		Probably Aquivalence

Tab. 6.2: Type of chemicals and their classification (Mackay *et al.* 1996a/b), vp = vapour pressure, Sw = water solubility, pKa = logarithmic anion constant, aquivalence stands in contrast to fugacity for substances which tend to migrate to water instead to air.

Some relevant limitations of level III models for LCA

The widespread limitations of level III models are documented extensively in the literature (e.g., Mackay 1991, SETAC 1995, Rippen 1996, Guinée *et al.* 1996). For the application in LCA we want to quantify the increase in the average exposure of human beings and of the biota. Using the Dutch USES system with the adaptations for LCA as described in Guinée *et al.* (1996), one can identify the following relevant limitations when applying it for LCA purposes:

- The available models are not suitable for all substance types relevant for LCA. If different models are used, this introduces inconsistencies in the fate analysis and limits the comparability of the fate factors.
- The unit world (described in the so-called 'country file') does not yet reflect all important emission and receiver areas relevant in LCA. The nesting of unit worlds could allow for a more site-dependent fate modelling for emissions where additional information is available (Brandes *et al.* 1996). This nesting is not considered in the model version that is used.
- The distribution of the substances in the compartment considered is assumed to be homogenous. The chosen compartments are, in many cases, too large or too small for our purposes, i.e., the exposures of humans and of terrestrial ecosystems could be reflected by an atmospheric compartment which reaches to a height lower than the first 1'000 m. The higher troposphere and stratosphere become relevant for not readily degradable substances as well. The quality of the model would be increased by not only a substance-specific compartment size but also by more compartments.
- The terrestrial biomass and the marine compartments are missing.

The desirable refinements of the model mentioned above will increase the demand for additional data for transfer and transformation parameters and for more specific information on the unit world, such as pH-values. We are compelled already now to model with many default values, QSAR[13]-estimations, and other parameters that have to be calculated beforehand. The widespread availability of data on substances (e.g., Rippen 1996, Reichmuth 1996, Voigt *et al.* 1995, Etienne 1996, Mackay *et al.* 1993, Howard *et al.* 1991) should be evaluated by experts in fate analysis in order to support, in a relevant manner, the many models available. In the next paragraph, not only the multi-media fate model that is used, but also its update is described in a compact manner. The update includes some of the refinements that have been mentioned here.

Short description of the Simplebox model

The fate analysis is performed with a multimedia fate model called Simplebox (version 1.0). It is a level III model of the so-called Mackay type and developed by RIVM (USES 1994). The version of Simplebox actually used is implemented in the *Uniform System for the Evaluation of Substances* (USES) version 1.0. It has been chosen for three reasons:

- Adequacy: The multimedia model is a level III-model which requires a minimum of input data to calculate the exposure data required. The output data obtained are concentrations in water, air, soil, and the intake through food due to emissions to air and to water.
- Availability: The system has already been adapted for LCA purposes in a co-operative effort of an LCA research group (CML) and the original model builder (RIVM) (Guinée *et al.* 1996).
- Perspective: The system is considered by the EU to be *the* appropriate tool for the first tier in risk assessment. It was updated and upgraded in 1997 to become the European Uniform System for the Evaluation of Substances (EUSES)[14]. Under these circumstances it is very likely that, in the future, both substance and fate data will be provided in a form that is already consistent with EUSES. The EUSES follows the approach prescribed in EEC (1996).

For the calculations we use only the distribution and intake modules from the USES tool provided by Simplebox. None of the other features, such as the estimation of emissions and of toxicity parameters, are used. The same holds for risk evaluation.

The fate model from USES used here distinguishes eight compartments: air, suspended particles, water, aquatic organisms, sediment, natural soil, and agricultural and

---

[13] Quantitative Structure-Activity Relationship.

[14] The new version Simplebox 2.0 is described in Brandes *et al.* (1996) and will form the multi-media fate model in EUSES. This version could not be considered anymore for the calculations made for this study. The main features of this model update are:

1. Nesting of regional scales in the continental scale
2. Temperature dependent partition coefficients and degradation rates
3. Two separate water compartments at regional and continental scales
4. Terrestrial vegetation compartment added
5. Soil depth derived from chemical-specific penetration depth
6. Water as bulk compartment, assuming thermodynamic equilibrium between dissolved phases and subphases
7. Default settings according to EU procedures for evaluation of substances

and several modifications in calculation routines, effect assessment, output presentation etc.
The changes 1-3 in the update are irrelevant for the fate factors of carcinogenic substances, but the updates 4 to 6 will improve the quality of the fate modelling. Point 7 was not made explicit in Brandes *et al.* (1996) and its consequences cannot therefore be foreseen here.

industrial soils (Figure 6.4). The model takes degradation, advection and diffusion processes into account. The formation of metabolites is not included. The advective flows to unit worlds in the neighbourhood are set equal to zero for LCA purposes. The chosen region is Europe. It is large enough to justify these assumptions for all fast degrading or non-mobile substances[15]. It follows that degradation and outflow via deep underground water are the only real sinks in the adapted model. Additionally, substances reaching the deeper sediment layers are not considered to be part of the system anymore. They are thus regarded as immobilised. These assumptions on sinks and immobilisation are questionable for some substances due to emerging knowledge on natural cycles in the environment. A model adaptation to consider substance-specific immobilisation mechanisms was not part of this case study.

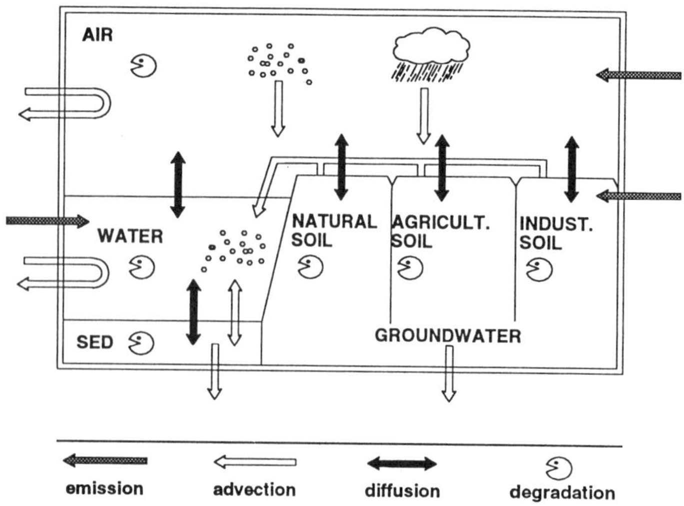

Fig. 6.4: Compartments and processes described in the regional distribution model Simplebox (USES 1994). The advection flows crossing the system border to the compartments air and water are set equal to zero.

The modelling is done on a regional scale. We did not use the continental model because we are interested here in concentration increases (and not in absolute concentrations because non-threshold behaviour of the effects is assumed). The model used here is linear; therefore background concentrations can be set to zero.

The intake module is described in Figure 6.5. It is clear that the food make-up consisting of fish, crops, cattle meat, and milk is only a rough approximation of the oral intake. The combination of surface and groundwater for drinking purposes is subject to wide variations even within Europe. Further information on the model used and on the adaptations made there for LCA-purposes can be found in USES (1994) and in Guinée *et al.* (1996). Information on the default data can also be found there.

[15] For substances with a travelling distance of more than 500 km some net advective losses could be assumed. In Subsection 6.3.5 we will correct for this fact by an adjusted population density.

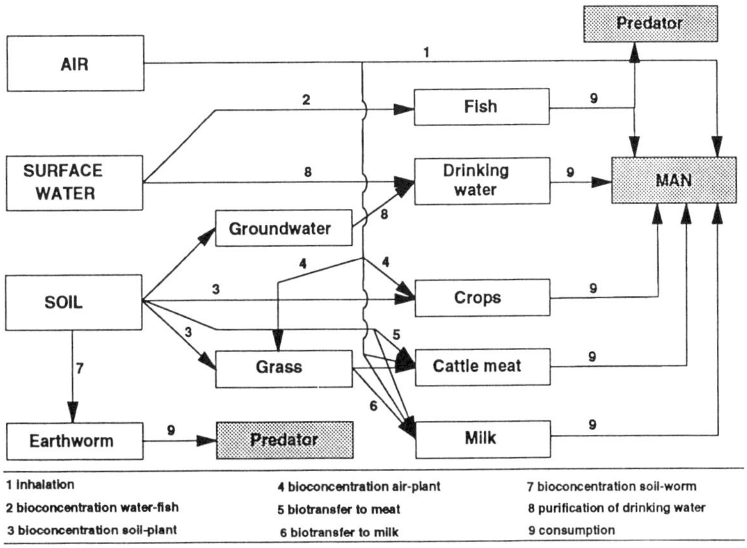

Fig. 6.5: Overview of the exposure routes for men and predators considered in the modelling (USES 1994).

6.2.3 Multimedia fate analysis of carcinogenic substances

Here, we describe the selection of the carcinogenic substances to be modelled, the input data for the calculation of their fate factors, the output data obtained and their validation and uncertainty analysis. After several model adaptations, the calculation used will be described in Subsection 6.2.5 and forms the basis for the calculation of the fate factors *Fijk* that will be used and that have been introduced in Subsection 6.1.3. As we rely on the Simplebox model in USES (1994) and on adaptations already made for LCA purposes (Guinée *et al.* 1996), we limit this subsection to the description of what we changed and added to this basis and how we proceeded to do so.

Selection of the substances

To operationalise the approach, we selected those substances from the U.S. EPA database on carcinogenic substances (IRIS 1996) for which an estimate for unit risks due to inhalation and/or oral intake exists. In addition, we considered substances with unit risk factors in an earlier EPA report (USEPA 1990), a German cancer report (LAI 1992), and the WHO guidelines (WHO 1987/1996a/b). The result of this compilation is a list of 104 substances (Appendix 6.7). The IARC classifies substances according to the available evidence on their ability to act as human carcinogens. (In Subsection 6.3.2 we will elaborate on this classification.) The compilation in IARC (1993b) makes it possible to assign the substances on this initial list according to the evidence on carcinogenity to one of the four Groups 1, 2A, 2B and 3. This classification is the starting point for the selection of substances considered in the fate analysis with highest priority given to Group 1 substances. Group 3 substances have lowest priority.

A comparison of the database produced by Guinée *et al.* (1996) with the list described above throws up 31 substances that are common to them both. We improved the comprehensiveness of the fate analysis by incorporating the physico-chemical information for an additional 21 substances contained in Mackay *et al.* (1993) and in Rippen (1996). It is possible to calculate additional fate factors by using the databases described in Voigt (1995), Voigt *et al.* (1995), and Reichmuth (1996). This effort can only be justified for substances that show up in the inventory table. The resulting compilation of 52 substances covers the list in Appendix (6.7) as follows:

7 out of 11 (64%)	Group 1 substances (carcinogenic to humans)
11 out of 15 (73%)	Group 2A substances (probably carcinogenic to humans)
20 out of 36 (56%)	Group 2B substances (possibly carcinogenic to humans)
14 out of 42 (33%)	Group 3 substances (not classifiable as to human carcinogenity)
52 out of 104 (50%)	

One has to be aware that this selection procedure is pragmatic. It means that 50% of the substances for which dose-response relationships are available are disregarded and that many other potentially carcinogenic substances without quantified dose-response relationships reported in the mentioned literature above are omitted. The disregarded substances can be included later after the collection of appropriate physico-chemical information. For the omitted substances, additional sources to establish dose-response estimates are given in Subsection 6.3.4.

The input data for the multimedia modelling

As already mentioned, we rely as much as possible on the data contained in USES (1994) and in Guinée *et al.* (1996). Appendix (6.1) includes a table that shows which of the substances we will use here are already included in Guinée *et al.* (1996). USES (1994) was designed as risk assessment software. Missing data on the physico-chemical behaviour of the substances is therefore either calculated with the help of knowledge on QSAR or approximated with default values. At least the default values are a reasonable worst case in terms of risk assessment. This overestimation of the exposure is an undesired effect for LCA purposes. Especially for the degradation time, there are often only default values given and these influence the fate factors in a relevant way. To improve the quality of the data to be used, we made use of measured data from Howard *et al.* (1991) and from Rippen (1996) where appropriate. The default values are therefore only used where they seem to be appropriate (e.g., time to half the initial quantity of substances by degradation with hydrolysis (DT 50 hydrolysis) in water) or where no appropriate data is available in the first place. Appendix (6.1) reports the changes made compared to Guinée *et al.* (1996).

The limitations of the model used here especially affect certain types of chemicals (see Table 6.2). Some of the substances contained in Appendix (6.1) therefore do not fulfil the requirements for being modelled with a model of the Mackay-type. The four metals of chromium VI, arsenic, nickel and cadmium are type 2 and 4 chemicals, respectively. Chromium VI is very active as it acts as an anion. RIVM entered these substances into the model by including mostly data on their physico-chemical properties and on their bioaccumulation and immobilisation (degradation) behaviour (Guinée *et al.* 1996). The results seem plausible (dominant intake by food), but the absolute intake is subject to a higher degree of uncertainty than is true for the other substances. Here, we stick to the given information in order to avoid introducing additional uncertainty through the choice of metal dispersion models with another set of assumptions about the unit world and the intake model (see, e.g., BUWAL 1996c) .

Pentachlorphenol and 2,4,6-Trichlorphenol are type 5 substances and do not fit into the model because phenols dissociate in water to form an equilibrium between the neutral molecule and its anion. One should therefore choose the Dow instead of the octanol-water partition coefficient Kow in order to consider the dissociated anions and cations. It is possible to correct Henry's coefficient for the different partitioning between air and water due to dissociation in the same way[16]. Surprisingly, the recalculation with the log(Dow) instead of log(Kow) and DH instead of KH only lead to moderate changes. Due to the lower octanol-water partition coefficient, the bioaccumulation factors are lower and lead to less intake by food. On the other hand, the lower Henry's coefficient leads to a higher concentration in water and compensates partly the lower bioaccumulation. The further calculations for Pentachlorphenol and 2,4,6-Trichlorphenol are based on the corrected octanol-water partitioning and Henry's constant.

The input data used for the fate analysis of the 21 additional substances are given in Appendix (6.2). Most data is taken from Mackay *et al.* (1993) which itself is based on a large survey of the literature and which has already been selected with an eye towards the application in multimedia modelling. The quality of this data is therefore rather good. Mackay *et al.* (1993) gives degradation times according to rough classes only. We have therefore taken the median of each class or the data contained in the fact sheets. Water solubility was set to 1E +06 mg/l if the substance was mentioned as being miscible[17]. A substance is considered to be readily biodegradable if it degrades by more than 70% within 28 days. All other input data were calculated by USES or taken as default.

The default values in USES (1994) have also been chosen for the meteorological conditions and the intake parameters. The LCA country file, which represents a rough approximation of the terrestrial part of Europe, has been used for the geo-

---

[16] The following steps are necessary to calculate the D_{ow}:

$\Sigma\,[\text{Phenol}] = [HA] + [A^-]$

$$D_{ow} = \frac{\Sigma\,[\text{Phenol}]_{oct}}{\Sigma\,[\text{Phenol}]_{aq}} = \frac{[HA]_{oct}}{[HA]_{aq} + [A^-]_{aq}} = \frac{[HA]_{oct}}{[HA]_{aq}} \cdot \frac{1}{(1 + 10^{pH-pKa})} = K_{ow} \cdot f$$

where $f = \dfrac{1}{(1 + 10^{pH-pKa})}$

$\log(D_{ow}) = \log(K_{ow} \cdot f) = \log(K_{ow}) + \log(f)$

In analogy for Henry's coefficient: $D_H = K_H \cdot f$

Choosing the example of 2,4,6-Trichlorphenol with $pKa = 6.15$, $\log(K_{ow}) = 3.72$ (Escher 1995) and $K_H = 8.251$ Pa·m³/mol and assuming an average European pH of water of 7 we get:
$\log(D_{ow}) = 3.72 - 0.91 = 2.81$, $D_H = 1.021$ Pa·m³/mol

Choosing the example of Pentachlorphenol with $pKa = 4.75$ and $\log(K_{ow}) = 5.24$ (Escher 1995) and $K_H = 24.73$ Pa·m³/mol and assuming an average European pH in water of 7 we get:
$\log(D_{ow}) = 5.24 - 2.25 = 2.99$, $D_H = 0.138$ Pa·m³/mol
Many thanks to Dr. André Weidenhaupt, technical chemistry ETHZ, who helped me to understand the necessary modifications and to calculate D_{ow} and D_H.

[17] It is assumed that the substance's density is equal to water. This assumption is a rough approximation without a relevant impact on the fate calculations.

graphic assumptions (Guinée *et al.* 1996), but it has been adapted in one respect for certain substances: the height of the atmosphere. This is explained in Subsection 6.2.5

The output obtained from the modelling

Most of the results offered by using USES are of little or no interest for the purpose at hand. The calculation has to be done twice per substance: in one run 1000 kg/d of the substance are emitted to the air and in the other run the same amount to surface waters (and not waste water because LCA inventorises emissions after treatment). The following minimum information was then taken from the resultant reports and listed in Appendix (6.3):

- the steady-state concentration in the regional model for air [mg/m³] and drinking water [mg/l]
- the human dose [mg/(kg·d)][18] due to food intake (fish, stem and root of plant, meat, and milk).

In the end, these three media are responsible for the exposure of humans towards carcinogenic substances. We can expect to get high concentrations for persistent chemicals and chemicals which do not change the compartment because, as input, we always assume the same emission for each substance.

USES (1994) was developed for risk assessment where emission flows and areas matter. But for our purposes, we need generic fate factors without them being identified with a given area or mass flow. The emission input data into USES (1994) can be understood as:

$$mij = \frac{M'ij}{A} \cdot \Delta t \qquad [\frac{kg}{m^2}] \qquad (6.3)$$

where $M'ij$ is the emission flow of substance i [kg/a] into the compartment j of the model world, A is the surface of the model world [m^2] and Δt indicates a time window expressed in years during the steady-state situation. The reader should note that the unit of mij is not time dependent anymore, but a pulse emission (distributed over the time Δt). This is one of the alternatives to transform the flux input into a mass input. (Guinée at al. (1996) provide also other solutions for this so-called 'flux-pulse problem'.)

The output of the model is the concentration increase due to mij during the time Δt.

$$\text{model output}ik = \delta Cik \cdot \Delta t \qquad [\frac{kg \cdot a}{m^3}] \qquad (6.4)$$

where δCik means the increase of the concentration in compartment k (here k = air). The increase in concentration in drinking water and in food intake can be written analogously. This output can be understood as the cumulated concentration.

The fate factor $Fijk$ represents all the calculations in the multimedia model:

$$Fijk \cdot mij = \text{model output}ik \qquad (6.5)$$

with (6.3) and (6.4) and resolved for $Fijk$ we can rewrite Equation (6.5) as

[18] The unit for the human dose expresses the daily pollutant intake [mg/d] normalised per kg body weight.

$$Fijk = \frac{\delta Cik}{\left(\frac{M'ij}{A}\right)} \tag{6.6}$$

Equation (6.6) shows that the magnitude of Δt is irrelevant because it drops out of the equation.

For the different receiving compartments *k* for the substance *i* emitted to the compartment *j* we can write the following relationships.

$$k = \text{air} \qquad Fij(air) = \frac{\delta Ci(air)}{\left(\frac{M'ij}{A}\right)} \qquad [\frac{m^2 \cdot a}{m^3}] \tag{6.6a}$$

$$k = \text{drinking water} \qquad Fij(water) = \frac{\delta Ci(water)}{\left(\frac{M'ij}{A}\right)} \qquad [\frac{m^2 \cdot a}{l}] \tag{6.6b}$$

$$k = \text{food} \qquad Fij(food) = \frac{\delta Ci(food)}{\left(\frac{M'ij}{A}\right)} \qquad [\frac{m^2 \cdot a}{kg \cdot d}] \tag{6.6c}$$

The m^3 for air represents the breathing air inhaled, the *l* are litres of drinking water, and the *kg·d* represents the specific pollutant intake by food per kg body weight and day.

In the calculations we used A = 3.56 E+12 m^2 (area assumed in the LCA country file) and $M'ij$ = 365'000 kg/a (equal to 1000 kg/d).

The results for *Fijk* are calculated for *j* = air or surface water and *k* = air, drinking water, or food, and are listed in Appendix (6.4).

Validation of level III models

Level III models have already been subjected to validation exercises (Rippen 1996, SETAC 1995, USES 1994). In principle, even the industrialisation process in different countries can be considered as a large scale experiment delivering data for the validation of the model, but a validation based on this real life data is problematic because:

- Emission inventories of specific substances to air, water, and soil for the same area are, in most cases, unavailable or of low quality.
- Concentrations in air, water, soil and food are, in most cases, not measured continuously and at the same time. Measurements usually exist only for the media with the highest concentration and for places where high concentrations prevail (urban areas).
- To account for the advection (transboundary flows) in the real world, models are required which are difficult to validate.
- The area chosen for the validation only partly reflects the unit world considered in the multimedia model because of site-specific singularities and variations.
- For persistent substances, the real world is not in a steady state, and for short-lived substances, the concentrations measured vary by several orders of magnitude depending on the distance from the source and other site-specific factors.

Macrocosms[19] have been used for validation purposes in order to circumvent some of these problems. The agreement between modelled and measured data is good when the physico-chemical data is of high accuracy (Rippen 1996). But the validation exercise reported in USES (1994), performed on the basis of an older version of USES, showed low validity for many different QSAR and the data calculated had uncertainty ranges larger than factor 10. The intake data, as far as it was measurable, showed surprisingly good results due to compensating factors. It has to be mentioned that the present version of USES (1994) already incorporates improvements of those elements where the validation exercise has revealed inaccurate estimations. A validation of HAZCHEM (another multi-media model of the Mackay type) shows good agreement for benzene and di-2-ethylhexylphtalate (DEHP) between the calculated and measured environmental concentrations, i.e., the calculated were in most cases within the range of measured concentrations[20] (cited in SETAC 1995).

A limited validation can be done by comparing different models for predicting fate factors. In SETAC (1995) such an exercise was done with CalTOX (California), ChemCAN (Canada), HAZCHEM (Europe) and Simplebox (Netherlands, integrated into USES). Trichlorethylene, benzo(a)pyrene, 1,4 dichlorobenzene, hexachlorobenzene, hexachlorbiphenyl, pentachlorphenol, atrazine, LAS, and lead were chosen for the test because of substantial differences in the substances' behaviour (but nonetheless fulfilling the requirements for all models). The chemical properties of the substances and the description of the unit world was provided as input to all models. The ratio between the maximum and the minimum values for a steady-state distribution was, for air, within a factor smaller than two (except for atrazine (3.4), LAS (85.4) and lead (76.4)), although the other modelling parameters were not even given the same values. For water, this ratio was in most cases, between 6 and 13 and for soil, lower than 10 (except lead with 110). SETAC (1995) mentions that lower factors are achievable when model parameters are made the same as well. This exercise showed that for certain substances (atrazine, LAS, lead), even similar models produce rather large variations in the results and thus generate rather uncertain fate factors. Thus, a careful selection of models being appropriate for the substances to be modelled and an uncertainty assessment are necessary.

In Subsection 6.2.5 some multimedia model fate factors are validated using real world data.

Uncertainty in data and modelling

The model is imprecise and generates uncertainty in the results. The following factors are mainly responsible for this outcome:

I The linearised and proportional nature of the exchange rate between compartments and accumulation within compartments does not reflect reality.

II The assumption of uniform concentrations within compartments is relevant for human exposure, but does not hold in reality.

---

[19] Macrocosms are miniature worlds which are used as test biospheres. Many parameters can be influenced and the response of a limited set of ecosystems can be observed. Controlled emission flows to macrocosms lead to measurable concentrations in the different compartments which can be compared with modelling results.

[20] But these concentrations themselves had spreads of one to two orders of magnitude!

III The substance-specific physico-chemical and degradation data are themselves subject to uncertainty due to weaknesses in the analytical techniques and to their variability (for degradation). Additional uncertainty occurs because some of the data is from QSAR and not from concrete measurements.

IV The Mackay-type models are inappropriate for some of the substances (see Subsection 6.2.2).

V The unit world is simplified compared to the real world and, therefore, of limited value to predict actual chemical behaviour.

It is difficult to determine the uncertainty associated with factors (I) and (V) with statistical uncertainty assessment. The fate varies by order of magnitudes depending on the local environmental conditions (V). However, this variation is not due to the weakness of the fate model; it is the result of a lack of information in life cycle inventories. A model refinement will be proposed in the next subsection to deal with the uncertainty resulting from the assumption about the dilution height in the atmosphere. Roorda *et al.* (1997) made an investigation to allow for a more location specific fate modelling. They chose four standard landscapes: agriculture on clay soils, sandy areas, pastures on peat soil and urban areas. The first results indicate a difference of about a factor 10 between the highest and lowest value of the calculated fate factors, i.e., the assumptions made for the definition of the unit world are sensitive parameters. In the new Simplebox 2.0 model (Brandes *et al.* 1996), a vegetation module was added leading to a change in air and soil concentrations up to a factor 2. The choice of unit world parameters that reflect European conditions is in contradiction to the assumption that LCA reflects global potential effects. The bias of the model in favour of geographic and meteorological conditions found in the northern temperate zone can be justified somewhat by the fact that dose response functions have the same bias[21].

Factor (II) generates a bias towards low concentrations for substances with short half-lives and high specific densities that are inhaled. The reason for this is that their concentrations follow a gradient and are above average just above the ground. Besides, atmospheric pressure is lower at higher altitudes and therefore less substance mass can be stored, assuming that the same concentrations are measured in parts per million (ppm).

Factor (III) is an uncertainty which can be assessed with statistical uncertainty analysis. Meier (1997) undertook a detailed one for 20 solvents that exhibit similar behaviour and dominant processes in the atmosphere. He estimates, on the basis of a sensitivity analysis for many parameters, that the relative uncertainty of the fate factors is of a factor of 1.5 (up and down). He concludes that the physico-chemical constants are reasonably correct while decay processes are more uncertain. Van de Meent (1995) used Simplebox 1.0 to calculate soil to air concentration ratios for 21 chemicals known to be hazardous in soil. He described 30 variables, such as physico-chemical constants, degradation times and parameters of the country file, by their individual distributions. The uncertainty factor for the ratios, expressed as the ratio between the likeliest and the 5-percentile value, was below 5.2 for more than 70% of the substances. The uncertainty factor for the other substances, mostly highly persistent agents, was as high as 10, 20, and in one case, even 58. Etienne

[21] This statement makes clear that results of 'Western Europe models' have to be critically questioned before they can be applied to other continents.

(1996) made a similar investigation with SimpleBox 1.0. He analysed the stochastic uncertainty of the air-water concentration ratio for eleven volatile compounds. After introducing distributions for the most input parameters, he ended with a squared geometric standard deviation σg^2 (he found almost a lognormal distribution, see Appendix (6.8)) of about 2 to 4 for all substances but ethylene oxide and 2-chloro-1,3-butadiene (both up to a factor 40). The substances (from metals to dissociating substances) analysed in this report are much more dissimilar than those analysed by Meier (1997), but similar to those looked at by van de Meent (1995). The pathways through drinking water and food were also important for the substances analysed here in this report. One therefore has to assume that the uncertainties in the set of fate factors that we have calculated are much higher than those resulting from Meier's analysis, but must be similar to those found by van de Meent.

Factor (IV) supports that the model should be applied exclusively to substances which fulfil the conditions of Mackay-type models (not fully fulfilled in this chapter) and that, for the other substance classes, other models would be used.

Based on the limited possibilities of validation with real world data, of macrocosms, and of comparisons with other models (see subsection above), and considering the factors mentioned above, a group of international model developers published their consensus view on the accuracy of chemical concentration estimates (SETAC 1995). These accuracy factors assume exactly known emission rates and well characterised degradation rates, i.e., the uncertainties are due to chemical properties and transfers between media. The following cases were distinguished for emissions to air and to water (SETAC 1995):

- The substance remains in the media to which it was discharged and the properties are well known. In such cases the uncertainty factor[22] is 2.
- The substance shows multi-media partitioning and its properties are well known. The concentration in the discharge medium then has an uncertainty factor of 3 in the primary sink medium, i.e., the medium it partitions firstly, an uncertainty factor of 6, and in the secondary sink medium of 12.
- If the substance shows multi-media partitioning and the properties are uncertain, then the concentration in the discharge medium has an uncertainty factor of 20, in the primary sink medium, i.e., the media it partitions firstly, an uncertainty factor of 100 and in the secondary sink medium of 500.

These estimates of uncertainty are the only reliable and generic reference that has been found on that subject in the literature.

First attempts at a reliability analysis of the data calculated here are described in Subsections 6.2.4 and 6.2.5. An overall evaluation is presented at the end of Subsection 6.2.6.

[22] With a confidence interval of 95%, the calculated value could be smaller or larger by a factor 2, i.e., $\sigma_g^2 = 2$ (Appendix 6.8).

6.2.4 Simplified dispersion modelling in the atmosphere

As mentioned in the previous subsections, particles and heavy metals do not fulfil the modelling requirements for the multimedia model that has been used in Subsection 6.2.3. Alternative methods to model the fate factors for emissions to air to exposure by inhalation will therefore be presented in this subsection. First, a statistical method will be introduced and applied. Second, the fate of diesel soot will be modelled. Finally, rough estimates for the fate of heavy metals in the atmosphere will be presented.

Statistical method with empirical data

Taking a closer look at the real world can be an alternative to modelling a unit world. For each substance, a certain amount is released to air, to water, and sometimes to soil, all of which lead to background concentrations in a large number of compartments. This real life experiment, the basis for a second approach to the calculation of fate data, is described here. It is used so as to profit from the availability of measured data in the hope that the resultant fate data is more accurate than the one from the model-based approach (real world test data!). This approach is practically limited to substances for which we have some knowledge on geogenic and anthropogenic emissions and for which a dense net of measurements of background concentration exists. With this information, we can calculate the fate factor Fik for various compartments k (adapted from Jolliet *et al.* 1997b, in this formula k = air) for each substance i :

$$Fik = \frac{Cik}{\left(\frac{M'i}{A}\right)} \qquad [\frac{m^2a}{m^3}] \qquad (6.7)$$

where Cik average concentration in compartment k (here k = air) [kg/m^3]
$M'i$ emission flow to air of substance i [kg/a]
A surface over which emission occurs [m^2]

Formula (6.7) is almost identical to (6.6) and the units that result from both of them are identical. The main difference is also the main limitation of this model: The measured concentration Cik cannot be attributed to emissions into only one compartment. This limitation is negligible if the largest amount of substance i is emitted to only one compartment (e.g., benzene to air)[23]. This assumption also makes it possible to deduce the fate factors for compartments other than the one into which the initial emission happened to occur.

Additional limitations are:

- Cik is only under certain assumptions the steady-state answer for the measured emission flow $M'i$. The emission flow $M'i$ either has to be constant over many years or the substance has to degrade within a short time. Jolliet *et al.* (1997b)

[23] Jolliet (1997) mentions that $M'i$ should not only cover the direct emission in compartment k, but also the inter-media transfer from other compartments to compartment k. This again implies an estimation of inter-media transfers.

corrected for this shortcoming by introducing a rate for the annual increase in the concentration of greenhouse gases.

- The measurement points for background concentrations are not dense enough to get a balanced dataset for concentration measurements. The existing points are often concentrated in urban areas or in places where clean conditions prevail. The distribution of measurements does not reflect the average distribution of the places where people stay. This might lead to an overestimate of the fate factors unless one compensates with, e.g., the lead-substance method proposed by Boström *et al.* (1994) (see also Subsection 6.2.1).
- Full data for the emissions to the compartments is often unavailable on a large scale. (If Cik is the background concentration, then $M'i$ has to take into account the full geogenic and anthropogenic flows.) Data availability is probably best for emissions to air and problematic for emissions to soil, surface and groundwater, and the sea.
- We have to budget for the import and export flows if area A is not the globe.

For all these reasons we have to be careful when using the statistical method based on empirical data. The analysis in this case study is limited to emissions to air and the resultant concentrations in air in order to avoid misinterpretations. The consequence is that we calculate only one of the six fate factors proposed in Subsection 6.2.3.

This empirical calculation is available for a set of only 20 of the substances in Jolliet *et al.* (1997b). Only the fate factor for particles might be relevant for the carcinogenic substances among this set. Jolliet *et al.* (1997b) give approximations for the fate factors for an additional 100 substances by using information on residence time and an estimation of the height of dilution[24]. This data are compared to the results of the multimedia modelling in the next subsection.

Some empirical fate factors *Fair,air* for carcinogenic substances

The procedure proposed above is demonstrated here as evidence of some typical carcinogenic substances emitted mostly to air (condition for the reliability). Data for Germany and Switzerland was chosen because both emission and background concentration data are available to the author (Tables 6.3/6.4).

The emission inventory for Germany dates from the time before 1989 and includes only the territory of Western Germany. Based on these emissions, we can calculate

---

[24] The approximation of steady-state fate factors was introduced into and applied to LCA by Hofstetter (1991) with the assumption of a constant dilution volume. Jolliet *et al.* (1997b) show that a better approximation is possible if the average residence time *and* the substance-specific dilution volume is considered as follows:

$$F_{ik} = \frac{\tau_{ik}}{V_{ik}} \quad [\frac{m^2 a}{m^3}]$$

where τ_{ik}: average residence time including both degradation and deposition rates [a]
V_{ik}: volume of dilution per unit surface [$m^3 m^{-2}$]

with $V_{ik}(\tau) = c \cdot \tau^b$ [$m^3 m^{-2}$] for $\tau < 60$ days
and $V_{ik}(\tau) = 10'000\ m^3 m^{-2}$ for $\tau \geq 60$ days

where $c = 30100$ and $b = 0.61$ (fitted from 6 data points)

The formula for V_{ik} is derived from a small sample of about 20 substances. The reliability is therefore questionable.

the area-specific mass flow per year. The measurement of background concentration is rather good thanks to the data provided by LAI (1992, 1995). The data is available for many different sites and conditions for the 1990's. Average concentrations in rural and urban areas still vary by a factor of between 10 and 20. Concentrations could be weighted according to the shares of people living in rural and urban areas if one adopted an exposure point of view. (According to LAI (1992), about 60% of the German population is living in urban areas.) This procedure would probably overestimate the fate factor because it assumes that the emissions are spread equally over the whole country. This is apparently not true. High emission densities occur in the same places as high concentrations. Table 6.3 shows the measurements that are already averaged. The last column of the table shows the range of values for the fate factor that have been calculated.

	Yearly emissions to air in Western Germany	Mass flow per area (A= 248577 km²)	Yearly average of background concentration in Germany (LAI 1992)		Averaged background concentrations in Germany from numerous measurements 1989-1994 (LAI 1995)				Range of calculated $F_{air,air}$
	(LAI 1992)		Urban	Rural	Urban living area	Rural	Traffic area	Industrial area	
	(1)	(2) = (1)/A	(3)	(3)	(3)	(3)	(3)	(3)	(3)/(2)
	t/a	mg/(m²a)	µg/m³	µg/m³	µg/m³	µg/m³	µg/m³	µg/m³	m²a/m³
2,3,7,8-TCDD	27 E-6	1.1 E-7	3-20 E-9	<3 E-9	4 E-9	5.2 E-9	2.3 E-9	20 E-9	21-180 E-6
Arsenic	16-68	0.06-0.27	5-20 E-3	<5 E-3	2.7 E-3	3 E-3	2.5 E-3	4.6 E-3	9-330 E-6
BaP	4.1-16.5	0.016-0.066	1-3 E-3	0.5-1 E-3	1.7 E-3	0.8 E-3	1.7 E-3	2.2 E-3	7-190 E-6
Benzene	47'200	190	5-10	<1	3.1	2	10	2.7	5-53 E-6
Cadmium	25.2-48.5	0.1-0.2	2-5 E-3	0.5-1.5 E-3	1.6 E-3	0.7 E-3	0.8 E-3	1.8 E-3	2.5-50 E-6
Diesel soot particles	70'000	282	5-10	0.5-1.5	7.2	3.7	8.7	4.5	1.8-35 E-6

Tab. 6.3: Fate factors for Germany using published data on emissions (80's) and on background concentrations (early 90's)

	Emissions CH ca. 1995 (soot 1992)	Mass flow per area (A= 41'293 km²)	Background concentrations in CH early 90's	Range of calculated $F_{air,air}$
	(BUWAL 1994, BUWAL 1995, Yetergil Kiefer 1997)		(BUWAL 1996a/b, GVF 1996, Yetergil Kiefer 1997)	
	(1)	(2) = (1)/A	(3)	(3)/(2)
	t/a	mg/(m²a)	µg/m3	m²a/m³
BaP	>0.1	>0.0024	0.00025 (rural), 0.0005 (urban	<100-<200 E-6
Benzene	2'740	66	2.6 (rural), 4 (urban)	39-61 E-6
Cadmium	2.5	0.06	0.0005	8 E-6
Soot (elemental carbon)	800-1000	19-24	2 (rural), 4.3 (urban)	83-230 E-6

Tab. 6.4: Fate factors for Switzerland using published data on emissions and on background concentrations

The same procedure has been used for Switzerland where the same data quality problems exist. Background concentrations are in part based on only a few measurements. The share of the urban population in Switzerland is about 68% (Yetergil Kiefer 1997). But averaging the background concentrations that are available again runs up against the problem that the measurements of emissions are biased towards the urban areas.

Before interpreting or comparing the results, we have to be aware of the fact that:

- The quality of the emission and the background data is poor. The data for Germany might be more reliable than the one for Switzerland.
- The geogenic or natural emission are not included in the emission estimates.
- Both areas are too small to disregard the advection flows into and out of the respective countries. It is known from other studies on conventional air pollutants (Stanners *et al.* 1995) that in most European countries, imports do not equal exports of pollutants. The smaller the country, the larger the influence of advection is likely to be. The Swiss results in particular seem to be severely affected by advection effects.

A comparison of the fate factors shows that the numbers for Switzerland are, for some substances, higher than those for Germany. This can be interpreted to mean that the Swiss emissions are probably not the only cause for the actually measured background concentrations (net import of pollutants). Apart from this remark, it can be said that the fate factors for the two countries indeed show similar values and that the fate factors for the different substances vary between themselves by factors of less than 100. A further comparison is done in Subsection 6.2.5.

Fate factor for diesel soot

Pagano *et al.* (1996) have shown that the mass of total suspended particles (TSP) is not, or at most only poorly, correlated with their mutagenic potential. The small particles with an aerodynamic diameter in the order of 100 nm are the relevant ones. Such particles are typical for the emissions from diesel- and gasoline-driven vehicles. Only PM1 or PM2.5 might therefore be relevant for a discussion of carcinogenity.

The secondary formation of particles contributes significantly to the total particle volume (Section 7.2). IPCC (1996) estimates that the natural emission of particles amounts to about 3'000 Tg/a world-wide. The primary anthropogenic emission amounts to an estimated 113 Tg/a and the secondary one to 256 Tg/a. According to the same source, it is clear that only about 13 Tg/a of soot (elemental carbon) are emitted from anthropogenic sources.

Particles contribute in a relevant manner to respiratory effects. Therefore, they are analysed in detail in Chapter 7. Subsection 7.2.2 will provide the necessary information to calculate the fate factors for the different-sized particles based on their residence time in the atmosphere and the mixing height.

The residence time of soot particles with diameters between 0.1 and 1 μm is dominated by the wet deposition rate. Based on Jaenicke (1978) and Roedel (1992), one can assume an average residence time of 5 days. Subsection 7.2.2 will suggest assuming an average height of the mixing layer of 800m and we will show there that these assumptions lead to a fate factor Fair,air = 17 E-6 m^2a/m^3 with an estimated squared geometric standard deviation σ_g^2 of 3 (Table 7.11).

The share of vehicles in Germany's fleet equipped with diesel engines is very high. This leads to heavy "house-made" pollution. The numbers derived at for soot in Table 6.3 should therefore confirm our results. The most current measurements (LAI 1995) suggest that the average background concentration is somewhere between 4 and 7 $\mu g/m^3$. This leads to a Fair,air = 14 - 25 E-6 m^2a/m^3. A Fair,air = 17 E-6

m^2a/m^3 seems, in this situation, to be a reasonable value and it will be used subsequently. All the other fate factors for diesel soot are set equal to zero because the inhalation path alone is important (LAI 1992, Cantor *et al.* 1996) and because diesel soot is normally not emitted directly to water and if it is, will not be transferred to air again. Polyaromatic compounds and heavy metals are covered separately.

Fate factor for heavy metals

Appendix (6.4) lists fate factors for heavy metals (As, Ni, Cr, Cd) although they do not fulfil the requirements needed for the model used, as has been mentioned previously. The reported values for Fair,air are obviously too low as they correspond to average atmospheric residence times of only a few hours. At least the fraction which is bound to particles will show much longer residence times in air.

The dry deposition velocities for arsenic, nickel, and chromium were taken from Pacyna *et al.* (1985). Cawse (1980) found that, for these metals, dry deposition may contribute only 20 to 40% to total deposition. The wet deposition velocity has been calculated on the assumption that τwet equals 5 days for all metals (same as for particles in Roedel (1992)). The dry deposition velocity for cadmium was set to zero due to lack of concrete information. The resulting fate factors are calculated and listed in Table 6.5.

	Dry deposition velocity V_p (Pacyna 1995)	$F_{air,air}$ (dry)	Dry deposition velocity V_p (Pacyna *et al.* 1985)	$F_{air,air}$ (dry)	$F_{air,air}$ (tot)	σ_g^2
	cm/s	m^2a/m^3	cm/s	m^2a/m^3	m^2a/m^3	-
	(1)	100/((1)·365·24 ·3600)	(2)	100/((2)·36 5·24· 3600)	100/(((2)+0.2)· 365·24·3600)	
Arsenic	0.1-0.4	32 E-6 - 8 E-6	0.2	16 E-6	8 E-6	4
Nickel	0.4-2	8 E-6 - 1.6 E-6	0.5	6 E-6	4.5 E-6	4
Chromium	0.3-0.9	11 E-6 - 3.5 E-6	0.4	8 E-6	5.3 E-6	4
Cadmium					16 E-6	8

Tab. 6.5: Calculation of the fate factors Fair,air from the deposition velocity. The wet deposition velocity is calculated by the ratio of the assumed dilution height of 800 m with the residence time due to wet deposition (τwet = 5 days) resulting at about 0.2 cm/s.

The resulting fate factors are more than one order of magnitude larger than what has been obtained with the multimedia fate model and close to what has been found empirically (see Tables 6.3 and 6.4). The geometric standard deviation has been estimated based on the range given for dry deposition and a similar assumption for the uncertainty of the wet deposition velocity.

6.2.5 Combination of the models for fate analysis

One of the shortcomings identified in Subsections 6.2.2 and 6.2.3 is the poor representation of the atmospheric compartment with a box of a fixed height of 1000 m. This limitation will be circumvented in a first step by introducing substance-specific mixing heights calculated with a model based on empirical data. The resulting fate factors will then be compared to the fate factors derived with other models in order to support the choice of the fate factors in Subsection 6.2.6.

Fate factors with substance-specific dilution height

As a pragmatic first step, we will calculate the specific dilution heights for each of the 52 substances. It would, of course, be better to partition the atmosphere into more than one compartment. However, this is feasible only if exchange rates between the compartments are known.

Substances with a residence time longer than about 1.4 days dilute, according to Jolliet *et al.* (1997b), not only within the lower 1000 m, but up to 10'000 m. A dilution height of 10'000 m is expected if the residence time is longer than 60 days. The basis for this estimate in Jolliet *et al.* (1997b) is small, but it seems reasonable that such a correlation exists. The following iterative procedure is proposed in order to include the relations given in Jolliet *et al.* (1997b) in the multimedia fate modelling:

Firstly, the average residence time per substance can be calculated with the multimedia model results listed in Appendix (6.4):

$$\tau_{i,air,air} = F_{i,air,air} \cdot V_{i,air} \qquad \text{where } V_{i,air} = 1000 \text{ m}^3/\text{m}^2 \tag{6.8}$$

The expected dilution height due to the resulting residence time can be calculated with (Jolliet *et al.* 1997b):

$$\text{if } \tau_{i,air,air} \geq 0.164 \text{ years} \qquad \text{then } V_{i,air} = 10'000 \text{ m}^3/\text{m}^2 \tag{6.9}$$

$$\text{else } V_{i,air} = c \cdot \tau_{i,air,air}^{\,b} \qquad [\text{m}^3/\text{m}^2] \tag{6.10}$$

with $c = 30'100$ m^3/(m^{2}a) ($14'000<c<64'000$) and $b = 0.61 \pm 0.37$

The results of the calculation of $V_{i,air}$ are listed in the second column of Appendix (6.5). From there, it can be seen that about a fourth of the substances dilute in the whole atmosphere (limited to 10'000 m). About half of the substances dilute from 1000 m up to 3000 m. The metals show a very low dilution height. This is incorrect, because metals in reality behave similar to particles, being adsorbed by them.

The new fate factors have been derived by changing the height of the atmosphere in the country file for each substance (Appendix 6.5). It is interesting to note that the fate factors from air to air, to water, and to soil always change by the same factor for each substance. This is consistent with the linearity of the Simplebox model. This multiplication factor is sometimes identical with the ratio between the old and the new dilution height. An independent, or a less than proportional behaviour, is found for metals, PAH, ethylene oxides, PCBs, dioxins, and some other substances. This indicates that their decay in air is not the dominant factor, but that adsorption processes at the surface and within the particles are. An initial emission to water, in contrast, changes the relation between the different fate factors.

The results from the first iteration can be used again to calculate $\tau_{i,air,air}$ and, from these, the second approximation of $V_{i,air}$. The result of this iteration is that convergence is good for all substances which are sensitive to the dilution height. The exception is PCB. The substances that are less sensitive to dilution height sometimes show a smaller convergence, but this has no influence on the fate factors. Only for PCB was it necessary to undertake a second iteration. Its result has been directly included in Appendix (6.5).

The proposed corrections of the dilution height have two important shortcomings:

- The relationship between residence time and dilution height is based on a small sample of empirical data with limited correlation ($R^2 = 0.82$). Other factors are omitted, even though they are important for the determination of the dilution height, such as the density of the substance.
- The atmospheric compartment gets larger for substances with a residence time longer than 1.4 days. This means that the realisation of a homogenous dilution is even less probable. The consequence is that the relevant average concentration 1 m above ground may be much different from the average concentration[25]. It is the concentration at ground level which is relevant for the real exchange behaviour between air, soil and water[26].

A comparison with other fate factors

The new results (Appendix 6.5) are compared for the 22 substances in the subset that is common with Jolliet *et al.* (1997b) (Table 6.6). 14 out of 22 substances show a ratio smaller than factor 2. Three substances show a factor between 2 and 10. Next to the heavy metals only 1,1,2,2 Tetrachlorethane is in poor agreement. This is due to a large difference in the assumptions about residence time, i.e., 700 days half live time according to Mackay *et al.* (1993) used in the multimedia model *versus* a residence time of only 38.4 days in Jolliet *et al.* (1997b). The fate factors for the four metals are not further discussed because it was already mentioned that the used multimedia fate model does not fit for these metals.

If we compare the fate factors calculated from empirical data with those from the multimedia model (Table 6.7), we notice that:

- The factors for benzene agree quite well. The calculation with the variable dilution height lowered the fate factor and it is now in good agreement with Jolliet *et al.* (1997b).
- A better agreement for dioxins had been expected. It is plausible that the measurements of background concentrations in Germany are biased towards higher

[25] The difference is already large between the 1.2 m above ground where children breath air and the height of 4.5m which, in Germany, is used for air quality measurements. A factor of almost two has been observed according to Greenpeace (1993) for diesel soot, PAH, NO and CO.

[26] More sophisticated models like Gaussian plume dispersion models for local dilution and Lagrangian trajectory models for long-range transport have been developed for this reason (see, e.g., ExternE 1995). These models allow for making more accurate predictions of ground level concentrations, but need more information than is available from LCI. This means that the partitioning of the atmosphere into several compartments is needed in the future to allow for a more accurate modelling of ground level concentrations and for keeping down the amount of information needed on the sources of emissions.

concentrations[27]. It is also clear that the relevant exposure path for humans is not inhalation, i.e., the intake by food is decisive.

- For BaP, the difference is small and may partly be explained by biased background concentration measurements.

Substance name (Jolliet *et al.* 1997b)	Residence time (Jolliet *et al.* 1997b)	Fate factor (Jolliet *et al.* 1997b)	Height of dilution (Jolliet *et al.* 1997b)	$F'_{air,air}$ (App. 6.5)	Ratio F (Jolliet *et al.* 1997b) to $F'_{air,air}$	Height of dilution (App. 6.5)
	(1)	(2)	(1)/(2)	(3)	(2)/(3)	eq. 8-10
	[days]	[m^2a/m^3]	[m^3/m^2]	[m^2a/m^3]	[-]	[m^3/m^2]
1,1,2,2-Tetrachloroethane	38.4	1.38E-05	7617	2.8E-04	0.05	10000
1,1,2-Trichloroethane	36.5	1.35E-05	7394	1.5E-05	0.88	9005
1,2-Dichloroethane	**52.6**	**1.56E-05**	**9236**	3.2E-05	0.49	10000
1,3-Butadiene	**0.1**	**1.54E-06**	**246**	2.5E-06	0.63	514
1,4-Dioxane	**1.5**	**3.85E-06**	**1038**	3.8E-06	1.01	1016
Acrylonitrile	2.4	4.69E-06	1411	6.5E-06	0.72	2356
Arsenic	11	8.46E-06	3547	3.7E-07	23.07	241
Benzene	9.4	7.97E-06	3236	7.9E-06	1.01	3148
Benzyl chloride	**4**	**5.72E-06**	**1924**	6.8E-06	0.85	2496
Bis-(Chloromethyl)ether	**0.04**	**9.03E-07**	**107**	3.8E-06	0.24	1029
Cadmium	11	8.46E-06	3547	5.3E-07	15.91	303
Chloroform	80.4	2.20E-05	10000	3.2E-05	0.70	10000
Chromium	11	8.46E-06	3547	5.0E-07	17.06	290
Dibenzodioxins and furans	4	1.10E-06	10000	9E-06	0.12	1696
Dibutyl phthalate	1.3	3.72E-06	983	4.8E-06	0.78	1414
Dichloromethane	**116.9**	**3.20E-05**	**10000**	2.3E-05	1.42	10000
Epichlorohydrin	**26.3**	**1.19E-05**	**6051**	6.6E-06	1.80	2358
Formaldehyde	1.2	3.58E-06	923	3.3E-06	1.08	894
Nickel	11	8.46E-06	3547	2.9E-07	29.00	210
Styrene	0.1	1.38E-06	207	2.0E-06	0.67	386
Trichloroethene	4.8	6.14E-06	2150	6.2E-06	0.99	2172
Vinyl chloride	**1.7**	**4.13E-06**	**1158**	5.7E-06	0.73	1908

Tab. 6.6: Comparison of the fate factors (emissions to air, concentrations in air) calculated by Jolliet *et al.* (1997b) with those in Appendix (6.5). The substances printed in bold type are calculated with degradation times because their residence times (including deposition) are unavailable. The fate factors printed in bold types can therefore be understood as maximum estimates.

Fate Factors $F_{air,air}$	Empirical factors for Germany (Table 6.3)	Empirical factors (Jolliet *et al.* 1997b) (Table 6.6)	Multi-media modelling with dilution height = 1000m (Appendix 6.4)	Multi-media modelling with var. dilution height (Table 6.6)
	m^2a/m^3	m^2a/m^3	m^2a/m^3	m^2a/m^3
2,3,7,8-TCDD	21-180 E-6	1.1 E-6	9 E-6	9 E-6
BaP	7-190 E-6		5.4 E-6	5.4 E-6
Benzene	5-53 E-6	8 E-6	25 E-6	7.9 E-6

Tab. 6.7: Comparison of the empirical fate factors and the fate factors from the multimedia model.

Are the fate factors more accurate now?

The Simplebox model (version 1.0) has now been adapted to include a substance specific atmospheric dilution. This introduces an additional uncertainty via the estimated relationship for the dilution height. Disregarding the real height profile of concentrations introduces a bias: concentrations for inhaled air as well as those for drinking water and for food are too low.

[27] The stations where air pollutants are measured are not evenly distributed, but sited at neuralgic places and next to research institutes. In general, this siting leads to a bias towards higher average concentrations.

The comparison with the data given in Jolliet *et al.* (1997b) suggests that the improvement in the quality of the data is relevant. This might be considered an artefact only. The same formula has been used in both cases to calculate the dilution height which is based on only a small set of empirical data. It is well-known that the atmosphere consists of different layers and that they mix well or badly depending on the meteorological situation. The exchange behaviour is determined to a large extent by the prevalent temperature gradient. We assume that the Formula (6.8) that is used to calculate the dilution height is, in general, more a source of uncertainty and does not improve the results. The small basis on which the formula rests is one of the reasons, but more important is the fact that we are interested mainly in concentrations close to the ground. Enlarging the volume that will mix is only increasing the error made by assuming a homogeneously mixed atmosphere. Consistent with this reasoning, we will use the formula here only for substances where the dilution height is smaller than 1000 m. The proposed model adaptation will reduce uncertainty for sure if this restriction is observed.

6.2.6 The results of fate modelling

The fate factors to be used are selected as follows:

- They are based on the results from Appendix (6.4).
- The model adaptation with a substance-specific dilution height has been used only for 1,3-butadiene, formaldehyde, styrene, 1,1-dichlorethylene, and aldrin. For these substances the results from Appendix (6.5) have been taken.
- The fate factor *Fair,air* for diesel soot particles is the one taken from the calculation in Subsection 6.2.4.
- The fate factors *Fair,air* for the heavy metals are the ones listed in Table 6.5.

The final compilation of the fate factors is given in Appendix (6.6).

The Figures 6.6 and 6.7 show the shares of the intake by air, drinking water and food for the substances that have been modelled[28]. This illustration is the visual translation of the data in the forbidding looking tables in the appendices and should help to clarify the meaning embedded in all that data. The substances are ranked according to their share of the intake by inhalation. It is obvious that the inhalation path is more important if the initial emission's compartment is air than if it is water and analogously for intake by drinking water.

But these two figures also illustrate the very important finding that there are a large number of substances where a large share of the intake occurs through impact paths via the non-emitting compartments. It is this finding which points to the relevance of the multimedia approach proposed here.

The inhalation path dominates the intake if the substance is emitted to air for more than half the substances. The other substances are dominated by the intake through

[28] For the transformation from fate factors to intake, we need information on the amounts of inhaled and absorbed air, of drinking water, and of body weight. USES (1994) assumes for inhalation an absorption of 75%. The average lung capacity was set at 20 m^3/day and the average water intake at 2 l/day. The average body weight was assumed to be 70 kg. With these numbers the daily intake by different paths can be calculated.

food. That is, drinking water can be disregarded as a path for emissions to air for all but three substances (Figure 6.6). It is interesting to mention here that for a few substances such as arsenic, cadmium, nickel, PAHs, PCBs, dioxins, and hexachlorobenzene, the fate factor to drinking water by emission to air is larger than by emission to water (Appendix 6.6). This is due to the assumption that drinking water is in part making use of groundwater. Groundwater is, for these substances, more polluted by dry and wet deposition from air than the surface water.

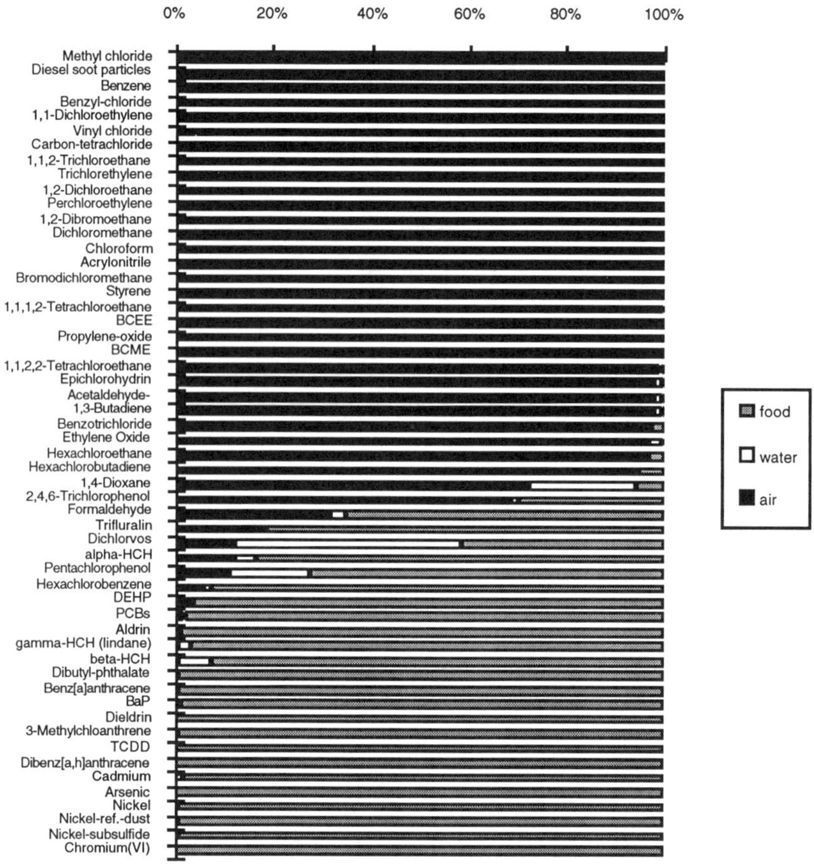

Fig. 6.6: Relative intake by humans for an emission to air based on the fate factors in Appendix (6.6) and on typical intake behaviour

For emissions to surface waters (Figure 6.7) the intake by drinking water is dominant for almost a third of the substances. Inhalation is the main intake path for the surprisingly high share of again one third of the substances. In these instances the substances diffuse after the initial emission to water into air. Intake by food is the dominant intake path for the last third of the substances (Figure 6.7).

Substance clusters are formed when the substances are ranked according to the share of intake by inhalation. Substances where the dominant intake path is by inhalation have a high vapour pressure and a low water solubility. Substances found in food are characterised by high octanol-water partition coefficients and are therefore prone to a high rate of bioaccumulation. High water solubility, low Kow and low Henry coefficients increase the probability for a relevant intake by drinking water.

A presentation of the absolute rather than relative values would reveal that the differences in the absolute intake are very large. They vary by up to six orders of magnitude. The qualitative grouping of the substances undertaken here is therefore an unsuitable basis for a quantitative fate analysis.

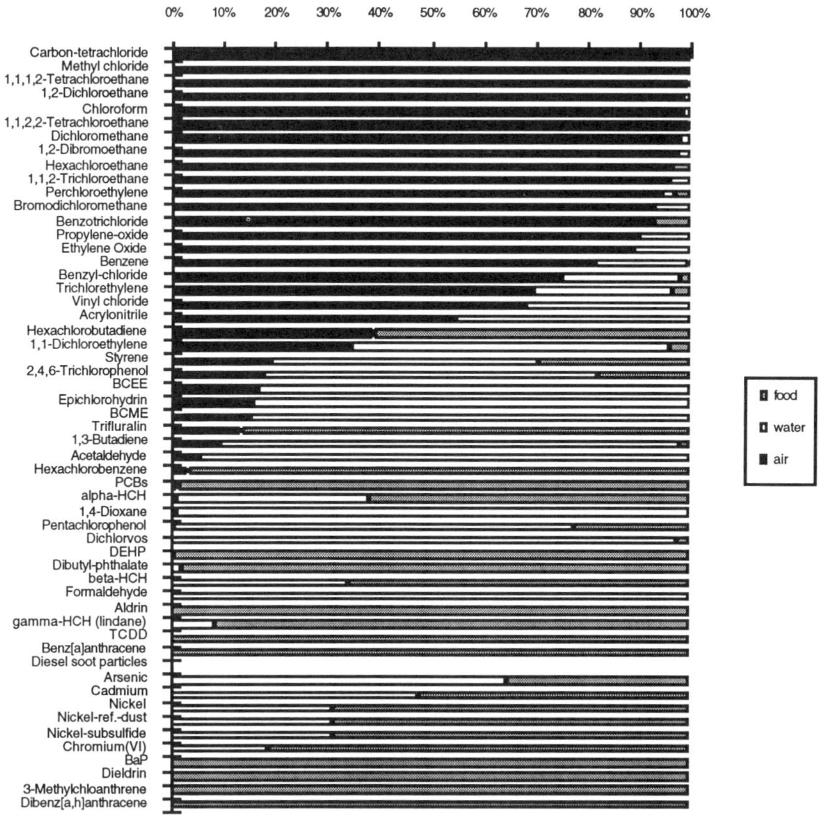

Fig. 6.7: Relative intake by humans for an emission to surface water based on the fate factors in Appendix (6.6) and on typical intake behaviour

Evaluation and conclusions

A multimedia fate model of the Mackay level III type has been chosen to calculate, for 54 carcinogenic substances[29], the fate factors for inhalation of air, for drinking water and for food for the substances' emissions to air and surface water, respectively. The model area is a kind of unit world reflecting average European conditions and abstracting from the high seas. The climate factors in this European world are averaged and constant, all humans breath outdoor air and eat a standard diet composed of fish, crops, cattle meat, and milk. The substance specific dilution height has been calculated for five substances with an assumed atmospheric dilution height lower than 1000 m (the default of the model used for the calculations) and then incorporated into the model. The model used for the dilution height calculations is based on a few substances only. The empirical relationships and the residence times have been taken from the literature. The fate factors *Fair,air* for soot and the heavy metals have been calculated based on measured residence times and dry deposition velocities and assumptions of the height of the mixing layer and wet deposition velocities. No metabolites have been taken into account.

To a certain extent it was possible to validate this multimedia model for fate factors from air to air (Table 6.6 and 6.7). All the other fate factors could not be validated in this investigation. The multimedia model chosen here will become a standard for substance risk assessment in Europe. This is a different purpose than the one we have used it for, i.e., we are not interested in whether NOEC's may become exceeded under certain conditions or not, we are interested rather in modelling, as accurately as possible, an average exposure to human beings. One has to keep in mind that the two purposes do not place the same demands on the model.

An earlier full-scale validation of the model has revealed considerable uncertainties and deviations from reality which partly have compensated each other in the integrated intake modelling.

The different intake paths within the damage function will be multiplied by effect factors. The uncertainty assessment therefore has to be done primarily for the intake paths which turn out to be the dominant ones. That is, high uncertainty of fate factors for negligible paths does not influence the reliability of the damage estimate.

A quantitative estimate of the uncertainty in the fate factors listed in Appendix (6.6) can be undertaken based on:

- the experts' judgement in SETAC (1995),
- the experience gained with the validation exercises undertaken here,
- the insights from the discussion in Subsections 6.2.2/3 of the accuracy of the model and model parameters that had been chosen, and
- the distribution and intake behaviour of the substances given in Figure 6.6 and 6.7.

Meier (1997) and Rabl (1996) state explicitly, based on their experience, that the distribution of the values that they assume to be stochastically spread can be approximated by a lognormal distribution. Van de Meent (1995) calculated probability

[29] We include here both nickel-subsulfide and nickel refinery dust as substances nr. 53 and nr. 54 although they are not modelled separately from elementary nickel.

distributions with a Monte Carlo Simulation which could, for most substances, be approximated with a lognormal distribution. SETAC (1995) makes this assumption implicitly. The fate factors are always positive and the distribution can be assumed to be oblique. Therefore the fate factors in Appendix (6.6) are assumed to be the mean value of a lognormal distribution with a geometric standard deviation σg. The estimates of σg^2 for the three fate factors are listed in Table 6.8. According to Appendix (6.8), the mean value multiplied and divided by σg^2 covers the confident interval of 95%.

The criteria used for assigning the substances to one of three uncertainty classes for emission to air and water is given in the first column in Table 6.8. The metals[30] and phenols are both placed into class with the highest uncertainty because they do not or only partly fit with the model restrictions. Other substances belong to the most uncertain class because they either showed poor accordance with the results from Jolliet *et al.* (1997b) (i.e., Tetrachloroethane) or were calculated with default degradation rates for relevant compartments (Appendix 6.1). In contradiction to SETAC (1995), we assumed in the case of the most uncertain class the same additional uncertainty factors for the first and second change of media as we did for the first two classes. We chose this procedure because most of the substances in this class with the largest geometric standard deviations have their main intake path via food; but this path is assumed to have a better quality than is suggested by the $\sigma g^2 = 500$ proposed by SETAC (1995). All other σg^2 in Table 6.8 are directly taken from SETAC (1995) (see also end of Subsection 6.2.3 for the details).

The estimated geometric standard deviations in Table 6.8 include both stochastic and systematic errors. The stochastic errors alone, relevant if the fate relative to a reference substance is determined, would result in smaller standard deviations. However, we do stay with the assessment of the absolute fate factors because our aim is the modelling of absolute potential damages.

Further work on the validation of multimedia fate models is necessary to improve the expert-based estimates made here (Table 6.8). Comparisons of model outcomes are currently ongoing (Jolliet 1997).

[30] The $F_{air,air}$ for the metals are an exception because they are modelled based on deposition velocities. Table 6.5 suggests a σ_g^2 of 4 which will be used here.

Criteria	Substances concerned (for emission to air)	σ_g^2 $F''_{air,air}$	σ_g^2 $F''_{air,water}$	σ_g^2 $F''_{air,food}$
• More than 95% of the total intake is inhaled, i.e., the substance shows only minor partitioning • The properties are well known • The substance is well suited for the chosen model	Methyl chloride, 1,1,1,2-Tetrachloroethane, 1,2-Dichloroethane, Chloroform, Dichloromethane, 1,2-Dibromoethane, Hexachloroethane, 1,1,2-Trichloroethane, Perchloroethylene, Bromodichloromethane, Ethylene oxide, Benzene, Benzyl-chloride, Trichlorethylene, Vinyl chloride, Acrylonitrile, Epichlorhydrin, Diesel soot particles, 1,1 Dichlorethylene, Carbon-tetrachloride, Styrene, BCEE, BCME, Acetaldehyde, 1,3-Butadiene	2	4	8
• The substance partitions • The properties are well known • The substance is well suited for the chosen model	Trifluralin, Hexachlorobenzene, alpha-HCH, Dichlorvos, DEHP, Dibutyl-phthalate, beta-HCH, Formaldehyde, Aldrin, gamma-HCH, 1,4-Dioxane, PCBs, Benz[a]anthracene, BaP, Dieldrin, 3-Methylchloanthrene, TCDD, Dibenz[a,h]anthracene	3	6	12
• The properties are uncertain or unknown, or • The substance is not well suited for the chosen model	Arsenic, Cadmium, Nickel, Nickel-ref.-dust, Nickel-subsulfide, Chromium(VI), Propylene-oxide, 1,1,2,2-Tetrachloroethane, Benzotrichloride, Hexachlorobutadiene, 2,4,6-Trichlorphenol, Pentachlorphenol	20 (§)	40	80

Criteria	Substances concerned (for emission to water)	σ_g^2 $F''_{water,air}$	σ_g^2 $F''_{water,water}$	σ_g^2 $F''_{water,food}$
• More than 95% of the total intake is by drinking water, i.e., the substance shows only minor partitioning • The properties are well known • The substance is well suited for the chosen model	Acetaldehyde, Dichlorvos, 1,4-Dioxane, Formaldehyde	4	2	8
• The substance partitions • The properties are well known • The substance is well suited for the chosen model	Trifluralin, Hexachlorobenzene, alpha-HCH, DEHP, Dibutyl-phthalate, beta-HCH, Aldrin, gamma-HCH, PCBs, Benz[a]anthracene, BaP, Dieldrin, 3-Methylchloanthrene, TCDD, Dibenz[a,h]anthracene, Methyl chloride, 1,1,1,2-Tetrachloroethane, 1,2-Dichloroethane, Chloroform, Dichloromethane, 1,2-Dibromoethane, Hexachloroethane, 1,1,2-Trichloroethane, Perchloroethylene, Bromodichloromethane, Ethylene oxide, Benzene, Benzyl-chloride, Trichlorethylene, Vinyl chloride, Acrylonitrile, Epichlorhydrin, Diesel soot particles, 1,1 Dichlorethylene, Carbon-tetrachloride, Styrene, BCEE, BCME, 1,3-Butadiene	6	3	12
• The properties are uncertain or unknown, or • The substance is not well suited for the chosen model	Arsenic, Cadmium, Nickel, Nickel-ref.-dust, Nickel-subsulfide, Chromium(VI), Propylene-oxide, 1,1,2,2-Tetrachloroethane, Benzotrichloride, Hexachlorobutadiene, 2,4,6-Trichlorphenol, Pentachlorphenol	40	20	80

Tab. 6.8: Estimated geometric standard deviations for the calculated fate factors. The mean values for the fate factors are given in Appendix (6.6). § see Table 6.5 for the heavy metals

6.3 Effect analysis

6.3.1 Overview

The most important information on the mechanisms of carcinogenesis, on the risk factors, and on the pathways analysed, have already been given in Section 6.1. In this section a quantitative effect analysis for the 55 chemical carcinogens identified in Section 6.2 will be performed.

The next subsection will use Cultural Theory (Chapter 3) to discuss how one could look at the interpretation of different degrees of evidence on human carcinogenesis. Subsection 6.3.3 will introduce straightforwardly the unit-risk concept used by WHO and U.S. EPA. Subsection 6.3.4 will explain the compilation of the unit-risk data base. From this the effect factor *Eik* for substance *i* and exposure path *k* can be calculated. The embedding of these effect factors in the damage function in order to calculate the incidence of cancer *Tijk* (tumour factor) will be shown in Subsection 6.3.5. The last subsection will end with a quantitative statement of the uncertainty.

6.3.2 Human carcinogens and the certainty of effects

Qualitative risk assessment and classification systems

Providing evidence of a causal link between agent and tumour incidence is a complex task and needs the consideration of all kinds of experimental results and epidemiological studies (see, e.g., Lewtas 1993). The International Agency for Research on Cancer (IARC) is one scientific body performing such qualitative risk assessments. It uses a classification system to group substances according to the evidence available on human or animal carcinogenity. The descriptions of these Groups are reproduced in Tab. 6.9.

Group	Description
1	The agent, mixture, or exposure circumstance is carcinogenic to humans.
2A	The agent, mixture, or exposure circumstance is probably carcinogenic to humans (a positive association has been observed between exposure and human cancer for which a causal interpretation is credible, but chance, bias, or confounding could not be ruled out with reasonable confidence; there is also sufficient evidence of carcinogenity in experimental animals).
2B	The agent, mixture, or exposure circumstance is possibly carcinogenic to humans (there is sufficient evidence of carcinogenity in experimental animals, but no adequate data on cancer in exposed humans).
3	The agent, mixture, or exposure circumstance is not classifiable as to its carcinogenity to humans (this Group applies if no other category is used).
4	The agent, mixture, or exposure circumstance is probably not carcinogenic to humans.

Tab. 6.9: IARC-Classification of substances (e.g., Vainio *et al.* 1991)

In addition to the IARC classification, there exist many other systems to classify carcinogenic substances[31]. A comparable and also frequently used system is the

[31] Becher *et al.* (1995) introduce a system to measure the suitability of the unit risk concept per substance. For each substance, they attribute one of the following notions: UR++ = unit risk is very suitable, UR+ = unit risk is suitable, UR- = unit risk is not suitable. This classification is not widely used and unavailable for many of the substances looked at here. Thus, it is dropped from any further

classification used by the Environmental Protection Agency (EPA) of the United States of America (Table 6.10).

Category	Description
A	Proven human carcinogen
B1	Limited evidence from human studies and sufficient evidence from animal studies
B2	Inadequate evidence from human studies and sufficient evidence from animal studies
C	Possible human carcinogen
D	Not classifiable as to human carcinogenity
E	Evidence on non-carcinogenity for humans
None	No data

Tab. 6.10: U.S. EPA-Classification of carcinogenic substances (USEPA 1986)

Group 1 from IARC corresponds to category A of EPA. 2A is similar to B1 and 2B to B2, but EPA category C is also similar to 2B. Group 4 is equal to EPA category E, and EPA categories D and *none* are covered by IARC Group 3.

Until 1993, IARC had tested 768 agents so far. Their classification is indicated in Table 6.11. 317 of them are thought to be, at least possibly, carcinogenic to humans and only one (Caprolactam) is probably not carcinogenic to humans. This 41% share of substances that are at least possibly carcinogenic is unlikely to hold for all the substances as yet untested[32]. The substances that have been tested so far are a biased sample because the most suspect substances were tested first.

IARC Classification	Number of agents
Carcinogenic to humans (Group 1)	60
Probably carcinogenic to humans (Group 2A)	51
Possibly carcinogenic to humans (Group 2B)	206
Cannot be classified as to its carcinogenity to humans (Group 3)	450
Probably not carcinogenic to humans (Group 4)	1
Total	768

Tab. 6.11 Overall evaluations of carcinogenity to humans in the IARC Monographs program (volumes 1-58) (IARC 1993b)

The relevance of these official classification systems will be discussed after an excursus on epidemiological studies.

The problems of epidemiological studies

One has to distinguish between three types of epidemiological studies: ecological (cross-sectional), cohort, and case-control studies. The use of ecological epidemiological studies for the deduction of cancer risks due to environmental pollutants is extremely difficult for many reasons. Four of the most important ones are mentioned here:

evaluation. Brusick (1991) presents the classification of the International Commission for Protection against Environmental Mutagens and Carcinogens. The proposed system includes in vivo as well as in vitro results and ends in agents' scores and a much more detailed classification system. The system is largely based on genetic tests to predict carcinogenity. These tests are not widely accepted and the classification is therefore not considered any further in this study. ECETOC (1996) presents the classification system used by the European Union.

[32] One should keep in mind that over 2800 compounds have been identified in ambient air in 1985 (USEPA 1990). Adams (1995) points out that we do not know much about the vast majority of chemicals: from millions of different chemical substances only 7000 have been tested, about 1500 have been found to be carcinogenic in animals, and only 60 have been definitely linked with cancer in humans.

- Cancer is a cumulative effect with a long latency time. Present exposures have therefore little to do with observed incidence rates.
- Lifestyle dependent factors such as smoking are much more important than ambient concentrations in air and water. To correct for these factors makes studies in many cases inconclusive.
- To assess the actual exposure (over centuries) is normally impossible. The technical means to measure a number of substances at ambient concentrations has only existed for a few years.
- The natural variation is normally larger than the effect to be observed. For example, the overall cancer risk is about 25% in the USA (and similarly in Europe); the calculated extra-risk for exposure to formaldehyde in urban ambient air is smaller than 0.008%. To differentiate between a risk of 25% and of 25.008% within a confidence interval of 95% is impossible for the sizes of populations that are available (Graham 1993).

Pershagen *et al.* (1993) give a good overview of epidemiological studies that assess the evidence on the link between outdoor air pollution and cancer. The authors adduce results from ecological epidemiological studies that show significantly higher risks for cancer of the bronchus and of the trachea in urban than in rural areas in Japan and 9 European countries. The significance of the risk is higher for women due to their lower baseline risk. The interpretation of these results has to reflect the fact that average tobacco consumption is higher in urban areas. Hemminki *et al.* (1994) review results from 7 cohort studies on lung cancer. A correction was made for smoking behaviour. The studies show a relative risk that is up to 1.5 higher for smokers living in urban versus those living in rural areas. For non-smokers the number of cases was generally too small to produce conclusive results. Van Kessel *et al.* (1992) show some correlation between specific industries and the risks of lung cancer, but state in their summary that *"...the value of ecological analysis is limited..."*.

Case-control studies give much more detailed information on long-term exposures and differences in lifestyle. From such studies much more reliable results can be expected. Pershagen *et al.* (1993) and Hemminki *et al.* (1994) review such studies and state that many of the studies do not provide evidence for a higher cancer risk due to outdoor air pollution. But the adjusted relative risk for urban populations that is based on cohort studies is confirmed in general, although some studies were inconclusive. Occupational studies that look at locations with known high concentration exposure deliver the most relevant quantitative information on causal relationships for cancer risk due to exposure to pollutants. The extrapolation of these results to low doses can only be undertaken based on assumptions about the cancer-causing mechanisms (see next subsection).

The sample size needed to detect significant causalities between environmental exposure to single substances and cancer cases is much too large for many different research designs for epidemiological studies. Only elevated exposure levels as in the case of occupational exposure allow for cohort and case-control studies with the hope for significant outcomes.

Causality, evidence and attitudes toward risk

We have seen that there are serious limitations on the evidence about a link between exposure to single substances and carcinogenity. The long latency time, the very small additional risk due to all the other risk factors, and well-known problems with the transfer of dose relationships from animals to humans and from high to low doses are all responsible for some of the most bothersome uncertainties in this assessment.

The information given in Table 6.11 should be a warning. It seems almost impossible to prove that a substance is not carcinogenic at high concentrations. The decision makers have to decide whether they would like to allocate their resources primarily to the protection against proven human carcinogens or extend it to substances on which there is less evidence. In other words, should the calculated risks estimated for IARC Group 1, 2A, 2B or 3, respectively, be added-up, weighted by a factor of evidence, or should a cut-off criterion be used[33]?

The answer to this question is considered to be a matter of the world view held by decision-makers (that can be collective ones too) and their management styles. The question can be approached by expert judgement, but in this book we argue that there can be multiple answers depending on the cultural perspective chosen. This approach has already been introduced in Chapter 3.

The question is whether the proven risks should be reduced with highest priority (risk reduction principle) or if all the substances possibly causing damage to human health should be managed, i.e., if the prevention principle should be applied. It has to be stated here that this differentiation is not based on different uncertainty factors related to the quantitative risk estimates. Rather, it is based on the inherent uncertainty if carcinogenic effects to humans occur at all.

A proposal for a way to introduce arguments for the in- or exclusion of substances when there is limited evidence for carcinogenic potential which makes use of specific cultural perspectives is proposed in Table 6.12[34]. The aim of this approach is to produce more consistent value choices within the whole impact assessment framework (see Section 3.4). It has to be mentioned here that in contrast to many other value-laden choices this one will not lead just to slightly different weightings of the different criteria. The consequence of introducing the cultural perspective here is that three different indicators will be constructed to assess carcinogenic substances.

[33] All the non-tested substances are missing here and are considered by the index for unknown damage (see Section 4.4).

[34] Swanson *et al.* 1997 chose another way to deal with the different levels of evidence. They assigned the highest hazard value to Group 1 substances and decreasing hazard values to the subsequent Groups. This can be judged as an attribution of weights of evidence. In a proposal for the relative risk-based environmental indicator methodology designed to aggregate the data from the Toxic Release Inventory (TRI), it is suggested to apply a weight of evidence as well. SAB (1997) agrees in principle with this step, but requests a policy judgement by U.S. EPA in order to take account of the highly subjective nature of these weights. These weights are highly subjective and supported only by one group of decision makers, if at all. Therefore, we discard the weight-of-evidence approach.

Cultural Perspective	Attitude and Argumentation	Choice
Individualist	The individualist prefers an adaptive management style which means that resources are spent for proven harm to human health at the moment of decision. The decision will immediately be adjusted if new evidence emerges so as to realise an optimal resource allocation. Risks which have not yet resulted in evident harm are accepted. Such an attitude makes it possible to consider Group 1 substances only because of the limited evidence for all other substances.	Group 1
Hierarchist	The hierarchist's management style is to control situations. He is therefore closest to the authoritative bodies in government and in international organisations. The responsibility for the group and towards the leader of the group demands finding a balance between evidence and probability. WHO (1987, 1996a) gives in its guidelines risk estimates for a small selection of Group 1, 2A and 2B substances. Substances from Group 3 are not included because this could lead to an unjustified cut-back of needs already expressed by society.	Groups 1, 2A, 2B
Egalitarian	The risk aversive and preventive management style asks for an attentive attitude towards risk management. Egalitarians are well aware that many substances in the inclusive Group 3 might in the coming decades be proven to be potent human carcinogens. The responsibility towards the others in the group (and coming generations) leads to the inclusion of all risk factors. Egalitarians may be ready to reduce the satisfaction of their needs in order to spend more resources on risk prevention than individualists or hierarchists would accept (however this is here not the important point).	Groups 1-3

Tab. 6.12: Different choices due to the world view and management style of different cultural perspectives (see also Chapter 3 for more detail on the Cultural Theory)

6.3.3 The unit-risk concept for the estimation of the dose-response relationship

In Section 6.2 we used different models to assess external exposure. In this subsection we are looking for a quantitative model to predict the incidence of cancer based on external exposure, i.e., the dose-response relationship. This relationship should be quantified so that it can satisfy the needs of LCA. It should be able to discriminate between single substances (including the common sum parameters measured at emission sources). The dose-response relationship should be valid in particular for human beings as we are interested in human cancers only.

WHO (1987) introduced a model that has since been known as the unit lifetime risk or unit risk concept. This model was already in use at that time within EPA under the name of "average relative risk model" (EPA 1983). The WHO model can be described as follows:

The unit risk factor for inhalation is an estimate of the probability that an average individual will develop cancer when exposed to a pollutant at an ambient concentration of one microgram per cubic meter ($\mu g/m^3$) for the individual's life (70 years).

All kinds of studies and experiments have been analysed to develop these unit risk factors (UR). For the estimates that are based on epidemiological data the following relation has been used (WHO 1987):

$$UR = \frac{Po(R-1)}{X} \quad (6.11)$$

where UR unit lifetime risk [tumour cases per μg/m^3]

Po background lifetime risk (from age/cause-specific death or incidence rates found in national vital statistics tables using the life table methodology, or it is available from a matched control population) [tumour cases]

R relative risk, being the ratio between the observed and expected number of cancer cases in the exposed population [-]

X lifetime average exposure; standardised lifetime exposure of the study population on a lifetime continuous exposure basis (in the case of occupational studies, X is calculated by a conversion of the occupational 8-hour, 240-day exposure over a specific number of working years) [μg/m^3]

The unit risk due to its dependence on *Po* is in principle dependent on the country-specific background lifetime risk. We will use unit risk factors from WHO Europe, U.S. EPA, and Germany; countries for whom it can be assumed that the respective populations have encountered at least a similar pattern of background lifetime risk.

Some additional important assumptions are necessary:

- The response is a function of *cumulative dose* or exposure. This assumption is a big help when the concept is applied to LCA where no information on the time pattern of doses is available. This also means that the carcinogen is supposed to be active throughout all stages of the cancer development process, an assumption which is not necessarily true.
- There is *no threshold dose* for genotoxic chemical carcinogens. This assumption has already been discussed in Section 6.1 and is supported by many scientific advisory bodies (WHO 1996a, IRIS 1996, LAI 1992). This no-threshold behaviour is consistent with the knowledge that most carcinogenic agents cause irreversible damage to DNA.
- The linear extrapolation of the measured dose-response curve towards zero gives a conservative upper-bound estimate if the unknown true dose-response function has a sigmoid shape. This assumption is discussed later.

As we have already mentioned, it is difficult to identify with epidemiological studies cancer risks due to environmental exposure. Occupational studies are mostly used for this purpose. These studies often suffer from multi-agent exposure and, in most cases, from incomplete knowledge about past exposures (long periods due to the long latency time).

Animal bioassays[35] of chemicals are used additionally to improve the knowledge base provided by epidemiological studies. These assays are sometimes used to estimate unit risk factors as well.

[35] These are in vivo-tests. In vitro-tests with animal or human cells are not used due to the high variability and uncertainty of the test results. The Ames test is one of the most famous in vitro-tests. It is widely used to test new substances for their mutagenic potential (Seidel 1996).

It is clear from this short introduction that the unit risk concept is based on several questionable assumptions. The following major sources of uncertainty should be kept in mind (USEPA 1990 and others):

- It is assumed that the *ambient levels* for each pollutant either *average out or remain constant.* Both assumptions are seldom met in reality. In most cases, concentrations are either increasing or decreasing.
- It is assumed that *people stay* put at the same place (characterised by constant exposure) for their whole lifetime, but people do move in many cases from rural to urban areas and *vice versa.*
- The cancer risk due to inhalation assumes continuos *outdoor* exposure, but on the one hand, people spend most of their time indoors. It is known that indoor exposure to tobacco smoke, radon, formaldehyde, and other VOCs is several times higher than out-of-doors. On the other hand, it is unclear to what extent trace metals and PICs[36] penetrate indoors (if there are no indoor sources). Fishbein *et al.* (1993) give estimates of the ratio of indoor to outdoor concentrations for several substances. Only suspended particles are lower indoors for up to 50% if there are no indoor sources. Higher indoor concentrations can be expected for most other carcinogenic substances, especially if there are also indoor sources for them. We assume for the time being that higher indoor concentrations are relevant only if LCAs are performed that include indoor pollution and that indoor concentrations are comparable to outdoor ones in all other cases, i.e., full penetration is assumed[37].
- All risks are assumed to be *additive*. Synergistic and antagonistic interactions are considered to be irrelevant. At a minimum, this assumption is inapplicable[38] in the case of smokers who experience synergistic effects in comparison to non-smokers due to urban air pollutants (e.g., Hemminki *et al.* 1994).
- The extrapolation to low ambient air concentrations from toxicity data or epidemiological studies that have made use of high exposure requires making assumptions about the slope of the curve. There exists the additional uncertainty when toxicity data from animal studies (mostly mice and rats) is transferred to the human model. A *non-threshold behaviour is assumed* in all of these cases. The linearised multistage procedure used by U.S. EPA leads to a plausible upper limit for the risk. Lutz (1997) concludes from a discussion of the linearity of several processes in carcinogenesis that a sublinear behaviour of the dose - mutation curve could be expected. This leads one to overestimate the unit risk factors for the linear extrapolations to low doses. LAI (1992) points out that supralinear (concave) dose - mutation functions could also be expected due to saturation effects. It concludes therefore that the unit risk concept with linear extrapolation does not produce a clear overestimation of the cancer risk. It makes use of several extrapolation models. ECETOC (1996) discusses a number of mathematical models and concludes that with rare exceptions they cannot be recommended. It recommends instead to perform the evaluation on a case-by-case basis. ECETOC's

[36] Products of Incomplete Combustion.

[37] If the unit risk factors are derived from epidemiological studies, the compatibility of exposure modelling and effect factor is much better because epidemiological studies are mostly based on outdoor measurements as well.

[38] Wilson (1971) even found that *"synergistic effects among chemical pollutants are more often present than not"*.

criticism is a valid one and should be considered, but it is not helpful for our purpose due to its failure to provide guidance on how to improve the possibilities for estimating dose-response relationships. USEPA (1990:ES-4) states: *"The estimate of cancer risk for each pollutant, considering the unit risk factor alone, is conservative; that is, while the actual risk may be higher, it is more likely to be lower and may even be as low as zero"*. This judgement is partly due to the fact that not only proven human carcinogens, but also the effects of probable and of possible human carcinogens, are included in the estimate.

- In most cases, a large number of assumptions are necessary concerning the endpoints and the effects of chemicals, the relevant exposure of humans, and the way substances interact inside the human body. Unit risk estimates are therefore subject to continuous update whenever new discoveries are made.

All these assumptions and limitations are accepted in the field of health policy and they are compatible with LCA philosophy and needs. We therefore continue to use the unit risk concept[39], but adapt it making use of Cultural Theory in such a way that it reflects the different degrees of evidence for the causalities (Subsection 6.3.2).

6.3.4 The compilation of the unit risk factors

For LCA we need consistent quantitative estimates of the carcinogenic potential of substances emitted through anthropogenic activities and that have been measured in the respective exhaust streams. We therefore need large databases with a large range of consistent assessments. IRIS (1996) contains the largest database for unit risks and slope factors[40] for carcinogenics. This database is continuously updated and published by the U.S. EPA. All the substances for which this database gives unit risk estimates are listed in Appendix (6.7). The list has been structured according to the IARC Group classification of the substances. The data are largely based on IRIS, however, it is completed with additional data from USEPA (1990), LAI (1992), and WHO (1987, 1996a,b)[41]. The values for the substances for which more than one source is available are given in Table 6.13. As a rule, the latest risk estimate has been used and, if two sources are published in the same year, the value from the more internationally-oriented organisation has been preferred, i.e., WHO before U.S. EPA. The estimate for vinyl chloride listed in WHO (1987) has been preferred because the year of the estimate in USEPA (1990) could not be identified.

[39] There are other concepts such as the *individual life time lost* introduced by Becher *et al.* (1995). The main difference is that not the risk, but that average hours life time lost are calculated. This system is not widely used and only little data for a few substances is available. The approach taken here ends up with a similar concept as we will see in Section 6.4. ILSI (1996) suggests to use the TD_{50} (dose with 50% tumour incidence) instead. It is not clear whether this preference is based on the data availability or the discussable extrapolation procedure to low doses in the unit risk concept. However, we stick to the unit risk concept in order to be able to use the information derived from epidemiological studies with humans.

[40] The slope factors for oral intake given in Appendix (6.7) are based on additional risk for cancer incidence per $mgkg^{-1}day^{-1}$, i.e., per mg substance intake per kg body weight each day.

[41] An inconsistency is introduced here into the data because WHO extrapolates with a linear model, LAI (1992) with several models, and U.S. EPA uses the multistage model, choosing the slope of the upper 95% confidence interval. The extrapolation chosen by EPA should lead to a slightly lower slope, but this bias cannot be seen in the data presented. See Wahrendorf *et al.* (1993) and Becher *et al.* (1995) for a detailed discussion of the differences between these extrapolation methods and the arguments for and against them.

Table 6.13 also gives an idea of the uncertainty that results if we start with estimates that are already averages and then look mainly at their changes over time. The ratios between the largest and the smallest values vary between 1.3 to 7 and their average is about 3. Yetergil Kiefer (1997) compiled a large number of estimates for benzene, BaP, and soot. She found only small variations for benzene and BaP of between a factor 2 to 3. The estimates for soot vary much more (factor 10 and more) because of the very different size fractions and compositions that have been used to derive them. More on uncertainty in estimates is given in Subsection 6.3.6.

Substance / Source	Vainio *et al.* (1991), Higginson *et al.* (1992), Hemminki *et al.* (1994), WHO (1987), and others	LAI (1992)	IRIS (1996), $=USEPA (1990)	WHO (1987)	WHO (1996a), £ = WHO (1996b)	This report
	Targets	$[\frac{1}{\mu g/m^3}]$	$[\frac{1}{\mu g/m^3}]$	$[\frac{1}{\mu g/m^3}]$	$[\frac{1}{\mu g/m^3}]$	$[\frac{1}{\mu g/m^3}]$
Acrylonitrile	Lung		6.8 E-5	2 E-5		6.8 E-5
Arsenic and inorg. comp.	Lung, skin, (liver)	4 E-3	4.3 E-3	4 E-3	1.5 E-3	1.5 E-3
Benzene	Leukaemia, hematopoietic system	9 E-6	8.3 E-6	4 E-6	6 E-6	6 E-6
Cadmium and comp.	Lung, prostate, kidney	1.2 E-2	1.8 E-3			1.8 E-3
Chromium VI	Lung		1.2 E-2	4 E-2	4 E-2	4 E-2
Diesel Soot Particle	Lung	7 E-5 #	2 - 10 E-5 $		3.4 E-5 £	3.4 E-5
Nickel	Lung		4.8 E-4	4 E-4	3.8 E-4	3.8 E-4
PAH as BaP	Lung	7 E-2	7 E-2	9 E-2	8.7 E-2	8.7 E-2
Trichlorethylene			1.7 E-6 $		4.3 E-7	4.3 E-7
Vinyl Chloride	Liver, blood vessels (brain, lung, lymphatic system)		4.1 E-6 $	1 E-6		1 E-6

Table 6.13: Evaluation of unit risk factors for potent human carcinogenics based on a selection of data in the literature
This risk estimate has to be divided by 0.7 if the particles are measured in elemental carbon in order to compensate for the non-carbon fraction (LAI 1993).

No risk data is reported for many of the carcinogenic substances listed in IARC (1993b). If emission data is available, there are at least six additional sources from which to derive or to calculate slope factors. Firstly, the IARC monographs provide a comprehensive overview on single substances and compound groups, including references to all available data. The publications from the International Agency for Research on Cancer (IARC) represent a broad consensus between experts. The second option is the Environmental Health Criteria Series, edited by the World Health Organisation. It is made up of nearly 200 reports on single substances, mixtures, compounds and methods (see, e.g., WHO (1996b) for an index to these reports). A similar compendium is established by the German Chemistry Society (BUA 1985). Each year, new evaluation reports are published to enhance the scope of the compendium. The Carcinogenic Potency Database (Gold *et al.* 1989/1997) can be used in case both of these widely supported report series provide insufficient quantitative support. The database can be used to estimate unit risks on the basis of rodent toxicity tests. It lists 975 chemicals already tested and the TD50 values[42] for 492

[42] TD50 stands for the daily dose at which the share of tumour-free animals is half as big as in the non-exposed control group after the animal-specific standard lifetime.

rodent carcinogens are given[43]. Only 3 PAH are listed in Appendix (6.7). McClure (1996) has developed a procedure to estimate the cancer potency of other PAHs. The equivalency factors developed by the NATO/CCMS-model can be used for other dioxins than 2,3,7,8-Tetrachlordibenzo-p-dioxin (Braun *et al.* 1992).

Table 6.13 and Appendix (6.7) contain the unit risk data as well as information on the type of cancer that is expected, i.e., the endpoint which is affected by a tumour. It is obvious from Appendix (6.7) that the cancer type is often unknown and is mainly identified for Group 1 and 2A substances. Subsection 6.4.2 will further elaborate on this topic.

6.3.5 Population density and estimates for cancer incidence

Two additional steps are necessary before one is able to estimate the incidence of cancer due to the external exposures that have already been calculated in Subsection 6.2. The unit risk is expressed as the lifetime risk for an average age assumed to be 70 years. The exposure is calculated on a yearly base. The unit risks therefore have to be corrected to harmonise these diverging assumptions. In addition, one also has to specify if people live in the areas that are exposed and how many of them do so.

The population density and its distribution is decisive for the number of people that are exposed to the constant emission of a substance. The population density ρ varies depending on the place of emission and of exposure. The following aspects should be considered before a model to calculate the population density is presented:

- The exposure by food nowadays depends very little on the sources of carcinogenic emissions in the neighbourhood or the region (because of national and international trade).
- The way drinking water management is practised today suggests that citizens do not drink water that contains the contaminants typical for the emissions of a city's industries.
- Only short-lived substances and substances emitted by mobile sources or low chimneys lead primarily to the local exposure of human beings.
- In 1990, less than one third of the populations in the USA, Latin America, Western Europe, Oceania and Japan lived in rural areas (Klein Goldewijk *et al.* 1995). The world-wide average is only 57%, but in Western Europe it is a low 22.3% and in Eastern Europe 39.3%. At least for the Western world we can therefore assume that people live at the place where they also emit.
- Pollutants with long atmospheric residence times emitted in Europe will also be spread over large areas outside of Western Europe, including the seas. An average wind speed of 5 to 10 m/s (430 to 860 km/day) can be assumed for long-range dispersion (Jones 1981).
- The average population density in Western Europe is about 160 P/km^2 (and varies between 80 and 395 P/km^2 if calculated per country). On other continents we have a different situation: Africa: 23 P/km^2, America: 18 P/km^2, Asia: 107 P/km^2, Oceania: 3 P/km^2, Russian Federation: 9 P/km^2, World: 42 P/km^2 (UNESCO

[43] An update of the database can be found under http://potency.berkeley.edu/cpdb.html.

1996). The average world-wide population density (including the seas) will be about 13 P/km^2 in 2000.

In Section 6.2 it had been assumed that the emissions occur in Europe. It is clear from the information given above that short-lived substances and substances with a low mobility will lead to the exposure of the densely populated Western Europe. However, even pollutants with atmospheric residence times of only a few days will already disperse over the seas and over the countries in Eastern Europe.

The population density is therefore modelled per substance dependent on their atmospheric residence times. Yearly averages could be calculated with a long range dispersion model, a data base on global meteorological data, and a map with actual population densities. A simpler model is proposed here due to the lack of this information. The travelling distance of pollutants is assumed to be proportional to their atmospheric residence time. The population density is set to zero if the pollutants are blown out to the seas or, for instance, to 9 P/km^2 if they are dispersed over the Russian Federation, i.e., it can easily become very low after a travelling time of only a few days.

Equation (6.12) is used to approximate the population density ρ as a function of the atmospheric residence time τ. α and β have been calculated on the assumption that ρ should equal the average European population density (160 P/km^2) if τ equals one day and that ρ should equal the average world-wide population density of 13P/km^2 if τ equals one year, i.e., full global dispersion is assumed after one year. It is furthermore assumed that substances with atmospheric residence times shorter than 7 hours will nevertheless expose not more than 300 P/km^2 (densely populated areas in Europe). The atmospheric residence time has been calculated with Equation (6.8). The dilution height has been set equal to 1000 m for all substances but particle soot (800 m), 1,3-butadiene, formaldehyde, styrene, 1,1-dichlorethylene, and aldrin (see Table 6.6).

$$\rho i = \alpha \cdot \tau i^{-0.5} + \beta \qquad \text{and} \qquad \rho i \le 300 \text{ E-6 P/m}^2 \qquad [\text{E-6 P/m}^2] \qquad (6.12)$$

where: ρi average population density for substance i [E-6 P/m^2]
τi atmospheric residence time for substance i calculated with Equation (6.8) [a]
α fitting constant = 8 E-6 P/m^2/a$^{0.5}$
β fitting constant = 5 E-6 P/m^2

Figure 6.8 visualises this fit. The relationship chosen is responsible for the decrease in the population density after 5 days of dispersion (= 2000 up to 4000 travelling km) to 73 P/km^2 and after 10 days (= 4000 up to 8000 travelling km) to 53 P/km^2. These numbers appear to be reasonable best estimates if we assume an emission source in central Europe and that the wind is dispersing the pollutants in a half circle only to the east of the emission source (and keeping in mind the world map of population densities). The argument that not only the population density decreases with higher residence time, but also the concentration, is not relevant in this case because a non-threshold behaviour was assumed. The squared geometric standard deviation is estimated to be a factor of three.

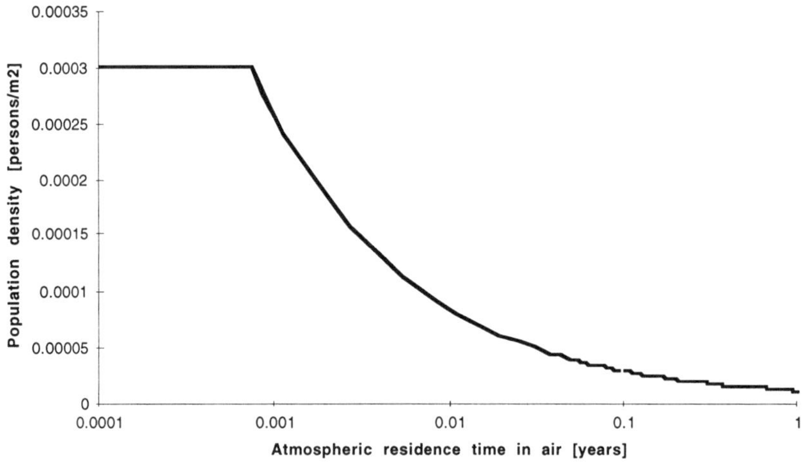

Fig. 6.8 Population density as a function of the atmospheric residence time of substances emitted in Western Europe according to Equation (6.12).

Now all elements are available to calculate the effect factor *Eik* of substance *i* due to the exposure path *k*:

$$Eik = \frac{\rho i}{LT} \cdot URik \tag{6.13}$$

where ρi population density (Equation 6.12) [P/m^{-2}]
LT assumed lifetime in *UR* = 70 [a/P]
$URik$ unit risk value of substance *i* and exposure by path *k* (*k* = air, drinking water, food) [tumour cases/conc.]

$$Ei(inhalation) = \frac{\rho i}{LT} \cdot URi(inhalation) \quad [\frac{\text{tumour cases}}{\mu g} \cdot \frac{m^3}{m^2 a}] \tag{6.13a}$$

$$Ei(drinking\ water) = \frac{\rho i}{LT} \cdot URi(drinking\ water) \quad [\frac{\text{tumour cases}}{\mu g} \cdot \frac{1}{m^2 a}] \tag{6.13b}$$

$$Ei(food) = \frac{\rho i}{LT} \cdot URi(food) \quad [\frac{\text{tumour cases}}{mg} \cdot \frac{kg \cdot day}{m^2 a}] \tag{6.13c}$$

The tumour incidence rate *Tijk* for substance *i* by the emission compartment *j* and the exposure path *k* can be written as the product of the fate factor *Fijk* from Equation (6.6) and the effect factor *Eik* (Equation 6.13):

$$Tijk = Fijk \cdot Eik = \frac{\delta Cik}{\left(\frac{M'ij}{A}\right)} \cdot \frac{\rho i}{LT} \cdot URik \tag{6.14}$$

The results of the calculation of *Tijk* are given in Appendix (6.9) per kg substance emission.

6.3.6 Uncertainty estimate

There are several sources of uncertainty which are added by the effect factor:

I Firstly, through the choice of the unit risk concept as such with the assumed *non-threshold* behaviour.

II Secondly, the modelling of the *population density* enters uncertainty due to the unequal distribution of human beings on earth.

III Thirdly, the unit risk estimates are uncertain due to the *high variability between the risk estimates* contained in the studies evaluated, the transfer from the animal to the human model, the extrapolation to low doses, etc.

IV Last but not least, the unit *risk factors are incomplete* for some substances, i.e., they are sometimes missing for oral intake and drinking water and sometimes for inhalation. Sometimes the missing path is indeed irrelevant because an effect only occurs in the lung, or because a substance cannot be absorbed if it is inhaled. But sometimes the path is missing due to a lack of toxicity data or due to inexistent investigations.

The uncertainty factor I can only be evaluated when compared to other assessment methods.

The population density (error source II) has been modelled by assuming that the emission occurs in Western Europe. The model allows for the calculation of the substance-specific population density as a function of the substance's atmospheric residence time. This density should nonetheless be changed if the damage functions are used for single countries or for regions with densities that diverge substantially from the average that has been used here. With no changes made and staying with the assumption of an emission in Europe, the squared geometric standard deviation is estimated to be a factor of 3.

The uncertainty in the single unit risk factors is different for each substance (error source III). A reliable estimate requires for each substance consultation of the fact sheets in IRIS (1996) or of the IARC monographs. Such a task was outside the scope of this investigation. It is known that the calculation of unit risks from epidemiological studies is much more certain than from animal studies. Animal bioassays make use of transfer and safety factors which produce uncertainty. It is therefore obvious that unit risks for IARC-Group 1 substances have a higher reliability than for Group 3 ones. In addition, it has to be considered that most data on oral intake are based on just a small number of epidemiological studies or animal bioassays because epidemiological studies mostly focus on the inhalation path[44].

In VDI (1991) and LAI (1992/1993) sets of independently calculated unit risk factors for the same substances are presented on a logarithmic scale. The number of data points is too small to test for the correct distribution function, but a normal distribution cannot be rejected. There are four reasons why we assume a lognormal distribution here (see Appendix 6.8). At the present time the dominant view is that unit

[44] It is not really clear how such epidemiological studies, e.g., in the cadmium industry, correct for additional Cd-exposure by drinking water and oral intake. No correction can lead to counting the risks twice.

risk factors are positively valued. Many toxicological processes can be linearised through a logarithmic presentation. An oblique distribution of the unit risk factors is not counterintuitive. And the data in VDI (1991) and LAI (1992/1993) could be normally distributed on a log-scale. The geometric standard deviations for lognormal distributions presented in Table 6.14 are rough estimates based on the evaluation in Table 6.13 and the discussion in Yetergil Kiefer (1997).

IARC-Group	σ_g^2 for inhalation	σ_g^2 for drinking water and oral intake
1	2	4
2A	3	6
2B	5	10
3	10	20

Tab. 6.14: Estimated geometric standard deviations (lognormal distribution) for the unit risk factors given in Appendix (6.7).

The incomplete set of unit risk factors (error source IV) can be evaluated by comparing the tumour incidence rates given in Appendix (6.9) with the information contained in Figures 6.6 and 6.7 where the dominant intake paths are identified. We can calculate a Potential Extrapolation Factor (PEF) if unit risk factors are missing for relevant exposure paths (e.g., more than 10% of total intake). The PEF in turn could be multiplied by the tumour incidence factor *Tijk* for those exposure paths for which unit risk factors are available. These PEFs are given in Table 6.15 for all the substances concerned. We call them *Potential* Extrapolation Factors because they are based on the assumption that the absorption of the substance (internal exposure) and its toxicokinetics and toxicodynamics are comparable for the missing paths. This error source (IV) is dominating all the other sources for 15 out of 55 substances (compare Table 6.14 and 6.15!). Potential errors of up to twelve (!) orders of magnitude may occur!

Substance name	PEF $T_{air, inhalation}$	PEF $T_{air, drinking water}$	PEF $T_{air,food}$	PEF $T_{water, inhalation}$	PEF $T_{water, drinking water}$	PEF $T_{water,food}$
Cadmium-	472			0.42 E 12		
Chromium(VI)	153'896			0.63 E 12		
Nickel	3'585			2.2 E 12		
Vinyl chloride				1.5		
1,3-Butadiene				11		
Benz[a]anthracene-	1'260			14'206		
Dibenz[a,h]anthracene	10'366			8'596'359		
Formaldehyde-	3.2			5'626		
Polychlorinated-biphenyls- (PCBs)	64			108		
2,3,7,8-Tetrachlordibenzo-p-dioxin, TCDD	9'548			10'611		
Acetaldehyde-				17		
Benzotrichloride-			35			13
Benzyl-chloride-			4'326		4.4	
Bromodichloromethane-		819			15	
Dichlorvos-		2.2				
gamma-Hexachlorocyclohexane (lindane)	128			11'423		
Styrene				5.2		
3-Methylchloanthrene	4'142			217'019		
Trichlorethylene				1.4		

Tab. 6.15: Potential Extrapolation Factors (PEF) for the tumour incidence factors reported in Appendix (6.9) due to a lack of unit risk factors for certain exposure paths

The non-existence of effect data for the relevant paths is symptomatic rather than accidental for the impact-pathway analysis. Here, we are in the comfortable situation that we know what is missing. There are at least three ways to deal with this situation:

1. The non-existence of a unit risk factor can be interpreted to meant that there is no knowledge on causalities. In this case, the tumour incidence rates are taken from Appendix (6.9) and the knowledge gap is assumed to be represented by the indicator for unknown damage (Section 4.4). Another version of this first approach consists in simply disregarding the substances listed in Table 6.15 when undertaking the assessment.
2. The epidemiological studies and the literature on animal tests can be screened in order to be able to derive additional unit risk factors for the substances listed in Table 6.15. One then assigns a higher error range to these additional effect factors and can include them in the assessment.
3. It is assumed that internal exposure, the toxicokinetics and toxicodynamics are the same for all paths, both the missing and the known ones. New unit risk factors can then be calculated and included in the assessment by making use of those that already exist.

Before we discuss these proposals further, we should recall what has been said earlier in this section. The evidence for human carcinogenity of substances is highest where epidemiological studies exist. These studies are mostly based on occupational exposure and focused on inhalation. Epidemiological studies have rarely monitored drinking water quality or even food contamination. Reliable data on oral intake is therefore often missing. A cursory review of the descriptions of a number of substances in IRIS (1996) shows that they contain often an indication for the carcinogenic potential of oral intake. But there is often no evidence given in support of this because there exist neither epidemiological studies nor animal tests. Seidel (1996) estimates from the risk to outdoor exposure to cadmium and dioxin the risk due to oral intake. He applies large multiplication factors to compensate for the omitted but relevant food intake paths. Ziqiang *et al.* (1996) give unit risk values for the ingestion pathway for several metals including cadmium and chromium. Due to lacking citations of the primary source we do not take their values[45], but see it as a support of our extrapolation approach.

In view of this situation, we reject proposal (1) because it fails to make use of information that is available. Proposal (2) seems appropriate when the decision to be made can be postponed until the resource-intensive task of surveying epidemiological studies and the literature is completed. We ourselves follow the proposal (3) in view of the time restrictions placed on this case study. As a consequence, we will apply a σg^2 of 20 for all the unit risk factors which are added in order to take into account the additional uncertainty from the assumptions on internal exposure and mechanisms.

The transformation factor from unit risk inhalation to oral slope factor will be calculated under the assumption that a person weighs 70 kg and inhales 20 m^3 per day on the average. This gives a transfer factor of 3'500 (70 kg times 1000 (to convert from µg to mg) divided by 20 m^3). This ratio of 3'500 results for many substances where both the inhalation unit risk *and* the oral slope factor are known. The transfer factors for the other extrapolations can be calculated analogously if one assumes that a person drinks two litres of water per day on the average.

---

[45] For the substances cadmium and chromium, their values are close to the results of our extrapolation.

The new unit risk factors are listed in Appendix (6.10) and Appendix (6.11) contains the full list of tumour incidence rates. The new factors are set in bold characters to facilitate their identification.

Reflection: This final adaptation is typical of situations where there is no relevant information to construct full damage functions for a large set of substances. Such situations are the rule rather than the exception. The constructivistic nature of the damage function approach requires making assumptions and rough extrapolations, but the interesting question is to the motives that made us adopt proposal (3). Was this a value choice which could be explained with Cultural Theory? Was the situation not similar to the classification of carcinogenic substances (Table 6.12)? Indeed there are arguments to follow proposal (1) which have an individualist touch, those for proposal (2) a hierarchist one, and those for (3) reflect an egalitarian point of view. However, the principle that guided us here was to find an adequate procedure to predict tumour incidence in the best manner possible and this is an aim shared by all three of the cultural perspectives identified here.

One consequence of these additional assumptions is that we shall speak from *potential* damage functions in order to underline the extensive use of models and model assumptions.

6.4 Life of Years Lost (YLL) and Years Lived Disabled (YLD)

6.4.1 Overview

With the information given in the preceding sections it was possible to calculate the cancer incidence rate due to specified substance emissions. In this section the question is how this incidence rate is translated into the proposed measure of the damage to human health, the Disability Adjusted Life Years (DALYs) (Section 5.4). This requires answers to questions such as: which type of cancer has to be expected, which share of tumour patients will die, how many potential life years are lost, how long will the patient feel ill due to tumour incidence and how is one to determine the severity of his or her disability?

These questions can be addressed with one of two approaches. In a first approach, medical experts are asked about the specific way such a tumour is built, how fast it will grow, how probable it is that someone will be cured by having recourse to the latest cancer treatment technology, and after how many years the tumour will lead to death if left untreated. This is akin to the bottom-up approach.

The other approach, and the one followed here, is an epidemiological one. Most countries, or at least certain districts within countries, have cancer registers where each case of cancer incidence and cancer death is registered with information on cancer type, age at diagnosis, and sometimes some additional information. Based on such registers, statistics can be made which show the survival rate of people after cancer has been diagnosed and age-specific mortality tables can be constructed for each cancer type.

6.4.2 Which cancer types have to be expected?

From Appendix (6.10) it is known which cancer types are caused by the different substances. Group 1 and 2A substances are the well tested ones, mostly supported by epidemiological studies and demonstrated effects in humans. The cancer type can be identified only if effects in humans can be detected. Animals normally develop tumours at other sites than humans do, so the transfer is not always possible. Very often, more than one endpoint is given. This is a typical situation. It is difficult to predict only one cancer type, especially if the substances are taken in by food and by drinking water. Many carcinogens do not act in organ-specific ways. The weakest organ in the body, probably already affected by other processes, will then most probably fail in the repair task and produce a tumour. Nevertheless, the identification of cancer types is important for the determination of the possibilities of treatment, survival rates and typical age of onset.

For reasons of simplicity we assume that the first mentioned site in Appendix (6.10) is also the most important one[46]. For pragmatic reasons we distinguish only those

[46] In the volume on the nuclear fuel cycle, ExternE (1995) used a set of about ten cancer types caused by radioactive radiation. The authors were in the favourable situation that the shares of these cancer types are known.

sites which are considered in Murray *et al.* (1996a) (see also Table 5.9) for the disability weights and which are represented in cancer statistics. The 'lymphatic and hematopoietic system' and the 'soft tissue sarcoma' are therefore not listed as separate cancer sites but added to the category of 'unspecified' ones. 'Nose' and 'nasal cavity' are merged into one category. The large category 'unspecified' will be modelled by the average over all cancer sites.

Furthermore, we assume that the substances causing cancer of the lung and of the nasal cavity through inhalation will not develop these cancers if taken in orally. It is assumed that they show average behaviour (i.e., unspecified). The final categorisation is given in Table 6.16.

Substances	Cancer site for inhalation	Cancer site for oral intake
Arsenic (inorganic), Bis(chloromethyl)ether- (BCME), Cadmium, Chromium(VI), Nickel, Acrylonitrile, Benzo[a]pyrene- (BaP), Diesel soot particles, Epichlorohydrin, alpha-Hexachlorocyclohexane (alpha-HCH), beta-Hexachlorocyclohexane (beta-HCH), gamma-Hexachlorocyclohexane (lindane), Bis(chloroethyl)ether- (BCEE)	Lung	Unspecified
Benzene	Leukaemia	Leukaemia
Nickel-refinery-dust, Nickel-subsulfide, Formaldehyde	Nasal cavity, nose	Unspecified
Vinyl chloride, Carbon-tetrachloride	Liver	Liver
Polychlorinated-biphenyls(PCBs)	Skin (melanoma)	Skin (melanoma)
Propylene-oxide, Benz[a]anthracene, Dibenz[a,h]anthracene, 1,2-Dibromoethane, 1,2-Dichloroethane, 1,4-Dioxane, 2,4,6-Trichlorophenol, Acetaldehyde, Benzotrichloride, Benzyl-chloride, Bromodichloromethane, Chloroform, Di(2-ethylhexyl)phthalate (DEHP), Dichloromethane, Dichlorvos, Hexachlorobenzene, Pentachlorphenol, 1,1,1,2-Tetrachloroethane, 1,1,2,2-Tetrachloroethane, 1,1,2-Trichloroethane, 1,1-Dichloroethylene, 3-Methylchloanthrene, Aldrin, Dibutyl-phthalate, Dieldrin, Hexachlorobutadiene, Hexachloroethane, Methyl chloride, Trichlorethylene, Trifluralin, 2,3,7,8-Tetrachlordibenzo-p-dioxin, TCDD, 1,3-Butadiene, Ethylene Oxide, Perchloroethylene, Styrene	Unspecified	Unspecified

Tab. 6.16: Cancer types caused by different substances through inhalation or oral intake, based on Appendix (6.10).

The task to attribute specific cancer sites to chemical carcinogens is difficult and sometimes impossible as we have already mentioned earlier. The assumed average behaviour may therefore best reflect the reality for certain causal agents. As we show later, the consequences of a wrong classification are limited because of the comparably small differences between the DALYs for the different cancer sites (Table 6.20).

6.4.3 Survival rate and Years of Life Lost

A large number of articles and statistics were reviewed to find accurate data, especially for survival rates and mortality tables (Levi 1986, Levi *et al.* 1986/89, SL 1991, HK 1991, Raymond *et al.* 1993, IARC 1993a, SK 1994, Griffiths *et al.* 1995, Coebergh *et al.* 1995, SC 1995, WHO 1995b, IARC 1995, Murray *et al.* 1996a/b, Schüler *et al.* 1997). If we use these sources, we make at least two important assumptions:

- Firstly, the average survival rates and mortality tables of the last decade are relevant for the prediction of the future health outcomes due to cancer sites.
- Secondly, the cancer cases due to environmental chemical carcinogenesis show the same characteristics as the average of all causes (physical, viral, and chemical).

The first assumption can partly be checked by comparison with older statistical data: Recent statistics show increasing survival rates and ages at death. The survival rate and age at death will therefore be underestimated slightly for future health outcomes. The second assumptions is only a first approximation. For instance, ExternE (1995) in the volume on the nuclear fuel cycle uses more specific data for cancer from radioactive radiation.

Survival rates are normally reported for distinct periods made up of a number of years, e.g., after 1, 5, and 10 years. The quality of the statistics varies because they are not always based on a cohort approach where one follows real individuals (Levi *et al.* 1986/1989) and where corrections are made for people moving to other districts or for death due to other causes, for instance. Other statistics base the survival rate on the registration of cancer incidence and of cases of cancer mortality (on an individual basis). The survival rates are normally reported either as *observed* or as *relative* rates. The relative rates correct for the fact that the probability to die from cancer increases with age. Relative survival rates are therefore higher than the observed ones. The former are therefore the relevant ones if one is interested in the additional cancer cases due to additional risk factors.

From data on survival rates we will derive the share of people which die due to the cancer incidence. As a measure for the share of people that die (i.e., not survive) we use the complement of the relative survival rate after 10 years. This is a choice. Survival rates after 15 years are sometimes also available. This choice is acceptable because the relative survival rate after 5 years is decreasing only slowly. Each cancer type has a different survival rate and these, in turn, vary from country to country. These variations reflect the different medical possibilities of diagnosis and of treatment of the different types of cancer, on the one hand, and the investments in screening programs and treatment facilities, on the other. It can be shown that the survival rates have been increasing for many decades because of improved treatment possibilities and the increased use made of the treatment facilities.

Some of the survival rates used here (Table 6.17) reflect the situation in Europe from 1978 to 1985, i.e., the situation in the twelve countries or their districts, respectively, which participate in the EUROCARE Study (IARC 1995). The averaged and weighted data for the relative survival represent therefore the lower estimates for the situation in 1997 because the survival rate may have increased in the last twelve years. One can assume that non-contributing countries might show lower survival rates due to the selection process of the EUROCARE study (availability of good data). As a consequence, these 'old' numbers are not corrected for improved health service in order to reflect the present situation in the whole of Europe. The same holds true for the data derived from Raymond *et al.* (1993) from the district of Geneva in Switzerland, which are used for the cancer types missing in the EUROCARE study (Table 6.17).

The decision to derive the share of dying people from the complement of the survival rate implies the assumption that the cases of incidence calculated in Section

6.3 have been diagnosed at the same time as the cancer incidence reported in the cancer registers. This assumption is theoretically relevant because the onset and detectability of a chronic illness such as cancer occur before symptoms show up, and normally before the illness is diagnosed. The survival period therefore starts relatively shortly after the first symptoms show up, while rodents in bioassays or humans (in case control or cohort studies) can be screened before the symptoms become obvious. This assumption, though, is of little practical relevance for our purposes because our focus is on the damage which occurs only after symptoms have appeared.

The data from IARC (1995) form a sound statistical basis for further analysis because of the large amount of cases that are included in this statistic. The data for liver and for skin cancer are based on a cohort study by Raymond *et al.* (1993) which included only a small number of cases. This data is less reliable.

t =	1-year $S_{1,m}$	3-year $S_{3,m}$	5-year $S_{5,m}$	8-year $S_{8,m}$	10-year $S_{10,m}$	*Death rate after 10 years*	Included cases	Source
	%	%	%	%	%	%	persons	
Leukaemia	52	34	27	20	16	*84*	21'360	IARC (1995)
Lung	29	11	8	7	7	*93*	167'086	IARC (1995)
Nasopharynx	67	44	38	32	29	*71*	1'078	IARC (1995)
All types	46	34	30	27	26	*74*	678'185	IARC (1995)
Liver	15		4		1	*99*	144	Raymond *et al.* (1993)
Skin (melanoma)	98		84		84	*16*	211	Raymond *et al.* (1993)

Tab. 6.17: Age adjusted relative survival rates for five cancer types and the average of all cancer types in Europe from 1978-1985 (IARC 1995), and 1970-1990 (Raymond et all. 1993)

With the death rate after 10 years known, it is possible to calculate the cancer deaths by making use of the tumour incidence rates given in Appendix (6.11). In a second step, we then calculate the potential years life lost (YLL) due to these deaths per cancer site.

The years of life lost (YLL) were derived from mortality data for Canada (SC 1995), USA (WHO 1995b), Hamburg (HK 1991) and the Saar region (SL 1991) in Germany, Geneva (Raymond *et al.* 1993) in Switzerland, and Switzerland (SK 1994) itself. For this purpose, the age-dependent death numbers from the aforementioned cancer statistics are used to derive the average number of years lost due to a premature death. For the life expectancy we used the standard life table reproduced in Table 5.7 (Murray *et al.* 1996a). In Section 5.4 we already discussed the questions of discounting and age-weighting. $YLL(a,r,K)$ means the years of life lost if someone dies at age a; the years are discounted by the rate r and the age-weighting is performed to the extent K (K=1 corresponds to a full age-weighting). The formulas to calculate $YLL(a,r,K)$ have been given in Section 5.4.6 and the relevant results are listed in the Tables 5.7, 5.10, and 5.11. From the statistics, we know the age at death a and the number of deaths registered at that age Tm,a. The weighted sum of these products is divided by the absolute number of death Tm due to tumour site m to calculate the average $YLLm(r,K)$ per death due to tumour site m. So far we have calculated only the incidence cases and therefore now have to correct with the complement of the 10-year survival rate $S10,m$ given in Table 6.17. This leads to:

$$YLLm(r,K) \text{ per cancer incidence} = (1 - S10,m) \cdot \frac{1}{Tm} \sum_a YLL(a,r,K) \cdot Tm,a \qquad (6.15)$$

The results are given in Table 6.18. We differentiate between the calculations for *YLLm(0,0)*, where neither discounting nor age-weighting has been applied, and *YLLm(0,1)*, where age-weighting has been used. The first columns for *YLLm(0,0)* and for *YLLm(0,1)*, respectively, show the range of results derived from the various statistics that have been used. This gives an idea on the variations between countries due to different living conditions and health systems. Almost no data is available for skin melanoma and for cancer in the nasal tract. Especially little empirical data was available for cancer in connection with the nose. Sometimes the calculation is based on only a small number of reported deaths and this explains the large variation in the estimates. The best estimate we deduced from the range of results is reported in the second column of each block. We have done so for each one of these cancer sites and for the weighted average for 'all sites'. The results in the third column are the years of life lost per incidence case and per cancer site that have been calculated according to Formula (6.15).

	Range YLLm(0,0) per cancer death	YLLm(0,0) per cancer death	YLLm(0,0) per cancer incidence	Range YLLm(0,1) per cancer death	YLLm(0,1) per cancer death	YLLm(0,1) per cancer incidence
Lung	15.5-18.4	17	15.8	8.4-12.4	11	10.2
Skin melanoma	14.3-26.1	20	3.2	11.5-21.5	16	2.6
Nasal, nose, nasopharynx	6-22	17	12.1	4-18	11	7.8
Liver	13.6-17	16	15.8	9.9-12.2	11	10.9
Leukaemia	13.8-21.4	19	16	8.5-16.2	14	11.8
All types	12.8-18.9	17	12.6	7.1-13.5	11	8.1

Tab. 6.18: Estimate for the years life lost (YLL), range calculated from (SC 1995), (HK 1991), (SL 1991), (WHO 1995b), (Raymond *et al.* 1993) and standard life expectancy table from Table 5.7 and 5.12 (Murray *et al.* 1996a)

More actual, detailed and sophisticated analysis of YLL per cancer type will be possible in the future, as soon as all the cancer registries are available electronically on the world wide web[47].

6.4.4 Disability weights and Years Lived Disabled

After having calculated the years life lost due to a tumour incidence, we address here the duration and severity of morbidity. For severity, we have already given the disability weights for the different cancer sites (Table 5.9) that are available from Murray *et al.*(1996a). It only has to be recalled here that the estimates are based on expert panels made up of health providers and that it was assumed that nowadays 90% of all cancer cases are treated in industrialised countries.

The duration of disease can partly be derived from statistical information on the survival rate (e.g., Table 6.17). From this information, it is possible to calculate the average time someone lives within a 10-year period. This can be done through a linearisation of the survival rate and the calculation of the integral (see, e.g., Yetergil Kiefer *et al.*(1997)). The additional information needed is how many of the surviving cancer patients are disabled after the 10-year period and what share of the surviving patients within the 10-year period are disabled at all. The information given in Murray *et al.* (1996a/b) on the average duration of the disease for each

[47] The cancer registry of Munich is already on the web: http://www.med.uni-muenchen.de/trm.

cancer site and on the age of the onset of disease has been used in the absence of other appropriate data (Table 6.19).

The calculation of the weighted years lived disabled can be done for the case of no discounting and no age-weighting (*YLD(0,0)*) by the simple multiplication of the disability weight *Dm* with the disease duration *Lm*:

$$YLDm\ (0,0) = Dm\ Lm \tag{6.16}$$

For the age-weighted years lived disabled (*YLD(0,1)*) a somewhat more complicated Formula (6.17) has to be used

$$YLDm(0,1) = Dm \left\{ \frac{Ce^{-\beta am}}{\beta^2} \{e^{-\beta Lm} [-\beta(Lm+am)-1] + \beta am + 1\} \right\} \tag{6.17}$$

where *am* is the age of disease onset, β is a parameter to determine the shape of the age-weighting and is set to 0.04, and $C = 0.1658$ is a correction factor.

The results of these calculations are given in Table 6.19. A first interpretation shows little differences between different cancer sites (factor 2.4 between smallest and largest YLD) and between YLD with and without age-weighting. The YLD with age-weighting are always smaller than without because the average age of onset is at an age where the age-weighting is already smaller than one (see Figure 5.4).

The age of disease onset given in Table 6.19 can in addition be used to cross-check the YLL calculated in Table 6.18. Two aspects have to be kept in mind: (1) the age of death is after the age of disease onset, and (2) the standard life expectancy at the average age of death is different from the addition of age-specific life expectancies because of the higher life expectancy with increasing age. Considering these two points, the agreement between the numbers given in the two tables is rather good.

	Average disability weights *Dm* (Murray *et al.* 1996a)	Age of disease onset *am* (Murray *et al.* 1996b)	Average duration of disease *Lm* (Murray *et al.* 1996b)	*YLDm (0,0)*	*YLDm (0,1)*
Mouth and oropharynx	0.096	59.4	4.3	0.41	0.36
Liver	0.239	64.3	1.77	0.42	0.34
Trachea, bronchus and lung	0.146	66.7	2	0.29	0.22
Melanoma and other skin	0.045	55.4	4.4	0.20	0.19
Lymphomas and multiple myeloma	0.060	58.5	3.8	0.23	0.20
Leukaemia	0.099	56.8	4.6	0.45	0.42
All sites	0.154	64.8	3.4	0.48	0.37

Tab. 6.19: Years lived disabled for different cancer sites with and without age-weighting.

6.4.5 Results and uncertainty

The DALYs per incidence case for the individual cancer types can now be calculated through addition of the YLLs and YLDs. They are shown in Table 6.20 for both the cases with and without age-weighting as introduced in Section 5.4. The small contribution of the YLDs (3-7%) to the DALYs is obvious, a result already suggested by Figure 5.6 where many cancer types ranked much higher if only deaths instead of DALYs were considered.

Making use of age-weighting causes a reduction of the YLLs by about 40%. This decrease changes little in the comparison of the different cancer sites, but it may have significant impacts if the results are compared to other diseases which occur at younger ages.

	YLLm(0,0)	YLDm (0,0)	DALYs m(0,0)	YLLm(0,1)	YLDm (0,1)	DALYsm(0,1)
Lung	15.8	0.29	16.1	10.2	0.22	10.4
Skin melanoma	3.2	0.20	3.4	2.6	0.19	2.8
Nasal, nose, nasopharynx	12.1	0.41	12.5	7.8	0.36	8.2
Liver	15.8	0.42	16.2	10.9	0.34	11.2
Leukaemia	16.0	0.45	16.5	11.8	0.42	12.2
All sites	12.6	0.48	13.1	8.1	0.37	8.5

Tab. 6.20: Summary of the DALYs without and with age-weighting for different cancer sites.

Another result is that the differences between the individual cancer sites are small except for skin melanoma. The uncertainty concerning the specific cancer sites that might be affected, especially for the oral intake, is therefore of limited relevance for the assessment.

The estimate for the square of the geometric standard deviation σg^2 for YLLs in Subsection 5.4.8 was 10% and for the uncertainty range for disability weights, a factor 2 has been found. This 10%-range for YLLs includes the uncertainty from the use of the standard life table and the age-weighting.

Here we have to additionally consider:

- the variation in the age-specific death distribution found in today's statistics
- the survival rate used to calculate the death rate from the incidence rate, and
- the fact that deaths in the statistics are not just cancer death due to environmental risk factors, but also due to smoking, diet and all other physical and virological factors. (There is no indication that cancers due to environmental risk factors occur earlier or later in life than cancers due to other risk factors[48]).

For all sites except those in the nose, a range of +/-30% can be estimated for the YLLs per cancer death. The survival rate is increasing with time. A variation of +/-20% of the death rate after 10 years seems reasonable. Using Equation (A6.3) in Appendix (6.8), we can calculate the total σg^2 for YLLm and arrive at a factor 1.4.

The YLDs are not only influenced by the uncertainty of the disability weights, but also by the age of onset and the average duration of the disease. The age of onset is of little relevance here and is rather accurate anyway. The σg^2 for the average duration of the disease is estimated to vary by a factor of 2. If the two uncertainty factors are combined, overall uncertainty is therefore a factor 2.7.

The YLDs make up a very small share – 3% to 7% – of the total DALYs as has already been pointed out above. This means that the high uncertainty of the YLDs does not get carried over to a correspondingly high uncertainty of the DALYs (less than 10%). It is pointed out in Appendix (6.8) that there is no easy procedure to add two logarithmic distributions on an algebraic level. As all distributions and standard deviations are estimated anyway, we take the easy way out and estimate directly the

[48] All major risk factors have latency times. Nevertheless, it could be argued that there is a higher probability that the relevant hits occur later in life because of the low concentration of environmental pollutants than, e.g., would be true in case of a heavy occupational exposure at the age of 20. The assumptions made here may therefore lead to upper estimates.

overall uncertainty for the DALYs $\sigma g^2 = 1.5$. The uncertainty of the attribution of the right cancer site is included in this estimate. The overall error factor for cancers of the nasal cavity and of the nose, for which the statistical basis is much smaller, is estimated to be $\sigma g^2 = 2$.

6.5 Results for the complete damage functions

6.5.1 Overview

This section summarises the substeps of the damage function described so far and links them together in order to determine the damage to human health due to emissions of carcinogenic substances to air or water. This linkage is first done in a purely mathematical form in order to clarify the different elements that make up the calculation. The linkage is then done for the mean values that have been calculated for the single steps in the appendices and in Section 6.4. Finally, the linkage is done for the estimates of the error ranges for all steps.

These new results are then compared with results from studies performed within the course of LCA or for other purposes.

6.5.2 The mathematical construction of the damage function

We started this chapter with Formula (6.2), first proposed in Section 6.1. It is repeated here to facilitate the demonstration of building the damage function:

$$\frac{DALYsij}{Iij} = \sum_k\{Tijk\cdot(YLLm + YLDm)\} = \sum_k\{Fijk\cdot Eik\cdot(YLLm + YLDm)\} \quad [a/kg] \qquad (6.2)$$

where			
	$DALYs$	Disability Adjusted Live Years	[a]
	I	emission, environmental intervention	[kg]
	T	tumour incidence cases	[cases/kg]
	YLL	Years Life Lost	[a/case]
	YLD	Years Lived Disabled	[a/case]
	F	fate factor (for exposure by air)	$[\frac{m^2\cdot a}{m^3}]$
	E	effect factor (for exposure by air)	$[\frac{1}{\mu g}\cdot\frac{m^3}{m^2\ a}]$
	i	carcinogenic substance	
	j	emission media (air or surface water)	
	k	exposure path (air, drinking water, or food)	
	m	cancer site	

The definition of the different elements are repeated here too in order to allow for a comprehensive overview. The fate factors can be calculated with Equation (6.6) where δCik is the calculated or measured concentration increase and $M'ij$ is the substance emission flow in area A:

$$Fijk = \frac{\delta Cik}{\left(\frac{M'ij}{A}\right)} \qquad (6.6)$$

$$k = \text{air} \qquad Fij(air) = \frac{\delta Ci(air)}{\left(\frac{M'ij}{A}\right)} \qquad [\frac{m^2 \cdot a}{m^3}] \tag{6.6a}$$

$$k = \text{drinking water} \qquad Fij(water) = \frac{\delta Ci(water)}{\left(\frac{M'ij}{A}\right)} \qquad [\frac{m^2 \cdot a}{l}] \tag{6.6b}$$

$$k = \text{food} \qquad Fij(food) = \frac{\delta Ci(food)}{\left(\frac{M'ij}{A}\right)} \qquad [\frac{m^2 \cdot a}{kg \cdot d}] \tag{6.6c}$$

The effect factors are calculated with Equation (6.13) where ρ is the modelled population density (Equation 6.12), *LT* is the assumed lifetime (70 *a*), and *UR* is the unit risk factor:

$$Eik = \frac{\rho i}{LT} \cdot URik \tag{6.13}$$

$$Ei(inhalation) = \frac{\rho i}{LT} \cdot URi(inhalation) \qquad [\frac{\text{tumour cases}}{\mu g} \cdot \frac{m^3}{m^2 a}] \tag{6.13a}$$

$$Ei(drinking\ water) = \frac{\rho i}{LT} \cdot URi(drinking\ water) \qquad [\frac{\text{tumour cases}}{\mu g} \cdot \frac{l}{m^2 a}] \tag{6.13b}$$

$$Ei(food) = \frac{\rho i}{LT} \cdot URi(food) \qquad [\frac{\text{tumour cases}}{mg} \cdot \frac{kg \cdot day}{m^2 a}] \tag{6.13c}$$

The years of life lost (YLL) are calculated with Equation (6.15), where *S10* is the survival rate after 10 years and *Rma* quantifies the number of deaths at age *a* due to cancer type *m*:

$$YLLm(r,K) \text{ per cancer incidence} = (1 - S10,m) \cdot \frac{1}{Rm} \sum\nolimits_a YLLm(a,r,K) \cdot Rm\,a \qquad [a] \tag{6.15}$$

We have shown in Section 5.4 that the *YLL(a,r,K)* can be written as follows if the discount rate is set at 0, *a* is the age of death, *K* stands for the age-weighting factor, β determines the shape of the age-weighting, *C* is a correction factor due to the age-weighting, and *L* is the standard life expectancy at age *a*:

$$YLLm(a,0,K) = \frac{KCe^{-\beta am}}{\beta^2} \{e^{-\beta L} [-\beta(L+am)-1] + \beta am + 1]\} + (1-K)\,L \qquad [a] \tag{5.4}$$

Finally, the YLD can be taken from Section 5.4 with *a* being the onset of the disease and *Lm* indicating the average duration of the disease period:

$$YLDm(0,K) = Dm \left\{ \frac{KCe^{-\beta am}}{\beta^2} \{e^{-\beta Lm} [-\beta(Lm+am)-1] + \beta am + 1\} + (1-K)\,Lm \right\} \qquad [a] \tag{5.7}$$

This list of the formulas involved in the different substeps helps in checking the units. It becomes clear that the different mass units have to be compensated by a multiplication of the tumour incidence factor by 10^9 for the exposure by air and drinking water, and by 10^6 for the exposure by food. A linkage of these single steps to one overall formula does not produce a greater insight and is therefore omitted.

6.5.3 The best estimates of the damage factors

Appendix (6.11) already lists the mean values of the tumour incidence factors *Tijk* per substance, emission media, and exposure path. The resultant damage in terms of DALYs can be calculated based on the results for the DALYs per cancer site given in Table 6.20 (see Equation 6.2).

The attribution of substances to cancer types is taken from Table 6.16 and the results of the final multiplication are given for the case without age-weighting (DALYs(0,0)) in Appendix (6.12) and with age-weighting (DALYs(0,1)) in Appendix (6.13). The results listed in Appendix (6.12) are visualised in Figure 6.9.

A meaningful interpretation of the results shown in Figure 6.9 is difficult because the normalisation per kg emission does not yet allow for links to reality. One main insight, for example, is that between dioxins and styrene there exists a difference of eleven orders of magnitude in damage potential to human health per kg emission. Six orders of magnitude of this difference come from the fate analysis. The other five orders result from the combination of the fate factors with the effect and the damage factors. A look at Appendix (6.10) shows that the unit risk factors vary by seven orders of magnitude and the calculation of the DALYs per tumour case add only a small additional variation. One can therefore conclude that the fate and the effect factors compensate each other very little when multiplied with each other, i.e., highly persistent substances have, in many cases, also high unit risk factors and *vice versa.* In addition, it can be seen that it does matter whether a substance is released to air or surface water. Furthermore, it is a characteristic of the substance whether higher damage potentials results from emission to air or to water.

The relevance of the different exposure paths for the damages to human health due to emissions to air (Figure 6.10) can be compared with Figure 6.6 where only the exposure was considered. The pictures are similar with minor exceptions. The same holds true for emissions to water (see Figures 6.11 and 6.7). If one takes only those substances where unit risk data from official guidelines have been used, the assumption made for all the other substances – that internal exposure is proportional to external exposure for all exposure paths – is confirmed. The values have to be the same for those substances for which we calculated unit risk factors for other exposure paths than those given in the guidelines. This is because the same assumptions on uptake have been made. We can therefore conclude that for emissions to air, the exposure path either by air or by food is the relevant one. For emission to water all exposure paths are of similar relevance.

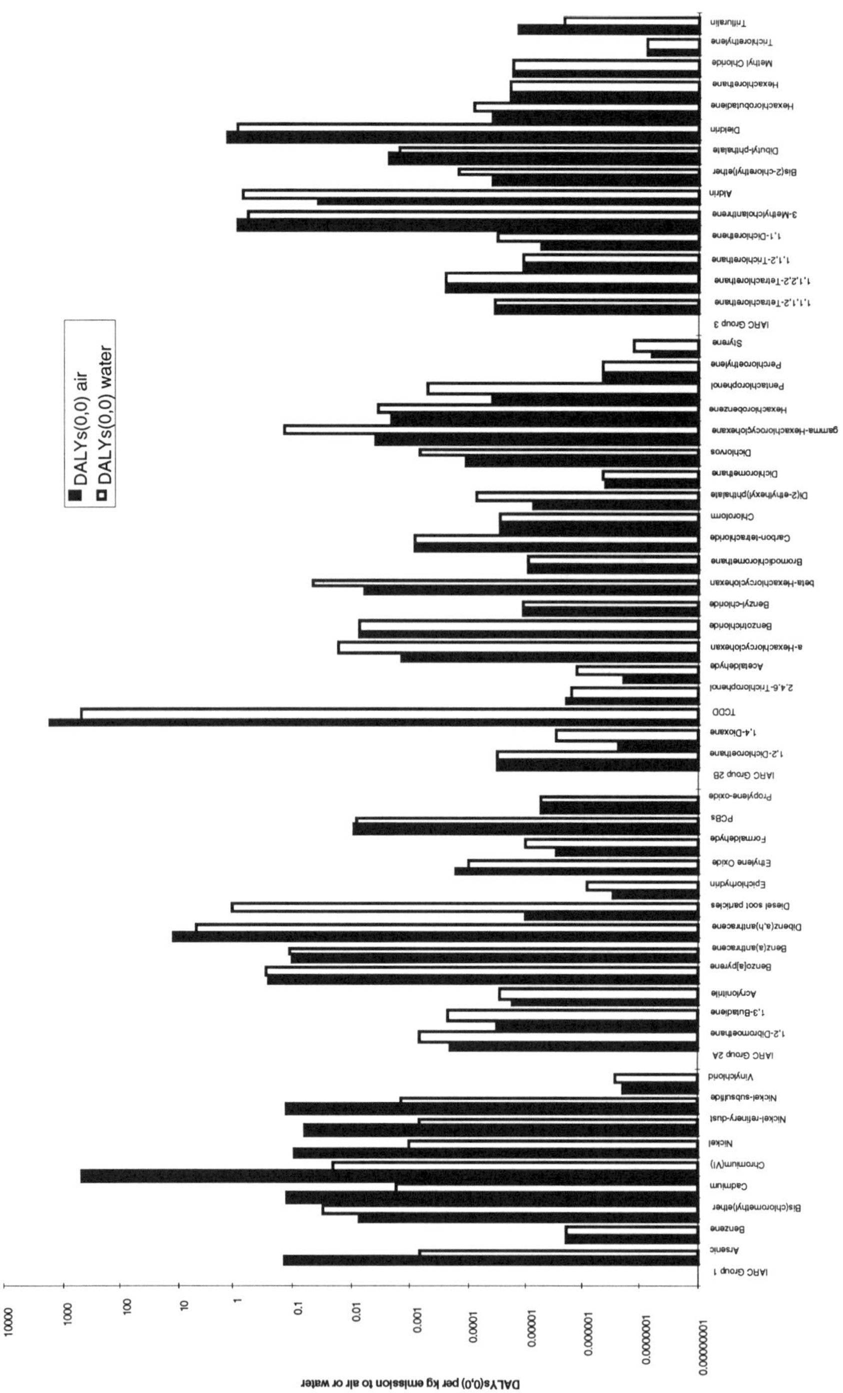

Fig. 6.9: DALYs(0,0) (no discounting and no age-weighting) per 1 kg substance emission to air and water respectively (results are given in Appendix 6.12)

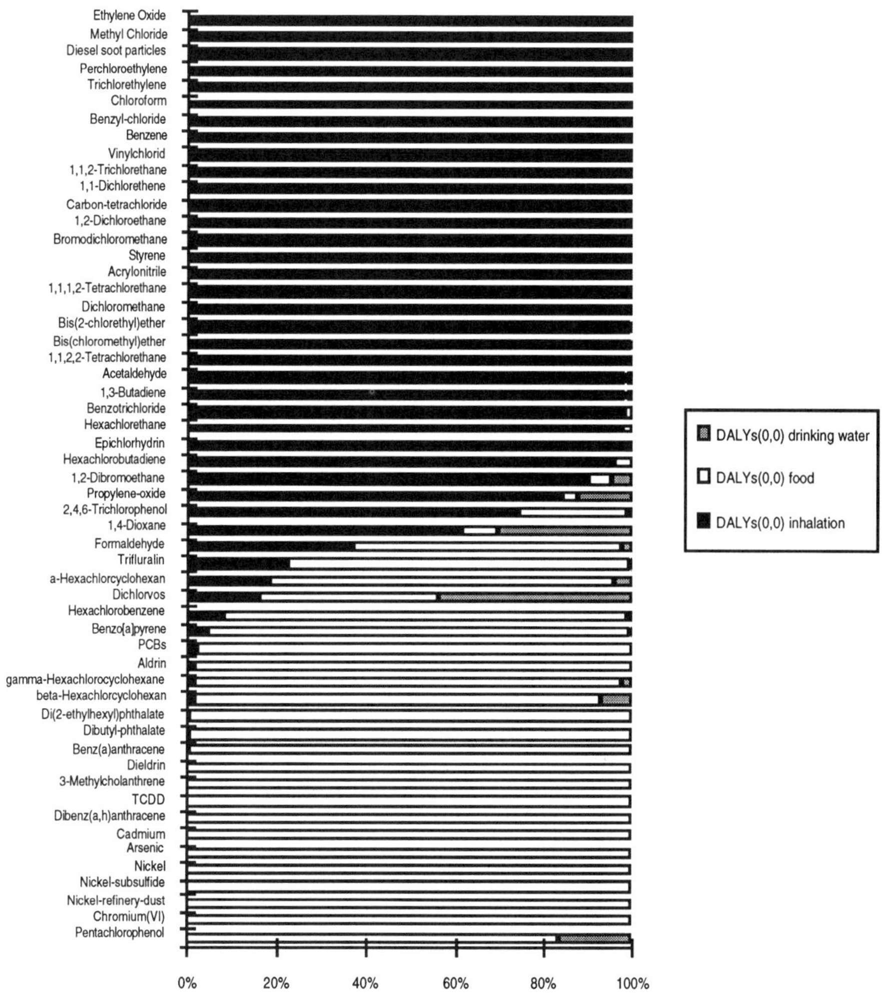

Fig. 6.10: Relative shares of the exposure paths (inhalation, drinking water and food) in the damage to human health due to emissions to air.

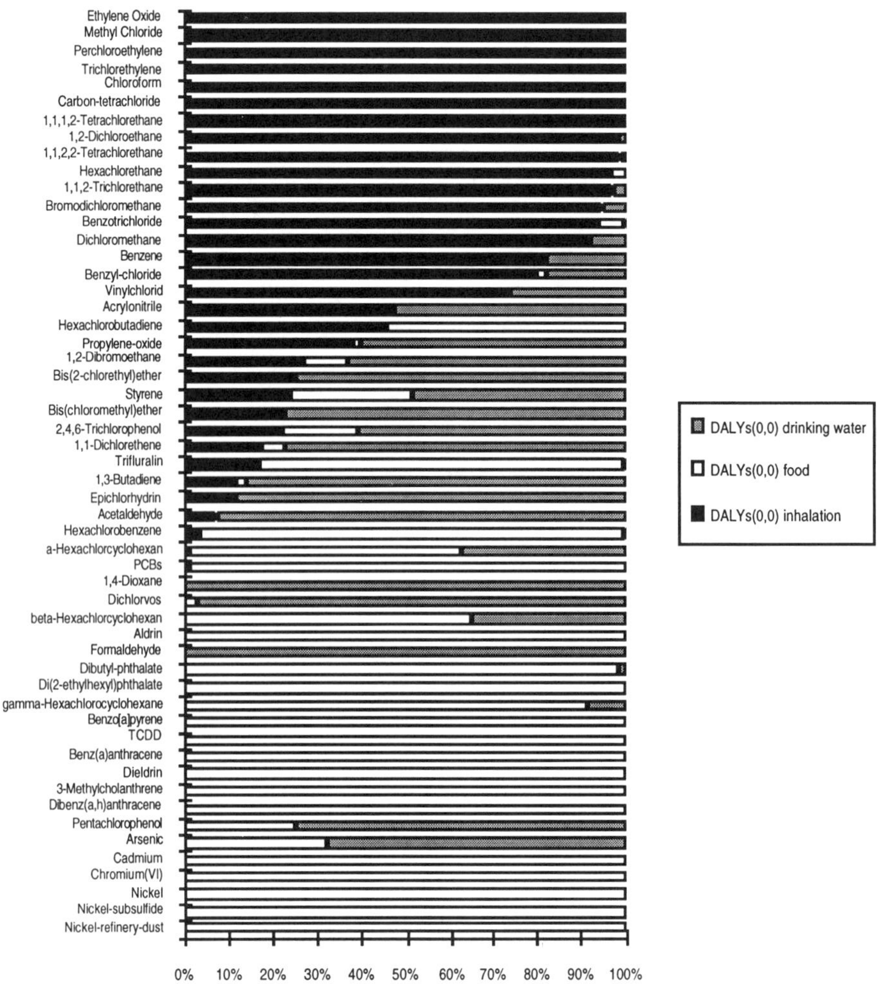

Fig. 6.11: Relative shares of the exposure paths (inhalation, drinking water and food) in the damage to human health due to emissions to water.

6.5.4 Cumulated error ranges for the estimates

Error estimates have been made for each substep in the calculation of the damage factor. We assumed lognormal distributions and estimated the (squared) geometric standard deviation σ_g^2. The range between the expectation value divided by σ_g^2 and the expectation value multiplied by σ_g^2 spans the confidence interval of 95% (Appendix 6.8). The error estimates can be found for the:

- fate factors in Subsection 6.2.6, Table 6.8
- population density in Subsection 6.3.5
- effect factors in Subsection 6.3.6, Table 6.14 and in the text
- DALYs in Subsection 6.4.5

These error estimates are presented again per substance in Appendix (6.14). For further analysis, we assume that the variables are independent[49]. The total geometric standard deviation for emissions to air and water and intake by inhalation, drinking water and food can be calculated (Appendix 6.15) by applying the rules on the arithmetic multiplication of lognormally distributed variables (Formula (A6.2) and (A6.3) in Appendix 6.8). Combining these values with the mean values for DALYs(0,0) given in Appendix (6.12), the lower (2.5%) and upper (97.5%) values of the 95% confident interval for DALYs(0,0) for emissions to air and to water can be calculated (Appendix 6.16).

Figures 6.12 and 6.13 show the graphical interpretation of these results. This quantitative error analysis reveals the huge variation in the width of the confidence interval for the different substances. Substances that fit well to the models used, and for whom sufficient information is available, show a confidence interval spanning about one (emission to air) to two (emission to water) orders of magnitude (e.g., benzene, bis(chlormethyl)ether, and vinylchloride). The damages due to, e.g., metal emissions, are much less certain. The confidence interval for them reaches a maximum with a range of 5 (!) orders of magnitude.

The results that are presented in Figures 6.12 and 6.13 correspond to the egalitarians' perspective, i.e., substances of IARC Group 1, 2, and 3, no discounting and no age-weighting. Assessment systems for hierarchists' disregard the 14 substances that are on the right of (but including) 1,1,1,2-tetrachlorethane (substances of IARC Group 3). Only the nine IARC-Group 1 substances are relevant for the individualists' perspective. The results for the individualists' perspective with the application of age-weighting are reported in Appendix (6.17). These DALYs(0,1) are lower than those for the other perspectives, but the geometric standard deviations remain unchanged. They are therefore not listed again.

It has to be noted that the error analysis undertaken here is based on estimates of the confidence intervals for mainly stochastic errors of single values. Unknown aspects, such as threshold behaviour instead of the assumed non-threshold behaviour, or a sensitivity to only one of the three exposure paths (inhalation, drinking water, and food) thought to be relevant, are not reflected in the calculated error ranges.

These probability distributions will be added up when the index for damages to human health due to a product alternative is calculated. The resulting probability distribution (no more lognormally distributed) will then be used in the dominance analysis which will be introduced in Subsection 8.1.4.

[49] This assumption might be wrong for certain fate and effect factors. A highly persistent and accumulating substance may show some dependence in the variation of the fate and effect factor. However, this dependence, though probable, cannot be considered due to a lack of information on covariance.

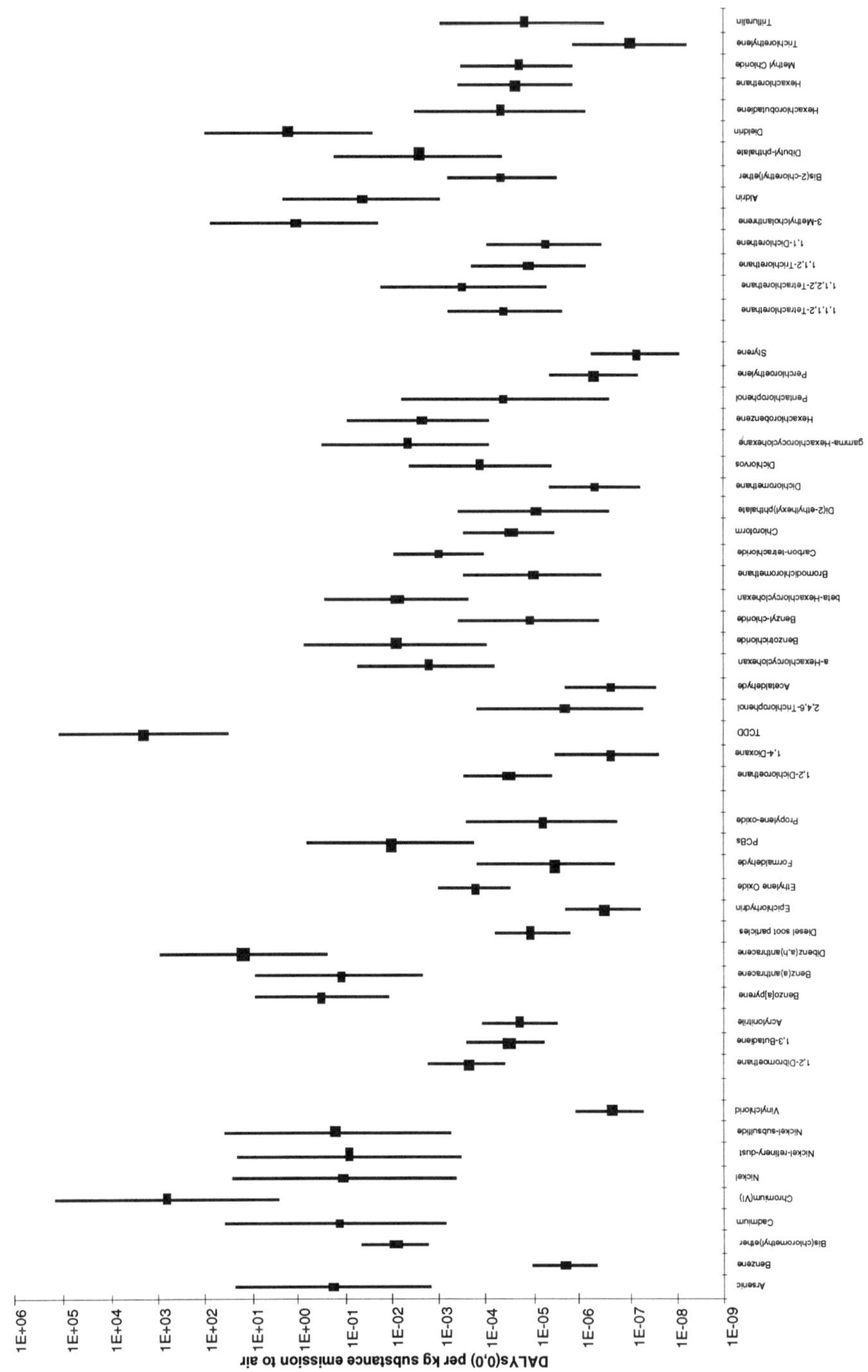

Fig. 6.12: 95% confidence interval for DALYs(0,0) per kg substance emission to air (numbers see Appendix 6.16)

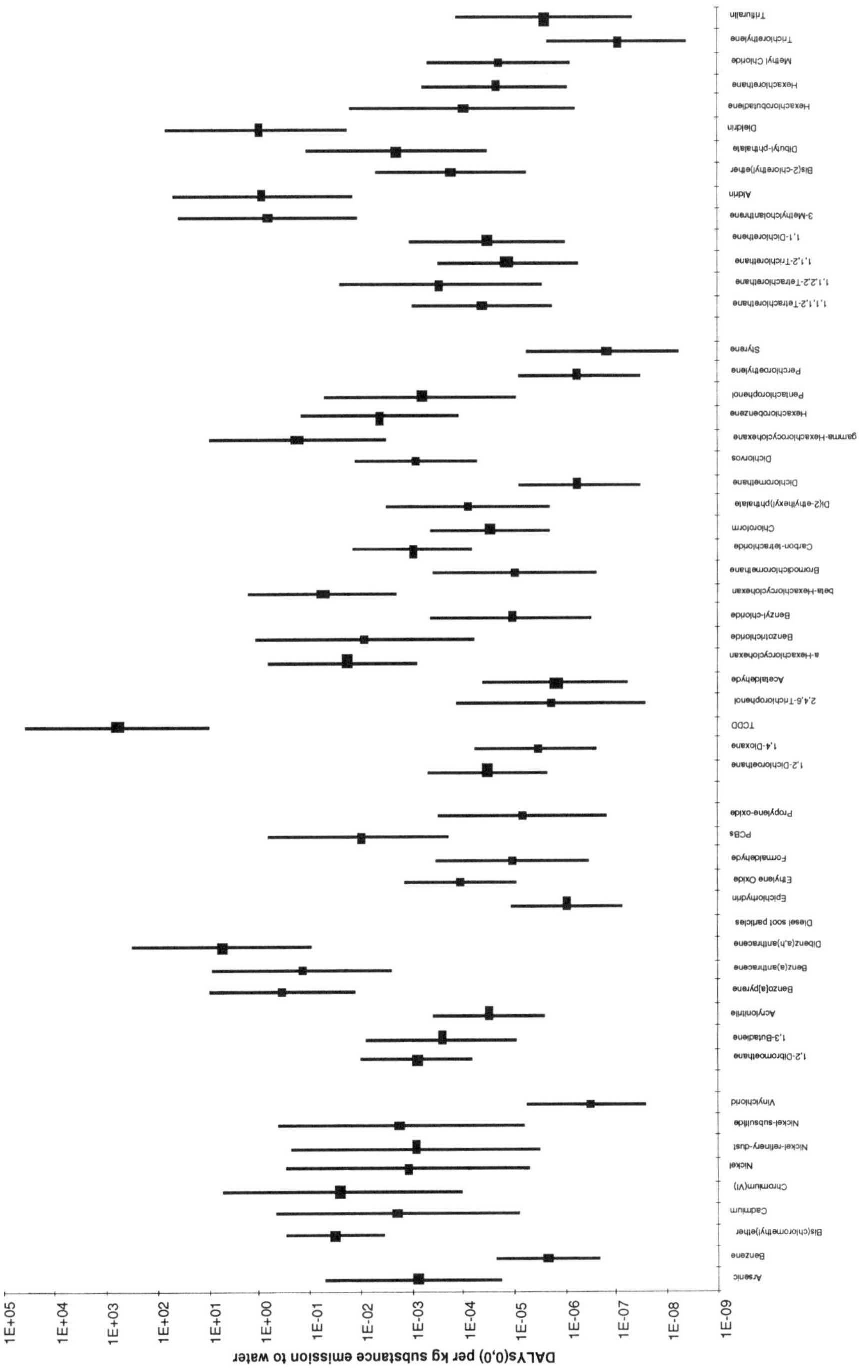

Fig. 6.13: 95% confidence interval for DALYs(0,0) per kg substance emission to water (numbers see Appendix 6.16)

6.5.5 Comparison with other cancer risk estimates

Review of cancer incidence estimates due to environmental risk factors

LAI (1992) estimated the cancer risks due to inhalation of air pollutants such as Polycyclic Aromatic Hydrocarbons (PAH), benzene, dioxins, cadmium, arsenic, diesel soot particles, and asbestos based on measured concentrations and on the unit risk approach. They found that the cancer risks of these substances lead in urban areas to 81 cancer cases per 100'000 inhabitants (if they are exposed during 70 years to the measured 1990 concentrations of Western-Germany). The same substances cause only 15 cancer cases per 100'000 inhabitants for a population benefiting from the air quality in rural areas. This amounts to 57 cancer cases per 100'000 inhabitants if one uses the German urban/rural distribution of inhabitants for averaging (LAI 1992). The same study found that other carcinogenic air pollutants such as vinyl chloride, chromium, nickel, and others increase these numbers by 45%. This results in a total of 118 and 22 cancer cases per 100'000 inhabitants for urban and rural areas respectively, and of 83 cases for the average German situation. This can be taken as an estimate for the total cancer risk due to inhalation of environmental air pollutants. This risk estimate has to be increased if additional indirect cancer risks due to air pollutants taken up through drinking water and food, and through direct water and soil pollution are to be incorporated in the risk estimate.

The number of 83 cancer cases per 100'000 inhabitants and a cancer incidence of 1.2 per 100'000 inhabitants and year (83 divided by 70 years) translate into an estimate of about 700 cases of cancer per year caused by air pollution if one proceeds on the basis of a population of about 60 millions (for the old Germany of 1989). This is about 2.5% of the total cases of lung cancer in Germany in 1989 (which affect more than 22'000 men and 5'500 women each year) (LAI 1992)).

USEPA (1990) made an estimate of the cancer risk in the United States of America due to the inhalation of air pollutants at the level of 1986 emissions. The best estimate arrives at 1'700 to 2'700 excess cases of cancer annually (7 to 11 per year per million inhabitants). This is the effect of 90 air pollutants emitted by 60 source categories. The detailed results are given in Table 6.21[50]. Twelve of these substances contribute to more than 90% of the total[51]. USEPA mentions that the approach used for the determination of cancer potency (unit risks) and some assumptions made about exposures, may have led to an overestimate. Potentially missing pollutants[52], non characterised sources, long-range transport and transformation could, in contrast, have caused an underestimation of the actual risk.

---

[50] It has to be mentioned here that the cancer risks due to Products of Incomplete Combustion (PIC) are largely based on benzo(a)pyrene-content and neglect, therefore, other aspects of particle mechanisms that are considered in LAI (1992).

[51] One cannot deduce from this statement that only these 12 substances have to be reported and assessed in LCA. USEPA (1990) analyses the average pollution mixture in the USA . LCI for single products will, in many cases, show rather different pollution profiles (i.e., patterns) with diverging major pollutants. This will result in differing priorities for process improvements.

[52] USEPA (1990) states that, in 1985, more than 2800 compounds were identified in ambient air. Only about 10% of them have been tested so far for mutagenity or carcinogenity. We know nothing about the nature of the other 2'500.

Both studies (USEPA 1990, LAI 1992) have used concentrations of air toxins found in the ambient air as the basis for their calculations. They also assumed that exposed persons breathe this outdoor air 24 hours a day, which is clearly not the case.

		Estimated annual cancer cases[a]	
Pollutant	EPA Classification[b]	Range	Point[c]
Acrylonitrile	B1	13-14	13
Arsenic	A	8-68	68
Asbestos	A	82-126	88
Benzene	A	143-181	181
1,3-Butadiene	B2	244-266	266
Cadmium	B1	6-16	10
Carbon tetrachloride	B2	31-47	41
Chloroform	B2	29-115	115
Chromium (hexavalent)	A	113-283	147-265[d]
Coke Oven Emissions	A	7-11	7
Dioxin	B2	2-125	2-125[e]
Ethylene dibromide	B2	25-68	68
Ethylene dichloride	B2	16-45	45
Ethylene oxide	B1-B2	5-6	6
Formaldehyde	B1	124-240	124
Gasoline vapours	B2	19-76	19-76[f]
Hexachlorobutadiene	C	9	9
Hydrazine	B2	6	6
Methylene chloride	B2	3-6	5
Perchloroethylene	B2	6-13	6
PIC[g]	-	438-1120	438-1120[h]
Radionuclides[f]	A	1-3	3
Radon[f]	A	2	2
Trichlorethylene	B2	5-13	7
Vinyl chloride	A	13-25	25
Vinylidene chloride	C	0.5-10	10
Miscellaneous[j]	-	15	15
Totals		1,366-2,909	1,726-2,706

Tab. 6.21 Summary of estimated annual cancer cases in the USA by inhaled air pollutants in 1986 (USEPA 1990)

Note: Values in this figure are not absolute predictions of cancer occurrence and are intended to be used in a relative sense only. The dose-response relationships and exposure assumptions have a conservative bias, but omissions due to uncharacterised pollutants (either directly emitted or secondarily formed) and emission sources, the long-range transport of pollutants, and the lack of knowledge of total risk from multi-pollutant exposures will offset this bias to an unknown extent.

a) These estimates are based on unit risk factors that may overstate the actual risk. The unit risk factors for arsenic, benzene, cadmium, and hexavalent chromium are maximum likelihood estimates. The unit risk factor for asbestos is a "best" estimate, very similar to the value that would be obtained if the maximum likelihood estimate was calculated. Unit risk factors for PIC have no classification. All other unit risk factors are upper-bound estimates.

b) For discussion of how EPA evaluates suspect carcinogens and more information on these classifications, refer to "Guidelines for Carcinogen Risk Assessment" (51 Federal Register 33992). The EPA classifications used in this report are:

A = proven human carcinogen

B = probable human carcinogen (B1 indicates limited evidence from human studies and sufficient evidence from animal studies but inadequate evidence from human studies)

C = possible human carcinogen

c) If a range is shown, it was considered unreasonable to select a point of estimate.

d) Range primarily reflects uncertainty with the exposure to hexavalent chromium from cooling towers. Some uncertainty to actual exposure to hexavalent chromium from all sources exists because the percent of total chromium that is hexavalent is still being evaluated for most sources.

e) Range reflects great uncertainty associated with exposure to dioxin from treatment, storage, and disposal facilities, and from municipal waste combustors. Other uncertainties associated with dioxin estimates include sampling method and extrapolation from tetrachlorinated dibenzodioxin (TCDD) to the other dioxin subspecies.

f) Range reflects different assumptions as to which portion of gasoline vapours is carcinogenic. The upper end of the range assumes all gasoline vapour is carcinogenic; the lower end assumes only the C6 and higher fraction of the gasoline vapour is carcinogenic.

g) PIC (products of incomplete combustion) is a group of pollutants that have not been very well defined and for which EPA has not developed a classification. It is composed of some pollutants, such as BaP, for which EPA has developed a classification. BaP is a B2 pollutant (probable human carcinogen).

h) Range reflects the use of two unit risk factors for diesel particulate.

i) From sources emitting significant amounts of radionuclides (and radon) to outdoor air. Does not include exposure to indoor concentrations of radon due to radon in soil gases entering homes through foundations and cellars.

j) Includes individual pollutants primarily from the TSDF study and the Sewage Sludge Incinerator study.

Schümann *et al.* (1989) in their interesting work report a risk estimate for Hamburg using a very fine grid resolution of 500 m times 500 m and applying site-specific background concentrations where available. The evaluation included 12 substances and used the unit risks published by EPA and WHO. The 28 expected cancer deaths per year for Hamburg were linked to BaP (38%), Dichlorethane (27%), Diesel exhaust (12%), Chromium (8%) and the other 8 substances. The high shares for Dichlorethane and BaP are surprising and probably reflect the specific industry mix and the district heating technologies used in Hamburg (in the mid-eighties).

Pruppers *et al.* (1996) calculated risk maps for accidents, radiation, and a few chemicals. For six carcinogenic substances (benzo(a)pyrene, benzene, ethylene oxide, vinylchloride, 1,2-dichloroethane, and acrylnitrile), they calculated background concentrations, exposure, and the resulting risk due to emissions included in the Dutch emission registry (Pruppers 1996) (Table 6.22).

	Emissions in the Netherlands, 1992 (Pruppers 1996)	Mortality risk range in the Netherlands due to Dutch emission sources (Pruppers *et al.* 1996)	Average mortality risk (own rough estimate from the given range)
	kg/a	Relative risk per year	Relative risk per year
Benzo(a)pyrene	2'402	10^{-5} - 10^{-8}	5 10^{-7}
Benzene	8'240'930	10^{-6} - 10^{-8}	5 10^{-8}
Ethylene oxide	115'371	10^{-7} - $<10^{-9}$	5 10^{-9}
Vinylchloride	207'632	10^{-8} - $<10^{-9}$	1 10^{-9}
1,2-Dichloroethane	636'069	10^{-8} - $<10^{-9}$	1 10^{-9}
Acrylnitrile	123'455	10^{-8} - $<10^{-9}$	1 10^{-9}

Tab. 6.22: Emissions of chemical carcinogenics and their resulting mortality risk in the Netherlands

Yetergil Kiefer (1997) assessed, for Switzerland, ambient concentrations of the three carcinogenic air pollutants benzo(a)pyrene, benzene, and diesel soot particles in air and calculated first cancer incidence cases (Tab. 6.23) and finally external costs in terms of monetary values. She used the concept of unit risks to estimate the incidence rate.

The EPS-System (Steen *et al.* 1992, Steen 1996) uses an approach that is similar to the one followed by Yetergil Kiefer (1997). The results are presented in terms of

ELU (Environmental Load Unit[53]) per kg substance emission. The carcinogenic damages due to As, Cd and Cr are calculated from Swedish data. They made global estimates for ethylene oxide (formed on the basis of ethene) and for PAH. One case of excess mortality was valued with 1 Mio. ELU's. Given an average of 35 years lost due to an excess death, it is possible to recalculate the underlying years of life lost from the impact indices calculated in Steen (1996) (Table 6.24).

	Inland emissions in Switzerland, 1992-1995	Cancer incidence 1994 Best case	Cancer incidence 1994 Central case	Cancer incidence 1994 Worst case
	t/a	Cases/year	Cases/year	Cases/year
Benzo(a)pyrene	>0.1	2	3	5
Benzene	2'740	1	3	5
Diesel soot particles (elemental carbon)	800-1000	6	36	201

Tab. 6.23: Cancer incidence due to the air concentration of three carcinogenic chemicals in Switzerland (7'019'000 inhabitants, concentrations due to inland emissions and imported pollution) (Yetergil Kiefer 1997)

	Emissions in Sweden, 1985	Impact index	Years life lost
	t/a	ELU/kg	a/t
Arsenic	40	10	0.35
Cadmium	5	1.2	0.042
Chromium	75	0.8	0.028
Ethene	n.a.	2.7	0.094
PAH	n.a.	8'800	310

Tab. 6.24: Emissions of chemical carcinogenics and years life lost in Sweden (Steen 1996), n.a. not applicable because the cancer risk estimation was made on the basis of world-wide emissions.

Doll *et al.* (1981) estimated that the share of cancers in Western industrial countries due to air and water pollution is 1-5% of the total cancer incidence. Their best estimate is 2%. This early estimate is not transferable to the German situation with its high shares of coal use for heating purposes and of diesel-engined cars, but it might be applicable to the Swiss situation. LAI (1992) cites case control studies from Poland and China; the estimates of the share of lung cancer due to air pollution vary between a low 4.3% and a very high 75%.

The risk from environmental pollution has to be seen in relation to other risk factors identified so far (Table 6.25). All estimates given here are made for the industrialised world or for the USA alone. The causal factors in developing countries are likely to differ from those in the industrialised ones. One of the most important conclusions to be drawn from these investigations is that *"cancer is indeed a preventable illness*[54]*. Nearly two-thirds of cancer deaths in the USA can be linked to the use of tobacco, diet, obesity, and lack of exercise - all of which can be modified through action, both at the individual and at the societal level"* (Harvard 1996). All studies find that the share of cancers due to environmental pollution is below 5%. In this sense, Ames (1990) is correct when he points to the misconceptions about the causes for cancers prevalent in society and in science. It is especially important in the valuation step of LCA to make clear that environmental pollution is responsible for only a very limited part of today's harm to human health[55]. Lutz (1997) has

[53] One ELU corresponds to the value of one ECU.

[54] This is true on a societal, but not on an individual, level.

[55] However, individuals judge the involuntary exposure (e.g., environmental pollution) as more important than the same voluntary exposure (e.g., smoking, alcohol), i.e., the reduction of involuntary

estimated that, for a hypothetical human being endowed with all the lowest risk factors from lifestyle and genetic heritage, only up to 10% of today's cancer incidence can be considered as endogenous, i.e., as inevitable or as attributable to general risk factors.

Risk factors	Causes of U.S. cancer incidence [%] (Möller *et al.* 1994)	Estimated percentage of total cancer deaths attributable to established causes of cancer in USA (Harvard 1996)	% of all cancer deaths in Western industrial countries (Doll *et al.* 1981) Best estimate	Range
Smoking, Tobacco	30	30	30	25-40
Adult diet/obesity	35	30	35	10-70
Sedentary lifestyle		5		
Occupational factors	4	5	4	2-8
Family history of cancer		5		
Viruses/Infection/other biological agents	10	5	10?	1-?
Prenatal factors/growth		5		
Reproductive factors		3	7	1-13
Alcohol		3	3	2-4
Socio-economic Status		3		
Environmental Pollution	2	2	2	<1-5
Ionising/ultraviolet radiation		2		
Prescription drugs/medical procedures		1	1	0.5-3
Salt/other food additives/contaminants		1	<1	-5-2
Industrial products			<1	<1-2
Geophysical factors			3	2-4
Other	18			
Unknown			?	?

Tab. 6.25: Estimates for the causes of human cancer from different sources

In the course of LCA studies other attempts were made to include carcinogenic effects. Tellus (1992) and BUWAL (1996e) are not discussed because they did not undertake a fate analysis. Gebler (1992) applied a simplified fate analysis and used a non-effect (threshold) oriented concept which can hardly be interpreted in terms of damage.

This short review takes into account a limited share of the relevant literature, which is extremely large due to the high importance of cancer as cause of death and the long research tradition. In a next subsection we will compare some of the estimates with the calculations made here.

Comparisons of the literature with own calculations

In order to limit the number of comparisons we select from the literature that has just been reviewed, those estimates for which emission data and damages in terms of incidence cases or mortality are given (LAI 1992, Pruppers *et al.* 1997, Steen 1996, Yetergil Kiefer 1997). The comparison follows a three-step procedure: firstly, the cases of incidence (or years of life lost) per kg substance emission are calculated from the underlying literature sources; secondly, the tumour incidence factors for the same exposure paths calculated here are taken from the appendices; and, thirdly, the value from the literature is divided by the one calculated here. The incidence rate for all relevant exposure paths for the assessed emissions is also given as supplementary information. It is, of course, impossible to discuss differences between factors when the literature sources used do not analyse relevant exposure paths.

exposure has a high relevance independent from the magnitude of voluntary exposure (see, e.g., Slovic *et al.* 1980).

The lifetime risk given in LAI (1992) has been recalculated for the comparison with the two assumptions that 60 million people in West Germany are exposed to the emissions listed in Tab. 6.26 and that they are only exposed during 1 year (division by 70 years) (see column (3) in Table 6.26). LAI (1992) considered only inhalation of emissions to air. *Tair,inhalation* in column (4) has therefore been chosen for the comparison. Column (5) shows the ratios between the two values. The discussion of this comparison can be supported with the data from Tables 6.3 and 6.7 for the fate factor and from Table 6.13 for the effect factor. The comparison based on the fate factors shows that the fate factors from LAI (1992) and from our own calculations are very similar for diesel soot, benzene, and cadmium. For all other substances the fate factors from LAI (1992) are substantially larger. The unit risk factors used by LAI (1992) are higher than those used in this case study for all the substances except for BaP (Table 6.13). It is therefore no surprise that the ratios for all the substances are larger than one. If one assumes that the more recent unit risk factors that have been used in this case study are also the more accurate ones, then we are still faced with the problem that the fate factors for dioxins, As, and BaP used in LAI (1992) are larger than those from the multi-media modelling exercise.

	Yearly emissions to air in Western Germany	Lifetime risk in Western Germany	Cancer incidence cases per kg emission	Cancer incidence $T_{air, inhalation}$	Cancer incidence $T_{air,inhalation+water+food}$	Ratio column (3) to own calculations
	(LAI 1992)	(LAI 1992)		Appendix (6.11)	Appendix (6.11)	
	(1)	(2)	(3)=(2)·600/70/(1)	(4)		(5)=(3)/(4)
	t/a	10^{-5} Cases	Cases/kg	Cases/kg	Cases/kg	-
Diesel soot particles	70'000	35	4.3E-6	6.1E-07	6.1E-07	7
Benzene	47'200	4.6	8.4E-7	1.2E-07	1.2E-07	7
2,3,7,8-TCDD	27 E-6	0.0007	2.2E-1	1.6E-02	2.7E-02	14
Arsenic	16 - 68	3.2	4E-4 - 1.7E-3	1.6E-05	1.2E-02	25-110
Cadmium	25.2 - 48.5	2.9	5.1E-4 - 9.9E-4	2.8E-05	9.8E-03	18-35
BaP	4.1 - 16.5	10	5.2E-3 - 2.1E-2	7.6E-04	2.0E-02	6.8-28

Tab. 6.26: Comparison of the estimates for cancer incidence due to air pollution from LAI (1992) with own calculations

The explanations for these differences have already been given in the comment to Table 6.7: the emissions used in LAI (1992) are likely to be underestimated and the concentrations measured are biased towards sites with high concentrations. Both reasons lead to overestimating the fate factors. The calculations for these substances made here are known to be poor. It has to be mentioned that for all three substances with poor agreement the intake through drinking water and food is important (dioxins and BaP) or even dominant (As). LAI (1992) omits the relevant intake by food. Would it not have done so, the metals would have been identified as the most dominant risk factors for cancer incidence cases caused by environmental chemicals.

One can use the average mortality risk in Pruppers *et al.* (1996) to calculate the incidence cases by multiplying it with the Dutch population and dividing with the emissions in the Netherlands (column (3) in Table 6.27). The factors thus calculated can be compared with the cancer incidence factors from Appendix (6.11). Column (5) in Table 6.27 shows the ratios between the two assessments. The ratio should be about a factor 2 because the population density in the Netherlands is about twice the assumed European population density. Taking this into account, the agreement is good for BaP, benzene, and vinylchloride, but differences of up to a factor 100 are found for ethylene oxide, 1,2-dichloroethane and acrylnitrile.

	Emissions in the Nether-lands, 1992 (Pruppers 1996)	Average risk (own rough estimate from Pruppers *et al.* 1996)	Average risk per kg emission	Cancer incidence $T_{air, inhalation}$ (App. 6.11)	Cancer incidence $T_{air,inhalation+water+food}$ (App. 6.11)	Ratio column (3) to own calculations
	(1)	(2)	(3) = (2)/(1) · 15'285'000	(4)		(5)=(3)/(4)
	kg/a	Relative risk per year	Mortality per kg	Cases/kg	Cases/kg	-
Benzo(a)pyrene	2'402	$5\ 10^{-7}$	3.2E-03	7.6E-04	2 E-2	4.2
Benzene	8'240'930	$5\ 10^{-8}$	9.3E-08	1.2E-07	1.2 E-7	0.77
Ethylene oxide	115'371	$5\ 10^{-9}$	6.6E-07	1.2E-05	1.2E-5	0.055
Vinylchloride	207'632	$1\ 10^{-9}$	7.4E-08	1.3E-08	1.3E-8	5.7
1,2-Dichloroethane	636'069	$1\ 10^{-9}$	2.4E-08	2.3E-06	2.3E-6	0.01
Acrylnitrile	123'455	$1\ 10^{-9}$	1.2E-07	1.0E-06	1E-6	0.12

Tab. 6.27: Comparison of the estimates for cancer incidence due to air pollution from Pruppers *et al.* (1996) with own calculations

The average concentrations given in Pruppers (1996) can be used to recalculate the fate factors (Formula (6.7) in Subsection 6.2.4). This recalculation shows that, for the three substances that least conform, the large differences are almost completely explained by the differences in the fate factors. The descriptions in Pruppers (1996) make it clear that a model that included wet and dry depositions, and degradation as well, was used for the calculation of the fate factors. The degradation times used by Pruppers (1996) were slightly smaller than those used here, but this difference cannot be the sole reason for the observed differences. In Pruppers *et al.* (1996), the wet deposition is the dominant process for the average residence time for ethylene oxide. This behaviour is probably poorly reflected in the multi-media modelling calculations that have been undertaken here.

This comparison shows that, for half of the assessed substances, large differences occur due to the use of different fate factors. A further evaluation of the two models that have been used would be necessary to come to a judgement on their respective qualities.

	Inland emissions in Switzerland, 1992-1995	Cancer incidence 1994 central case	Cancer incidence cases per kg emission	Cancer incidence $T_{air, inhalation}$	Cancer incidence $T_{air,inhalation+water+food}$	Ratio column (3) to own calculations
	Yetergil Kiefer 1997#	Yetergil Kiefer 1997		Appendix (6.11)	Appendix (6.11)	
	(1)	(2)	(3)=(2)/(1)	(4)		(5)=(3)/(4)
	t/a	Cases/year	Cases/kg	Cases/kg	Cases/kg	-
Benzo(a)pyrene	>0.1	3	<3.0E-02	7.60E-04	2.00E-02	<39
Benzene	2'740	3	1.1E-06	1.20E-07	1.20E-07	9.1
Diesel soot particles	800-1000	36	3.6E-05	6.10E-07	6.10E-07	59

Tab. 6.28: Comparison of the estimates for cancer incidence due to air pollution from Yetergil Kiefer (1997) with own calculations (# from BUWAL 1994/1995 and personal communication from BUWAL)

Yetergil Kiefer (1997) made a direct estimate of the cancer incidence cases in Switzerland due to pollutants in the air. Pruppers *et al.* (1996) differentiated between the risks due to inland and to imported pollution, Yetergil Kiefer starts instead from measured concentrations. Her estimates therefore not only reflect the emissions in Switzerland, but also the net contribution of imports minus exports. The high ratios in column (5) in Table 6.28 can largely be explained by the effect of this net contribution and the high population density in Switzerland. Yetergil Kiefer also used slightly higher unit risk factors for BaP and diesel soot particles for her central case than had been used in the calculations made here. It also has to be mentioned that the estimate of BaP-emission was identified as the lowest possible and that the Swiss EPA (BUWAL) is in the process of correcting it.

As mentioned above, Steen (1996) estimated cases of excess death before monetarising them. He used Swedish concentrations and emission estimates for the metals As, Cd, and Cr VI. The applied unit risks are somewhat higher for As and lower for Cd and Cr VI than the factors used in this case study. He assumed that the death rate from incidence cases is 50% and that a premature death causes a loss of ten life years. Both of these assumptions are lower than those used in Subsection 6.4.3. In addition, he makes the assumptions that Sweden's emission exports equal its imports and that the concentration measurements used are representative. All these points may partly explain the differences found for As, Cd, and Cr VI as expressed by the ratios calculated and reported in column (3) (Table 6.29). Another source of a systematic lower estimate than our calculations is the population density which is in Sweden much lower than the average in Europe. If Steen had not only considered inhalation, but also intake by food, his damage estimates would have been considerably higher.

	Years life lost, own recalculations from Steen (1996)	$DALYs(0,0)_{air, inhalation}$ Appendix (6.12)	Total $DALYs(0,0)_{air}$ Appendix (6.12)	Ratio Steen (1996) to own calculations
	(1)	(2)		(3) = (1)/((2)·1000)
	a/t	DALYs per kg emission to air	DALYs per kg emission to air	-
Arsenic	0.35	2.60E-04	1.60E-01	1.4
Cadmium	0.042	4.50E-04	1.30E-01	0.09
Chromium	0.028	5.60E-03	5.30E+02	0.005
Ethene	0.094	not available	not available	
PAH	310	1.20E-02	2.70E-01	1.2

Tab. 6.29: Comparison of the estimates for years life lost due to air pollution from Steen (1996) with own calculations

The estimate by Steen (1996) for ethene cannot be checked because no damage estimates have been made here so far for metabolites. Ethene is assumed to form ethylene oxide (Törnqvist 1994) which, however, has been assessed in the preceding sections. Including carcinogenic metabolites is a further step towards an improvement of the damage estimates (see Section 6.7).

The estimate of Steen (1996) for PAH is very crude and uncertain because he based it on global concentrations and emissions. For PAHs, he included the oral intake path in his analysis. This has been considered in the calculation of the ratios in column (3) (Table 6.29). The agreement between these two estimates is very good, but probably the result of mere chance.

Conclusions from these comparisons

The differences found between the risk estimates reported in the literature and those calculated here are sometimes small and sometimes very large. The explanations for this can be summarised as follows:

- The unit risk concept has been used to model the dose-effect relationship for all the risk estimates compared here. These unit risks factors vary only within a small range; they therefore cannot be the cause for the major differences.
- The fate factors vary widely and are subject to uncertainty in all the studies that have been reviewed. LAI (1992), Yetergil Kiefer (1997), and Steen (1996) use ambient air concentration measurements and only Steen (1996) calculates the normalised risk factors per kg substance emission. A review of the concentration measurements, averaging procedures, emission estimates, and of the emission budgeting underlying these measurements would be necessary to improve the basis for the empirical calculation of fate factors (Subsection 6.2.4). Pruppers *et al.* (1996) used a simplified fate model which showed good accordance with the calculations made here for only half of the substances compared. Fate modelling should therefore generally be improved.
- The risk estimates in the literature are based on the inhalation of air pollutants. Other paths are mostly neglected or excluded from consideration by definition. The results that have been presented in this case study are a significant improvement upon this situation.
- All the studies used for the comparisons use only one country for the analysis. The population densities used in those studies therefore do not represent the average population density a kg of substance emission will be faced with when being distributed all over Europe. For all but Sweden, this leads to an overestimate of the receptor density.
- The studies reviewed consider survival rates and years of life lost only if monetarisation translates the incidence cases into damages (Steen 1996, Yetergil Kiefer 1997). None of the existing studies used a comparably detailed approach as the one laid out in Section 6.4.
- The carcinogenic potential of metabolites has been disregarded in this case study. Ethylene oxide formed from ethene is one relevant example that should be considered in a future assessment.
- The numbers found in the literature are sometimes lying outside of the 95% confidence interval which has been estimated and calculated for this case study (Appendices 6.14/15/16). This observation cannot be interpreted further without a detailed evaluation of the data that has been used in the studies reviewed here.

These observations on the comparisons made here lead us to the overall conclusion that there is no need to replace or change elements used for the operationalisation of this case. More general conclusions will be given in Section 6.7.

6.6 Index for Manageability of Cancer

6.6.1 Recalling the preliminary proposal

After the detailed description of the index for known damage due to chemical carcinogenesis a second index for manageability will be assessed here. The index for manageability is based on the index for the magnitude of damage derived in Section 6.5, but enhanced by three additional indicators for: the possibilities to and the ease with which to reduce the assessed damage, for the excess of an environmental problem compared to a political target level or a sustainable level, and for the success of already introduced policy measures. The index is calculated as follows:

$$Mp,c = Rp,c \cdot Xp,c \cdot Sp,c \cdot Dp,c \qquad (6.17)$$

with Mp,c cultural perspective dependent index of manageability
Rp,c indicator for the ease of damage reduction [-]
Xp,c indicator for the excess of the target damage [-]
Sp,c indicator for the success of regulation [-]
Dp,c outcome of the damage assessment for human or ecological health measured in the
respective damage units
p index for environmental problem
c index for the three cultural perspectives (individualists, egalitarians and hierarchists)

This index has been explained and discussed in detail in Section 4.5. The parameters used for the index are those set out in Table 4.12 or if not from there, then those that will be estimated here in Subsection 6.6.2.

The application of this index for manageability to chemical carcinogenesis is just a feasibility test and nothing more. The important feature of this test is that there is a quantification of the index; the emphasis is not on the value of the index which will result from this test. There is a large body of literature on cancer prevention, cancer treatment, and policy measures. This literature has not been reviewed systematically and the selection of papers in support of the quantification of the index may therefore turn out to have been arbitrary.

6.6.2 Determination of the index of manageability for chemical carcinogenesis

Indicator for damage reduction

The damage assessment that has been presented in Sections 6.2 through 6.5 does not consider different scenarios for the future development of the world. The present state of the health sector formed the basis for the estimates of survival rates, of the age of onset, and of the disease history. The consideration factor *fc* has therefore to be set equal to one for all three cultural perspectives.

The relative reduction of DALYs per kg substance emission due to chemical carcinogenesis has to be estimated in the next step under the assumption that additional financial expenditures and legislative effort (*Ec*) is provided. The following most important measures may be considered to reduce damage due to chemical carcinogenesis (at a given emission level):

1. Food could be produced only in areas with clean air, water, and soil so as to lower the intake of carcinogenic substances by humans.
2. Drinking water could be produced only from clean sources of water to lower the intake of carcinogenic substances by humans.
3. The inhaled air could (at least in cities) be filtered by wearing a filter towel protecting mouth and nose to lower the inhalation of carcinogenic substances by humans.
4. R&D efforts could be enlarged to isolate cancer suppressing agents as, e.g., those that have already been identified through epidemiological studies in green tea.
5. Methods and instruments for the detection of tumours at an early stage of development could be developed. Such methods could be used in improved health screening programs.
6. Additional R&D efforts could lead to improvements in cancer treatment that would raise survival rates after detection and that would lower disabling consequences due to tumour growth and side-effects of treatment methods.
7. Risk factors (behaviour) found to act synergistically with environmental pollution, such as smoking (Hemminki *et al.* 1994), could be constrained by law.

Measures (1) and (2) appear unrealistic given the few places where such conditions still exist, the high costs induced by such a limitation[56], and the legislative effort that would be needed to convince the agriculture sector to adopt only organic farming techniques[57] in non-polluted areas. Measure (3) might have costs that are lower than the set limit of *Ec*. However, such a measure can be only introduced on a voluntary base under present societal conditions. The damage reduction achieved overall is therefore likely to be very small. Measures (4) and (6) could lead to very large reductions of damage at given emissions. However, whether new findings will

[56] With two litres of drinking water per day, more than 700 litres are needed per year and per person. This measure alone might exceed the maximum additional expenditure possible under E_0.

[57] This is a necessary condition because pesticides and heavy metals in synthetic fertiliser are both carcinogenics as well.

revolutionise the medical possibilities of tumour suppression and treatment is highly speculative. The same holds partly true for measure (5), although improved health screening programs improve early detection in any case.

Lung cancer is a relevant cancer site for chemical carcinogenesis. Lung cancer has a long latency period, but progresses quickly once it has reached the stage where it can be detected. It can be assumed that screening intervals would have to be substantially shorter than 6 months to detect lung cancer at an early stage in order to be effective because experiments with semi-annual screenings did not reduce mortality in a significant way. Primary prevention (less exposure) is considered to be the only efficient management strategy for lung cancer (Tomatis *et al.* 1993).

Graham (1993) estimated costs per life year saved for various strategies to prevent and treat cancer. He considered only screening for and treatment of colorectal and breast cancer and he estimates that the costs would reach $1'000 to $10'000 per life year saved. Prohibition of products, renovation of homes with high radon levels, and the setting of more stringent emission standards would cause costs of $10'000 to $100'000 per life year saved. Germany could mobilise expenditures of $4 billion per year if it would spend $50 per person and year. This amount would be sufficient to save between 40'000 and 4 million life years per year in Germany (assuming costs of $1000 to $100'000 per life year saved). About 2 million years of life are lost in Germany due to cancer if the average YLL is taken from Table 6.18 and if an average death rate of 200 persons per 100'000 population is assumed. This expenditure would therefore result in a calculated damage reduction of between 2% and 100%, depending on the costs that are assumed. That is, full reduction would seem to be achievable. The lower costs of $1000 per life year saved hold only for colorectal and for breast cancer both of which occur frequently and are well understood. The linearity that is assumed in this calculation therefore does not apply and its applicability to chemical carcinogenesis due to environmental pollutants is questionable.

Brown *et al.* (1996) estimate that in the year 1990 more than 110 $ per inhabitant were spent on medical care for cancer in the United States of America. The 50 $ or 100 $ set as the additional unit effort *Ec* (see Table 4.10) would therefore permit a significant increase in screening and treatment activities. The legislative effort would be relevant for the measures (1) and (2) listed above but were rejected as being unrealistic. Measure (7) has already been implemented in part in some countries where smoking in public buildings and places is forbidden. Further restrictions with respect to sales outlets, a higher minimum age for buying tobacco products, higher taxes, restricting smoking at work, etc. may yet be introduced through additional laws and decrees.

For individualists, we assume that they invest the unit effort in measures (4) to (6). They do this in such a way that not all groups of society can profit equally from it. Damage reduction will therefore be highest in high-income groups. The damage reduction possible with effort *Ec* in this case is estimated to be 20%.

Egalitarians establish a social health screening program that also covers those groups which are at present insufficiently covered by the medical care scheme. Measures (4) to (6) will be taken within the budget restrictions. Measure (7) will be implemented to some extent. However, the indirect benefit of lower incidence rates due to environmental pollutants will be very small compared to the direct effect in the form of reduced health damages of less smoking. A reduction of 30% seems to be achievable.

Hierarchists spend more money (doubling today's medical care budget for cancer) and implement measures (4) to (7). They will spend reasonable amounts on research and may therefore realise new detection and treatment techniques within the latency time of about 20 years. This would allow them to considerably reduce the assessed damage. A 50% damage reduction potential seems possible under this scenario.

It is clear that these are all rough estimates in order to quantify the indicator. The discussion of these measures and the arguments in support of them and their effectiveness could be significantly improved if the knowledge of health care providers on these subjects could be systematically made use off.

Indicator for excess of the target damage

The quantification of the indicator for excess of the target damage requires determination for the present and the target level for the impacts due to environmental pollutants causing cancer. A long list of estimates for cancer cases due to environmental pollutants exists:

- USEPA (1990) estimated 7 to 11 incidence cases per million inhabitants due to the inhalation of air pollutants in 1986 (US American conditions).
- LAI (1992) arrived at 12 incidence cases per million inhabitants due to the inhalation of air pollutants in 1990 (Western German conditions).
- Törnqvist *et al.* (1994) found 27 incidence cases per million inhabitants due to the inhalation of air pollutants (Swedish conditions).
- Yetergil Kiefer (1997) estimates that the incidence is somewhere between 2 to 41 cases per million inhabitants due to the inhalation of air pollutants in 1994 and reports that the best estimate is 9 incidence cases per million inhabitants (Swiss conditions).

All these estimates include only emissions to air and exposure through inhalation, but for many substances, this is not the relevant exposure path as shown in Section 6.5. Sagunski *et al.* (1991) mention that exposure through food and, in part, through drinking water and soil, are significant as well. The numbers given by sources in the literature quoted above therefore serve as lower estimates only. In Subsection 9.2.1 and Appendix (9.1) extrapolations for Europe based on the results in Appendix (6.16) and emission estimates will be made. These calculations result in the high number of about 300 cases per million due to emissions to air[58].

Both Goedkoop (1995) and Müller-Wenk (1997) suggest setting a sustainable level for *T* at 1 premature death per year and per million inhabitants in the absence of an explicit political target. WHO (1987) calculates concentrations where carcinogenic substances potentially cause 1 premature death per year per million inhabitants. However, this is done without proper substantiation and the premature deaths due to different carcinogenics are additive. Yelokhin *et al.* (1996) report an acceptable risk for new objects of 10^{-6} accidents a year which they say agrees with international

[58] This number results if one assumes that one cancer case equals to 15 DALYs and that the concerned population equals 600 million.

practice. Lacking any further information on target levels, we continue the calculation with this target damage.

In order to get the best estimate of the target damage excess factor *N/T*, it is assumed that the damage from carcinogenic pollutants by all exposure paths is lower than the best estimate from our extrapolation, i.e., $N = 200$ premature deaths per year and per million inhabitants. It is considered that deaths due to environmental pollutants will, in general, lead to less years of life lost than from accidents and that we used steady-state incidence rates rather than actual rates. With Formula (6.18) we can calculate the indicator for the target damage excess factor X_c. *Xindividualist* is calculated to be 1.7, *Xegalitarian* and *Xhierarchist* are both 2.9.

$$X_c = \left(\frac{N}{T}\right)^{g_c} \qquad [-] \qquad (6.18)$$

The result of these calculations lets us conclude that we are far away from the envisaged sustainable level. The highly subjective nature of the determination of the sustainable level has a large influence over the outcome. Thus, the setting of sustainable levels may be done equally well based on cultural perspectives. (This problem does not occur if long-term policy levels have been determined.) In addition, the subjective setting of gc in Table 4.12 (0.1 for individualists and 0.2 for hierarchists and egalitarians) has a huge influence on the resulting target damage excess factor X_c.

Indicator for regulatory success

The decision tree shown in Figure 4.9 is used to determine the value of the indicator for regulatory success Sc. Chemical carcinogenesis has been known for decades and can be considered to be well understood, although there are questions still open on the explanation of mechanisms and of influencing factors.

The problem of chemical carcinogenesis is not regulated as such. However, many carcinogenic substances are regulated because of their known carcinogenic potential. The WHO guidelines (WHO 1987) listed some of the most potent carcinogens to motivate individual countries to set standards. Improvements have been achieved by limiting emissions of heavy metals and PAH's from metal refining industry and coking plants. The use of cadmium is regulated as well and the concentration of benzene in petrol has already been limited in some countries.

Some loads have definitively been declining in established market economies due to large investments in highly efficient electrostatic filters for power stations for the treatment of flue gases, to billions of dollars invested in the reduction of BaP from coking plants, and to process improvements in many other economic sectors. It is doubtful that this is also true for developing countries.

The last question in the decision tree (Figure 4.9) addresses the accordance with long-term policy targets. They do not exist for carcinogenic substances as a class. They may exist for certain specific carcinogenic substances, but it cannot be assumed that the existing targets, or the sustainable levels, will be met if we recall the high target damage excess factor, and remember the continuing large growth in traffic and the lack of an overall strategy.

This discussion suggests that the parameter $s1_c$ has to be attributed to indicator S_c, i.e., 0.9 for individualists and 0.8 for egalitarians and hierarchists.

Aggregation of the indicators to an index

The values of the three indicators *R, X, S* are summarised for each of the three cultural perspectives in Table 6.30 based on the preceding discussion. These three indicators are multiplied with each other and then multiplied with the index for the magnitude of damage caused by substance *i* emitted to compartment *j* per unit intervention. The index for magnitude of damage is measured in DALYs according to the procedure described in Sections 6.1 to 6.5. The DALYs per substance, emission compartment, and cultural perspective are listed in Appendices (6.16) and (6.17).

Cultural perspective	Individualists	Egalitarians	Hierarchists
R (Ease of reduction)	0.8	0.7	0.5
X (Target damage excess factor)	1.7	2.9	2.9
S (Regulatory success)	0.9	0.8	0.8
M (Manageability)	$1.22 \cdot \frac{DALYs_{ij}}{I_{ij}}$	$1.62 \cdot \frac{DALYs_{ij}}{I_{ij}}$	$1.16 \cdot \frac{DALYs_{ij}}{I_{ij}}$

Tab. 6.30: Composition of the index for manageability *M* from the three indicators for each cultural perspective and from the index for the magnitude of damage from chemical carcinogenesis

6.6.3 Discussion

For a comprehensive discussion, it would be necessary to calculate the index of manageability for several other environmental problems. Unfortunately, no other indices of manageability have been calculated so far.

One should keep in mind that the index of manageability presented here is built on the rough assumptions made above, and very much influenced by, the default values suggested in Section 4.5. Further investigations are necessary to collect the relevant information to improve the values for the indicators and to validate the default values that have been suggested here.

The index shows a difference of 40% in the weighting of the damage between egalitarians and hierarchist. The index for individualist lies in between and is close to the magnitude of damage ($DALYs_{ij}/I_{ij}$). It was the intention behind the design of the index of manageability for individualists that its value would be more stable than for the other perspectives, i.e., close to one. This is just a reflection on the little relevance of the whole index for individualists. The values of the index for the egalitarians and the hierarchists can vary between 0.3 and 3 times the magnitude of damage[59].

An interpretation of the index of manageability is not possible without looking at the individual indicators of which it is comprised. Relevant damage reductions of up

[59] This range was assumed when the index was designed, see Appendix (4).

to 50% are possible within the given additional effort *Ec* (50 to 100 $ per person per year plus changes in legislation). The target damage excess factor is still very large at the present time although the first regulative measures have already shown their effects. But there exist no indications that a damage level of 1 premature death per year and per one million inhabitants will be reached in the year 2025.

The index of manageability has the same unit as the index for the magnitude of damage, i.e., DALYs per kg substance emission. However, this equality of units does not imply that the two indices can simply be added. For the combination of the indices see Section 4.6.

6.7 Remaining aspects, the main assumptions, and conclusions

Bringing the example of chemical carcinogenesis to an end

In order to recall the many assumptions and observations made, the indications given, and outcome of the result this final section:

- points to two aspects, the time dimension and carcinogenic metabolites, which have been so far neglected,
- provides a concise list of limitations and assumptions connected with the results of the damage assessment, and
- contains some conclusions.

There is no claim that these concluding remarks will be the definitive treatment of the topic of chemical carcinogenesis, nor that all aspects relevant to Life Cycle Impact Assessment will have been addressed. The service to the reader is the presentation and discussion of one possibility to quantify damages to human health due to a selection of 55 potentially carcinogenic substances. There are other ways to deal with the damage assessment of carcinogenics and there is no doubt that each of the proposed steps in the impact pathway analysis can be improved by making use of additional expert know-how from the different scientific fields. That is also true for the feasibility test of the preliminary proposal for an index of manageability. Chemical carcinogenity served, in this book, as an example to work out some elements proposed in the methodological framework (Chapters 3 to 5). The modelling and linkage of all substeps, rather than the elaboration of the single substeps, is the added value from the elaboration in this chapter.

The time dimension

Little has been said so far about the time of occurrence of the damages. The occurrence of an emission[60] at time $t = 0$ will not immediately lead to an exposure situation as assumed in Section 6.2. The exposure by air through inhalation will only be slightly delayed compared to the delay in case of an emission that follows the other paths of drinking water and of food, especially. The stochastic behaviour of the cancer mechanisms and the varying amount of promoting and progressing agents and conditions lead to a delay between the initiation and the appearance of tumour symptoms. This time is called latency time. Higginson *et al.* (1992) mention a latency time of 20 years as typical, but this is an average from several cancer sites and conditions . A similar latency time has also been observed in the context of epidemiological studies based on occupational exposures. Pilkington *et al.* (1997) confirm for selected cancer types a latency time of 15 to 20 years, but report a shorter period of five to ten years for acute myeloid leukaemia caused by benzene exposure. Longer latency times than 20 years are known for some other risk factors such as asbestos.

[60] This time again is very difficult to determine in LCA because the emission can occur from infrastructure production decades before or from landfilling decades after the use phase (Hofstetter 1996a).

As discussed in Subsection 6.4.3, there is in additional delay of several years between the appearance of a tumour and the occurrence of premature death.

These time delays can be very long. Latency time is a minimum of 20 years and 50 or more years may pass during the accumulation in the food chain and the survival time after tumour incidence. That is why the damages to human health reported here usually do not occur during the use-phase of the product. This time delay should be considered in LCA if the time dimension is included in the valuation and interpretation. In LCA *sensu stricto* discussed here, one can disregard it. For the same reason, DALYs used here disregards time preference and therefore the discount rate is set to zero.

Secondary formation and metabolisation of carcinogenic substances

Several potentially carcinogenic substances are formed from precursor substances, i.e., they are formed through decay or synergistically from primary emissions. USEPA (1990) calculated that for formaldehyde, the secondary production exceeds primary emissions. The information in Table 6.21 suggests that formaldehyde accounts for at least 5% of total cancer cases due to inhalation of ambient air at the concentrations that are prevalent in the USA. Törnqvist (1994) analyses the formation of ethylene oxide in mammals (including humans) subsequent to the inhalation of ethene and concludes that, at an average ethene level of 1.8 mg/m^3 in Sweden, about 13 cancer deaths and about twice as many cases of disease are caused annually. The uncertainty in this estimate is due to the uncertain rate of conversion of ethene to ethylene oxide. Törnqvist *et al.* (1994) think that an additional 5 incidence cases occur in Sweden from the inhalation of propene and its transformation to propylene oxide. However, IRIS (1996) fails to include both ethene and propene on its list of potential cancer risks. Atkinson *et al.* (1994) describe the short atmospheric lifetime of benzo(a)pyrene and other PAH and their transformation to mutagenic nitro-PAH and other nitropolycyclic aromatic compounds. They conclude that health risk assessments of combustion emissions should include atmospheric transformation products.

It is therefore important to add models for the formation of secondary pollutants in the atmosphere wherever possible, i.e., as it will be done in Section 7.2 for ozone formation. Ethene and propene itself should be considered to be carcinogenic if evidence for the metabolisation of ethylene oxide and propylene oxide is adduced and if the conversion rates can be estimated. Damage factors for ethene and propene should be added to the list of carcinogenic substances. The usefulness of additional atmospheric transformation models for PAH has to be questioned. In most cases, only BaP is measured in combustion emissions and considered in epidemiological studies for PAH risk factors. In this case, it makes little sense to add uncertainty through the use of submodels for the calculation of ambient concentrations *and* unit risk factors for single PAH, nitro-PAH, and other substances.

For LCA purposes we are interested in estimates which are as accurate as possible for the carcinogenic potential of substances emitted from processes that include the risks from all subsequently formed metabolites. The use of the references cited above would make it possible to include the formation of carcinogenic secondary pollutants in the assessment, but carcinogenic metabolites could not be included in this case study.

Recalling somc assumptions

In order to be able to position and discuss the results from the damage assessment developed in this case study, it is necessary to recall some of the main assumptions that had to be made in this chapter:

- It is assumed that emission measurements for single substances are available.
- Only carcinogenic effects in humans are assessed. No other effects to humans and no effects at all on ecosystem health are analysed in this chapter.
- It is assumed that only information on the magnitude of the emission and of the receiving media, i.e., air and surface water, is available. It is assumed that no specific information on time, place or condition of release is available. Average European conditions are therefore assumed for all substances.
- The three main steps in the impact pathway analysis – fate analysis, effect analysis, and damage assessment – are all based on average European conditions concerning geographical factors, meteorological factors, exposure conditions including intake parameters, the states of health of the populations, and confounding stress factors. The demographic factors are assumed to correspond to a modelled standard which will probably be achieved in Europe in the near future.
- For the population density, it is assumed that the emissions occur in central Europe and that the substances dilute as a function of their atmospheric residence times in an easterly direction. Therefore, a substance-specific population density has been modelled.
- It is assumed that the exposure can be modelled by inhalation of outdoor air, by drinking water, and by eating a simplified meal as a proxy for food intake. Inhalation of indoor air is approximated by the inhalation of outdoor air. Intake of soil by young children is assumed to be negligible compared to food intake. Dermal transfer is not considered in the assessment.
- The application of a multimedia fate model of the Mackay type is suitable for lipophil substances. The fate analysis of other substances such as metals therefore suffer from limited model accuracy. A homogenous mixing within the eight model compartments is assumed. This assumption causes substance-specific rather than systematic errors. The missing compartment for the oceans leads to a bias towards higher concentrations in water because the residence time assumed for sweet water is longer than in reality. The missing terrestrial biomass enters a bias towards higher air concentrations because the absorption on biomass surfaces is not modelled.
- No sophisticated uncertainty assessment of the multi media modelling used is available. The assumptions on uncertainty that have been used are therefore largely based on expert judgements.
- The substances that are considered are all assumed to be genotoxic carcinogens acting as initiators. The process of initiation is assumed to follow a stochastic behaviour resulting in a non-threshold behaviour.
- The selection of substances for the assessment has occurred pragmatically based on the availability of input data for the fate and effect analyses. The list should therefore be expanded when potentially carcinogen substances are emitted which have not yet been assessed.

- The unit risk factors used are based on the assumption of full additivity between and within substances, i.e., the cumulative dose is taken as reference, no threshold dose is assumed and, for most substances, a linear interpolation has been used between zero risk/exposure and effect information for concentrations found in occupational exposure studies or animal experiments. Many authoritative bodies think that extrapolating in this manner produces estimates at the upper limit.
- Equal absorption and effect rates were assumed if there were no unit risk factors available for exposure paths found to be relevant in the fate analysis. In this case, values for known unit risk factors found in the literature were used.
- The evidence about carcinogenity to humans varies from substance to substance. It was assumed that the minimum of evidence that is required to define a substance as carcinogenic is a value choice that depends on the cultural perspective used.
- The relevant tumour type could only be identified for a few substances. Several cancer types have been observed for many substances and there are often no observations available from epidemiological studies. An arithmetic average of all cancer types was assumed in the later case.
- The cancer "history" due to chemical carcinogenesis was assumed to be the same as for the average of all risk factors together, i.e., the survival rate and the age pattern of tumour onset was assumed to be the same as reported in the cancer registries.
- The years of life lost were calculated based on a theoretical standard life table reflecting the conditions in Japan today, the country with the highest life expectancy.
- It was assumed that the application of the age-weighting – to correct for different values of life years at different ages – is a value judgement whose outcome depends on the cultural perspective held.

More detailed sets of assumptions and limitations of the models used have been reported in the Sections 6.1 to 6.6. The consequences of these assumptions for the assessment have, in most cases, not be tested by sensitivity analysis. The models or the knowledge required for the making of alternative assumptions are, in many cases, unavailable. The error ranges calculated in Subsection 6.5.3 do not reflect the uncertainty introduced by the assumptions that have been explicitly stated.

The index of manageability that has been calculated is built on rather rough estimates and less on an in-depth analysis. Default values which have been developed here have been used for many parameters without it being possible to subject them to a validation so far. The resultant value for the index of manageability should not be considered as a reliable estimate, but should rather be taken as proof that an operationalisation of such an index and its quantification are possible.

Conclusions

The specific damages due to one kilogram emission to air or surface water for 55 carcinogenic substances have been modelled here based on the assumptions presented above. The differentiation according to cultural perspectives led to three sets of results:

The *individualist* considers only those substances for which the best evidence is available (IARC Group 1) to be carcinogenic. From epidemiological studies it is known that these nine substances cause cancer. The remaining 46 substances are disregarded or included based on the evidence for other effect types. The damage is measured on the basis of age-weighting (see Section 5.4). The resulting damage factors are supplemented by lower and upper estimates of the 95% confidence interval and are listed in Appendix (6.17).

The *hierarchist* includes in addition all substances for which sufficient evidence of carcinogenity exists from experiments with animals (IARC Groups 1, 2A and 2B). This subset of 41 substances excludes only the 14 substances of Group 3. It was assumed that the hierarchist would not want to use age-weighting. The resulting damage factors can be found listed in Appendix (6.16).

The *egalitarian* applies the precautionary principle and includes therefore substances of IARC Group 3 as well, although the evidence on their cancerogenity to humans is inadequate. It was nevertheless possible to derive unit risk factors for these additional 14 substance based on animal experiments. The perspective of an egalitarian prohibits the use of age-weighting. Appendix (6.16) lists the resulting damage factors with lower and upper estimates for the 95% confidence interval.

This outcome confirms that value judgements can be made more compatible with one value system if the same perspective is applied in each situation, and, it is an advantage if the analysis is performed for more than one perspective. Thus, this chapter can be considered as a successful demonstration of the methodology described in Chapters 3 to 5.

The modelling of the magnitude of damage in Sections 6.2 to 6.5 makes explicit how the construction of damage functions (or the slope in the today's relevant range) can work. The word *construction* underlines the constructivistic nature of the approach. Many elements from epidemiological studies and from top-down analyses are included for single steps. But the linkage of the many submodels keeps the flavour of an inductive stochastic model where many assumptions are necessary to allow for predictive power of the whole modelling framework.

This last observation implies that validation is only possible to a limited extent. The overall validation by comparison with other studies which estimate effects from emissions of carcinogenic substances either showed differences whose origin can be explained or it revealed the limitations of earlier estimates that looked only at single exposure paths. Nevertheless, this comparison is of little relevance for the validation because all studies made use of the unit-risk concept to estimate the dose-response relationship. Some main flags to recall the quality of the results are:

- The metals with high and accurate estimates for the unit risk factors are linked with a poor fate modelling. The relevant oral intake path assumed equal absorption through inhalation and through food. These extrapolations have to be applied with caution.

- The modelling of the water compartment disregards the function of the open sea as a large sink with little relevance for drinking water production. A bias towards overestimating the carcinogenic potential of drinking water can therefore be expected.
- The 95% confidence interval given for the results reflects the estimated uncertainty of the average exposure and effect factors. The influence of many of the decisive assumptions that have been made above is not reflected in the quantitative uncertainty assessment.

From all these comments it can be concluded that the methodology developed in Chapters 3 to 5 can be successfully applied to and operationalised for the construction of damage functions. However, the quality of the damage factors derived is generally poor and has to be improved. This chapter should therefore be seen as a demonstration and is not to be taken as a reflection of the quality of the method proposed.

The calculation of the index of manageability in Section 6.6 has given an idea of the problems of quantification. It has become clear that it requires improvement by using more information from the relevant fields before the index can be used as part of the valuation framework. However, the feasibility of this approach has been demonstrated even though this part of the construction of the index of manageability is one of the least developed parts of the methodological framework presented in this book.

7 Damage to Human Health from Respiratory Effects

The choice of impact categories for operationalisation has been justified in Subsection 4.3.6. In this chapter we operationalise the impact category 'respiratory effects in human beings'. Effects in humans due to the different acting agents are assessed through the construction of damage factors. Damage factors are composed of the fate factors to calculate exposure due to emissions (Section 7.2), of the effect factors to determine expected effects in humans (Section 7.3), and of the disability adjusted life years lost due to the assessed effects (Section 7.4).

In a further section the results are compared to assessments reported in the literature (Section 7.5). The index for manageability is calculated in Section 7.6 before final conclusions are drawn for this case study to operationalise the approach introduced in Chapters 3 through 5.

The structure of this chapter is the same as for Chapter 6 in order to facilitate accessibility for the readers, but in contrast to Chapter 6, the emphasis is placed primarily on the quantitative operationalisation of the damage factors. Competing models and the models actually used are only briefly introduced. In addition, the focus of the chapter is on those elements that are different from the ones used in Chapter 6.

7.1 Introduction

This first section identifies the effects that will be analysed and gives a short introduction to the newly defined impact category 'respiratory diseases'. An important choice is made in Subsection 7.1.2 where also further limitations of the chosen approach are addressed. Subsection 7.1.3 is a kind of readers' guide, where the steps of damage assessment required to calculate the *magnitude of known damage* are summarised.

7.1.1 Respiratory diseases – evidence, endpoints and thresholds

Historical developments of evidence

The early environmentalist, Edward I, who reigned in Surrey from 1272-1307, banned the use of sea coal in London. One of the stated reasons for this measure was that burning it damaged human health. His successor, Edward II, strengthened this ban with the order that persons who fouled the air with smoke from burning coal should be tortured! A more liberal successor, Richard II (1377-1399), approached the problem by taxing coal (Wilson 1996).

After this "success" story from the early millennium little further attention was paid to the problem. The phase of industrialisation and the resultant improvement of welfare covered up much of the shadowy side of this development. The London smog period from December 5th to 9th, 1952, was the event most responsible for turning renewed attention to the health effects of air pollutants. The fivefold increase in the death rate that was observed during that event corresponded well with the concentration measurements of SO_2 and of smoke. The causal link between air pollution and the acute effects that had been observed was recognised and the British parliament, for instance, enacted the clean air act that forbade the burning of soft (brown) coal in the centre of London (Wilson 1996).

Lave *et al.* (1970) were among the first to report on the association between air pollution variables and death rates, finding the strongest association for particles. They did not make use of threshold assumptions. Therefore, their regression analysis and their findings were disputed up to the 90's.

In more recent years, a large body of epidemiological studies came to the conclusion that respirable particles are associated with the increased occurrence of respiratory problems such as bronchitis, chronic cough, persistent anatomic lung disease, fatale illness, and acute mortality. These studies are extensively reviewed, e.g., in Schwartz (1994), ExternE (1995), Concawe (1995/1996), Künzli *et al.* (1996), BUWAL (1996a), Dockery *et al.* (1996), Pope *et al.* (1996), and Pilkington *et al.* (1997). The association of particles with chronic mortality is still the subject of a large debate. The most powerful studies on this topic were performed in the USA by Dockery *et al.* (1993) and Pope *et al.* (1995b). The correlation between air pollution and chronic diseases is much more difficult to establish due to the many confounding factors which have to be known and which have to be measured over decades for the study population.

The missing evidence from toxicology

Animal toxicology is not yet able to reproduce or explain the effects of particles at ambient air concentrations. Two testable hypotheses are suggested by Brain (1996:IV): *"First, the particles commonly used in contemporary human chamber or animal studies may be non-representative of 'wild' urban ambient particles. Second, the healthy young animals studied may not be representative of those humans most susceptible to increased mortality in urban areas."* The suggested effects of SO_2, O_3, CO, NO_x, and probably other substances as well, at ambient concentrations, are not seen in animal studies or human chamber experiments. It may well be that the cocktail of substances at low concentrations leads to synergism which show up only in epidemiological studies. Recent toxicological studies using high concentrations of urban air mixtures showed short-term effects in the same magnitude as observed in epidemiological studies[1].

[1] Personal communication with C. Braun-Fahrländer, Institut für Sozial- und Präventivmedizin der Universität Basel (15-12-1997)

Endpoints

The effects summarised within the category of respiratory effects cover a wide range of diseases in connection with the lung, the bronchus, and the throat, i.e., the respiratory system. The following distinctions are made (Van Loveren *et al.* 1993, Dockery *et al.* 1994, Künzli *et al.* 1996):

Respiratory symptoms:	Runny or stuffy nose Sinusitis Sore throat Wet cough Head cold Hay fever Burning or red eyes Wheezing Dry cough Phlegm Shortness of breath Chest tightness, discomfort, or pain Nausea Headache
Lung:	Decline of lung function Lung inflammation Hyperreactivity and alterations in lung clearance
Bronchus:	Chronic bronchitis Reduced bronchial responsiveness

Decline in capacity
Asthma attacks
Pseudo croup
Acute and chronic mortality

The symptoms in this large set are often difficult to distinguish from each other. Many epidemiological studies, and also health statistics (Murray *et al.* 1996b), group the respiratory diseases into the two broad classes of *chronic obstructive pulmonary disease* (COPD) and of asthma. In this book, the term *respiratory effects* is used for the effects on the respiratory system mentioned in the list given above.

This new impact category will replace the impact categories 'winter smog' and 'summer smog' in Goedkoop (1995). In the framework of Heijungs *et al.* (1992), it will replace the category 'photochemical oxidant formation' for the damages to human health. The category 'human toxicity air' in Heijungs *et al.* (1992) included so far all effect mechanisms. Therefore, the new impact category does not just replace some equivalency factors.

No observed threshold

The epidemiological studies performed in the 90's suggest that there is no safe level of air pollution. There is a threshold at the *individual level* where most people show no effects at ambient concentrations, but there is good evidence that at the population level no such threshold exists, i.e., some vulnerable persons show adverse effects even at low background concentrations. The evidence is especially good for particles and it is getting better that this is also true for ozone. Pilkington *et al.* (1997) recommend that quantification of *all* respiratory effects should be made on a no-threshold basis. Best correlation was found when a constant percent increase of effects at all concentrations was assumed (GVF 1996). For small increases, e.g., in mortality, such a correlation leads to an approximately linear relation between effects and concentrations. For large increases, e.g., in respiratory symptoms, an over proportional increase in symptom cases with high concentrations occurs.

The assumption of such a no threshold behaviour increases the accurate prediction of potential effects because each kg of a pollutant that is emitted will potentially increase the health risk (if receptors inhale the substance). However, in contrast to the case of carcinogenity (Chapter 6), the slope factor increases with rising concentrations and in Section 7.3 we will suggest a pragmatic procedure to find the slope in the relevant part of the function.

7.1.2 The dilemma of causality

The failure of toxicological studies with animals and humans to produce evidence for health effects in case of exposure to lowly concentrated single substances seriously limits the evidence of causality between single substance exposure and observed effects. There is a lot of evidence to suggest a relation between air pollution as such and health effects, but the attribution of health effects to single substances is vague.

Two approaches – the epidemiological and the toxicological – that can be used to find a way of operationalising the causal attribution of health effects to single substances – are presented here.

The epidemiological approach

Subsection 6.3.2 and Section 7.3 discuss the different types of epidemiological studies and the criteria they have to fulfil in order to reliably quantify causal relationships. The epidemiological approach to solving the causality problem is mostly based on proper study design where all relevant confounding factors, such as lifestyle (smoking, eating behaviour), weather conditions, extraordinary events (festivities, strikes), and exposure to a set of substances are considered.

The correlation between the observed health effects and single substances can be tested once the control for all confounding factors is assured. It is then suggested that those substances with high correlation are the causal factors. The evidence for causalities can be increased if a set of epidemiological studies is performed at different places with different confounding factors and exposure profiles. Pilkington *et al.* (1997) consider this to be a feasible way to attribute observed effects to single pollutants. GVF (1996), however, rejected this procedure. GVF (1996) instead monetarised the external costs of health damages due to total traffic. GVF (1996) argued that the best correlation between health effects and air pollution can be identified for exposure to particles. They therefore selected particle exposure as a reference substance for air pollution and attributed all effects to it.

The toxicological approach

As already mentioned above, toxicological experiments do not produce effects at ambient concentrations because: the type of pollutant (normally single substance exposure) used is not the same as those present in ambient air, and the test animals or persons do not belong to the groups of sensitive or already weakened individuals. Besides, toxicological studies cannot reproduce the long-term, decade-long, exposure to pollutants that is causing chronic diseases. The toxicologically derived no observed adverse effect level (NOAEL) therefore cannot serve as a yardstick for deciding whether ambient concentrations of pollutants cause damage or not.

However, the following hypothesis could make it possible to use toxicological data: the effect levels or NOAELs determined in single pollutant exposure studies are a good proxy for the relative harmfulness of a pollutant and its contribution to the epidemiologically observed health effects.

Under the assumption that this hypothesis holds true, i.e., that synergistic effects are caused predominately by substances with low effect levels, one can attribute the observed health effects according to

Health effect of i per kg =

$$\frac{1}{\text{total emission } i} \cdot \text{total health effect} \cdot \frac{\frac{\text{concentration } i}{\text{effect level } i}}{\sum_i \frac{\text{concentration } i}{\text{effect level } i}} \tag{7.1}$$

where the term 'total' refers to a defined study region, 'emission' refers in this case to emissions to air, 'concentration' stands for concentration in inhaled air due to emissions within the study area, i stands for substances that show respiratory effects and 'effect level' refers to the concentration that shows respiratory effects on humans or animals in toxicological studies.

This formula is different from the one used by the well known approach of critical volumes (BUWAL 1984). Firstly, the effect level and not a politically derived standard level is used here. Secondly, a rather homogenous health endpoint, i.e., respiratory effects, is chosen as a base for the effect level. Thirdly, the lifetime and distribution of the substances, i.e., the fate, is correctly considered. And, as a last point, the relative shares are related to epidemiologically observed health effects.

Substance	Year of evaluation	No-Effect Level (NEL)	Effect Level (EL)
Aluminium	1982	0.1-2.7 mg/m^3	
Cobalt	1983	0.03 mg/m^3	
Piperazine	1985	0.3 mg/m^3	
Vanadium	1983		0.06 mg/m^3
Sulphur dioxide	1985		1 ppm (2.7 mg/m^3)
Coal dust	1986		2 mg/m^3
Nitrogen dioxide	1986		0.5 mg/m^3
Cotton dust	1986		0.3-0.5 mg/m^3
Terpenes	1987		125 mg/m^3
Ozone	1987		0.24 mg/m^3
Diisocyanates and polyisocyanates	1988		1 ppb
Titanium dioxide	1989		0.2-2.8 mg/m^3
Paper dust	1990		<5 mg/m^3
Attapulgite	1991		2.7 mg/m^3
Talc, asbestos-free and with low quartz content	1992		1 mg/m^3

Tab. 7.1: No-Effect and Effect Levels reported for substances for which the critical effects are effects on the respiratory system (Hansson 1997)

Table 7.1 gives a compilation of substances for which the critical effects are effects on the respiratory system (Hansson 1997). This compilation is based on thorough reviews of the results for 278 substances that have been evaluated by the Swedish Criteria Group in the context of setting occupational exposure limits. Anonymous

(1994) gives an overview of the substances tested and of the results that have been published in the Swedish journal *Arbete och Hälsa.*

An additional 6 substances were identified as belonging to this group, however no effect levels were derived for them. It should be noted that only substances for which the critical effects are respiratory effects are listed in Table 7.1, i.e., a substance is not listed here if it causes effects on the nervous system at a concentration of 1 mg/m^3 and effects on the respiratory system at concentrations of 3 mg/m^3. This is a shortcoming that conflicts with the intention to build damage factors per effect type.

The choice of the epidemiological approach

The toxicological approach presented above may appear attractive. It would provide an opportunity to consider the many ingredients in the air pollution cocktail that potentially contribute to respiratory diseases. However, the operationalisation of this procedure requires:

- a comprehensive evaluation of toxicity experiments with respiratory effects as endpoints, and
- the measurement of emissions and concentrations within a defined study area with known health effects of all substances found to cause respiratory effects.

Moreover, one has to assume that the hypothesis of proportionality that was set as a prerequisite for this approach will be proven to be true.

On the other hand, the epidemiological approach suffers from limited possibilities to prove causalities, to show correlation with several dozens of substances, and to attribute health risks among pollutants with identical emission sources (and with that of the same course of emission and concentration). However, the epidemiological approach, in contrast to the toxicological approach, can profit from a large body of literature and has already been applied in several externality studies (ExternE 1995, ESEERCO 1995, GVF 1996). The most recent of these sources has prepared new risk factors including a wider range of pollutants in order to serve a forthcoming externality study of transport systems (Pilkington *et al.* 1997).

Two reasons let us opt for the epidemiological approach: firstly, it is readily available and can be adapted with little effort and, secondly, it is directly based on expert knowledge in epidemiology and the health sciences while the toxicological approach would be based on a non-tested hypothesis without support from toxicologists.

7.1.3 Overview on the calculation of the damage factors

The damage factors to be assessed in this chapter have as a common characteristic the causation of respiratory diseases in human beings, i.e., they reflect the new impact category 'respiratory diseases in human beings'. The way of thinking in its construction is again a top-down procedure, i.e., after having observed health effects, the exposure causing them and finally the emission of pollutants are analysed. The bottom-up procedure is chosen here to calculate the damage factors for the reasons already explained in Chapter 6 :

- It is assumed that the emission *Ii* of substance *i* can be measured in kg and that the substance is emitted to air under average European weather, meteorological, and emission conditions. Only those substances are included which in epidemiological studies showed a significant correlation with health effects or which contribute to the formation of substances that have such an effect.
- The fate analysis (Section 7.2) derives fate factors *Fi* for substances *i* which are emitted to air and lead to an exposure by inhalation. The fate of precursor emissions, their distribution, and the subsequent formation of secondary pollutants causing respiratory effects are reflected in only one fate factor. The fate factors transform emissions into external exposure that cause respiratory effects under European conditions. Pilkington *et al.* (1997) found that exposure to $PM_{2.5}$, PM_{10}, nitrates, sulphates, ozone, CO, SO_2, and NO_2 causes respiratory effects. This leads us to consider $PM_{2.5}$, PM_{10}, TSP, NO_x, NH_3, CO, VOCs, and SO_x as primary pollutants.
- The effect factor *Eim(c)* describes the relationship between exposure to substance *i* and health endpoint *m* for the cultural perspective *c*. The endpoints considered are coughing, lower respiratory symptoms (wheezing), asthma attacks, bronchodilator usage, chronic bronchitis, respiratory hospital admissions, respiratory symptoms, acute and chronic mortality due to COPD, emergency room visits for COPD, asthma and croup, restricted activity days, and minor restricted respiratory days (Section 7.3).

The product of the fate and of the effect factors result in the respiratory disease factor *Rim(c)*:

$$Rim(c) = Fi \cdot Eim(c) \qquad \text{[respiratory health impacts/kg]} \qquad (7.2)$$

- Each health endpoint m causes a disability, and some of them, mortality. The duration and severity of morbidity and years of life lost per premature death will be assessed by the years lived disabled (YLDm) and years of life lost (YLLm) per health endpoint *m* (Section 7.4).
- The linkage of all elements in the damage function in Section 7.5 makes it possible to calculate disability adjusted life years (DALYs) per kg substance emission *i* for the cultural perspective *c* (Equation 7.3).

$$\begin{aligned}\frac{DALYs_i(c)}{Ii} &= \sum_m \{Rim(c) \cdot (YLLm(c) + YLDm(c))\} \\ &= \sum_m \{Fi \cdot Eim(c) \cdot (YLLm(c) + YLDm(c))\} \qquad \text{[a/kg]} \qquad (7.3)\end{aligned}$$

Equation (7.3) describes the damage per kg pollutant emission to air due to respiratory effects as a function of the cultural perspective *c*. Equation (7.3) describes the slope of a function and not a concentration dependent function. The ambient concentration is normally not known in LCA. We will therefore assume the same average ambient concentration as the one that has been observed in the area for which the underlying epidemiological study has been undertaken.

7.1.4 Manageability of respiratory diseases

The determination of a manageability factor for respiratory diseases will be presented in Section 7.6 by following the method that has been described in Section 4.5. Only a limited effort is made to arrive at a high quality for the index of manageability as the aspect of feasibility is the guiding principle for this application.

The index of manageability is based on the index for the magnitude of damage which is presented in Section 7.5.

7.2 Fate analysis (from emissions to external exposure)

7.2.1 Introduction

The aim of this section is to calculate accurate fate factors which relate the primary emission of substances to the concentrations in inhalation air for those substances that have been identified to cause respiratory diseases. The inhaled substances are the ones which have been shown in epidemiological studies to be related to morbidity or mortality assigned to the respiratory tract. These are:

- Particulate matter PM_{10} and $PM_{2.5}$
- Nitrate and sulphate
- SO_2
- O_3
- CO, and probably
- NO_x

The primary emissions that cause exposure to these substances are $PM_{2.5}$, PM_{10}, TSP, NO_x, NH_3, CO, VOCs, and SO_x. They are considered as primary pollutants in the fate analysis. A set of methods has been used to derive best estimates for the fate factors. Subsection 7.2.2 approaches the problem by working with models for the residence time and the height of the mixing layer for particles in the atmosphere. Subsection 7.2.3 makes use of measured or calculated concentrations for given areas due to known emissions. In Subsection 7.2.4 best estimates are made and listed in Table 7.11. Another 118 fate factors for precursors of ozone creation are calculated in Subsection 7.2.5 by making use of the so-called 'umbrella principle'.

7.2.2 Calculating fate factors for particles from residence times

As already suggested in Subsection 6.2.4, it is possible to calculate fate factors based on the volume of the mixing layer of air per unit surface *Vik* and the average residence time τik for substance *i* in compartment *k* (Jolliet *et al.* 1997b). The average height of the mixing layer *Hik* is therefore the second parameter that has to be known besides the residence time (see Equation (7.4)).

$$Fik = \frac{\tau ik}{Vik} = \frac{\tau ik}{Hik} \qquad [\frac{m^2 \cdot a}{m^3}] \qquad (7.4)$$

For the purpose of this chapter only fate factors for emission to air to concentration in inhaled air are relevant (Fair,air). The many limitations mentioned in Subsection 6.2.4 are therefore largely irrelevant here. The following aspects are important when Equation (7.4) is used to calculate fate factors:

- The residence time has to be averaged for all meteorological conditions and include all processes which influence decay and deposition.
- The height of the mixing layer has to be averaged with respect not only to different weather conditions and to the meteorological differences between different

countries. It is also necessary to make reasonable assumptions with respect to the substance distribution within the mixing column. This is especially important because we are most interested in concentrations near the surface (inhalation air).

- The approach is more appropriate for substances which do not form metabolites in a complicated interaction of atmospheric chemistry and for substances which have a residence time that is long enough that they will be mixed homogeneously within the mixing layer.

This last recommendation limits the applicability of the formula to particles. SO_2 and NO_x are transformed to a relevant extent into sulphates and nitrates respectively, and VOC contributes to ozone formation. The approach presented in Equation (7.2) is therefore used here only for particles.

In a next step, reliable data for τi and Hi have to be collected for particles[2]. Before we present best estimates for these parameters, one should be aware of the complexity of aerosol physics and chemistry. Aerosol can be composed of solids or fluids. One speaks of particles starting at a size of 0.001 μm and the range ends at about 100 μm. The smallest ones are sometimes the size of larger gas molecules or viruses. The largest correspond to dust and sea salt aerosols. Primary emissions from technical processes usually cover the range from 0.01 to 1 μm. Larger particles are primarily emitted by non-combustion emission sources such as mining and ore processing.

There are four classes of particles measured in monitoring: TSP (total suspended particles), BS (black smoke), PM_{10} (particle matter < 10 μm), $PM_{2.5}$ (Particle matter < 2.5 μm). The reliable measurement of the quantities of $PM_{2.5}$, or even more of PM1, is still a difficult task today.

The residence time

The simple model to explain aerosol behaviour in the troposphere distinguishes between three modes: the Aitken mode, the accumulation mode, and the large aerosols (Ackermann 1997).

The *Aitken nuclei mode* includes the primary emission of particles smaller than 0.05 μm and secondary particles formed by the chemical transformation of gases (e.g., SO_x to sulphate). This mode tends to coagulate with larger particles of the accumulation mode. Coagulation is by far the most important sink for the fraction of ultrafine particles.

Particles from the accumulation mode are between 0.05 μm and 2 μm in diameter. In addition to coagulation, they are formed by gas-to-particle conversion processes known as heterogeneous nucleation and by condensation of gases onto pre-existing particles in the accumulation mode. Their atmospheric lifetime is dominated by wet deposition.

Coarse particles with a diameter larger than 2 μm have a shorter resident time due to a higher sedimentation velocity.

---

[2] I am grateful to Alfred Trukenmüller from IER, University Stuttgart, for his valuable provision of such data sources.

This description makes it clear that the particles' residence time in air depends on their size and the prevailing meteorological conditions. For the average residence time as a function of the particle radius, Jaenicke (1978) determined the approximation equation:

$$\frac{1}{\tau tot} = \frac{1}{\tau wet} + \frac{1}{c} \cdot \left(\frac{r}{R}\right)^{-2} + \frac{1}{c} \cdot \left(\frac{r}{R}\right)^{2} \quad [1/s] \qquad (7.5)$$

where c constant = 1.26 E+08 s ≈ 4 years
R normalisation radius = 0.3 μm
τwet partial lifetime for wet deposition = approx. 5 days (Roedel 1992)
r particle radius

The partial lifetime for wet deposition is the decisive value in Equation (7.5). Jaenicke (1978) discusses a range of published data indicating a τwet of between 8 and 21 days. Roedel (1992) corrected this value to 5 days which is the one used here. For particle sizes of between 0.1 μm and 2.5 μm (accumulation mode), the residence time varies between 4.5 and 5 days. Ultrafine particles coagulate to larger particles and therefore have a slightly higher residence time. (Using Equation (7.5) shows that, e.g., a particle with 0,01 μm diameter needs on the average 9 hours to coagulate with a larger particle of the accumulation mode.) A coarse particle of 10 μm diameter is already dominated by the sedimentation process. This gives an average residence time of about 2.5 days. Particles with a diameter of 100 μm would have a residence time of 0.05 days according to the approximation formula given above.

Dockery *et al.* (1994) found for North American situations that about 55% of TSP are PM_{10} and that PM_{10} is made up of $PM_{2.5}$ to about 60% . There is some evidence that these mass distributions between TSP, PM_{10}, and $PM_{2.5}$ do not apply in European conditions. Harrison *et al.* (1997) report for the surroundings of Birmingham (UK) a share of $PM_{2.5}$ in PM_{10} of 83 % for winter time and of 42% for summer time. The winter time data is more relevant because less geogenic particles are to be expected. From BUWAL (1996a:31), it is clear that the composition of TSP is highly dependent on the degree of urbanisation and the precise geographical conditions, i.e., for Zurich the PM_{10}/TSP ratio found was as high as 0.81. BUWAL (1996b) reports a series of PM_{10}/TSP ratios for three Swiss cities falling within a range of 0.60 to 0.86. POST (1996) presents a figure with a typical particle mass distribution over their diameters. Best estimates for these distributions are 0.8 for the PM_{10}/TSP ratio and 0.75 for the $PM_{2.5}/PM_{10}$ ratio. This last ratio corresponds well with the other data quoted here and is therefore taken as the representative concentration profile for Europe as a consequence of anthropogenic emissions (Table 7.2).

The size distribution in Table 7.2 represents the profile measured in the atmosphere. Besides primary particles emitted by anthropogenic sources, it also includes particles emitted by natural sources as well as particles formed secondary.

As we are interested in the fate factor transforming emissions into concentrations, it is necessary to recalculate the profile for the emissions. Due to the low atmospheric residence time of coarse particles, a much larger share than 20% has to be emitted to cause a share of 20% in the concentration measurements. If we assume that the mixing height is the same for all particle sizes then Equation (7.4) shows that the fate factor *F* is proportional to the residence time τ. The share *Se* of the emission profile can therefore be calculated by dividing the share *Sc* of the concentration profile with τ (Equation 7.6).

		>10µm (20 µm)	2.5-10 µm (8 µm)	<2.5 µm (0.4 µm)
τ_{tot}	Equation (7.5)	1.04 days	3.11 days	4.95 days
TSP	POST (1996)	20 %	20 %	60 %
PM_{10}	POST (1996)		25 %	75 %
$PM_{2.5}$	POST (1996)			100 %

Tab. 7.2: Share of three particles size classes (POST 1996) and of the residence time of the single fractions (ttot) by applying Equation (7.5) from Jaenicke (1978). A residence time due to wet deposition of 5 days is assumed (Roedel 1992). The size in the brackets indicates the average particle size taken to calculate the residence time.

$$Se = Sc/F \sim Sc/\tau \tag{7.6}$$

The shares of the different particle size classes again have to add up to 100%. Therefore, the results of Equation (7.6) have to be standardised (Table 7.3). This new profile based on the emissions[3] can now be used to calculate the average residence time for the three most frequently reported particle classes.

		>10µm (20 µm)	2.5-10 µm (8 µm)	<2.5 µm (0.4 µm)	average τ
τ_{tot}	Equation (7.5)	1.04 days	3.11 days	4.95 days	
TSP	POST (1996)	51%	17%	32%	2.6 days
PM_{10}	POST (1996)		35%	65%	4.3 days
$PM_{2.5}$	POST (1996)			100%	5 days

Tab. 7.3: Calculation of the average residence time τ for three particles classes by considering their relative composition during emission (recalculated with Equation (7.6) from Table 7.2) and of the residence time of the single fractions (τ_{tot}) by applying Equation (7.5) from Jaenicke (1978). A residence time due to wet deposition of 5 days is assumed (Roedel 1992). The size in the brackets indicates the average particle size taken to calculate the residence time.

These results are a rough approximation because:

- Equation (7.5) is only an approximation formula
- the residence time of 5 days for wet deposition (Roedel 1992) used for the calculation is highly dependent on the exact meteorological conditions (precipitation rate) and varies accordingly within a wide range
- the average size distribution for the different primary particle classes TSP, PM_{10} and $PM_{2.5}$ is unknown and varies largely dependent on geographical situation and sources of emission

Renoux (1996) cites newer studies by Jaenicke where typical residence times of 8 days are reported for the lower troposphere, of 3 weeks for the middle troposphere, and of 200 days for the tropopause. For our purpose of looking at inhalation it is

[3] If the available European emission inventories would provide this information no such recalculations would have been necessary. Berdowski *et al.* (1997) assume 0.7 for the PM_{10}/TSP ratio (0.49 according to Table 7.3) and calculate 0.57 for the $PM_{2.5}/PM_{10}$ ratio (0.65 according to Table 7.3). This is judged to be a reasonable agreement and the values in Table 7.3 are chosen for the further calculations.

sufficient to consider the lower troposphere when calculating an average residence time. This way of proceeding covers the overwhelming share of all particles.

In Houghton *et al.* (1996) the IPCC estimates the global anthropogenic emissions of dust and soot (113 Tg/a for primary particles) and the resulting global mean column burden (2.4 mg/m^2). From that, it is possible to derive a global average residence time for anthropogenic primary particles of about 4 days.

The average residence times in Table 7.3 are taken as best estimates for the mean values for τi. A factor of 1.6 is chosen for the squared geometric standard deviation σg^2 in order to make sure that the residence time of 8 days is within the 95% confidence interval of the assumed lognormal distribution of the error interval (see Appendix 6.8).

The height of the mixing layer

Gaussian dispersion models differentiate between six diffusion categories which show different mixing heights from 200 m to 1600 m (Panitz *et al.* 1989). The mixing layer is normally thicker during the day time and in southern Europe and thinner during the night and in northern Europe (BUWAL 1996d). The shares of the different heights of mixing layers was compiled, e.g., by Päsler-Sauer (1989) for different years and sites. The mixing height can be determined from sodar data (Beyrich 1997).

Van Jaarsfeld (1995:52) mentions that it is not the average, but the highest mixing height between emission source and receptor which is relevant for the modelling of concentrations. This is obviously true because particles which have been transported up to a height of 1200 m will not be recollected when, during night time, the mixing height falls to 400 m. Due to these day - night instabilities and diffusion mechanisms, a small share of particles is mixed in the whole troposphere. However, it is assumed here that this share is small and that the only relevant sink is the deposition to ground (Roedel 1992:378ff). In order to make use of the information about the changes in mixing height, one would need the average maximum mixing height per trajectory, i.e., per air package containing the particles. For two reasons this average maximum height is too high: (1) it will take some time before the maximum height is reached and (2) the concentration profile will show higher concentrations in the lower layers. Therefore, an average mixing height between 800 m and 1200 m may be a reasonable choice.

Other modellers apply a fixed height of 800 m for the mixing layer (Derwent *et al.* 1988/1989, Metcalfe *et al.* 1989) which was considered as a reasonable average under all conditions (Jones 1981). These models proved to provide modelled concentrations close to measured data. 800 m are therefore taken as a reasonable best estimate for the mixing height in Europe.

For Hik in Equation (7.4) we therefore use the mean value of 800 m and assume a lognormal distribution with a (squared) geometric standard deviation σg^2 of factor 1.5.

The fate factor

The fate factors for three groups of particles can be calculated using the data presented above and Equation (7.4). The mean values and the resulting (squared) geometric standard deviation σg^2 are listed in Table 7.4. The latter is calculated with Equation (A6.3) from Appendix (6.8).

	>10µm (20 µm)	2.5-10 µm (8 µm)	<2.5 µm (0.4 µm)	average τ for particles	σ_g^2 of τ	average H of mixing layer	σ_g^2 of H	fate factor $F_{particle,air}$	σ_g^2 of F
						m		m^2a/m^3	
TSP	51%	17%	32%	2.6 days	1.6	800	1.5	8.9 E-6	1.9
PM_{10}		35%	65%	4.3 days	1.6	800	1.5	14.7 E-6	1.9
$PM_{2.5}$			100%	5 days	1.6	800	1.5	17.1 E-6	1.9

Tab. 7.4: Calculation of the fate factor for particles emitted to air and inhaled by air of three different classes TSP, PM10, and, PM2.5 applying Equation (7.4).

It has to be noted that the assumed independence of τ and H is in reality not given. Short residence time will be linked to small mixing height and *vice versa*. It may therefore well be that the standard deviation is much smaller than the one calculated here by assuming independent parameters.

The fate factors presented here will be re-evaluated in Subsection 7.2.4 after additional attempts to calculate fate factors are described in Subsection 7.2.3.

7.2.3 Statistical methods with empirical and modelled data

A different approach to the one presented above makes use of the real world, seen as an experiment. The ratio between measured or calculated concentrations and known emissions can be interpreted as a fate factor (Jolliet *et al.* 1997b). The description of the method has been already provided in Subsection 6.2.4 and the Equation (6.7) there is rewritten here as:

$$Fik = \frac{Cik}{\left(\frac{M'i}{A}\right)} \qquad [\frac{m^2a}{m^3}] \qquad (6.7)$$

where Cik average concentration in compartment k (here k = air) [kg/m³]
$M'i$ emission flow of substance i [kg/a]
A surface over which emission occurs [m²]

Jolliet *et al.* (1997b) calculated a number of fate factors using this method. They are listed in Table 7.5. Jolliet *et al.* additionally presented the results calculated by a multi-media fate model (Guinée *et al.* 1996) in order to provide a wider view. However, one should keep in mind the arguments from Subsection 6.2.2 that the proposed multi-media model is not well suited for most of the substance classes discussed here and that it calculates with a height of 1000 m for the mixing layer.

The validity of the values in Table 7.5 cannot be checked because little is known about the averaging principles for the measured concentrations and the estimation procedure for the emissions that have been used in their calculation. The fate factors for CO, SO_2 and NO_x correspond rather well within the different geographical scales that had been chosen for the analysis. The results for both NO_x and SO_2 that have been calculated with USES are slightly lower than those determined with the statistical method. This outcome should be considered as accidental rather than as a sign of reliability; modelling the fate of these substances with USES required numerous assumptions and the USES model was not developed for them.

Pollutant	Fate factor [m^2a/m^3]	Reference
CO (R)	1.90E-05	Jolliet 1994
CO (G)	1.70E-05	Jolliet *et al.* 1997b
SO_2 (R)	3.10E-06	Jolliet 1994
SO_2 (C)	3.00E-06	Talabardon 1995
SO_2 (G)	5.10E-06	Jolliet *et al.* 1997b
SO_2 (USES)	2.80E-06	Guinée *et al.* 1996
NO_x (R)	6.70E-06	Jolliet 1994
NO_x (C)	4.00E-06	Talabardon 1995
NO_x (G)	3.40E-06	Jolliet *et al.* 1997b
NO_x (USES)	2.70E-06	Guinée et al 1996
Particles (R)	8.00E-05	Jolliet 1994
Particles (G)	6.00E-06	Jolliet *et al.* 1997b
VOC-->O_3 (G)	1.20E-04	Jolliet *et al.* 1997b

Tab: 7.5: Comparison of the fate factors for different scales of the statistical method and for the multi-media fate model USES (see Section 6.2.2 for an introduction). (R): Regional scale (Switzerland), (C): Continental scale (Europe), (G): Global scale (World). (USES): fate factors calculated by Guinée (Guinée *et al.* 1996), using the risk assessment model USES.

The situation for particles is different because the listed fate factors diverge by more than a factor 12. Jolliet *et al.* (1997b) explain this outcome with the choice of only small particles at the global scale whereas no size distinction was made at the regional level. This reasoning is insufficient to explain the difference. A much more reasonable explanation is that at the regional scale, Switzerland, the country that is modelled, is a net importer of particles and that the natural background concentration of about 5 $\mu g/m^3$ (GVF 1996) has probably not been subtracted from the measured concentration. Both these factors lead to an overestimation of the value for the fate factor. From Jolliet (1997) it is known that the global average is based on the assumption of 70% marine, 29.27% non-urban continental, and 0.63% urban continental areas. The share of the urban area is set much too low for those substances with a residence time of several days because an area that is larger than just the urban one will show 'near to urban' concentrations (Hoek *et al.* 1997). However, this explains the lower fate factors at the global scale only partly. Another explanation is that the uncertainty is large when natural plus anthropogenic emissions are estimated at the world level.

The fate factors presented in Table 7.5 cover most of the substances that are relevant for the generation of respiratory diseases. Sulphate and nitrate, the two secondary particles formed from SO_2, NO_x and NH_3, have not yet been considered. In addition, one would like to have single fate factors for all the hydrocarbons and for NO_x that contribute to ozone formation in the lower troposphere. Finally, a more transparent calculation procedure than the one used for the fate factors reported here would increase the possibility of estimating their uncertainty. These are the reasons for providing additional analyses below. However, it adds little to the demonstration of the approach itself; it is therefore done in a pragmatic manner.

EMEP modelling results for Europe

Extensive modelling of acidifying gases is done in Europe through the European Monitoring and Evaluation Programme (EMEP) (Sandnes 1993, Krüger *et al.* 1994, Barrett *et al.* 1996). The underlying chemistry in this model is presented in Figure 7.1. It can be seen that several mechanisms contribute to the formation of nitrates and sulphates. Ammonia, especially, is an important contributor to the formation of nitrates. Ammonia is the limiting factor in the formation of nitrates and sulphates at many locations. This explains their high concentrations in areas with intensive agriculture (which is a main source for ammonia).

The percentages given in Figure 7.1 indicate the assumed composition of the primary emissions and the shares which are deposited locally. The reader should consult Krüger *et al.* (1994) and Barrett *et al.* (1996) who provide detailed model descriptions and additional information on modelling assumptions. It seems especially appropriate for large scale modelling which includes transboundary pollution.

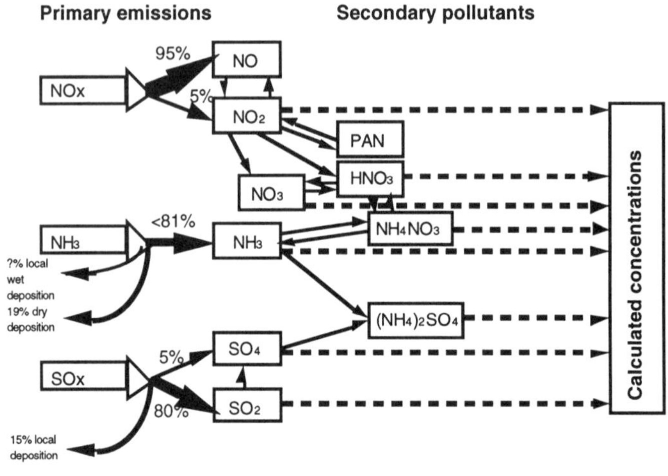

Fig. 7.1: The chemistry in the EMEP-model for emissions of NO_X, NH_3 and SO_X (after Krüger *et al.* 1994)

Complete emission estimates for 1995 in Europe, the surrounding seas, and parts of North Africa as well have been included in EMEP (1997). The modelling results are available only in the form of maps with iso-concentrations. Rough estimates for the average concentrations were made for a subpart of about 60% of the total area covering 23·35 grid cells with an area of 150·150 km each. The relevant concentrations given in Table 7.6 have been taken from the maps for those substances that EMEP (1997) have calculated. For the ammonium-compounds it was assumed that the ammonium originated from ammonia while the sulphate and nitrate parts were assumed to originate from SO_2 and NO_2, respectively. Thanks to these assumptions it was possible to derive separate fate factors for nitrates from ammonia and from NO_x and for sulphate from ammonia and from SO_2 (Table 7.6).

	Emissions 1995	Specific emission flow	Averaged modelled concentration	Fate factor
	(1)	(2) = (1)/ (10.8 E12 m^2)	(3)	(3)· E-9/(2)
	Mt/a	kg/m^2a	$\mu g/m^3$	m^2a/m^3
NOx	20.9	1.9 E-3	6	3.1 E-6
NH_3	7.0	0.6 E-3	1.2	1.9 E-6
SO_2	30.7	2.8 E-3	5	1.8 E-6
SO_4(part)			0.3	
$(NH_4)_2SO_4$			4.5	
$(NH_4)NO_3$			1.1	
NO_3(part)			6.6	
SO_2 -> SO_4 part	30.7	2.8 E-3	0.3	0.1 E-6
SO_2 -> $(NH_4)_2SO_4$	30.7	2.8 E-3	(§) 3.3	1.2 E-6
SO_2 -> sulphates	30.7	2.8 E-3		**1.3 E-6**
NH_3 -> $(NH_4)_2SO_4$	7.0	0.4 E-3	(#) 1.2	**1.9 E-6**
NH_3 -> $(NH_4)NO_3$	7.0	0.4 E-3	(#) 0.33	**0.5 E-6**
NOx -> $(NH_4)NO_3$	20.9	1.2 E-3	(¶) 0.77	0.4 E-6
NOx -> NO_3 (part)	20.9	1.2 E-3	6.6	3.4 E-6
NOx -> nitrates	20.9	1.2 E-3		**3.8 E-6**

Tab. 7.6: Calculation of the fate factors with Equation (6.7) by using roughly averaged concentrations from the calculations with the EMEP model and from emission reported in EMEP (1997).
(§) It is assumed that the sulphate part originates from SO2
(#) It is assumed that the ammonium part originates from ammonia
(¶) It is assumed that the nitrate part originates from NO_X.

ECOSENSE modelling results for Europe

A similar chemical scheme which is based on Derwent *et al.* (1988) has been employed in the work of ExternE (1995) and is implemented in the software called ECOSENSE.

The modelling area covers the EUROGRID with 1'161 (43 times 27) grid cells that cover an area of 10'000 km^2 (100 · 100 km) each. A large share of the European countries from Portugal to Finland are therefore within the modelling area. About one third of the area covered is made up of the sea areas surrounding South, West and North Europe.

The emission data from Corinair for the year 1990 has been used for modelling the concentrations in the grid cells. The average concentrations resulting from these emissions were calculated[4] for each grid cell by making use of a windrose trajectory model (WTM). The results for the 1161 grid cells were used to calculate the average concentration by applying a simple weighting per area. The results from this procedure and the final calculation of the fate factors are given in Table 7.7.

[4] I am very grateful to Dr. Wolfram Krewitt from IER, Stuttgart (Germany) who provided the calculation results.

The main observations concerning the results in Tables 7.6 and 7.7 are:

- The average concentrations are very low. This is due to the fact that only about 70% of the area covered is land surface and that the sparsely populated areas in Scandinavia are included.
- The concentrations of sulphates and nitrates do not correspond to the (world-wide average) proportion found in composition analysis of particles where much more sulphate than nitrate is found (Ackermann 1997). Spengler *et al.* (1996) have data from measurements in California, which has a population and a traffic density comparable to the European situation, and these confirm high shares of nitrate. Furthermore, the sulphate concentrations in Europe have been decreasing since 1975 (Arends *et al.* 1997).
- The fate factors are lower estimates because a net export from Europe to the East has to be expected[5] and because the concentrations on the surface may be higher than the average ones.
- The comparison of the fate factors in Tables 7.5 to 7.7 shows a fairly good agreement for all substances (a range of factor 2).

	Emissions 1990	Specific emission flow	Averaged modelled concentrations	Fate factor
	(1)	(2) = (1)/ (1161 E10 m^2)	(3)	(3)· E-9/(2)
	Mt/a	kg/m^2a	$\mu g/m^3$	m^2a/m^3
NOx	16.2	1.4 E-3	2.4	1.7 E-6
SO_2	28.2	2.4 E-3	7.5	3.2 E-6
H_2SO_4			1.02	
$(NH_4)_2SO_4$			2.85	
$(NH_4)NO_3$			1.39	
NO_3(part)			3.19	
SO_2 -> H_2SO_4	28.2	2.4 E-3	1.02	0.4 E-6
SO_2 -> $(NH_4)_2SO_4$	28.2	2.4 E-3	(§) 2.07	0.9 E-6
SO_2 -> sulphates	28.2	2.4 E-3		**1.3 E-6**
NH_3 -> $(NH_4)_2SO_4$	6.2	0.5 E-3	(#) 0.78	**1.6 E-6**
NH_3 -> $(NH_4)NO_3$	6.2	0.5 E-3	(#) 0.31	**0.6 E-6**
NOx -> $(NH_4)NO_3$	16.2	1.4 E-3	(¶) 1.08	0.8 E-6
NOx -> NO_3 (part)	16.2	1.4 E-3	3.19	2.7 E-6
NOx -> nitrates	16.2	1.4 E-3		**3.5 E-6**

Tab. 7.7: Calculation of the fate factors by Equation (6.7) using calculations with the WTM implemented in ECOSENSE.
(§) It is assumed that the sulphate part originates from SO2
(#) It is assumed that the ammonium part originates from ammonia
(¶) It is assumed that the nitrate part originates from NO_x.

The rough estimates of the concentrations in Table 7.6 may be wrong by a factor of 2 when compared to the results reported in Table 7.7 that are based on the detailed averaging done by adding up the average concentration for each grid cell. The fate factors for NO_x and SO_2 in Table 7.7 have therefore a higher quality. However, the model and the data used by EMEP (1997) may be more accurate than those used for

[5] E.g., Shannon (1997) shows for North America that the travelling distance for SO_2 is about 500 km and for SO_4 about 1'000 km. This means that emissions in Central and Eastern Europe will contribute to the pollution level eastern from the EMEP area.

calculating the factors reported in Table 7.7 and the measured data for sulphate concentrations in Europe are closer to Table 7.6 than 7.7 (Arends *et al.* 1997).

United States of America results for fate factors

The statistical method with empirical data needs a large study area in order to decrease errors due to import and export characteristics. For this reason, additional calculations for the United States of America are presented in Table 7.8.

When interpreting or using this data, one has to be aware that Spengler *et al.* (1996) included dust from road use, from construction activities and from agricultural tilling in their estimate. These emissions may partly take the form of particles larger than PM_{10} and fail therefore to be reflected in the measured concentrations; this leads to an underestimate of the fate factor. The measured PM_{10} concentration may be biased towards monitoring sites in urban areas and does include sulphate and nitrate components originating from NO_x and SO_2. These factors lead to an overestimate of the fate factor.

	Emission 1990	Specific emission flow	Averaged measured concentration	Source	Fate factor
	(1)	(2) = (1)/ (9.364 E12 m^2)	(3)		(3)· E-9/(2)
	Mt/a	kg/m^2a	$\mu g/m^3$		m^2a/m^3
PM10	42	4.5 E-3	28	Spengler *et al.* (1996)	6.2 E-6
TSP	8	0.85 E-3	48	Newell (1997)	56 E-6
CO	63	6.7 E-3	7000	Newell (1997)	1 E-3
NO_x	20	2.1 E-3	44	Newell (1997)	21 E-6
SO_2	21	2.2 E-3	24	Newell (1997)	11 E-6

Tab. 7.8: Calculation of the fate factors with Equation (6.7) using emission and concentration data from the sources cited.

The average measured concentrations reported by Newell (1997) include anthropogenic and natural sources and the monitoring sites are biased towards urban areas. The emissions, on the other hand, are lower estimates of the anthropogenic emissions. These two effects lead to an overestimate of the fate factors.

Ozone formation due to NO_x and VOC

The chemistry of ozone formation is very complex as it depends on the presence of precursors and meteorological factors and due to the short lifetime of ozone under certain conditions. The main influencing factors are the presence of OH-radicals and the availability of light energy (see, e.g., Fabian 1992). The number of OH-radicals in the lower troposphere is directly dependant on the primary emissions of NO_x and VOC. The exact composition of the anthropogenic NMVOC-emissions is not well known. Eliassen *et al.* (1982) estimate that NMVOC is made up of 30% ethane, 20% *n*-butane, 20% ethene, 10% propene and 20% *o*-xylene on a volume-by-volume basis. An interpretation of the UK emission data provided by Derwent *et al.* (1996) suggests however that these substances represent only one sixth of the total NMVOC emissions on a mass basis and about a quarter on a ozone formation basis. Natural emissions are made up mostly of isoprene and the various terpenes. The latter probably do not contribute to ozone formation because the terpenes react rapidly with both OH-radicals and ozone. Isoprene is emitted in large amounts from forests and causes high background concentrations.

Ozone concentration is highest in rural areas and not closest to the emission sources. This is different from the situation for all primary emissions where concentrations are highest next to the emission sources. (This observation is important because the correlation between high concentrations and high population densities is, for this reason, smaller for ozone than for primary pollutants). The main reason for this behaviour lies in the scavenging effect of NO. 95% of the NO_x-emissions are in the form of NO which is later oxidised to NO_2. So-called smog episodes occur when the ambient temperature is elevated and solar radiation is intense during daytime. If these conditions persist, the ozone concentration will increase with each additional sunny day. Derwent *et al.* (1996) model an air package which starts with an ozone concentration of 30 ppb in Vienna and whose concentration increases during its travel through Germany to the UK. The ozone concentration in the air package when it arrives over South England adds up to more than 100 ppb.

The derivation of a generic fate factor for ozone is problematic because:

- Ozone is formed or depleted very efficiently depending on the ambient conditions.
- Averaging the concentrations over summer *and* winter months, day- *and* night-time, and morning *and* afternoon periods is a difficult task.
- In some regions, ozone formation is NO_2-limited and VOC-limited in others. In yet other regions, the limiting factor changes with the season or the weather condition, i.e., while an additional emission of NO_x will increase the formation of ozone in some regions, it will not affect the concentration in other places or even contribute to ozone scavenging[6].

These are the reasons why we limit ourselves here to using models and not measurements in order to improve the averaging procedure and to estimate ozone formation due to marginal precursor emissions. A paper by Rabl *et al.* (1997a) suggests that one can rely for this purpose on the consequences of the reduction of precursor emissions modelled by Simpson (1992 and 1993). Simpson used the large amount of measurement data for the summers of 1985 and of 1989 to calibrate the EMEP Model. He covered all of Europe, including parts of the former Soviet Union, and used a time resolution of 6 hours to calculate daily peak concentrations during the six summer months due to yearly emissions of NO_x and VOCs. This study on the effect of emission reductions makes it possible to calculate a kind of marginal fate factor.

[6] The ratio of VOC to NO_x concentrations amounts to a factor 10 in the densely populated Northwest Europe but to about a factor of 30 in the other European countries. I.e., VOC is the limiting factor in the Northwest and NO_x in the other regions of the continent (Simpson 1993).

The following limiting conditions have to be considered when using the results in Table 7.9:

- The winter time ozone reduction has been assumed to be negligible. This underestimates the fate factors.
- The EMEP model calculated 6 hr-peak concentrations. To calculate fate factors for 1-hr or 24-hr ozone formation one has to multiply by factor 1.3 or divide by factor 1.5, respectively (Rabl *et al.* 1997a).
- The modelled concentration concerns the boundary rather than the surface layer. This overestimates the fate factors (Simpson 1993). Ozone production in the free troposphere is not considered here.
- Similar recalculations based on an improved model (Simpson *et al.* 1997:23) show that a 50% cut of NO_x emissions results in a smaller reduction in ozone concentration of about 5% (instead of 7%). This is due to the larger *in*crease in the ozone concentration in the VOC-limited UK (up to 22%) than modelled earlier.
- Calculations with the Harwell model show that the emissions of NO_x and VOC in Europe contribute significantly to the ozone formation outside of Europe (Rabl *et al.* 1997a). This additional ozone formation is not considered here and leads to an underestimation of the fate factors.

Emission scenario		Emission Mt/a (*)		Ozone reduction April to September (#)		Ozone reduction per Mt precursor emission (¶)	Fate factor (in ppb) (‡)	Fate factor
NO_x	VOC	NO_2	VOC	%	ppb	ppb·a/Mt	ppb·m^2·a/kg	m^2·a/m^3
100%	100%	22.4	24.5	0	0			
50%	100%	11.2	24.5	7	3.92	0.18	1225	2.5 E-6
100%	50%	22.4	12.25	6	3.36	0.14	960	1.9 E-6

Table 7.9: Fate factors for ozone formation (average of daily 6-hr peak concentrations) from NO_x and VOC
(*) Emissions for 1989 from Table 1 in Simpson (1993)
(#) Percentage reduction from Table 6 in Simpson (1993), baseline ozone concentration over Europe is assumed to be 56 ppb (Simpson 1992 and 1993)
(¶) It is assumed that the reduction in ozone concentrations occurs only in summer time
(‡) Modelling area ≈ 7 Mio. km^2 (estimated from Simpson 1992)

Another version of the EMEP model has been used in Annex E in Barrett *et al.* (1996). The baseline scenario there is based on emissions expected in the year 2000. From that, a 30% reduction of NO_x and VOC, respectively, has been assumed for two reduction scenarios. The resultant ozone reduction is much smaller than what is to be expected from the calculations in Table 7.9 and the reduction of NO_x turns out to be twice as effective as a comparable VOC-reduction (see Table 7.10). More recent calculations in Simpson *et al.* (1997:B2) for an emission cut of 40% resulted for NO_x in a much smaller, and for VOC in a slightly larger, reduction. A short communication with David Simpson failed to clarify the source for these large differences. However, the following changes were made in the model (Simpson *et al.* 1997):

- update of the initial concentrations,
- update of the chemistry used,
- increase of the deposition velocity to remove more ozone in order to reproduce measured concentration data,
- modifying the photolyses rates to get more pronounced peaks in the Mediterranean, and
- replacing the annual meteorology with a 5-year meteorology (1989, 1990, 1992, 1993, 1994).

As mentioned before, a decrease in precursor emissions may well lead to increased ozone concentrations (in Northwest Europe) and *vice versa* (Pryor 1998). Therefore, the large differences between the different model versions can partly be explained.

Emission scenario	Reduced emission (*)	Ozone reduction April to September (#)	Ozone reduction per Mt precursor emission (¶)	Fate factor (in ppb) (‡)	Fate factor
	Mt/a	ppb	ppb·a/Mt	ppb m^2a/ kg	m^2a/m^3
-30% NO_X	5.8	0.62	0.05	370	0.74 E-6
-30% VOC	5.3	0.33	0.03	220	0.44 E-6

Table 7.10: Fate factors for ozone formation from NOx and VOC (Barrett et al. 1996)
(*) Emissions for 2000 from Table E1 in Barrett *et al.* (1996)
(#) Reduction from Table E2 and E3 in Barrett *et al.* (1996)
(¶) It is assumed that the reduction in ozone concentrations occurs only during the summer
(‡) Modelling area ≈ 7 Mio. km^2

7.2.4 Best estimate for the fate factors

Subsections 7.2.2 and 7.2.3 have presented several sets of fate factors calculated with different methods and for different modelling areas. These calculations could be further improved by performing our own modelling exercises. However, we consider the data provided in this section to be of sufficient quality to present first estimates for the effects of air pollution on respiratory diseases.

The following principles are applied for the selection of the fate factors for the calculations that will follow:

- The fate factors should be appropriate for European conditions.
- Preference is given to fate factors for which the underlying assumptions are known.
- Average fate factors that assume a proportional relation between emissions and concentration have been used for all but ozone creation. In this instance, the marginal fate factor was considered most appropriate in order to reflect the non-linear atmospheric chemistry of ozone formation.

The fate factors presented in Table 7.11 can be considered as best estimates, given the many assumptions that are necessary for their calculations. Major errors are probably avoided because of the number of different approaches that have been used to arrive at the fate factor estimates.

Emitted substance	Target concentration	Fate factor (m^2a/m^3)	σ_g^2
CO	CO	100 E-6 (a)	4
TSP	TSP	9 E-6 (b)	2
TSP	PM_{10}	4.4 E-6 (c)	3
PM_{10}	PM_{10}	15 E-6 (b)	3
$PM_{2.5}$	$PM_{2.5}$	17 E-6 (b)	3
SO_x (as SO_2)	SO_2	3.0 E-6 (e)	2
SO_x (as SO_2)	SO_4 and $(NH_4)_2SO_4$	1.3 E-6 (d)	2
NO_x (as NO_2)	NO_2	2.5 E-6 (f)	2
NO_x (as NO_2)	NO_3 and $(NH_4)NO_3$	3.6 E-6 (d)	2
NO_x (as NO_2)	O_3	1.5 E-6 (g)	4
NH_3	$(NH_4)_2SO_4$	1.7 E-6 (d)	2
NH_3	$(NH_4)NO_3$	0.6 E-6 (d)	2
NMVOC	O_3	1.5 E-6 (g)	4

Tab. 7.11: Fate factors for emissions to air to concentration in inhalation air with their estimated squared geometric standard deviation (24-hr average concentration for all but ozone; daily 6-hr peak concentration for ozone)
(a) According to United Nations (1996) the emissions in EMEP Europe added up to about 100 Mt in 1990. From different sources an average concentration of about 0.5 to 1 mg/m^3 can be estimated. One can calculate a fate factor of 59 to 117 m^2a/m^3 with Equation (6.7) (area 11.7 E12 m^2) The fate factor reported for the USA (Table 7.7) of 1000 E-6 is much higher than the value of 19 E-6 in Jolliet *et al.* (1997b). Without further analysis we chose an intermediate value within the span of our own calculations due to the limited relevance of CO .
(b) Rounded values are taken from Table 7.4. The high values in Tables 7.5 and 7.8 are artefacts because natural background was not considered, net export was omitted and biased concentration measurements may cause additional errors. The lower values in Table 7.5 and 7.8 are within the confidence interval.
(c) According to Table 7.4 it can be assumed that 49 % of TSP is PM10.
(d) Averaged value from Tables 7.6 and 7.7 which show very good agreement.
(e) Weighted average from Tables 7.5, 7.6, and 7.7 with more confidence in Table 7.7.
(f) Averaged value from Tables 7.5, 7.6 and 7.7
(g) Results from Table 7.9 appear to be more reliable than those from Table 7.10. The results of the latest calculations from EMEP (1997) are considered by a lower fate factor for NO_x. The high uncertainty is reflected in the high factor for σg^2.

7.2.5 The umbrella principle for individual VOCs

The fate factor for VOCs to form ozone (Tables 7.9/10) did not differentiate between the ozone forming potentials of single hydrocarbons. The reactivity of single hydrocarbons varies widely and should be considered when the mixture of VOC emissions is known or if, e.g., one wants to support the decision on the choice between solvents.

Such a differentiation can be undertaken by applying the concept of Photochemical Ozone Creation Potential (POCP). The POCP expresses the incremental ozone concentration per incremental emission for VOC specie *i* normalised by the ratio for ethylene. Ethylene serves as the reference substance and is one of the most reactive VOCs. The unit is without dimension and the POCPs are normally given as a percentage of the one for ethylene.

Heijungs *et al.* (1992) list POCPs derived from three scenarios: the trajectory from Germany to Ireland, from France to Sweden, and within the UK. It is integrated over 9 days of travelling time. The values are taken from United Nations (1991) and ranges are given for a model run of 11 days. Derwent *et al.* (1996) have published new POCPs for trajectories from Poland and Austria to the UK. The results are considered to be typical for Northwest Europe, but not for the other regions in Europe. The weather condition assumed (easterly winds) are not typical for European weather conditions. Changes for several substance parameters occurred when compared to earlier modelling exercises (Derwent *et al.* 1991). The change for ethylene led to changes for all other POCPs. The model in Derwent *et al.* (1996) has been updated with the implementation of a Master Chemical Mechanism that explicitly treats the degradation of 120 VOCs (Jenkin *et al.* 1997). The POCPs were calculated for the 5 day standard trajectory from Vienna to Germany, France and the UK. Extensive validation led to good agreement of the new model with measurements and with the results from other international models.

The concept of *umbrella principle* is used to describe this approach because the fate factor is calculated for only one sum parameter (here NMVOC) or substance in a first step. This represents the shaft of the umbrella. The umbrella is formed by the many single substances which contribute to ozone formation. The relative activity of the umbrella substances has to be known. In our case, these are the POCPs. To link the shaft with the umbrella, it is necessary to express the umbrella substances in relation to the shaft substance. In Heijungs *et al.* (1992) the average POCP for NMVOCs is given with 41.6%. Derwent *et al.* (1996) published a detailed emission inventory for the UK. From the total NMVOC emission in the UK and the resulting total POCP-weighted emission (Table 6 in Derwent *et al.* 1996), it is possible to calculate the average POCP for NMVOC (59.2%). This can then be used for the new POCPs in Jenkin et al (1997) as well, according to Michael E. Jenkin[7], because he suspects that this will not change very much anyway.

A small selection of relevant precursors listed in United Nations (1991), Derwent *et al.* (1996), and Jenkin *et al.* (1997) is presented in Table 7.12. The fate factors for the single hydrocarbons can be calculated with:

$$F_i = \frac{POCP_i}{POCP_{NMVOC}} \cdot F_{NMVOC} \qquad [m^2a/m^3] \qquad (7.7)$$

	POCP	POCP	POCP	Fate factor	Fate factor	Fate factor	σ_g^2
	Heijungs *et al.* (1992)	Derwent *et al.* (1996)	Jenkin *et al.* (1997)	Heijungs *et al.* (1992)	Derwent *et al.* (1996)	Jenkin *et al.* (1997)	
Substance	%	%	%	m^2a/m^3	m^2a/m^3	m^2a/m^3	-
Toluene	56	77	64	2.0E-06	2.0E-06	1.6E-06	5
n-Butane	41	60	35	1.5E-06	1.5E-06	8.9E-07	5
Ethylene	100	100	100	3.6E-06	2.5E-06	2.5E-06	5
o-Xylene	67	83	105	2.4E-06	2.1E-06	2.7E-06	5
Propylene	103	108	112	3.7E-06	2.7E-06	2.8E-06	5
NMVOC (all)	41.6	59.2	(*) 59.2	(#) 1.5E-06	(#) 1.5E-06	(#) 1.5E-06	4

Tab 7.12: Example for the umbrella principle applied to ozone creating hydrocarbons by use of three different sets of models.
(*) Assumption that the average POCP of NMVOCs has not changed from Derwent *et al.* (1996) to Jenkin *et al.* (1997)
(#) Generic fate factor for NMVOC from Table 7.11

[7] Personal communication from Michael E. Jenkin, AEA Technology plc, on October 21, 1997.

The main difference between the older results in Heijungs *et al.* (1992) and the new results in Derwent *et al.* (1996) and Jenkin *et al.* (1997) is the changed fate factor for ethylene as has already been mentioned. The differences identified at the level of POCPs are smaller due to the division by the average POCP for all NMVOCs. Derwent *et al.* (1996) report that their POCPs have an uncertainty range of at least 5 percentage points. The range given in Heijungs *et al.* (1992) suggests deviations with a factor 2 or 3. This range is smaller when representative European conditions are used for the calculations. In order to reflect the additional uncertainty introduced by the umbrella of POCPs, the squared geometric standard deviation is estimated to be a factor of 5 (Table 7.12). Based on the most recent data reported by Jenkin *et al.* (1997), we calculated fate factors for, about 120 single VOCs which are listed in Appendix (7.1). They are representative for climatic conditions typically found in North-western Europe.

7.2.6 Summary

The fate analysis has made use of five types of models:

- A model that relates average residence times to average mixing volumes.
- A model that relates measured average concentrations to measured emissions.
- A model that relates modelled average concentrations to measured emissions.
- A multi-media model that models the fate of a unit emission.
- A model that relates modelled reductions in concentrations to assumed reductions in emissions.

The umbrella principle for hydrocarbons that contribute to ozone creation has, in addition, been introduced. Eight air pollutants have been identified in Subsection 7.1.3 as contributing through inhalation to respiratory diseases. More than 100 primary pollutants have been identified to contribute to the formation of these inhaled pollutants and, for each primary emission, one to three fate factors have been developed. The outcome of these calculations is listed in Appendix (7.1).

7.3 Effect analysis

7.3.1 Introduction

This section's aim is to determine the effect factors *Eim* which relate observed health effects on endpoints *m* to exposure to substances *i*. This, togcthcr with the fate factors calculated in the previous section, provides the basis for the calculation of the respiratory effects per kg emission of primary pollutants (Equation 7.2).

The decision to use the epidemiological approach has been explained in Subsection 7.1.2 and it is the starting point for this section. The next subsection provides therefore a further discussion of epidemiological studies. A set of endpoints for respiratory effects which are mentioned in the literature have been listed in Subsection 7.1.1. However, the choice of endpoints that in the end can be used is influenced by the availability of studies and two additional requirements: endpoints should be quantifiable and they should not overlap with other endpoints in order to prevent double-counting of effects (see Subsection 7.3.3). Subsection 7.3.3 also addresses the suggestion that effects are dependent on the ambient concentration of pollutants and proposes a simplifying linearisation in order to circumvent the use of concentration-dependent effect factors (i.e., dose-response *functions*).

Epidemiological studies have a very limited power to prove causality. This uncertainty about the strength of the evidence found on the relationships between emissions and the endpoints for respiratory effects is reflected in the application of the three cultural perspectives already introduced in Chapter 3.

Subsection 7.3.5 presents the calculation procedure to derive the health effects of respiratory diseases in a non-aggregated manner for each primary pollutant.

7.3.2 Epidemiological studies and their basic assumptions

Criteria for causation

When using epidemiological studies to estimate dose-response relationships, it is necessary to make use of some criteria to assess their validity. Künzli *et al.* (1996) have selected from Hill (1965) a list of criteria that appear to be relevant for our purpose:

- The exposure as an assumed risk factor has to occur *before* effects are observed.
- The *biological plausibility* should be given. This criterion depends on the state of knowledge. There are some cases in which epidemiological results stimulated toxicological research that then lend support to the plausibility of the identified relationship.
- The *consistency* of the results from a large set of studies with similar objectives, but different approaches and study areas, supports the interpretation of the results.
- Results should be *coherent*, i.e., if a risk factor increases the occurrence of cough, one should also observe an increase in the demand for medicine to cure cough.

In addition, one should only use articles that have appeared in peer-reviewed journals, studies with a study design that is both adequate and transparent, and studies that make use of a multivariate statistical analysis.

Type of study

Ecological epidemiological studies that do not correct for confounding factors are of little use when small additional risks should be observed. The reasons for this judgement have already been laid out in Subsection 6.3.2. This stricture also applies to the case of respiratory diseases due to air pollution.

Cohort studies deliver the best evidence because all confounding factors are known on an individual level for a long study period. Two such studies on the effect of air pollution on chronicle mortality could be identified (Dockery *et al.* 1993, Pope *et al.* 1995b).

A large number of so-called *time-series* studies are available. A large number of European studies were published in 1996 using the time-series approach and the APHEA-protocol. (APHEA stands for 'short term effects of **air p**ollution on **hea**lth'.)[8] They analyse short term changes in, e.g., mortality or hospital admission due to changes in ambient air pollution concentrations. The results are valid indications for short term effects as the studies correct for confounding factors, but this type of study in general underestimates the real effects as they fail to consider any long-term effect.

A fourth type of study, the *cross-sectional studies*, observes the prevalence of health effects during a certain time period, e.g., one year, and adds information on the individual level with respect to lifestyle factors and pollution history. Without further information it is, in principle, not possible to differentiate whether a factor is causing health effects or even a consequence of them. This study design can, for instance, be used to derive chronic prevalence data (Künzli *et al.* 1996).

Some basic assumptions

The outcome of the specific case-studies should be interpreted in light of a number of underlying assumptions that are recalled here once again. The following assumptions are made for almost all the studies that are used in the subsequent assessment (partly from ExternE 1995):

- It is assumed that personal exposure can be approximated by the measurement of ambient concentrations.
- From that, it follows that it is assumed that people breathe outdoor air during 24 hours although it is known that they spend more than 22 hours indoors. Colome *et al.* (1992) shows that, indoors, the concentration of PM_{10} is lower than outdoors and that personal samplers show inhalation concentrations that are closer to indoor than to outdoor concentrations. Monn *et al.* (1996) show that both the use of gas stoves and smoking increase the PM_{10} concentration indoors above the values outdoors.

[8] For the APHEA publications see Bachárová *et al.* (1996), Ballester *et al.* (1996), Dab *et al.* (1996), Katsouyanni *et al.* (1996), Pönkä *et al.* (1996), Ponce de Leon *et al.* (1996), Schouten *et al.* (1996), Schwartz *et al.* (1996), Spix *et al.* (1996), Sunyer *et al.* (1996), Touloumi *et al.* (1996), Vigotti *et al.* (1996), Wojtyniak *et al.* (1996), and Zmirou *et al.* (1996).

- Epidemiological studies also assume that variations over time in the pollutant concentration can be taken care of by an integration over time (relevant only for long-term studies).
- It is assumed that people spend no time outside of the study region and that the concentration within defined gridcells is homogenous. This assumption reflects the low density of monitoring stations and the fact that personal samplers are almost never used.

These four assumptions do not limit the usefulness of these studies for our investigation. To the contrary, they fit perfectly with the modelling used in the fate analysis to predict generic outdoor exposure. However, these assumptions give an idea of those confounding factors which have remained unconsidered. It is this which may prove to be of relevance.

- As mentioned earlier, the assumption of thresholds based on the London smog episodes has been withdrawn. That is, it is assumed that there is no safe level. For this reason, the regression analysis is performed with a Poisson regression.
- There is much less reliable information available on chronic or delayed than on acute effects that occur on the same day or only a few days after the occurrence of high concentrations. This lack is the result of the effort required to conduct cohort studies. This situation introduces a bias, i.e., chronic effects are underestimated.
- Confounding factors which are controlled are mostly lifestyle factors and weather conditions (temperature, humidity and, sometimes, wind speed). ExternE (1995) mentions that controlling these factors is difficult and that when it is done, it is done in such a way that the resultant effects of air pollution is just a lower estimate. However, unmeasured confounding factors are likely to be detected in the future although this may or may not alter the outcome. Jenkins *et al.* (1996) argue, for instance, for the inclusion of physical exercise in the confounding factors, an element which has not been considered so far.

Further discussion on relevant assumptions, limitations, and results of epidemiological studies on respiratory diseases due to air pollution is provided in the reviews by van Loveren *et al.* (1993), Schwartz (1994), Dockery *et al.* (1994), Brunekreef *et al.* (1995), ESEERCO (1995), ExternE (1995), Bertollini *et al.* (1996), Künzli *et al.* (1996), GVF (1996), Concawe (1996), Dockery *et al.* (1996), Pope *et al.* (1995a/1996), and Pilkington *et al.* (1997).

In light of this large body of review literature, we turn directly to the exposure-effect relationships suggested by this study.

7.3.3 The dose-response relationships for respiratory effects

The review articles and reports mentioned above give an excellent overview of available studies fulfilling the high quality standards posited by the reviews' authors. The reviews published before 1996 do not include the large body of literature from the APHEA study. Only Pilkington *et al.* (1997) review both the large American literature and the APHEA results. GVF (1996) reviews the literature in order to quantify total health effects due to air pollution and uses this as a base for calculating the share of health effects due to traffic. Dockery *et al.* (1996) and Pope *et al.* (1996) review the literature from the perspective of epidemiologists interested in the relative risks reported in several studies. Pilkington *et al.* (1997) review the available literature in order to calculate health damages attributable to single substances emitted to air. Donnan *et al.* (1997) provide the background to the choice and calculate exposure-response slopes. The data they derived has been used by Pilkington *et al.* (1997). Both studies chose an European bias wherever possible.

This survey suggested that the reviews by Donnan *et al.* (1997) and Pilkington *et al.* (1997) would serve our purpose best. The same exposure-effect slopes will also be used in the forthcoming study on external costs in transportation (ExternE Transport) and are used in the update of the external costs of different energy supply systems (ExternE 1997). Using them will therefore improve the comparability of results. However, the meta-analysis of the APHEA studies by the APHEA's authors was still in preparation when Donnan, Pilkington and Hurley prepared their own reports. They therefore decided against performing their own proper meta-analysis and chose instead to work with typical or representative exposure-response slopes, i.e., those whose values are close to the average of those available. They expect that this procedure will lead them to choose data that is close to the one to be published in the forthcoming APHEA meta-analysis.

A number of assumptions have to be made in order to present exposure-effect slopes. They are taken from Pilkington *et al.* (1997).

Particles

The epidemiological evidence on the adverse acute health effects of air polluted with particles is very substantial indeed. There is strong, but much less widespread, epidemiological evidence on chronic health effects.

The literature contains a wide variety of measurements for particles defined either as total suspended particles (TSP), PM_{10} (inhalable particles), black smoke (BS), sulphates, or finer fractions such as $PM_{2.5}$. When necessary, the recalculations were made using the relationships given by Dockery *et al.* (1994). Sulphates are assumed to result in particles smaller than 2.5 μm ($PM_{2.5}$). Nitrates have a higher solubility and it is assumed that they are better represented by PM_{10}. No European studies for $PM_{2.5}$ are available. Therefore, the exposure-response slopes for PM_{10} have been multiplied by a factor of 1.67 in order to be valid for $PM_{2.5}$ (Dockery *et al.* 1994).

Ozone

The overall evidence strongly supports the view that the acute health effects of ozone can be quantified and that they should be added to those of particles.

The characterisation of ozone in epidemiological studies is done in several ways (1-hr daily maximum, 5-, 6-, 8-, 24-hr daily averages). A conversion factor of 1.25 has been applied to convert per cent changes in health effects at a 1-hr daily maximum to a 6-hr daily average ozone concentration. (The same metric has been used for the fate analysis in Section 7.2.)

Sulphur dioxide (SO_2)

APHEA results establish a clear association between SO_2 and acute mortality. Whether this association is causal is still unclear, because it could also be explained with the insufficient measurements of fine particles, especially of sulphates. However, Pilkington *et al.* (1997) recommend assuming that the relationship is causal and adding the estimated impacts to the effects due to particles and ozone.

Carbon monoxide (CO)

There is little epidemiological evidence concerning CO. Pilkington *et al.* (1997) recommend on present evidence that only the relation between CO and congestive heart failure, but not the one between it and mortality, should be used. They propose to use the latter in a sensitivity analysis.

Associations with 1-hr maximum concentrations of CO are upscaled by a factor of 2 and those with 8-hr daily average concentrations by a factor of 1.5 in order to convert them to daily average ambient concentrations. (The same metric has been used for the fate analysis in Section 7.2.)

Nitrogen dioxide (NO_2)

APHEA reports a positive association between NO_2 and both mortality and respiratory hospital admissions. However, this association could be caused by particles as well or NO_2 could act as a surrogate for some mixture of traffic-related pollution. Pilkington *et al.* (1997) suggest using NO_2 only for the sensitivity analysis. Exposure-response slopes for 1-hr maximum levels of NO_2 are converted by a factor of 1.67 to 24-hr average concentration. (The same metric has been used for the fate analysis in Section 7.2.)

Bias for Western European studies

Epidemiological studies on populations in Western Europe were preferred over studies for populations and situations in Eastern Europe or on other continents if they were of high quality. The review by Pilkington et al (1997) showed that the exposure-response slopes for particles are lower in East Europe, but higher in North America compared to those for Western Europe[9]. The values found for the exposure-response slopes for ozone are generally higher for areas within Europe than for North America.

The use of a scaling procedure made it possible to use both European and North American results in a consistent manner; the American results were scaled down for particles and scaled up for ozone.

Uncertainty estimates

Pilkington *et al.* (1997) assume a lognormal distribution for the wanted values of the exposure-response slopes. For each function they determine a qualitative characterisation described with the four levels 'A', 'A?', 'B', or 'B?'. The question mark indicates that a function has been chosen in analogy, for instance for nitrates

---

[9] However, a re-analysis of the East European data considering delayed effects showed that similar exposure-response slopes as in Western Europe will result (personal communication from Dr. Regula Rapp/University Basle referring on an expert meeting in February 1998)

by treating them as PM_{10}. They then assigned a numerical value range for the geometric standard deviation at each level:

A = high confidence, roughly corresponding to $\sigma g = 2.5$ to 4
B = medium confidence, roughly corresponding to $\sigma g = 4$ to 6

For the squared geometric standard deviation – spanning a 95% confidence interval – we use the following estimates:

A: $\sigma g^2 = 6$
A?, B: $\sigma g^2 = 16$
B?: $\sigma g^2 = 36$

These ranges may be too large because the notation in Pilkington *et al.* (1997) also includes uncertainties in the fate modelling and the monetary valuation. Especially the upper range is not realistic in most cases. However, the exposure-response slope is considered to be the element introducing most of the uncertainty, therefore, we stay with the assumptions made above.

Presentation of the exposure-response slopes

Pilkington *et al.* (1997) give the slope factor of the exposure-response function for all endpoints but mortality. The E-R slope provides a quantified expression for the number of additional cases per year and per person with health effects *m* if the exposure concentration is increased by 1 $\mu g/m^3$. For mortality, only the per cent increase of death cases is given.

No effect dependency from exposure concentration

Pilkington *et al.* (1997) assume independence of the slopes from ambient concentrations, without providing a detailed justification, however. They just take the slope at the ambient concentration in the study region where the epidemiological investigation had been undertaken. But it is the percent increase in effects which is found to be constant at all levels of concentrations. A per cent increase of health effects for a 10 $\mu g/m^3$ increase in concentration below 10% can well be approximated by a linear relationship for the range of concentrations that are relevant in Europe. But such a linear relation is questionable when it is applied to vulnerable risk groups such as asthmatics and children or for minor effects such as symptom days where percent increases of health risks are larger than 10%.

Yet we will accept here in this study the simplifying assumption made in Pilkington *et al.* (1997). In a future, improved impact assessment, however, one should make use of an exposure-response function that is dependent on concentration. In such an improved version, one could calculate average European effect factors by calculating weighted averages based on frequency distributions of the concentrations in Europe. One could also calculate site-dependent effect factors for emissions in urban or rural areas by following an emission package during its trajectory under average weather conditions and then model the absolute concentrations during such a trip. A weighted average effect factor for different emission conditions and areas can then be calculated with this information on the concentration. Such calculations are already possible by using the more site-dependent tools developed within the studies that attempt to calculate externalities (see, e.g., ExternE 1995, ESEERCO 1995).

Table 7.13 lists all exposure-response relationships that Pilkington *et al.* (1997) found to be relevant. The original reference is listed for each endpoint and the groups affected are also mentioned. The relationship given is the slope of the linearised exposure-response function and is normalised for a concentration increase of 1 μg/m^3 and for 1 person.

We use here an example from Dab *et al.* (1996) for respiratory hospital admission due to particles in order to demonstrate the procedure used to derive the slopes of the exposure-response functions. The following information is known from Dab *et al.* (1996):

Population in the study area (Paris):	6'140'000	people
Daily hospital admissions for all respiratory causes:	79	admissions per day
Relative Risk (RR)	1.045	per 100 μg/m^3 PM_{13}

On the basis of this information it is possible to calculate the absolute risk. Dab *et al.* (1996) and many other epidemiological studies use Poisson regression to calculate the relative risk (RR). Equation (7.8) is used in order to determine the per cent increase per 1 μg/m^3 increase in particle concentration:

$$\% \text{ increase per } \mu g = exp(\frac{ln(RR)}{\Delta c}) = \exp(\frac{\ln(1.045)}{100\ \mu g/m^3}) = 0.044\% \qquad (7.8)$$

$$\text{absolute risk per } \mu g = \% \text{ increase per } \mu g \cdot \frac{\text{yearly baseline risk}}{\text{study population}}$$

$$= 0.044\% \cdot \frac{79 \cdot 365}{6'140'000} = 2.07\text{ E-6} \qquad (7.9)$$

The base for the percentage increase is the baseline risk. 79 daily respiratory hospital admissions times 365 days per 6.14 million inhabitants result in an absolute risk of 0.0047 to be admitted to a hospital per year. This baseline risk is increased by 0.044% through the exposure to an increase in the particle concentration of one additional μg/m^3. This results in an absolute individual risk of 2.07 E-6 hospital admissions per year per μg/m^3.

In the example above, no correction has been made for the difference between the measured concentration of PM_{13} and the one of PM_{10} used in the fate analysis. However, the effect factors for $PM_{2.5}$ and for sulphates are derived by multiplying the absolute risk per μg/m^3 for PM_{13} by 1.67 to correct for the higher share of potent fine particles in one μg $PM_{2.5}$ than in one μg PM_{13}.

The other exposure-response slopes listed in Table 7.13 have been calculated in the same way. Donnan *et al.* (1997) provide detailed reasoning and description of all the slopes that have been calculated.

Pollutant	Endpoint	Reference	Affected population group	E-R slope (*)	Cultural bias	σ_g^2
PM_{10}	Bronchodilator usage	Dusseldorp *et al.* 1995	Adult asthmatics	0.163	E, H, I	16
		Roemer *et al.* 1993	Asthm. children	0.078	E, H, I	16
	Cough	Dusseldorp *et al.* 1995	Adult asthmatics	0.168	E, H, I	6
		Pope *et al.* 1992	Asthm. children	0.133	E, H, I	6
	Lower respiratory symptoms (wheeze)	Dusseldorp *et al.* 1995	Adult asthmatics	0.061	E, H, I	6
		Roemer *et al.* 1993	Asthm. children	0.103	E, H, I	6
	Chronic bronchitis	Dockery *et al.* 1989	Children	1.61 E-3	E, H, I	16
		Abbey *et al.* 1995	Adults	4.9 E-5	E, H, I	6
	Chronic cough	Dockery *et al.* 1989	Children	2.07 E-3	E, H, I	16
	Restricted activity days (RAD)(#)	Ostro 1987	Adults	0.025	E, H, I	16
	Respiratory hospital admissions	Dab *et al.* 1996	All	2.07 E-6	E, H, I	6
	Acute Mortality (AM)	Spix *et al.* 1996, Verhoeff *et al.* 1996	All	0.04%	E, H, I	16
	Chronic Mortality (CM) †	Pope *et al.* 1995b	Adults > 30a	0.386%	E, H, I	16
	ERV for COPD	Sunyer *et al.* 1993	All	7.2 E-6	E	36
	ERV for asthma	Schwartz 1993, Bates *et al.* 1990	All	6.45 E-6	E	36
	ERV for croup in pre school children	Schwartz *et al.* 1991	All	2.91 E-5	E	36
$PM_{2.5}$, Sulphates	Bronchodilator usage	Dusseldorp *et al.* 1995	Adult asthmatics	0.272	E, H, I	16
		Roemer *et al.* 1993	Asthm. children	0.129	E, H, I	16
	Cough	Dusseldorp *et al.* 1995	Adult asthmatics	0.280	E, H, I	6
		Pope *et al.* 1992	Asthm. children	0.223	E, H, I	6
	Lower respiratory symptoms (wheeze)	Dusseldorp *et al.* 1995	Adult asthmatics	0.101	E, H, I	6
		Roemer *et al.* 1993	Asthm. children	0.172	E, H, I	6
	Chronic bronchitis	Dockery *et al.* 1989	Children	2.69 E-3	E, H, I	16
		Abbey *et al.* 1995	Adults	7.8 E-5	E, H, I	6
	Chronic cough	Dockery *et al.* 1989	Children	3.46 E-3	E, H, I	16
	Restricted activity days (RAD)(#)	Ostro 1987	Adults	0.042	E, H, I	16
	Respiratory hospital admissions	Dab *et al.* 1996	All	3.46 E-6	E, H, I	6
	Acute Mortality (AM)	Spix *et al.* 1996, Verhoeff *et al.* 1996	All	0.068%	E, H, I	16
	Chronic Mortality (CM) †	Pope *et al.* 1995b	Adults > 30a	0.643%	E, H, I	16
	ERV for COPD	Sunyer *et al.* 1993	All	1.2 E-5	E	36
	ERV for asthma	Schwartz 1993, Bates *et al.* 1990	All	1.08E-5	E	36
	ERV for croup in pre school children	Schwartz *et al.* 1991	All	4.86E-5	E	36
Nitrates	Bronchodilator usage	Dusseldorp *et al.* 1995	Adult asthmatics	0.163	E, H	36
		Roemer *et al.* 1993	Asthm. children	0.078	E, H	36
	Cough	Dusseldorp *et al.* 1995	Adult asthmatics	0.168	E, H	16
		Pope *et al.* 1992	Asthm. children	0.133	E, H	16
	Lower respiratory symptoms (wheeze)	Dusseldorp *et al.* 1995	Adult asthmatics	0.061	E, H	16
		Roemer *et al.* 1993	Asthm. children	0.103	E, H	16
	Chronic bronchitis	Dockery *et al.* 1989	Children	1.61 E-3	E, H	36
		Abbey *et al.* 1995	Adults	4.9 E-5	E, H	16
	Chronic cough	Dockery *et al.* 1989	Children	2.07 E-3	E, H	36
	Restricted activity days (RAD)(#)	Ostro 1987	Adults	0.025	E, H	36
	Respiratory hospital admissions	Dab *et al.* 1996	All	2.07 E-6	E, H	16
	Acute Mortality (AM)	Spix *et al.* 1996, Verhoeff *et al.* 1996	All	0.04%	E, H	36
	Chronic Mortality (CM) †	Pope *et al.* 1995b	Adults > 30a	0.386%	E, H	36
	ERV for COPD	Sunyer *et al.* 1993	All	7.2 E-6	E	36
	ERV for asthma	Schwartz 1993, Bates *et al.* 1990	All	6.45 E-6	E	36
	ERV for croup in pre school children	Schwartz *et al.* 1991	All	2.91 E-5	E	36

Ozone	Asthma attacks (AA)	Whittemore *et al.* 1980	All	4.29 E-3	E, H, I	36
	Minor restricted activity day (MRAD)[¶]	Ostro *et al.* 1989	Adults	9.76 E-3	E, H, I	16
	Respiratory hospital admissions	Ponce de Leon *et al.* 1996	All	3.54 E-6	E, H, I	6
	Symptom days	Krupnick et al 1990	All	0.033	E, H, I	6
	Acute Mortality (AM)	Sunyer et al 1996	All	0.059%	E, H, I	16
	ERV for asthma	Cody *et al.* 1992, Bates *et al.* 1990	All	1.32 E-5	E	36
SO_2	Respiratory hospital admissions	Ponce de Leon *et al.* 1996	All	2.04E-6	E, H	6
	Acute Mortality (AM)	Anderson *et al.* 1996, Touloumi *et al.* 1996	All	0.072%	E, H	16
NO_2	Acute Mortality (AM)	Sunyer *et al.* 1996, Anderson *et al.* 1996	All	0.034%	E	36
	Respiratory hospital admissions	Ponce de Leon *et al.* 1996	All	1.4 E-6	E	16
CO	Acute Mortality (AM)	Touloumi *et al.* 1994	All	0.00145 %	E	36

Tab. 7.13: Exposure-response slopes for human health impacts from air pollution on the respiratory system (Pilkington *et al.* 1997).
(*) The exposure response (E-R) slope is for Western Europe and is expressed in units of cases/(year-person-$\mu g/m^3$), except for mortality which is expressed as a percentage increase per $\mu g/m^3$.
E, H, I stand for egalitarians, hierarchists, and individualists, respectively, and indicate that only decision makers with the respective cultural perspective would accept the health effect as causal to the environmental pollutant mentioned (see Section 7.3.4).
(†) Since Pilkington *et al.* (1997) the concerned group was corrected to include only adults above the age of 30 years (personal communication of Joseph Spadaro, Ecole des Mines de Paris, 27 May 1998).
(#) Assumes that all days in hospital for respiratory admissions (RHA), congestive heart failure (CHF) and cerebrovascular conditions (CVA) are also restricted activity days (RAD). Also assumes that the average stay for each adult is 10, 7 and 45 days respectively. Thus, net RAD = RAD - (RHA·10) - (CHF·7) - (CVA·45).
(¶) Assumes asthma attacks (AA) are also minor restricted activity days (MRAD), and that 3.5% of the adult population (80% of the total population) are asthmatic. Thus, net MRAD = MRAD - (AA·0.8·0.035).

No disease specific baseline risk has been chosen for the mortality, but the per cent increase in deaths is reported directly and has to be related to the mortality rate of the respective area and population group. The cases of acute mortality are included in the chronic mortality and are therefore not additive.

The numbers for chronic mortality from Pope *et al.* (1995b) include the deaths due to lung cancer. However, the adjusted relative risk ratios between the most and the least polluted areas was only 1.03 for deaths from lung cancer alone, but 1.31 for cardiopulmonary deaths. The mistake we make with the use of the risk ratio for all causes is therefore relatively small. The information in the article by Pope *et al.* (1995b) unfortunately does not allow for a subtraction of cancer deaths[10].

In order to take into account the population group that is specifically affected, one has to know the share of the different groups within the entire population (Table 7.14).

[10] The final analysis in Section 7.7 will show that carcinogenic effects from particles have a negligible size of effects compared to respiratory effects. Therefore, a further separation of carcinogenic effects from the relative risk ratios would not alter the outcome.

Population group	Children	Adults	Adults 30+	Elderly 65+	Asthmatics	Asthmatic children	Adult asthmatics
Share in total population	20%	80%	57%	14%	5%	1%	4%

Table 7.14: Shares of the different population groups used in epidemiological studies
shares for children and adults from Pilkington *et al.* (1997)
value for 'Adults 30+' from Murray *et al.* (1996a)
value for asthmatics from WHO (1996a)

The exposure-response slopes for mortality are given in Table 7.13. They are listed as percentage increases compared to the background mortality, the quantities of which have still to be defined. We suggest using the average mortality rate for established market economies in 1990 that are provided in Murray *et al.* (1996a). The available data has to be corrected for the mortality due to injuries. Table 7.15 provides a comparison of this data with the Swiss and the World mortality rates. The comparison shows that the injury-corrected mortality rates are rather similar. We have chosen to use the rate of 0.84 %/a if the whole population is the baseline, and of 1.42%/a if only the adults above 30 years of age are concerned for further calculations.

	Established market economies 1990 (Murray *et al.* 1996a)		World 1990 (Murray *et al.* 1996a)	Switzerland 1994 (Stat. Jahrbuch 1996)
	adults 30+	all	all	all
Total inhabitants [millions]	459	798	5267	7.019
Total mortality [thousands/a]	6840	7121	50467	61.987
Injuries [thousands/a]	325	445	5084	4.845
Mortality without injuries [1'000/a]	6515	6675	45383	57.142
Mortality rate [%/a]	**1.42**	**0.84**	**0.86**	**0.81**

Tab. 7.15: Calculation of the injury adjusted background mortality rate for three different areas.

Additional exposure-response slopes for cardiovascular diseases are reported in Table 7.16 even though we will focus in this chapter only on respiratory effects. This information is given so as to motivate further work on other health effects.

Exposure-response slopes have a background similar to the one of the unit risk factors for carcinogenity. Unfortunately, until now, no organisation, such as WHO or U.S. EPA, has felt obliged to publish consensus lists for such exposure-response slopes for a number of pollutants[11]. The following arguments may explain this unsatisfactory situation:

- The number of epidemiological studies and their qualities have increased only recently. Establishing a new compilation needs time, however.
- The non-terminal endpoints are not yet defined sharply enough to allow for an international compilation.
- There is little experience with occupational studies and partly no support from toxicological ones.

[11] Each, of course, has its own compilation, but no generally agreed upon master list has been published so far. WHO will publish such a first list for particles including several endpoints in the course of the new European air quality guidelines. A draft of this list was published and used in IVM (1997).

Pollutant	Endpoint	Reference	Affected population group	E-R slope (*)	Cultural bias	σ_g^2
PM10	Congestive heart failure	Schwartz *et al.* 1995	>65a	1.85E-5	E, I, H	16
	Cerebrovascular hospital admissions	Wordley *et al.* 1997	all	5.04E-6	E, I, H	16
	Ischaemic heart disease	Schwartz *et al.* 1995	>65a	1.75E-5	E	16
PM2.5, Sulphates	Congestive heart failure	Schwartz *et al.* 1995	>65a	3.09E-5	E, I, H	16
	Cerebrovascular hospital admissions	Wordley *et al.* 1997	all	8.42E-6	E, I, H	16
	Ischaemic heart disease	Schwartz *et al.* 1995	>65a	2.92E-5	E	16
Nitrates	Congestive heart failure	Schwartz *et al.* 1995	>65a	1.85E-5	E, I	36
	Cerebrovascular hospital admissions	Wordley *et al.* 1997	all	5.04E-6	E, I	36
	Ischaemic heart disease	Schwartz *et al.* 1995	>65a	1.75E-5	E	36
CO	Congestive heart failure	Schwartz *et al.* 1995	>65a	5.55E-7	E, I	16
	Ischaemic heart disease	Schwartz *et al.* 1995	>65a	4.17E-7	E	16

Tab. 7.16: Exposure-response slopes for human health impacts from air pollution on the cardiovascular system (Pilkington *et al.* 1997)
(*) The exposure response (E-R) slope is for Western Europe and is expressed in units of cases/(year-person-$\mu g/m^3$), except for mortality which is expressed as a percentage increase per $\mu g/m^3$.
E, H, I stand for egalitarians, hierarchists, and individualists, respectively, and indicate that only decision makers with the respective cultural perspective would accept the health effect as causal to the environmental pollutant mentioned (see Section 7.3.4).

The first two points are arguments that speak for starting now the work on such a compilation. The third point will be addressed in more detail in the next subsection. It is certainly a good reason to introduce now a system to classify the evidence that is already known from carcinogenic chemicals (Section 6.3).

7.3.4 Evidence of causality in the light of Cultural Theory

Epidemiological studies are an excellent methodology to reveal associations between ambient air pollution and adverse health effects as has been suggested in Subsection 7.3.2. However, in LCA we are especially interested in causal relationships and not in epidemiological associations.

In this subsection additional information is given on the evidence for the assumed causal relationships that have been quantified in Table 7.13. Using the arguments of Subsection 6.3.2, this will make it possible to suggest how the different cultural perspectives might deal with the different qualities of the available evidence.

This necessarily short discussion relies partly on the arguments in the previous subsection and the information collected by Donnan *et al.* (1997). We will focus here mainly on the criteria of biological plausibility and of the quantity and the consistency of the available studies because all other criteria defining high-quality epidemiological studies are met already.

Many epidemiological studies that use PM_{10}, fine particles, black smoke, or sulphates as causal factors reveal an association between respiratory effects and the exposure to these particles. Seaton *et al.* (1995:176) suggest *"..that such ultra-fine particles are able to provoke alveolar inflammation, with release of mediators capable, in susceptible individuals, of causing exacerbations of lung disease.."*. Oberdörster (1995) confirms this hypotheses by citing test results with rats and fine

Teflon particles. Peters *et al.* (1997) confirmed in a re-analysis the association of increased plasma viscosity with air pollution. This is another element that supports the inflammation theory. Two additional hypotheses are presently being discussed in the scientific community (Brändli *et al.* 1997). The particle chemistry hypothesis refers to the composition of the particles: The oxidants, carcinogenics and iron which they contain are transported into the bronchial tree by piggy-backing on the fine particles and are deposited there on the mucous membrane and the alveolus. A last hypothesis refers to the synergistic effect of several pollutants that causes acute and chronic inflammation of the respiratory tract (e.g., bronchitis). Such effects decrease lung capacity through the resultant increase in resistance to air flows and this in turn leads to shortness of breath and aggravates the seriousness of already existing cardiopulmonary problems.

The first hypothesis of particle overload is the most attractive and believed by many, but it has not yet been proven for any of these particles in human beings. Nevertheless, the large number of supportive epidemiological studies and the existence of a concrete hypothesis for the toxicological mechanisms involved suggests that the evidence for the association of fine particles and respiratory effects should be taken rather seriously.

Not many studies exist that identify an association between nitrates and health effects even though nitrates are a very relevant share of the particle mass, especially in Europe[12]. If the first hypothesis presented above turns out to be true after all, then the nitrates in fine particles contribute equally together with the other particles and the sulphates to health effects. In contrast, nitrates would play a limited role if any one of the other two hypotheses is confirmed. The evidence for a causal relationship between nitrates and respiratory effects is therefore clearly smaller than for other particles.

The link between ozone and respiratory effects is not only supported by a large number of epidemiological studies, but also by human chamber experiments and by animal tests. In addition, the epidemiological studies of acute effects can profit from summer smog episodes with their characteristically large increases in concentration and where the change in effects is less affected by other pollutants. Therefore, the evidence for health effects due to ozone is of a high quality.

The link between the number of emergency room visits (ERV) for COPD, asthma, and croup due to all kind of particles (ERV for asthma is also caused by ozone) is based on different and many non-European sources. Pilkington *et al.* (1997) suggest using this data only for sensitivity analysis due to the contamination of it by different health systems. They think that the data is of low quality because of the lack of high quality studies that are representative for Europe.

The association of SO_2 with health effects is supported by many epidemiological studies. However, SO_2 may act as a surrogate for sulphates and it is therefore not fully clear whether SO_2 alone can cause adverse effects as well. Pilkington *et al.*

[12] The composition of particles depends on the availability of precursors. In Europe a lot has been done already to reduce the emission of dust from power plants and heating systems. Emissions of sulphur dioxide have already been decreasing for more than 10 years, but the emissions of NO_x and of ammonia, the precursors for nitrates, are not yet under control, mainly due to increasing road traffic and the practice of high density breeding of animals in agriculture.

(1997) refer to the APHEA studies where the size of the apparent SO_2-effect was independent from the background concentrations of ambient particles. Therefore, there is limited evidence available for this link.

Only a small number of good epidemiological studies consider CO and show a positive association with health risks. The epidemiological evidence for it therefore has be rated low. The toxicological mechanisms are only known to work at much higher concentrations than are normally encountered.

Last but not least, a positive association between NO_2 and health effects has been found in many epidemiological studies. However, NO_x is understood to be a surrogate for many other substances and particles, especially those emitted by traffic. The causal evidence is therefore low. One may argue that additional effects correlated with NO_2 should be included in the analysis in order to have a proxy for the many other substances for which no impact pathway analysis has been performed so far.

The degree of evidence needed to trigger precautionary actions is a question epidemiologists are discussing as well (Botti *et al.* 1996). Some of them demand that the burden of proof should now be reversed so that one has to prove that air pollution does not cause health effects. Others claim that today's ambient concentrations are too low to have any noticeable effects, or that - a more fatalistic view - pollution standards that would ensure no risk to the entire population would have to be set at an unrealistic level since measurable effects in a sensitive subgroup of the population are always to be expected, even for low levels of pollution (Botti *et al.* 1996). This short review of current arguments and the discussion in Subsection 6.3.2 suggest that causality is a subjective metric influenced largely by the world view of the decision maker.

We suggest relying on the classification of views introduced in Chapter 3 and applied so far in all steps where world view dependency has been identified. The classification in Table 6.12 suggests that individualists accept only causal relationships that are supported with highest degree of evidence while egalitarians defer much more to the precautionary principle and accept also weak evidence for causality. Hierarchists stand somewhere in between.

Tables 7.13 and 7.16 indicate in the column 'Cultural bias' those cultural perspectives that may be thought of as accepting the causality of the relationship as given. Only egalitarians consider as evident all the listed exposure-response slopes. Individualists, however, consider that causality is only proven for fine particles, sulphates, and ozone and disregard the effects revealed by emergency room visits due to the limited transferability of the findings to European conditions.

7.3.5 Emission-response relationships for respiratory effects due to air pollutants

Table 7.13 so far lists only slopes of the exposure-response function (E-R slope). Two additional steps are necessary before one is able to quantify the respiratory diseases per kg of the emitted pollutant: The effect factor *Eim(c)* has to be determined first and, secondly, the fate and effect factors have to be combined into the respiratory disease factor (*Rim(c)*).

The effect factor *Eim(c)* for substance *i*, endpoint *m*, and cultural perspective *c* can easily be calculated by multiplying the E-R slope with the number of people exposed per area (Equation 7.10). The average European population density[13] amounts to 80 persons per km^2. The composition of the population has been listed in Table 7.14 and is used here to correct for the fact that for some endpoints or slopes only certain risk groups are concerned.

$$Eim(c) = S \cdot \rho \cdot E\text{-}R\ slope\ im(c) \qquad [cases/(a \cdot m^2 \cdot \mu g/m^3)] \qquad (7.10)$$

where ρ — population density = 8 E-5 [persons/m^2]
E-R slope im(c) — exposure-response slope of substance *i* and endpoint *m* for the cultural perspective *c* [cases/(a·person·$\mu g/m^3$)]
S — share of population concerned [-]

Equation (7.10) and its dimension are valid only for the E-R slopes for morbidity. The slopes for mortality need to be multiplied in addition with the baseline mortality (Table 7.15).

Making use of Equation (7.2) it is possible to calculate the respiratory disease factor *Rim(c)* for substance *i*, endpoint *m* and cultural perspective *c*. The result has to be multiplied by 10^9 in order to get results per kg and not per μg of the emitted substance.

$$Rim(c) = Fi \cdot Eim(c) \cdot 10^9 = Fi \cdot S \cdot \rho \cdot E\text{-}R\ slope\ im(c) \cdot 10^9 \quad [cases/kg] \qquad (7.11)$$

Equation (7.11) can be used to calculate for the three cultural perspectives – the egalitarians, hierarchists and individualists – the respiratory effects that are characterised by the 15 endpoints mentioned in Table 7.13 for the about 120 substances listed in Appendix (7.1). These simple multiplication result in a large amount of numbers due to all the combinations possible. It is possible to later present more manageable aggregated results by using the aggregation rule for the different endpoints that will be defined in Section 7.4. However, the information that is necessary at this stage to calculate, e.g., the number of symptom days due to the emission of 1 kg hexane under European conditions, is now all available[14].

---

[13] This population density is not just the terrestrial density for a selection of highly populated European countries. One has to take into account the fact that the fate factor for particles includes exposure above sea and in the less populated East European countries. The fate factors for the other substances are based on the ECOSENSE model (area = 11.61 E12 m^2) and the EMEP model (adapted area = 10.8 E12 m^2). Use of the detailed maps of the models and of present population data (UNESCO 1996) suggests as the best estimate 80 persons per km^2 for the average population density. This density corrects for the fact that pollutants emitted in Europe spread out over the sea and the less populated areas outside Western Europe.

[14] The fate factor can be found in Appendix (7.1) and amounts to 1.2 E-6 $m^2a/m3$ with a squared standard deviation of factor 5 (lognormal distribution). The E-R slope can be taken from Table 7.13 for

7.3.6 Summary

This section provided the discussion of and the data for exposure-response slopes for pollutants that contribute to respiratory effects in human beings. The following limitations and assumptions have to be kept in mind when the exposure-response relationships are used to build up the damage functions:

- The approach used is based on epidemiological studies, i.e., substances found to cause respiratory effects in toxicological tests only have been excluded and the toxicological mechanisms of substances showing associations between exposure and respiratory effects are sometimes not yet fully understood.
- There is no authoritative organisation which evaluates the epidemiological studies that are available and that could suggest best guesses as done for unit risk factors (Section 6.3). The exposure-response slopes that have been chosen have been selected by English health experts as the basis for European externality studies (Pilkington *et al.* 1997, Donnan *et al.* 1997). The missing authoritative voice is thus partly compensated for by taking into account the very similar purpose for which the externality studies have collected them in the first place.
- The epidemiological studies on the relation between air pollution and respiratory effects that are available reveal large differences in the strength of the relationships. They offer therefore a good deal of room for subjective judgement through the selection of only a subpart of the available studies for further consideration.
- The selection of the slopes presented in Table 7.13 has a Western European bias and tends to favour average values for average conditions.
- The selection of the health endpoints that have been reviewed is biased towards economically valuable effects (but which is not a prerequisite for the use of the DALYs' approach) and tries to prevent double counting of health outcomes.
- The epidemiological studies show that on the societal level no thresholds can be defined, i.e., that there are individuals sensitive enough to show effects even at the very low concentrations prevalent in rural areas. This observation holds true for all the causal factors that have been evaluated, i.e., for particles (including sulphates and nitrates), ozone, SO_2, CO, and NO_2.

The quantitative information that is relevant here is contained in Table 7.13 and the calculation procedures used are represented by Equations (7.10) and (7.11).

---

symptom days due to ozone exposure and has a value of 0.033 cases/(a-person $\mu g/m^3$) with a squared standard deviation of factor 6 (lognormal distribution). The population density in Europe is 8 E-5 persons/m^2. The share of the population concerned is S = 1, i.e., all the people are potentially concerned. Using Equation (7.11) results in the respiratory disease factor of 3.2 E-3 symptom days per kg hexane emission. All three cultural perspectives consider this factor as relevant. The squared standard deviation can be calculated with Equation (A6.3) of Appendix (6.8) if it is assumed that the multiplied lognormal distributions are independent. In this example the calculation results in the factor $\sigma_g^2 = 11$.

7.4 Years of Life Lost (YLL) and Years Lived Disabled (YLD)

7.4.1 Introduction

The data and the information presented so far make it possible to calculate the respiratory disease factors *Rim(c)*. The next step is to determine the consequences from these respiratory effects for human health and well-being in terms of Years Lived Disabled (YLD) and Years of Life Lost (YLL).

To that purpose, we ask questions such as how long a disability will persist, how serious one judges the disability to be, or how many years are lost through premature death due to respiratory effects for each of the 15 health endpoints considered in Table 7.13. These questions will be addressed in Subsection 7.4.2 for endpoints leading to disability and in Subsection 7.4.3 for mortality endpoints.

The results will be summarised in the last Subsection, 7.4.4, where the uncertainty involved is also discussed. It is important to mention here that this section is based on a small database and may be substantially improved by additional input from health experts.

7.4.2 Disability weights and Years Lived Disabled

The 13 respiratory effects quantified in Section 7.3 which lead to years lived disabled are listed in Table 7.17. The task of this subsection is to estimate the time during which these effects persist, the degree of disability caused by these effects, and to calculate finally from that the *YLD*. The disability weights are based on Murray *et al.* (1996a) and some of the relevant data has already been provided in Table 5.9. However, there are no disability weights available for many of these effects which therefore have to be gained through interpolation.

It is assumed that bronchodilator usage, asthma attacks, cough, wheeze, and symptom days have a duration of one day. For some endpoints like cough, wheeze, and symptom days this assumption is supported by the findings of the underlying epidemiological studies. For asthma attacks, it is not clear whether the consequences of the attack last for more than one day or not.

The disability weights are taken from Murray *et al.* (1996a) and are listed in Table 5.9. However, the endpoints are not identical. The weights are therefore estimated here in order to be able to demonstrate the fruitfulness of the approach. In principle, it is necessary to determine the weights with the help of a panel made up of health experts.

We assume that both bronchodilator usage and asthma attacks are equally serious. The disability weight of 0.061 suggested by Murray *et al.* (1996a) concerns cases of asthma, not the asthma attacks we are interested in here. We estimate that the correct disability weight is 0.1 for both endpoints by comparing them with the seriousness of other diseases.

Cough, wheeze and symptom days are considered to be comparable with asthma cases and the disability weight is set equal to 0.05.

Chronic bronchitis is quantified here as incidence rate whereas other studies use data on prevalence (GVF 1996). Donnan *et al.* (1997) mention that chronic bronchitis in adults will last for about 40 years when considering a time lag between exposure and effect. In addition, they note that, in children, chronic bronchitis is best understood as an episodic event although they do not indicate the average duration for such episodes. ESEERCO (1995), for instance, assume for the same endpoint the duration of a full year, but tax the illness as not very serious. We fix the duration at six month because bronchitis is called 'chronic' after a minimum duration of 3 months and because it is assumed that the onset of summer helps cure the illness. Murray *et al.* (1996a) suggested a disability weight of 0.392 for obstructive pulmonary disease (COPD). This is a very heavy weight, indicating that most activities are restricted. Even Parkinson's disease is considered less debilitating than that. But it does not seem reasonable to assume that a person with chronic bronchitis suffers such a serious disability during 40 years. It is, for instance, assumed in GVF(1996) that from 22'000 cases of chronic bronchitis due to emissions from traffic, only 10 cases each year will become invalidating. In addition, it can be assumed that the illness starts with a slight cough and will lead to more serious effects only decades later. It is therefore assumed here that an average disability weight of only 0.05 for the whole period of 40 years is fully appropriate. This assumes that the patients have periods when their illness has relatively little consequences and that only a few of them will suffer for shorter periods with consequences for whom the high disability weight appropriate for COPD would be justified.

For chronic cough, the same duration as for chronic bronchitis in children is assumed for the time being and a disability weight of 0.05 will be used.

A restricted activity day (RAD) is defined as a day during which a study subject has been forced to alter his/her normal activity (Donnan *et al.* 1997). For adults RADs include work loss days and for children days away from school. More severely restricted days are those when it is necessary to stay in bed. Minor restricted activity days (MRAD) involve neither work loss nor bed disability. These types of endpoints are not very frequently used in health statistics, but are perfect for economic valuations. We apply a disability weight of 0.05 for MRADs and of 0.1 for RADs in the absence of more precise information on the relevant health states.

Respiratory hospital admissions have an average duration of 10 days (Donnan *et al.* 1997). In the absence of any detailed knowledge about the precise cause for admission, we assume a chronic obstructive pulmonary disease (COPD) as cause with a disability weight of 0.392 (Table 5.9).

Emergency room visits are only very short stays, but may cause disability lasting several days. Lacking detailed data, we assume here a disability during 3 days for COPD, asthma, and croup. The disability weight already chosen for asthma attacks was taken for all three endpoints.

		Duration Lm	Duration Lm	Disability weight Dm	YLD (0,1)	YLD (0,0)	σ_g^2
		days	years	-	years	years	-
Bronchodilator usage		1	0.0027	0.1		2.7E-04	2
	adults				3.3E-04		2
	children				2.5E-04		2
Asthma attacks (AA)		1	0.0027	0.1	3.1E-04	2.7E-04	2
Cough		1	0.0027	0.05		1.4E-04	2
	adults				1.7E-04		2
	children				1.3E-04		2
Lower respiratory symptoms		1	0.0027	0.05		1.4E-04	2
(wheeze)	adults				1.7E-04		2
	children				1.3E-04		2
Symptom days		1	0.0027	0.05	1.6E-04	1.4E-04	2
Chronic bronchitis	adults		40	0.05	1.8E+00	2E+00	3
	children		0.5	0.05	2.4E-02	2.5E-02	3
Chronic cough	children		0.5	0.05	2.4E-02	2.5E-02	3
Minor restricted activity day (MRAD)		1	0.0027	0.05	1.1E-04	1.4E-04	2
Restricted activity days (RAD)		1	0.0027	0.1	2.2E-04	2.7E-04	2
Respiratory hospital admissions		10	0.0274	0.392	8.6E-03	1.1E-02	2
ERV for COPD		3	0.0082	0.1	6.5E-04	8.2E-04	3
ERV for asthma		3	0.0082	0.1	9.5E-04	8.2E-04	3
ERV for croup in pre-school children		3	0.0082	0.1	7.7E-04	8.2E-04	3

Tab. 7.17: Rough estimates for the duration of disability and the disability weight during that time. The Years Lived Disabled (YLD(0,0)) are calculated by multiplying of *Lm* with *Dm*. There is no discounting and no age-weighting. But for YLD(0,1) an age-weighting according to Equation (5.7) has been applied.

We can work with Equation (5.7) for the calculation of *YLD* with age-weighting. The duration of the disability *Lm* and the disability weight *Dm* are both known. What we miss is the age at the onset of the disability. What we need is an age-distribution for each of the health effects due to the fact that we are not looking at one patient alone but at the whole society. Murray *et al.* (1996b:670ff) provide such age-distributions for the prevalence of COPD and asthma. We assume the same age-distribution as reported for COPD for the health effects MRAD, RAD, respiratory hospital admissions, and ERV for COPD, i.e., these are all effects which typically occur in the older part of the population. Asthma attacks, symptom days, and ERV for asthma are grouped together and described by the age-distribution of the prevalence of asthma. Two additional age-distributions have been created for the asthmatics by separating them into children and adults. The following health effects were subsumed in the children's group of asthmatics: chronic cough, chronic bronchitis, ERV for croup, bronchodilator usage, cough, and wheeze. For the group of adults we have included cough, wheeze, chronic bronchitis, and bronchodilator usage. These assumptions on the age-distributions make it possible to calculate YLD(0,1) that are representative for the established market economies.

The resulting YLD(0,1) are close to the YLD(0,0) because the age-weighting factor falls below 50% only after the age of 80 (see Figure 5.4) and because the age-distribution for asthmatics is spread over all the age-groups. The factor for children alone is smaller than for adults alone due to a very low age-weighting for young children below 5 years of age.

7.4.3 Years of Life Lost

The two health endpoints from Table 7.13 that have remained undiscussed so far are acute and chronic mortality. One has to differentiate between them because they have a different morbidity history. Acute mortality occurs predominantly in older people that almost certainly already suffer from serious ill health. The precise mechanism of action has not (yet) been established (ExternE 1995). Chronic mortality, on the other hand, is due to different mode of actions such as COPD, including chronic bronchitis, and it does not need a non-respiratory illness as a precondition for its onset. People belonging to this group generally die at higher ages than those succumbing to acute mortality.

We found the following estimates for years of life lost in the literature:

- ExternE (1995) finds, for acute mortality, that the death distribution is strongly skewed to the right with a median of weeks or of a few months at most and a mean of about 12 months. The years of life lost through chronic mortality are estimated somewhat arbitrarily to be equal to 12.5 years.
- GVF (1996) consider total mortality only which they find to be dominated by chronic mortality. GVF (1996) assume that people dying from chronic mortality lose the number of years that correspond to the standard life expectancy of their age-class. Lacking more detailed data, they assume that the age-distribution of respiratory mortality is similar to the age-distribution of all deaths. With these assumptions and Swiss data, they calculate a loss of 12.7 potential life years per death. They acknowledge that the standard life expectancy table would be different if mortality due to respiratory effects would have been excluded. However, the difference is thought to be smaller than 0.5 years and is therefore neglected.
- Rabl *et al.* (1997a) cite Hurley *et al.* (1997) who have an estimate for YLL for acute mortality. Both sources assume a median for YLL of 2.5 months with a geometric standard deviation of 5. The calculated mean of this distribution comes to about 9 months and is accepted as a working hypothesis.
- Rabl (1997) estimates the median for acute mortality to be 64 days with a squared geometric standard deviation of 4. The arithmetic mean for acute mortality is therefore derived to be 0.5 years. The years of life lost due to chronic mortality were calculated by the direct use of the relative risk derived in the epidemiological study. The resulting amount of 21.9 ECU/year per person and per $\mu g/m^3$ PM_{10} can be retransformed to years of life lost with the information that one year lost is valuated with 84'000 ECU and by applying the E-R slope based on Pope *et al.* (1995b) given in Table 7.13/15. The result of this recalculation is an average of 8 years of life lost per premature death due to long-term PM_{10} exposure.
- Metroeconomica *et al.* (1996:synthesis report p.35) report a best estimate for YLL for acute mortality of 15 months with a likely range from 1 month to 3 years. Their best estimate for chronic mortality is 3 years with a range from 1 to 6 years.

Epidemiological studies unfortunately do not provide detailed data on the age-distribution of the deaths and detailed information on the combination of illnesses is not given either. We chose the mortality statistics from WHO (1995b) as the basis for a recalculation of the YLL and selected, for this purpose, the deaths due to respiratory diseases (ICD-9 310-329). This age-distribution is now specifically valid for respiratory effects. We choose the data for the United States of America because there are the large number of almost 200'000 cases listed for the year 1990. The required standard life expectancy for each age-group has already been listed in Table 5.7 for the case without age-weighting and in Table 5.12 for the one with age-weighting. These calculations yield a YLL(0,0) of 13.2 years for the former and a YLL(0,1) of 8.4 years for the latter. The large influence of the age-weighting is due to the large number of deaths occurring at ages above 75.

The choice of a working hypothesis for this study has a certain arbitrariness to it given the lack of more reliable data. For YLL, due to acute mortality, we chose the value suggested by Hurley *et al.* (1997). The squared standard deviation takes into account the fact that the uncertainty is extremely large at the individual level, but less so at the societal one. We think that for chronic mortality, both our own calculations and the numbers in GVF (1996) and ExternE (1995) are too high because the coexistence of other illnesses has been neglected. Somewhat arbitrarily, we chose as best estimate 50% of the value produced by our own calculation. It is assumed that for both acute and chronic mortality, the relation between YLL(0,0) and YLL(0,1) is the same as the one produced by our own calculations. The data chosen is presented in Table 7.18.

	YLL(0,0)	**YLL(0,1)**	σ_g^2
	years	years	-
Acute mortality	0.75	0.48	5
Chronic mortality	6.6	4.2	3

Tab. 7.18: Working hypothesis for Years Life Lost (YLL) due to acute and chronic mortality due to air pollution with squared geometric standard deviation for an assumed lognormal distribution. YLL(0,0) stands for a calculation without discounting and no age-weighting, YLL(0,1) is based on an age-weighting (Section 5.4).

7.4.4 Results and uncertainty

The YLDs and YLLs per case given in Tables 7.17 and 7.18 make it possible to calculate aggregated health effects due to the exposure to any one of the substances listed in Table 7.13. We aggregate for presentation purposes the YLDs and YLLs with:

$$DALYs = YLDs + YLLs \qquad [a] \qquad (7.12)$$

The basic data needed for the subsequent calculations is listed in Appendix (7.2). It encompasses the shares of the population affected by an effect (Table 7.14), the baseline mortality rate (Table 7.15) relevant for the determination of mortality endpoints, the exposure-response slopes (Table 7.13) including the estimate of their standard deviations, and the YLDs and YLLs per case including their standard deviations (Tables 7.17/18).

The results of these calculations are listed in Appendix (7.3) and include the DALYs per person-year and $\mu g/m^3$. The lower and upper estimates for the 95% confidence interval are listed as well in order to indicate the uncertainty behind these results. This interval was calculated for each endpoint by applying Equation (A6.3) in

Appendix (6.8), using the geometric standard deviations for the E-R-slopes and the DALYs for each case.

These intermediate results lend themselves well for a first discussion. The relevant results from Appendix (7.3) are summarised in Table 7.19.

- No differentiation between different cultural perspectives has to be made for PM_{10}, $PM_{2.5}$, sulphates, and ozone. The endpoints for which there is limited evidence turned out to be negligible anyway. SO_2 and nitrates have the same DALYs for both egalitarians and hierarchists; individualists do not consider them to be a causal factor anyway. NO_2 and CO are only included in an impact assessment if it is carried out with an egalitarian bias. Neither hierarchists nor individualists believe that these two pollutants have an impact on the respiratory system.
- Maximally, three endpoints for each pollutant are relevant for the aggregated DALYs. In the case of primary and secondary particles, chronic mortality and chronic bronchitis in adults contribute about 60% and 30%, respectively, to the total DALYs (best estimate). For SO_2, NO_x, and CO, the contribution of acute mortality is dominant by far. Only for ozone do the symptom days dominate the best estimate; acute mortality and asthma attacks come next. One can therefore conclude that a re-analysis of the epidemiological studies and an assessment of the health damages due to endpoints should concentrate on these five endpoints.
- The share of the different endpoints varies between the low, best, and high estimates because the standard deviation is different for each endpoint. This explains, for instance, that the symptom days due to exposure to ozone dominate the DALYs in the lower, but not in the upper, estimate.

This assessment of the results suggests that we use those results that are printed in bold in Table 7.18 for the next step in the calculation. This will facilitate the presentation of results in the next section.

Some concluding remarks should be made with respect to the uncertainty in the step of damage assessment. The assumptions in this step added uncertainty because:

- rough assumptions had to be made concerning the duration of morbidity episodes
- preliminary values for the disability weights instead of weights determined by health experts had to be used, and
- poor data for life years lost due to premature death caused by respiratory effects had to be used.

However, the main influencing factor on the DALYs uncertainty distribution is the large uncertainty in the value of the E-R-slopes as expressed in their very high squared geometric standard deviations (Table 7.13). This means that the uncertainty introduced in this section is large, but then disappears because we assume independence between the E-R-slopes and the DALYs for each case. Nevertheless, it is advisable that improvements in the preliminary DALYs per case are achieved in the future through the involvement of health experts. This requires a comparably small effort for the removal of one of the weak elements in the impact pathway analysis.

Finally, one should note that the distribution that results from the addition of all endpoints affected by the same air pollutant is no more lognormal. But one can still assume that the distributions can be approximated by lognormal distributions because only a few of the endpoints are dominant and we have only assumed the distributions, but not derived them. The squared geometric standard deviations are estimated on the basis of the resultant lower and upper values of the aggregated DALYs per pollutant, both of which are listed in Table 7.19.

Endpoint		$\Sigma\sigma g^2$	DALYs(0,1) low	DALYs(0,1) best estim.	DALYs(0,1) high	DALYs(0,0) low	DALYs(0,0) best estim.	DALYs(0,0) high
Chronic bronchitis		8.2	8.6E-6	7.1E-5	5.8E-4	9.6E-6	7.8E-5	6.4E-4
Chronic Mortality (CM)		19.7	6.7E-6	1.3E-4	2.6E-3	1.0E-5	2.1E-4	4.1E-3
Total PM10	**E, H, I**	**15.0**	**1.7E-5**	**2.3E-4**	**3.6E-3**	**2.2E-5**	**3.1E-4**	**5.2E-3**
Chronic bronchitis		8.2	1.4E-5	1.1E-4	9.2E-4	1.5E-5	1.2E-4	1.0E-3
Chronic Mortality (CM)		19.7	1.1E-5	2.2E-4	4.3E-3	1.7E-5	3.4E-4	6.8E-3
Total PM2.5/ Sulphates	**E, H, I**	**15.0**	**2.7E-5**	**3.8E-4**	**6.0E-3**	**3.5E-5**	**5.1E-4**	**8.6E-3**
Chronic bronchitis		19.7	3.6E-6	7.1E-5	1.4E-3	4.0E-6	7.8E-5	1.5E-3
Chronic Mortality (CM)		42.4	3.1E-6	1.3E-4	5.6E-3	4.9E-6	2.1E-4	8.8E-3
Total Nitrates	**E, H**	**34.0**	**7.4E-6**	**2.3E-4**	**8.0E-3**	**9.6E-6**	**3.1E-4**	**1.1E-2**
Asthma attacks (AA)		38.5	3.5E-8	1.3E-6	5.1E-5	3.0E-8	1.2E-6	4.5E-5
Symptom days		6.8	7.7E-7	5.3E-6	3.6E-5	6.8E-7	4.6E-6	3.2E-5
Acute Mortality (AM)		24.7	9.6E-8	2.4E-6	5.9E-5	1.5E-7	3.7E-6	9.2E-5
Total Ozone	**E, H, I**	**15**	**9.6E-7**	**9.9E-6**	**1.6E-4**	**9.3E-7**	**1.1E-5**	**1.9E-4**
Acute Mortality (AM)		24.7	1.2E-7	2.9E-6	7.2E-5	1.8E-7	4.5E-6	1.1E-4
Total SO2	**E, H**	**24.7**	**1.2E-7**	**2.9E-6**	**7.2E-5**	**1.9E-7**	**4.6E-6**	**1.1E-4**
Acute Mortality (AM)		50.8	2.7E-8	1.4E-6	7.0E-5	4.2E-8	2.1E-6	1.1E-4
Total NOx	**E**	**50.8**	**2.8E-8**	**1.4E-6**	**7.0E-5**	**4.3E-8**	**2.2E-6**	**1.1E-4**
Acute Mortality (AM)		50.8	1.2E-9	5.8E-8	3.0E-6	1.8E-9	9.1E-8	4.6E-6
Total CO	**E**	**50.8**	**1.2E-9**	**5.8E-8**	**3.0E-6**	**1.8E-9**	**9.1E-8**	**4.6E-6**

Tab. 7.19: Low, best, and high estimates for DALYs per (a·person·$\mu g/m^3$). $\Sigma\sigma g^2$ for the aggregated (bold) numbers per pollutant are estimated based on the low and high estimates approximating the distribution with a lognormal one. The low and high estimates span a 95% confidence interval for each endpoint. The background data used here is listed in Appendices (7.2) and (7.3).

7.5 Results for the full damage functions

7.5.1 Introduction

With the information provided so far it is possible to calculate the damage factors, i.e., the health damages in terms of disability adjusted life years (DALYs) per kg primary emission. The necessary algebraic relationships are presented in Subsection 7.5.2.

The final results are discussed in Subsection 7.5.3 and listed in Appendix (7.4). The discussion is continued in Subsection 7.5.4 with the review of a number of different studies and the transformation of their results to make them comparable with our own and thus validate them. Extrapolating the results to Europe will give an estimate of health impacts from air pollution calculated by this bottom-up approach. In the final paragraph, we will discuss the elements that contribute most to the sensitivity of the results in this and the other evaluated studies.

7.5.2 The mathematical construction of the damage function

The basis for the mathematical construction has already been laid with Equation (7.3):

$$\frac{DALYs_i(c)}{I_i} = \sum_m \{R_{im}(c) \cdot (YLL_m(c) + YLD_m(c))\}$$

$$= \sum_m \{F_i \cdot E_{im}(c) \cdot (YLL_m(c) + YLD_m(c))\} \quad [a/kg] \qquad (7.3)$$

where			
	$DALYs$	Disability Adjusted Live Years	[a]
	I	emission, environmental intervention	[kg]
	R	respiratory disease factor	[cases/kg]
	YLL	Years Life Lost	[a/case]
	YLD	Years Lived Disabled	[a/case]
	F	fate factor for exposure by air	$[\frac{m^2 \cdot a}{m^3}]$
	E	effect factor	$[\frac{cases}{\mu g} \cdot \frac{m^3}{m^2\ a}]$
	i	pollutant causing respiratory effects	
	m	endpoint	
	c	cultural bias	

Equation (7.3) can be reformulated slightly for practical reasons by inserting for $E_{im}(c)$ the relation presented in Equation (7.10) and by aggregating *YLL* and *YLD* to *DALYs* according to Equation (7.12):

$$\frac{DALYs_i(c)}{I_i} = \sum_m \{Fi \cdot Eim(c) \cdot (YLLm(c) + YLDm(c))\}$$

$$= Fi \cdot \sum_m \{Eim(c) \cdot (YLLm(c) + YLDm(c))\}$$

$$= Fi \cdot \sum_m \{10^9 \cdot S \cdot \rho \cdot E\text{-}R \text{ slope } im(c) \cdot DALYm(c)\}$$

$$= Fi \cdot 10^9 \cdot \rho \cdot \sum_m \{S \cdot E\text{-}R \text{ slope } im(c) \cdot DALYm(c)\} \quad (7.13)$$

Equation (7.13) now reflects the structure already introduced in Subsection 7.4.4. The expression in the brackets aggregated over all endpoints has already been calculated and displayed in Table 7.19. The population density ρ is the one estimated for Europe and is set equal to 8 E-5 persons per m^2. The factor 10^9 compensates for the fact that the damage is in the end assessed per kg and not per µg. The fate factor *Fi* is reported for more than 120 substances in Appendix (7.1).

The details concerning the individual parameters, their definitions and derivations, can be found in the Sections 7.1 to 7.4 and 5.4.

7.5.3 The damage factors

The results of the calculations according to Equation (7.13) and the already mentioned sources for the input parameters are presented and discussed here. Appendix (7.4) lists all the results for each primary pollutant, a list of damage factors for over 120 substances that are emitted to air.

The results for the individualist's perspective are presented in Table 7.20a. The evidence for exposure to SO_2, NO_2, and CO is considered as insufficient by this perspective and exposure to these substances is not thought to harm human health by respiratory effects (Table 7.13, Subsection 7.3.4). There are therefore no DALYs listed for these substances in Table 7.20a. However, it is accepted that emissions of SO_x and of NO_x contribute to the formation of sulphates and of ozone, respectively. Both substances are therefore considered to contribute as causal agents to respiratory diseases.

Primary Pollutant	Secondary Pollutant	$\Pi\sigma_g^2$	DALYs(0,1) low	DALYs(0,1) best estimate	DALYs(0,1) high
		-	a/kg	a/kg	a/kg
TSP	PM_{10}	19	4.3E-6	8.0E-5	1.5E-3
PM_{10}	PM_{10}	19	1.5E-5	2.7E-4	5.1E-3
$PM_{2.5}$	$PM_{2.5}$	19	2.7E-5	5.1E-4	9.5E-3
SO_x (as SO_2)	Sulphates	16	2.4E-6	3.9E-5	6.4E-4
NH_3	Sulphates	16	3.1E-6	5.1E-5	8.3E-4
NO_x (as NO_2)	O_3	21	5.7E-8	1.2E-6	2.5E-5
NMVOC	O_3	23	5.1E-8	1.2E-6	2.8E-5

Tab. 7.20a: Damage factors due to respiratory effects for the individualist's perspective including age-weighting per kg pollutant emission to air under European conditions. The lower and upper values for DALYs span a confidence interval of 95% with an assumed lognormal distribution. $\Pi\sigma_g^2$ indicates the geometric standard deviation over all steps of the impact pathway.

As suggested in Section 5.4, it is assumed that individualists weight the importance of one year life lost differently depending on the age at which death occurs, i.e., an age-weighting is applied. It has been pointed out in Subsection 1.2.6 that LCA *sensu stricto* does not differentiate between different time dimensions. The correct treatment of time preferences within this type of LCA is therefore to avoid discounting (=> DALYs(0,1)).

Primary Pollutant	Secondary Pollutant	$\Pi\sigma g^2$	DALYs(0,0) low	DALYs(0,0) best estimate	DALYs(0,0) high
		-	a/kg	a/kg	a/kg
TSP	PM_{10}	19	5.9E-6	1.1E-4	2.0E-3
PM_{10}	PM_{10}	19	2.0E-5	3.7E-4	7.0E-3
$PM_{2.5}$	$PM_{2.5}$	19	3.8E-5	7.0E-4	1.3E-2
SO_x (as SO_2)	SO_2	27	4.1E-8	1.1E-6	2.9E-5
SO_x (as SO_2)	Sulphates	16	3.3E-6	5.4E-5	8.8E-4
SO_x (as SO_2)	*SO_2 + Sulphates*	*16.5*	*3.3E-6*	*5.5E-5*	*9.1E-4*
NH_3	Sulphates	16	4.3E-6	7.0E-5	1.1E-3
NH_3	Nitrates	36	4.1E-7	1.5E-5	5.5E-4
NH_3	*Sulphates + Nitrates*	*19*	*4.7E-6*	*8.5E-5*	*1.7E-3*
NO_x (as NO_2)	Nitrates	36	2.4E-6	8.7E-5	3.2E-3
NO_x (as NO_2)	O_3	21	6.1E-8	1.3E-6	2.7E-5
NO_x (as NO_2)	*NO_2 + O_3 + Nitrates*	*36*	*2.5E-6*	*8.9E-5*	*3.2E-3*
NMVOC	O_3	23	5.5E-8	1.3E-6	3.0E-5

Tab. 7.20b: Damage factors due to respiratory effects for the hierarchist's perspective without age-weighting per kg pollutant emission to air under European conditions. The lower and upper values for DALYs span a confidence interval of 95% with an assumed lognormal distribution. $\Pi\sigma g^2$ indicates the geometric standard deviation over all steps of the impact pathway. The numbers in *italic* are the sum per primary pollutant if more than one secondary pollutant causes respiratory effects.

Hierarchists think that there is insufficient evidence that exposure to CO and NO_2 will cause respiratory effects. They therefore disregard these damage factors (Table 7.20b). But NO_x emissions contribute to the formation of nitrates and of ozone and thereby lead to respiratory diseases. These emissions are therefore included in the damage assessment. There is no need for age-weighting and for discounting (given the type of LCA performed) according to the world view of hierarchists (=> DALYs(0,0)).

Egalitarians consider all the calculated damage factors to be causal. They apply neither age-weighting nor discounting (DALYs(0,0)). The corresponding results are listed in Table 7.20c and presented in Figure 7.2.

The highest damage factors can be attributed to the different classes of particles, $PM_{2.5}$, PM_{10}, and TSP (Figure 7.2). A second group with somewhat lower factors is made up of SO_2, ammonia, and NO_x. A look at Table 7.20c reveals that almost 100% of their damage is due to the secondary particles of sulphate and nitrate formed from them. The direct effects of the primary pollutants and the effect of secondary ozone are very small. The damage factors for CO and NMVOC are lower by about two orders of magnitude than those for the other pollutants. This means that they will only acquire a dominant influence on the damage to human health by respiratory effects if they are emitted in an amount that is more than 100 times higher than the one of particles, SO_x, NH_3, or NO_x .

Primary Pollutant	Secondary Pollutant	$\Pi\sigma_g^2$	DALYs(0,0) low	DALYs(0,0) best estimate	DALYs(0,0) high
		-	a/kg	a/kg	a/kg
CO	CO	64	1.1E-8	7.3E-7	4.7E-5
TSP	PM_{10}	19	5.9E-6	1.1E-4	2.0E-3
PM_{10}	PM_{10}	19	2.0E-5	3.7E-4	7.0E-3
$PM_{2.5}$	$PM_{2.5}$	19	3.8E-5	7.0E-4	1.3E-2
SO_x (as SO_2)	SO_2	27	4.1E-8	1.1E-6	2.9E-5
SO_x (as SO_2)	Sulphates	16	3.3E-6	5.4E-5	8.8E-4
SO_x (as SO_2)	*SO_2 + Sulphates*	*16.5*	*3.3E-6*	*5.5E-5*	*9.1E-4*
NH_3	Sulphates	16	4.3E-6	7.0E-5	1.1E-3
NH_3	Nitrates	36	4.1E-7	1.5E-5	5.5E-4
NH_3	*Sulphates + Nitrates*	*19*	*4.7E-6*	*8.5E-5*	*1.7E-3*
NO_x (as NO_2)	NO_2	54	8.0E-9	4.3E-7	2.3E-5
NO_x (as NO_2)	Nitrates	36	2.4E-6	8.7E-5	3.2E-3
NO_x (as NO_2)	O_3	21	6.1E-8	1.3E-6	2.7E-5
NO_x (as NO2)	*NO_2 + O_3 + Nitrates*	*36*	*2.5E-6*	*8.9E-5*	*3.2E-3*
NMVOC	O_3	23	5.5E-8	1.3E-6	3.0E-5

Tab. 7.20c: Damage factors due to respiratory effects for the egalitarian's perspective without age-weighting per kg pollutant emission to air under European conditions. The lower and upper values for DALYs span a confidence interval of 95% with an assumed lognormal distribution. $\Pi\sigma_g^2$ indicates the geometric standard deviation over all steps of the impact pathway. The numbers in *italic* are the sum per primary pollutant if more than one secondary pollutant causes respiratory effects.

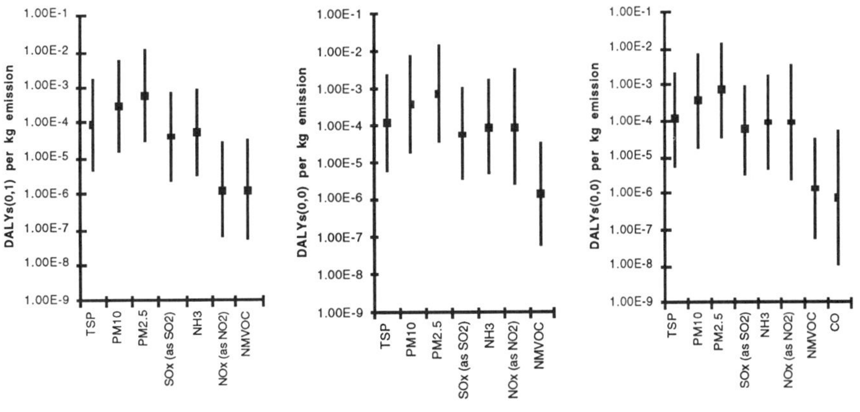

Fig. 7.2: Damage factors for the individualist's, hierarchist's, and egalitarian's world view (from left to right) in DALYs per kg substance emission to air under European conditions. The ranges shown for the factors indicate the 95% confidence interval assuming a lognormal distribution.

Figure 7.2 shows not only the best estimate of the damage factors, but the 95% confidence interval as well. The confidence interval is not the outcome of measurements in this case. but serves as an indicator for the uncertainty introduced through all steps in the impact pathway analysis where each time estimates of uncertainty had to be used. A look at Figure 7.2 reveals that the damage factors for primary and secondary particles are comparably certain or uncertain, i.e., the highest estimate is about 400 times higher than the lowest one. The exceptions are NO_x and CO. For NO_x, where the nitrates are the dominating risk factor, the ratio is about four times as large as for the other pollutants. For CO, the overall ratio between the highest and lowest estimate is about 4000 because not only the epidemiologically derived exposure-response slope, but also the fate factor, are very uncertain.

Looking at the Equation (A6.3) in Appendix (6.8) reveals that the largest σ_g in a chain of multiplicative elements will influence most the overall σ_g. The most uncertain element in Equation (7.13) is the exposure-response slope. These uncertainties in the slopes contribute most therefore to the total uncertainty. The uncertainty of DALYs per case and of the fate factors have about the same influence on the uncertainty.

It is important to mention here that the uncertainty in the damage factors for the different particles, for SO_x, NH_3 and NO_x are not independent of each other. All of these four air pollutants will show a lowered or an increased damage factor if the exposure-response slope for exposure to particles that has been derived from epidemiological studies turns out to have been either too high or too low. The fate factors are, to a large extent, independent of each other. It follows from this discussion that, when the data presented here is used in an impact assessment, the corresponding uncertainty distributions should be entered into the quantitative uncertainty assessment as dependent factors.

The damage factors for the 118 volatile organic compounds are not discussed here in detail. Their values are listed in Appendix (7.4). The absolute value is, e.g., for methane 100 times lower and for the very reactive subgroups such as alkenes, dienes, and aromatics about a factor two higher than the average value for NMVOC.

7.5.4 Comparison with other respiratory risk estimates

The results derived in the previous subsection are compared here with other published assessments in order to position them correctly. Unfortunately, the data in the literature is almost always presented in a way that precludes a direct comparison with the results in Appendix (7.4). There are four reasons for this state of affairs:

- It is still unusual to present health damages in terms of DALYs. Most existing studies either do not report damage-oriented indicators or calculate monetarised damages and thus present endpoints in monetary units.
- The current impact assessment systems for LCA use other impact categorisations than we do here, i.e., they group impacts either into the categories 'human toxicity' and 'summer smog' (SETAC 1993b) or into 'winter smog' and 'summer smog' (Goedkoop 1995). No system is known that allows directly for the grouping of respiratory effects.
- Most impact assessment systems for LCA are not based on epidemiological studies and therefore take into account no-effect levels instead of accounting for effects. The very different nature of the assessment principles preclude a sensible interpretation of the comparative findings.
- Studies using the damage cost approach are those that are most similar to the assessment presented here. However, such damage cost assessments are in most

cases site-dependent and are therefore unavailable for average European conditions (ESEERCO 1994, ExternE 1995).

Due to this limited basis for comparisons we calculate first damages due to the 1995 emissions in Europe in order to check whether the order of magnitude compares reasonably well with known death rates and total DALYs. Secondly, we recalculate damage factors from the data in existing studies so as to make them comparable to our own results.

Extrapolation to Europe

Table 7.21 shows the total damage due to the respiratory effects of air pollution in an area covering Europe and some parts of Africa and Russia. The emission data used include emissions from some natural sources such as volcanoes and the seas (sulphur in sea spray). The population in the area covered is estimated to be 700 millions inhabitants. However, more people than that are exposed to these emissions because of the long-distance transport of the pollutants. We start with the DALYs(0,0)/kg from Tab. 7.20c, thereby assuming an egalitarian perspective, and calculate the resulting DALYs per year given the areas' assumed emissions. We present these DALYs in terms of per capita in order to allow for additional interpretation.

The sum of the DALYs for all pollutants falls somewhere within a range going from 300 thousand to 150 millions. Is this a little or a lot? There are 700 million life years lived per year for the assumed population of 700 million in the model area. Murray *et al.* (1996a) calculate, based on various health statistics, that about 160 million DALYs per year are lost in the established market economies. This amounts to 200'000 DALYs per million inhabitants. The best estimate in Table 7.21 is equivalent to about 9'000 DALYs per million inhabitants which amounts to somewhat less than 5 % of the DALYs lost from all causes according to Murray et al (1996a). The upper estimate, however, is about the same as the total number of DALYs per year, i.e., this seems unrealistically high. The upper estimate is therefore almost certainly wrong[15]. The lower estimate amounts to about 0.2 % of the total DALYs, which is much lower than one would have expected based on epidemiological studies.

If we take into account that almost all DALYs in Table 7.21 are caused by primary and secondary particles and use the findings from Table 7.19, i.e., that about two thirds of the DALYs result from chronic mortality (6.6 YLL), we can recalculate an estimate for the death rate per million inhabitants (last column in Table 7.21). The resulting number of premature deaths amounts for the best estimate to about 900 people per million inhabitants. This number can be compared to the mortality rate in established market economies of 8'400 per million inhabitants (Table 7.15), i.e., about 10 % of the yearly deaths is attributed to air pollution. This share is very high but in the range found by Pope *et al.* (1995b).

To conclude this upscaling exercise, we can see that the best estimate is higher than one would expect, but not so much higher that it falls outside an explainable range. To the contrary, the upper estimate is an unrealistic worst case scenario. The upper estimate can at most be nine times higher than the best estimate if we keep in mind

[15] The only reason that we do not state that it is wrong is that we compare steady state results with a actual data, i.e., if the observed chronic mortality and bronchitis will rise in future then the higher estimate is not *a priori* wrong.

the almost 10 % share of deaths due to air pollution. In this case, all the reported deaths would have been caused by air pollution.

	European Emission 1995	Reference for emissions	Lower estimate	Best estimate	Upper estimate	DALYs standardised (best estimate)	DALYs transformed to premature death (best estimate)
	kt/a		DALYs/a	DALYs/a	DALYs/a	DALYs/ (Mio. P·a)	death/ (Mio. P·a)
SO_x as SO_2	30724	EMEP (1997)	101'688	1'677'000	27'800'000	2'396	242
NO_x as NO_2	20903	EMEP (1997)	51'676	1'863'000	67'509'000	2'661	269
NH_3	6973	EMEP (1997)	32'678	592'000	11'786'000	846	85
NMVOC	19398	EMEP (1997)	1'061	25'000	578'000	35	4
CO	73522	EMEP (1997)	834	54'000	3'463'000	77	8
CH_4	>31'000	United Nations (1996)	>17	>396	>9'000	1	0
PM_{10}	5'100	Berdowski *et al.* (1997)§	102'800	1'910'647	35'511'363	2'729	276
Total			290'754	6'122'228	146'656'374	8'746	883

Tab. 7.21: Damage assessment for respiratory effects (DALYs(0,0)) due to 7 air pollutants emitted in 1995 in EMEP-Europe, i.e., from North Africa to the European part of Russia to Iceland.
§ emissions in Europe without European part of Russia

Comparison with the LCA valuation method EPS

The Swedish EPS-system was developed before 1992 (Steen *et al.* 1992) and minor updates were made in Steen (1996). This valuation method for LCA is based on a damage-oriented approach and applies monetary values to aggregate damages to different health endpoints (Table 7.22). For comparability reasons these monetary values per kg substance emissions are transformed in Table 7.22 into DALYs. We use the equivalence of 100'000 ECU for one DALY. Steen (1996) allocates this sum to *"a painful morbidity or severe suffering"*. ExternE (1995) derives a value for a statistical life of between 2.5 to 4.4 million ECU. The value of a statistical life year can therefore be approximated with 100'000 ECU.

The interpretation of the comparison of the transformed results from Steen (1996) and the results from this study (Table 7.22) requires additional information. The numbers from Steen are in all cases much lower than our own results with the exception of the result for ethene. For CO, the explanation is clear because the mortality endpoint has not been considered by Steen. For dust, Steen considered only acute mortality and arrived at only one month lost per case. In our study, however, the largest shares are due to chronic bronchitis and to chronic mortality. For NO_x and SO_x, Steen does not consider the formation of secondary pollutants, which are the only relevant contributions in our assessment. The much lower values in Steen (1996) can therefore be explained by two omissions on the part of Steen: the formation of secondary particles and of chronic impacts. Furthermore, he assumed threshold behaviour for many impacts which may lead to additional deviations from our no-threshold approach.

Pollutant	Endpoint	ECU per endpoint Steen (1996)	ECU/kg Steen (1996)	DALYs/kg Transformation by 100'000 ECU = 1 DALY	DALYs/kg this study
CO	Nuisance	100	3.00E-05	3E-10	
	Morbidity	100000	3.00E-04	3E-09	
			3.30E-04	*3.3E-09*	*7.3E-7*
Dust	Premature mortality	1000000	4.00E-04	4E-09	
	Irritation of resp. tract	1000	7.00E-05	7E-10	
			4.70E-04	*4.7E-09*	*1.1E-4*
Ethene	Moderate nuisance	100	5.00E-04	5E-09	
	Premature mortality	1000000	2.70E+00	2.7E-05	
			2.70E+00	*2.7E-05*	*2.1E-6*
NO_x	Irritation of resp. tract	1000	2.80E-04	2.8E-09	
			2.80E-04	*2.8E-09*	*8.9E-5*
SO_x	Moderate nuisance	100	2.90E-03	2.9E-08	
	Morbidity	10000	2.88E-02	2.88E-07	
	Mortality	1000000	6.00E-04	6E-09	
			3.23E-02	*3.23E-07*	*5.5E-5*

Tab. 7.22: Transformation of damage factors from Steen (1996) into DALYs(0,0) for the comparison with own results in this study.

For ozone creation by ethene, Steen (1996) reports a value which corresponds reasonably well with our own assessment, i.e., his value is higher by factor eight. A look at the details of Steen's analysis reveals that his high value is not due to ozone formation, but due to carcinogenic effects which in our assessment do not belong to respiratory effects. For respiratory effects due to ozone formation, Steen (1996) only considers above threshold situations which then results in the low number of $5\ 10^{-9}$ DALYs/kg.

This comparison shows that the large deviations between the values reported by Steen (1996) and those from our own assessment can be explained by the missing impact paths and endpoints in Steen's study and the threshold behaviour assumed by him.

Comparison with European externality studies

A large number of externality studies have been undertaken during the last years by the members of the ExternE team (ExternE 1995). We will choose only two of its recent applications for a comparison with our own results because many of the elements used by these studies such as exposure modelling, exposure-response functions and the valuation are similar, if not equal, for all the studies. In addition, two other European studies that have been undertaken outside the ExternE team will be discussed.

IER/ETSU/EdM (1997) describe the damage costs of incineration plants with different levels of technology (mostly end of pipe). From this study, we take the damage costs they calculated for the macro pollutants. The study covered three sites: Paris, Stuttgart and Birmingham. We choose just the damage costs per kg emission for the two sites with the lowest and with the highest average damage costs (Table 7.23).We then again transform these results by assuming that 100'000 ECU equal one DALY(0,0).

For PM_{10}, SO_2 and NO_x, the best estimates from our study are about three times lower than the best estimates from IER/ETSU/EdM (1997) for their site with the lowest damage costs. The main reason for this difference is the value of 2.6 Mio ECU applied by IER/ETSU/EdM (1997) to each premature death independent of the estimated YLL. The implied YLL amount to about 26 years per death which is 4 times more than what we have assumed for chronic mortality and about 35 times more for acute mortality. Correcting for this difference the results from our study would be close to the average damage costs estimated by IER/ETSU/EdM (1997) for the site with the lowest damage costs. Minor reasons for deviations are slight differences in the exposure-damage slopes and the higher importance given to morbidity effects by the DALYs in comparison to monetarisation.

	Costs from damages to human health (IER/ETSU/EdM 1997)		Transformation from monetary values to DALYs (100'000 ECU = 1 DALYs)		This study
	ECU/kg		DALYs/kg	DALYs/kg	DALYs/kg
	Low	High	Low	High	Best estim.
PM10	144	614	1.4E-3	6.1E-3	3.7E-4
SO_2	17	39	1.7E-4	3.9E-4	5.5E-5
NO_x	34	86	3.4E-4	8.6E-4	8.9E-5
O_3 via NO_x §	2.5	2.5	2.5E-5	2.5E-5	1.3E-6
O_3 via NMVOC §	2.5	2.5	2.5E-5	2.5E-5	1.3E-6

Tab. 7.23: Comparison of the transformed damage costs from IER/ETSU/EdM (1997) with the results from this study. The upper and lower numbers of IER/ETSU/EdM (1997) stand for the best estimates for three incineration sites.
§ the numbers of IER/ETSU/EdM (1997) include damages to crops

For ozone, the situation is different. Our estimate is twenty times lower than the one from IER/ETSU/EdM (1997). One reason is the different fate factors applied by the studies. The fate factor used by IER/ETSU/EdM (1997) is based on the assumption that ozone formation by NO_x and NMVOC takes place during the whole year while we have assumed that this occurs only in summer time. Acute mortality was again valued with 2.6 Mio. ECU which is 35 times higher than our assumption of 0.75 years of life lost. The resultant difference in the valuation is partly compensated by the fact that their exposure-response slope is about 8 times lower than our own. Therefore, a difference of about factor 9 between IER/ETSU/EdM (1997) and our study can be explained by different assumption in the fate, effect, and damage analysis. The rest may be due to the inclusion of crop damages by IER/ETSU/EdM (1997), the effect of which we could not disaggregate.

The summary judgement is that results from the study by IER/ETSU/EdM (1997) and from our own correspond very well if the effectively lost YLL are taken instead of the value of statistical life and if newer findings from epidemiological studies are included in the assessment.

A comprehensive study for green accounting (Metroeconomica *et al.* 1996) was performed by partly the same institutes as IER/ETSU/EdM (1997) with the goal to calculate external costs for Germany, Italy, The Netherlands, and the UK. They assessed acute mortality with 1.25 and chronic mortality with 3 YLL (converted at a rate of 115'000 ECU/YLL), i.e., they changed the valuation method. They based their assessment on background concentration measurements. It is therefore difficult to relate the results to kg emissions per pollutant. However, the number of premature death per year arrived at were for:

Italy: 1'205 premature deaths per million inhabitants (85% chronic mortality)
Netherlands: 2'221 premature deaths per million inhabitants (86% chronic mortality)
UK: 643 premature deaths per million inhabitants (67% chronic mortality)

The numbers for Germany cannot be used because only SO_2 has been assessed. The numbers for premature deaths listed can now be compared with the data in the last column of Table 7.21, i.e., the average death rate of 905 premature deaths per million European inhabitants. From that, we can see that our own results fall within the range of UK and Italy, but are smaller, by a factor 2.5, than those for the Netherlands. Of course, the UK may benefit from fresh air blowing in from the sea and an effective transport of their own pollution to countries to the East of them, i.e., UK is not representative of the European situation. But then Metroeconomica *et al.* (1996) write that the Italian figures, for instance, are higher than the total number of deaths from respiratory effects in Italy (i.e., smoking would make no contribution to respiratory effects!). And they also conclude that for Italy and the Netherlands *"Likewise, ...the estimated number of deaths is considered too high and uncertain"* (Metroeconomica *et al.* 1996:41).

From that second study, we see that others end up with damage figures comparable to our own if they extrapolate from single pollution sources to the country level and they also feel that their numbers may be too high when the modelled death rates are compared with the data in health statistics.

A third European study (IVM 1997) has evaluated the costs and benefits of emission reduction measures in urban areas. The authors have used exposure-response slopes that are similar to ones used here, but did not consider chronic bronchitis in adults, an effect which has turned out to be a relevant endpoint in our own study. They used a value of statistical life lost for mortality endpoints. However, for acute mortality, they used this value only for the upper estimate and for the others assumed that only a few days of life are lost which they then did not value.

Table 7.24 lists the emission reduction within 36 (PM_{10}) to 151 (SO_2) European cities and the resultant health benefits calculated by IVM (1997). We normalised the total benefits with the reduction of emissions in order to calculate benefits per kg of avoided emissions. The benefits are transformed into DALYs (always lower and upper estimates) by setting 1 DALY(0,0) equal to 100'000 ECU and, finally, compared the result with the "egalitarian" DALYs(0,0) from this study. The comparison shows that our best estimates for SO_2 and NO_x are within the ranges given by IVM (1997) and for PM_{10} smaller by a factor 9 than IVM's lower estimate. The main difference in this case is explained by the assumption used by IVM (1997) that the full value of a statistical life is lost with each death. The resultant overestimate is partly compensated with the omission of chronic bronchitis as an endpoint. The remaining difference may well be caused by the geographic situation that is far different from the average one, i.e., by the special focus on urban areas. The population density in urban areas is much higher than the average one we have assumed. In light of these explanations, it seems that the results of the two studies are reasonably in accordance.

	Emission reduction (IVM 1997)		Population in analysis (IVM 1997)	Lower estimate (IVM 1997)	Upper estimate (IVM 1997)	Lower esti– mate	Upper esti– mate	Lower estimat e	Upper estimat e	Best estimate own study
	t/a	%	Mio	Mio. ECU/a	Mio. ECU/a	ECU/ kg	ECU/ kg	DALYs/ kg	DALYs/ kg	DALYs (0,0) /kg
PM_{10}	15'000	50	35	5007	51246	334	3416	3.3E-3	3.4E-2	3.7E-4
SO_2	50'000	10	75	85	3783	2	76	1.7E-5	7.6E-4	5.5E-5
NO_x	70'000	8	74	408	5900	6	84	5.8E-5	8.4E-4	8.9E-5

Tab. 7.24: Comparison of health benefits due to emission reductions calculated by IVM (1997) with own results by transforming external costs to DALYs(0,0) with 1 DALY = 100'000 ECU.

A recent Swiss study has assessed health costs due to traffic (GVF 1996). The study's goal orientation made it possible to work with PM_{10} as an indicator for air pollution. The authors attributed all the health risks to particles. The external costs are estimated to amount to 1.6 billion Swiss Francs per year. They used about 60'000 Swiss Francs as the value of a statistical life year lost which is taken here as being equivalent to one DALY. From that, it can be calculated that the DALYs caused by traffic amount to 27'000. Primary and secondary PM_{10} emissions in Switzerland from traffic can be estimated to be about 10'000 to 20'000 t/a. Therefore, the resulting damage factor lies between 0.0027 to 0.0014 DALYs/kg PM_{10}. This value is four to eight times higher than our best estimate. The higher value in GVF (1996) can be explained with their 12.7 YLL per case compared to the 6.6 years used in our study (only for chronic mortality) and the higher population density in Switzerland. In addition, GVF (1996) in principle includes effects from other air pollutants as well, but this does practically not alter the damage factor.

An US American externality study

ESEERCO (1995) is a comprehensive externality study assessing the effects of some macro and micro pollutant based on epidemiological studies in order to compare different energy supply systems. Lower and upper values from the different examples calculated in that study are displayed in Table 7.25. The lower numbers are from sites with low population densities downwind from the source of emission or with good dispersion from high stacks. We transformed the dollar values to DALYs(0,0) assuming one DALY = 100'000 $.

The comparison shows that even the highest values from ESEERCO (1995) are much lower than our own numbers. A detailed analysis of assumptions made by ESEERCO (1995) shows that acute, but not chronic mortality, was included. In addition, it seems that the formation of secondary particles from NO_x has not been included, but this is the dominant effect of NO_x. These two reasons explain the much lower values in ESEERCO (1995). The numbers contained in ESEERCO (1995) may be largely due to chronic bronchitis which the study assessed in a similar way to us. However, the details ESEERCO (1995) provides do not allow checking up on this hypothesis.

ESEERCO (1995) explains its choice to neglect chronic mortality with the low number of studies, the high probability that important confounding factors had not been controlled for, and the failure to identify the mechanisms that lead to the significantly higher results. So it is mainly a question of evidence which may have emerged after Pope *et al.* (1995b) had published their findings.

	Costs from damages to human health (ESEERCO 1995)		Transformation from monetary values to DALYs (100'000 $ = 1 DALY)		This study
	$/kg		DALYs/kg	DALYs/kg	DALYs/kg
	Low	High	Low	High	Best estim.
Particles	2.6	15	2.6E-5	1.5E-4	3.7E-4
NO_x	0.5	1.1	5.0E-6	1.1E-5	8.9E-5
SO_x	0.035	0.8	3.5E-7	8.0E-6	5.5E-5

Table 7.25: Comparison of the transformed damage costs from ESEERCO (1995) with the results from this study. The upper and lower numbers in ESEERCO (1995) stand for the best estimates for several facilities and different sites in the USA.

What do we learn from these comparisons?

Some insights from these comparisons should be stated here, although the final conclusions are made in Section 7.7. The main reasons for differences between the different studies are (order represents size of effect from high to low):

- the inclusion of chronic mortality or exclusion motivated by only few studies available,
- the different valuation principle concerning the way mortality is accounted for; some studies apply one statistical value of life per case, others opt for the YLL approach,
- the inclusion of secondary particles,
- the inclusion of chronic morbidity, and
- the higher value for disabilities by non-monetary health indices like DALYs compared to the monetary valuation.

For all these points, we remain committed to the choices we have made in this study:

- chronic mortality and morbidity are included because the few studies available are of high quality,
- the very short life period lost by acute mortality and the limited duration of life lost by chronic mortality is considered by replacing the concept of life lost with the one of life years lost[16],
- secondary particles are included as important source for particles, and
- we are convinced that the less serious endpoints such as symptom days or the first years of chronic bronchitis are systematically undervalued in monetarisation exercises.

Taking into account these positions, there is one point left: the extrapolation to the European level (Table 7.21) and the results in Metroeconomica *et al.* (1996) indicate clearly that our best estimate generates a death rate that is higher than the one that can be found statistically. This implies that the exposure-response slopes for the chronic endpoints are too high by a factor 2 to 10. This leads to the conclusion that important confounding factors have not been controlled for in the epidemiological

[16] This choice is as well supported by the Science Advisory Board of the U.S. EPA (Schmalensee 1996), which suggests calculating the benefits of the Clean Air Act based on a life years saved instead of a life saved approach.

studies which have been used here. The real values may therefore lie somewhere between our lower and the best estimate, while the upper estimate can be disregarded as unrealistic in sensitivity analyses.

7.6 Index for manageability

7.6.1 Recalling the preliminary proposal

A second index for manageability will be assessed here on the basis of the detailed description of the index for known damage due to respiratory effects initiated by air pollution (Section 7.5). It will be composed by three indicators for:

- the possibilities to reduce the assessed damage and the ease with which this can be done
- the extent to which an environmental problem exceeds a political target or a sustainable level, and
- the success of already introduced policy measures.

The index is calculated as follows:

$$Mp,c = Rp,c \cdot Xp,c \cdot Sp,c \cdot Dp,c \tag{7.14}$$

with Mp,c cultural perspective dependent index of manageability
Rp,c indicator for the ease of damage reduction [-]
Xp,c indicator for the excess of the target damage [-]
Sp,c indicator for the success of regulation [-]
Dp,c outcome of the damage assessment for human or ecological health measured in the respective damage units
p index for environmental problem
c index for the three cultural perspectives (individualists, egalitarians and hierarchists)

This index has been explained and discussed in detail in Section 4.5. The parameters used here are those set out in Table 4.12. Those that cannot be taken from there will be estimated here in Subsection 7.6.2.

The assessment of the index for manageability is not more than a feasibility test to gain experience with this new type of indicator. This application here for respiratory effects is the second one after its application to carcinogenity in Section 6.6. Time constraints have made it necessary to study only a very limited amount of additional literature. The basis for the calculation of the index is therefore even smaller than in the application to carcinogenity. The index of manageability for respiratory effects should therefore be considered as preliminary only.

7.6.2 Determination of the index of manageability for respiratory effects

Indicator for the ease of damage reduction

In order to derive the indicator for damage reduction, two questions have to be asked and the quantified answer has to be found:

- Do we need to consider this indicator at all, i.e., is this aspect not already considered in the damage assessment?

- If it is not yet considered: how much can the potential damage due to a given exposure be reduced with a given financial and legislative effort?

No attempt was made in Sections 7.3 and 7.4 to consider (cultural perspective-dependent) scenarios of measures that could reduce effects on and damage to health. The assumption there was that we do with the measures and health systems that actually exist in Europe or in established market economies. We have therefore to consider this indicator here and set the consideration factor $fc = 1$ for all three cultural perspectives.

The second question to the damage reduction potentials can only be answered by having specific measures in mind. We have argued in Section 4.5 that these measures start at a given background concentration level, i.e., no emission reduction measures are taken into account because the emission has already occurred. The following measures could be taken:

(1) Coast side, country side, and mountain side concepts: One could make it attractive to inhabitants to move to places with significantly lower background concentrations than those that they experience now. In the case of country and mountain side concepts this requires that the polluting activities do not move!

(2) Indoor concepts: It can be assumed that particle concentrations are lower indoors than outdoors if there are no indoor sources for them. For ozone the indoor concentration is much lower and it could be recommended that people stay indoor during afternoons in the summer.

(3) Protection of the respiratory tract from particles and ozone by wearing filter towels. Filter towels would filter out particles and transform ozone to oxygen.

(4) One could offer oxygen stations during smog periods in urban areas (already done in Mexico city).

(5) New treatments could be developed and disseminated, e.g., bronchodilator.

(6) Synergistic acting risk factors such as smoking could be limited or even eliminated through regulations.

These proposals will now be quickly discussed, keeping in mind that the measures have to be financed within a yearly budget of not more than 100$ per individual and have to be implemented with not more than 2 new laws and one change in the constitution. Measure (1) would require expenditures that are much higher than the set limit and is therefore unrealistic. Measures (2) and (3) cause little costs but restrict the behaviour of human beings in a significant way. Such measures could only be introduced on a voluntary basis with the result that only a (small) share of the population will be protected. The indoor concept would have limited success because human beings today already spend more than 21 hours a day indoors. Measure (4) may be a possibility to manage acute smog situations in urban regions. Its costs are relatively high and the damage reduction will be relatively small as both chronic morbidity and mortality have been identified as the main source for damages. Measure (5) is speculative. We do not know a treatment today that significantly reduces the risk of chronic morbidity and mortality. Similarly, little is known about synergistic acting activities and causal factors. Measure (6) therefore only has a limited potential for damage reduction.

In the absence of further information on possible measures and their effective performance, we make rough estimates of the damage reduction potentials of these measures for each of the three cultural perspectives:

- Individualists may inform the population about measures (2) and (3) (indoor concept and filters) and invest in oxygen stations to lower the "visible" acute effects of smog episodes (4). If new treatment methods become available, they will support such systems, however, only a small share of the population will have access to them. The potential reduction in damages within the budget limit of 50$ per inhabitant and year is estimated to amount to 10%. This estimate takes into account that the chronic diseases, although they are the relevant ones, will not be reduced by much by these measures.
- Hierarchists will use information campaigns to implement measures (2) and (3). At the same time, they will invest a lot in the development of new treatments (5). They will ban and regulate if knowledge on synergistic effects becomes available (6). Oxygen stations will possibly be installed, but are not a main strategy because their efficiency is considered to be too low. If ones speculated that such a management style will enable the detection of new treatment methods for chronic diseases, considerable damage reduction could be achieved thanks to large time lags and very long histories of disease. A reduction by 40% seems optimistic, but is thinkable in light of the limited knowledge we have today on the involved toxicological mechanisms.
- Egalitarians would invest in (5) and put effort into legislation if synergistic acting agents are known. They would inform the population about precautionary measures such as the use of filters and staying indoors during smog periods. However, egalitarians would probably invest much more in pollution prevention and pay less attention to such 'end of pipe' measures. The success of their measures (damage reduction, not emission reduction) will fall somewhere between those achieved by individualists and hierarchists and is estimated to amount to 20%.

The reader is reminded that the estimates are rough, sometimes arbitrarily chosen. Their role is to serve primarily as a demonstration of the approach on hand of a more concrete than purely abstract example.

Indicator for the excess of target damage

The target damage excess factor indicates how far away we are from a target level and is formed by the ratio of actual (N) to target level (T). The exponent *gc* is set to 0.1 for individualists and to 0.2 for egalitarians and hierarchists in order to correct for the fact that there is a saturation effect after a certain excess rate (Equation 7.15).

$$Xc = \left(\frac{N}{T}\right)^{gc} \qquad [-] \qquad (7.15)$$

In accordance with Subsection 6.6.2, we set the sustainable level for T at one premature death per year and per million inhabitants in the absence of an explicit political target.

Metroeconomica *et al.* (1996) estimated the premature deaths due to air pollution in three European countries and arrived at levels of between 640 and 2200 premature deaths per year per million inhabitants. Our own – probably upper – estimate for premature deaths per year per million inhabitants due to respiratory effects was 900 (Table 7.21). The share of the statistical death rate which is due to respiratory diseases is in the United States about 9% if only endpoints of the respiratory system (ICD-9 310-329) are considered (WHO 1995b). Assuming a death rate of 8400 per year per million inhabitants (Table 7.15), this results in a lower estimate of 750 deaths per year per million inhabitants due to respiratory effects. Many of these deaths are caused by lifestyle factors such as smoking.

For pragmatic reasons, we assume that the "true" death rate due to air pollution causing respiratory diseases is 900 deaths per year per million inhabitants and that such a death causes about half of the average YLL per case compared to the average for all causes of death. The corrected death rate due to the actual air pollution (N) is therefore set at 500 premature deaths per year per million inhabitants. The discrepancy between this result and the number in WHO (1995b) is pragmatically explained: many chronic mortality cases are in official death statistics probably reported under other causes of death and we probably include other causes of death in this assessment of deaths due to respiratory endpoints.

With $N = 500$, $T = 1$, and $gc = 0.1$ and 0.2, respectively, we arrive with Equation (7.15) at an indicator for the excess of target damage for individualists of $Xind = 1.9$ and for both egalitarians and hierarchists of $Xeg/hier = 3.5$. The reader is reminded that the magnitudes of the target level T and the exponents gc are largely subjective choices. The rough estimate of N is much less important for the sensitivity of the result than the settings of the other factors!

Indicator for regulatory success

The determination of this third indicator is guided by the decision tree that has been presented in Figure 4.9. Effects of air pollution on the respiratory system have been known for decades already, but only recently has the evidence grown that on the societal level there is no safe level of concentration, i.e., a threshold characteristic cannot be observed anymore. In addition, the American cohort studies proved only recently that a large amount of long-term effects complement the known short-term ones. This makes especially the primary and secondary particles into a major health concern. The extent of the environmental problem has therefore only recently become fully apparent and the exact mechanisms at work are still only fragmentarily understood. Consequently, regulatory policies are just now introducing new, much lower, air pollution standards while emission standards are still rarely adapted to the new knowledge. Emissions of SO_2 have been successfully reduced and with that concentrations of sulphates, but this has not yet happened for primary particles, NO_x and ammonia.

These considerations and the fact that measures to reduce loads significantly have not yet been taken make clear that regulation has not yet succeeded. The success factor S is therefore set equal to 1 for all three cultural perspectives. The fact that smog episodes of the severity observed in the 50's in London do not occur anymore does not alter our opinion. The acute health effects that have been of concern in these past smog episodes make up only a small, irrelevant share of the health effects that have been identified in this chapter.

Aggregation of the indicators to an index

The values of the three indicators *R, X, S* are summarised in Table 7.26 for each of the three cultural perspectives using the results from the preceding discussion. These three indicators are multiplied with each other and then multiplied with the index for the magnitude of damage caused by substance *i* emitted to air per unit intervention. The index for the magnitude of damage is measured in DALYs according to the procedure described in Sections 7.2 to 7.5. The DALYs per substance are listed in Appendix (7.4).

Cultural perspective	Individualists	Egalitarians	Hierarchists
R (Ease of reduction)	0.9	0.8	0.6
X (Target damage excess factor)	1.9	3.5	3.5
S (Regulatory success)	1	1	1
M (Manageability)	$1.7 \cdot \frac{DALYs_i}{I_i}$	$2.8 \cdot \frac{DALYs_i}{I_i}$	$2.1 \cdot \frac{DALYs_i}{I_i}$

Tab. 7.26: Composition of the index for manageability *M* from the three indicators for each cultural perspective and from the index for the magnitude of damage from respiratory diseases.

7.6.3 Discussion

The index for manageability has values for all cultural perspectives that are consistently larger than 1. This says that the manageability of respiratory effects due to air pollution is low. The difference between egalitarians and individualists is about 65%, the index for hierarchists lies in between. The indicators for the ease of reduction and for the target damage excess factor are dominant. It is the high target damage excess factor that is responsible for the index being larger than 1. The target level *T* has been defined on the level of damages. This makes for a large overshoot factor if the index for the magnitude of damage is large and *vice versa*. However, thanks to the high roots of 5 and 10, respectively, there is no proportionality between the indicator for the excess of target damage and the index for the magnitude of damage.

A further appreciation of the present state of the index of manageability will be provided in Subsection 9.2.2.

7.7 Main assumptions and conclusions

The modelling of the impact pathway in the form introduced in Section 4.3 is an extensive undertaking requiring huge amounts of data and making strong assumptions about the modelling principles. The most subjective choices have been modelled explicitly by introducing cultural perspectives. However, the many assumption that have still to be pondered further are summarised here. Overall final conclusions will be drawn in Section 9.2.

Recalling some assumptions

The main assumptions made in this chapter have been the following:

- It is assumed that the primary emissions can be measured. This is especially difficult for fine particles.
- The times and places of release are assumed to be typical for today's conditions in Europe. All emissions have been treated as if they had been released in the 1990's within Europe. The population distribution is assumed to be congruent with the distribution of concentrations and the population density used is representative for Europe including sea-side and lower populated areas in the east.
- The fate analysis is based on measured and modelled data. It is assumed that yearly averages of the fate factors can be estimated based on this data. Additional assumptions on present background concentrations and European meteorological conditions have to be made because the secondary formation of particles and ozone is included in the assessment, i.e., it was, e.g., assumed that the formation of ammonium nitrates or of sulphate nitrates is always possible to the same degree that occurs at the European average[17].
- We assumed that the formation of ozone from 120 different hydrocarbons can be modelled for the whole of Europe with the five day trajectory from Vienna to the UK, that the model for the chemical transformations is able to represent typical conditions, and that the model for ozone formation is representative for the air that is actually inhaled by people.
- The determination of the effects due to ozone is also based on the assumption that anthropogenic ozone is formed only in summer time.
- It is assumed that the observed health effects are caused by the pollutants for which there seems to exist sufficient evidence from epidemiological studies (cultural differences). Other pollutants that are found in toxicological studies at high concentrations to also cause respiratory effects have not been considered, however.
- The exposure-response relationships are adapted to the conditions that prevail in Western Europe. It is known that these relationships are different from those that prevail in Eastern Europe and in the U.S.A.
- The exposure-response relationships are intended to reflect only respiratory effects in human beings due to air pollutants. However, the numbers for mortality may

[17] IER (1997) showed that even within Germany large differences may exist and justify a more site-dependent assessment.

include other causes of death. This has to be considered when other impact categories are assessed in order to avoid double-counting. We have not considered the effects from the pollutants used in this study on the fauna and flora.

- It is assumed that, on the societal level, no safe level for the exposure to air pollutants can be found, i.e., a no-threshold behaviour is assumed.
- It is assumed that the exposure-response relationships are controlled for all confounding factors. One can never be certain that this requirement has been met. Even in cohort studies there may be confounding factors that are as yet unknown, but which influence the outcome very much[18].
- It is assumed furthermore that the exposure-response relationship can be linearised and that the slope at present concentrations can be taken to calculate marginal health damages due to air pollution.
- The DALYs per endpoint are estimated based on information provided by epidemiological studies and by reviews of such studies. Many more assumptions have been inspired by, although they are not based on, the 'bible' of DALYs (Murray *et al.* 1996a).
- The population structure for the damage analysis is assumed to be equal to the standard distribution observed for the Japanese population. The share of people concerned by a specific endpoint are determined on the basis of current European data.
- We assumed that the fate factors, the exposure-response slopes, and the DALYs due to respiratory effects would approximate lognormal distributions if a large enough amount of measurements and assessments would ever become available. The standard deviations are estimated individually for each factor. This assumption was made in order to be able to present a fully quantitative uncertainty assessment reflecting best the uncertainty range of the single factors. In order to be able to present the final damage factors as lognormal distributions as well, it was assumed that the addition of lognormal distributions did not significantly alter the shape of the distributions.
- The indicators constituting the index for manageability were estimated based on Section 4.5 and little additional information from literature. It is more a feasibility test than an assessment.

[18] Advent, the time these lines are written, suggests that one could ask whether epidemiological studies have ever tried to control for the different frequency of candle usage. It is known that fog episodes are correlated with high pollutant concentrations and with high health effects. If fog is as well correlated with a more depressive mood in the population or with an increased use of candles one could find an association between air pollution and health effects that is causal to depressions and candles. However, candle soot is probably to course to be a health risk factor.

Conclusions

The assumptions presented above have enabled us to model the respiratory effects due to eight ambient air pollutants, which in turn can be linked causally to the emissions of over 120 single substances. Damage factors quantifying the DALYs per kg substance emission have been derived in this chapter for these primary pollutants. Differentiating according to cultural perspectives has led to three sets of results:

- *Individualists* do not consider as causal all the associations between exposure and response and justify this position with a lack of evidence. Therefore for them, CO-emissions are not causally related to respiratory effects and the damage factor for NO_x emissions is set very low. All other damage factors are little affected by the exclusion of certain epidemiological studies due to their untrustworthiness because the remaining studies still exercise a dominant influence. Individualists assume an age-weighting with a factor lower than 1 for very young children and for older people. Respiratory effects dominate in the older part of population. Most damage factors are therefore slightly lower with age-weighting. The resultant damage factors are presented in Table 7.20a and for the approximately 120 hydrocarbons in Appendix (7.4).
- *Hierarchists* accept the evidence from additional studies and the assumption that nitrates can be treated like PM_{10}. The damage factors for NO_x and ammonia accepted by them are therefore higher than those accepted by individualists. It is assumed that hierarchists do not use age-weighting which is consistent with the argumentation in Section 5.4. The resultant damage factors are presented in Table 7.20b and for the approximately 120 hydrocarbons in Appendix (7.4).
- *Egalitarians* accept all epidemiological studies as long as experts consider them to be of high quality. The only change compared to hierarchists is their acceptance of a damage factor for CO. Again, no age-weighting is applied. The resultant damage factors are presented in Table 7.20c and for the approximately 120 hydrocarbons in Appendix (7.4).

Subjective choices supported by the distinct world views of the three archetypes have been necessary in the effect analysis, the damage analysis, and the indicators for the index of manageability. All other assumptions have to be made in order to be able to model a complex reality, i.e., the assumptions concerned rules for averaging and simplified the boundary conditions for the modelling. They therefore increase the uncertainty, but not subjectivity, of the findings.

Some conclusions independent of the cultural perspectives are:

- The respiratory health effects due to exposure to particles are dominated by chronic mortality and chronic bronchitis. These endpoints therefore dominate the whole damage assessment.
- The respiratory effects due to primary particles ($PM_{2.5}$, PM_{10}, TSP) and secondary particles (sulphates, nitrates) are the absolutely most relevant impact pathways for respiratory effects. The respiratory effects make up a very relevant share of all the effects generated by air pollutants and may well dominate most of the other impact categories focusing on human health.

- The plausibility checks and comparisons revealed that the best estimates for the damage factors are plausible. The upper estimates actually produced here seem to be unrealistically high and therefore should not be used in sensitivity analyses.
- Other mechanisms than those stimulated by primary and secondary particles will dominate only in processes or product chains where high amounts of CO are built up through incomplete oxidation and/or with processes releasing NMVOC in relevant amounts.
- The resultant damage factors have to be considered as interdependent due to the dominant influence of primary and secondary particles, i.e., if it turns out that the exposure-response slope is overestimated, then all damage factors will become smaller too. This means that the uncertainty distributions of the damage factors for primary particles, for SO_2, NH_3, and NO_x have to be entered as dependent parameters if they are used in an LCA with quantitative uncertainty assessment.
- The dominant source of uncertainty in our study is the exposure-response slopes that have been used, at least if the high uncertainty ranges taken from Pilkington *et al.* (1997) are confirmed in the future. The uncertainty in fate modelling and in damage analysis is much smaller, but could be lowered further by drawing upon the knowledge of experts for chemistry and the physics of the atmosphere and for health.
- The index of manageability has been calculated only on the basis of many preliminary and rough assumptions. The manageability is generally considered to be low due to a very high excess of target damage and the limited means that are available to prevent respiratory effects in the present exposure situation.

Finally, we refer to the critical remarks in Section 6.7 concerning the constructivistic nature of the approach that has been chosen here and the fact that only a limited effort of validation has been possible within this study.

8 Perfection of the Framework

In this chapter, we develop further methodological elements and applications of the framework before turning to a discussion of the results and the concluding chapter. A preliminary structure for the combination and the aggregation of the submodels of the ecosphere and their indices had been suggested in Section 4.6. In Section 8.1 we will now present a graphical dominance analysis which will make it unnecessary in many product comparisons to aggregate all the indices to one overall "eco-index". Section 8.2 will address the role of Cultural Theory in the modelling of the technosphere and show why uncertainty is reduced when the value choices are made in a coherent manner. A last section will explore the role of the framework as a meta-method within LCA and related life cycle tools (Section 8.3).

8.1 Graphical dominance analysis

This section's aim is to propose a tool for the graphical interpretation of the comparison of product alternatives. This procedure avoids having to make a final choice of one weighting set for the four indices of manageability adjusted damages to the safeguard subjects and of the unknown damage. This method was originally developed as part of an industry project (Braunschweig *et al.* 1997). It will be adapted here to the aggregation problem identified in Subsection 4.6.2 (case 2). The presentation is made easier by the use of a fictitious example comparing three alternative products which provide the same functional unit.

8.1.1 Four indices as the starting basis

In Subsection 4.6.2 we differentiated between two aggregation levels. On the first level, there are seven indices: an index for known damage and for manageability for each of the three safeguard subjects and the proxy index for unknown damage (see also Figure 4.10).

Earlier, it was suggested that the indices for known damage and for manageability to the so-called Manageability Adjusted Damages ($MADs_c$) be aggregated separately for each safeguard subject by making use of a panel-based procedure:

$$MADs_c = w \cdot D_c + (1-w) \cdot M_c \qquad \text{[respective damage unit]} \qquad (8.1)$$

where:
- D outcome of the damage assessment per safeguard subject
- M index of manageability [a]
- $MADs$ manageability adjusted damages
- w weighting factor between 0 and 1 for the share of the index for known damage in the MADs

c index for the three cultural perspectives (individualists, egalitarians and hierarchists)

The result of this first aggregation step consists, on the one hand, in MADs for human health, for ecological health, and for resource use for each of the three cultural perspectives and, on the other hand, in the proxy for unknown damage. These four indices form the starting basis for the second aggregation step, the subject of this section.

This second step is only necessary for product comparisons if these four indices do not show a high correlation, i.e., if they are independent from each other. This precondition may not be fulfilled *per se* because, e.g., the LCIA and its four indices will be based for the time being on the same inventory table, and the fate and effect data are sometimes the same or derived from the same toxicity tests for both damages to human and ecological health. This question will be discussed in more detail in Section 9.5.

The graphical dominance analysis presented in this Section is based on the assumption that not only one product will dominate all the others independent of the weightings of the indices that are used. This precondition means that even if there would be a correlation between the indices, it is not strong enough for only one alternative to dominate the others. If this precondition is not met, the decision maker is faced with the trivial case where only one product alternative scores best independent of the (positive) weighting of the four indices. It is clear that in such cases a graphical dominance analysis is unnecessary.

8.1.2 The "mixing triangle" or "mixing tetrahedron"

Decision making is made easier if one can represent the decision problem in an easy-to-understand graphical representation. Such a tool should indicate, for all possible weighting sets, which one of the alternative products is the dominant one in terms of the least harm to the environment. The weighting sets can be restricted to take into account positive weights only if one accepts that positive scores for the four indices always represent undesired impacts on what has been defined as the environment. The graphical dominance analysis fulfils this by providing the information at which weighting set one product alternative dominates the others in terms of the lowest environmental impacts.

The distance between a point within the body of a tetrahedron to each of the four corners can be interpreted as a representation of the relative importance of the properties represented by the four corners. In our case, the corners represent configurations of the four indices where one of them has a weight of 100% in turn. The tetrahedron is the geometric visualisation of the location of all possible sets of weights for the four indices.

Explaining graphical dominance analysis is made easier if we can operate in two-dimensional space, i.e., a simple mixing triangle. For this purpose, we have to characterise our product alternatives with just three, instead of the four indicators used here, to measure the environmental quality of a product.

Figure 8.1 introduces the main characteristics of the mixing triangle as it is used in, e.g., chemistry, geology and metallurgy. Each point within the triangle represents the relative weights of the characteristics mentioned in the corners. These relative weights always add up to 100%. In the case presented in Figure 8.1 we have chosen to measure the environmental quality of products with the manageability adjusted damages (MADs) for human health and for ecological health, and the index for unknown damage. (The MAD for resources has been omitted for didactic reasons only.)

These are the technical characteristics of the visual presentation, but there is also the important point of the content of this representation. What exactly is meant when a weight of 50% is given to human health and one of 40% to ecological health? A first possibility would be that decision makers have in mind all damages to human and ecological health respectively within given geographical boundaries, e.g., Europe or world. A second possibility would be that decision makers base their weighting on the number of damage units, i.e., one manageability adjusted DALY versus one manageability adjusted unit of damage to ecological health. As in every weighting situation, we may distinguish the following typical options:

1) Direct weighting of the indices measured with their units derived in chapters 4 and 5:

$$EI_C = WHH \cdot MADs_C HH + WEH \cdot MADs_C EH + WU \cdot U \tag{8.2}$$

2) Normalisation of the MADs and of the unknown damage according to the total steady-state MADs in a given area during a defined period of time, e.g., in Europe during one year:

$$EI_C = WHH \cdot NoMADs_C HH + WEH \cdot NoMADs_C EH + WU \cdot NoUDs \tag{8.3}$$

3) Scaling of the indices according to the highest score of a product alternative.

$$EI_C(A) = WHH \cdot \frac{MADs_C HH(A)}{max_{A \ldots N}(MADs_C HH)} + WEH \cdot \frac{MADs_C EH(A)}{max_{A \ldots N}(MADs_C EH)} + WU \cdot \frac{U(A)}{max_{A \ldots N}(U)} \tag{8.4}$$

where:

EI	Eco-Index calculated from the weighted average of the indices representing the environmental harm of a product
W	relative weight
U	proxy indicator for unknown damage [a]
$MADs$	manageability adjusted damages
$NoMADs$	normalised manageability adjusted damages
$NoUDs$	normalised unknown damages
HH	human health
EH	ecological health
$A \ldots N$	product alternatives A to N, where N depends on the number of products in the comparison
c	index for the three cultural perspectives (individualists, egalitarians and hierarchists)

In order to determine which of these three options is best, it will be necessary to make experiments with decision makers. In the fictitious example presented here we have chosen option (1), because option (2) requires the normalisation of the unknown damage[1], which is both difficult and data intensive, and option (3) entails an undesirable additional dependence on the set of alternatives.

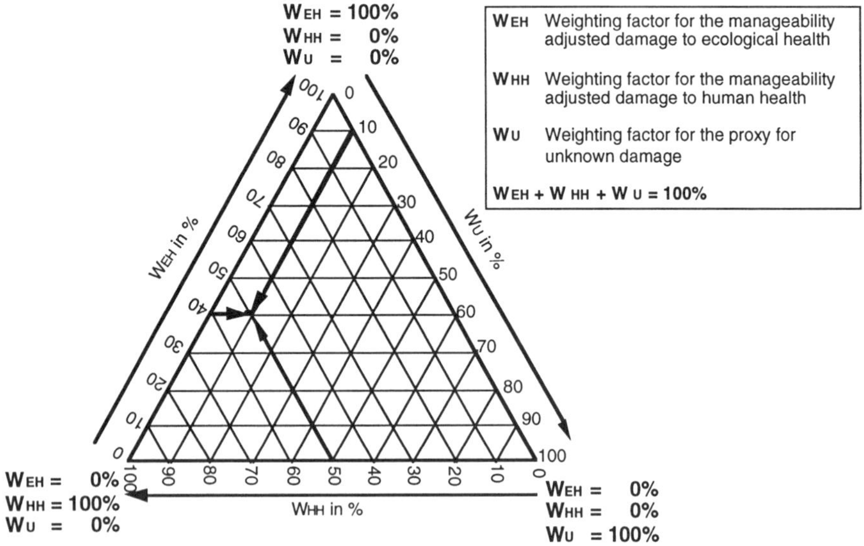

Fig. 8.1: The principle of the mixing triangle. Example: The weighting point where human health is weighted with 50%, ecological health with 40% and, consequently, the unknown damage with 10% can be found as indicated (based on Braunschweig et al. 1997).

But within option (1) it will still be necessary to provide the decision makers with information on total damages in a given area during a given period of time in order to improve their ability to differentiate between reasonable and unreasonable weighting sets.

8.1.3 Lines of indifference

Now that we have introduced the concept of the weighting triangle and have fixed the units of those indices which will be weighted, we can apply the triangle to a fictitious example.

If it is possible to find the weighting triples for which the eco-index of two products will be equal (Equation 8.2), then all other weighting triples will allow a ranking of alternatives. Braunschweig *et al.* (1997) have shown that all the weighting triples that lead to the same eco-index for two product alternatives (EI(A) = EI(B)) are found on a straight line in the triangle[2]. If more than two products are compared, the lines

[1] This problem has already been discussed in Subsection 4.6.2. The normalisation value for $MADs_c$HH can be estimated based on the estimates for the total DALYs in established market economies: DALYs(1,1) = 99 Mio. and DALYs(0,0) = 161 Mio, both related to a population of 798 million (Murray *et al.* 1996a). Between about 5% and 35% of these total DALYs can be attributed to environmental causes (see Chapters 5.2, 6.5.5, 7.5.4). It will be possible to make a better estimate for the $NoMADs_c$HH as soon as all relevant causal relationships between environmental interventions and DALYs have been established.

[2] The eco-index itself does not have the same magnitude on that straight line, but at each point on the line the two products compared have the same eco-index.

for the pair-wise product comparisons cross in just one point (see Figure 8.2). These lines can therefore be calculated by determining the points where the straight lines cross the border of the triangle by using Equation (8.2) and the condition that all weights together should equal 100%.

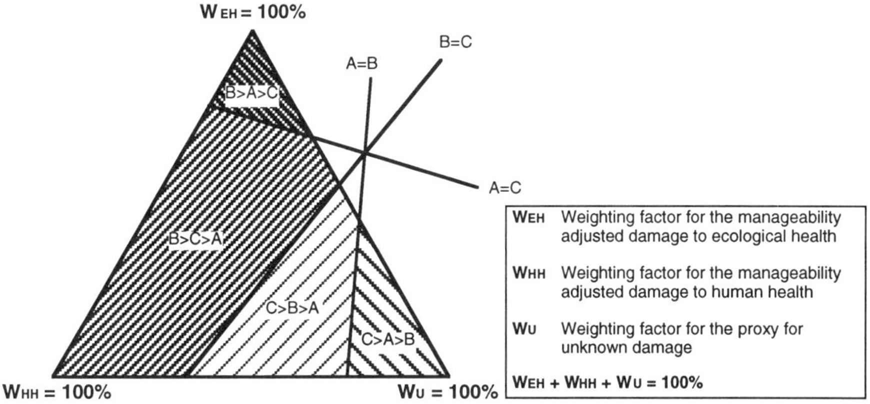

Fig. 8.2: The lines of indifference in the weighting triangle and the sub-areas with their specific ranking orders (based on Braunschweig *et al.* 1997).

In the fictitious example shown in Figure 8.2, all lines of indifference cross the triangle. Four sub-areas characterised by a different ranking of the product alternatives can be identified. First experiences with this procedure undertaken in Braunschweig et al. (1997) have demonstrated that, in practice, some of the alternatives will be dominated independently from the weighting set that is adopted (here product (A)). This is equivalent to saying that the lines of indifference do not cross within the triangle.

A first interpretation of Figure 8.2 allows the observation that there are no weighting triples where product A is best. Product C will rank highest if the unknown damage is weighted higher than about 50%; in all other cases product B scores best.

In Chapters 6 and 7 it was stated that the indicators are assessed as ranges rather than as exact numbers or point estimates. The high levels of imprecision and of variability found in the parameters used to calculate the indices have to be made transparent to the decision maker(s).

8.1.4 Areas with the same dominance order

To identify the areas where one product alternative dominates the others *significantly,* one has to define the level of probability that is thought to be significant for determining that product alternative A dominates alternative B. This threshold should be set by decision makers. In their absence, we use a 90% probability for the illustration in Figure 8.3. This is the step where the information on the probability distributions of the indices (see, e.g., Sections 6.5 and 7.5) is used to find the weighting sets which lead to significant differences between product alternatives.

This procedure generates areas with a significant dominance that are smaller than the dominance areas in Figure 8.2. The white area in Figure 8.3 indicates weighting sets under which the product alternatives are thought to cause comparable environmental impacts. For decision makers this may suggest that only other characteristics of the products should be used for decision making, i.e., the environmental dimension is irrelevant for the decision or that an additional and improved product should be included in the comparison.

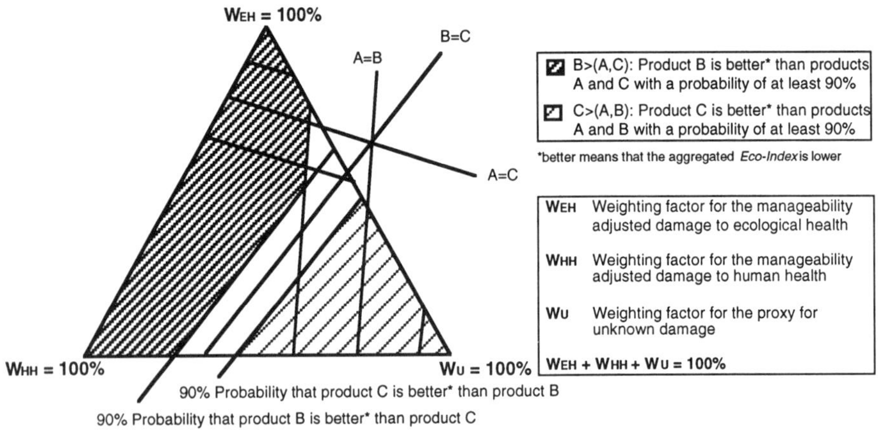

Fig. 8.3: Areas of significant dominance (90% probability) of one product (based on Braunschweig *et al.* 1997)

So far, it has been shown how the comparison of products can be supported graphically. The only choices that had to be made for this purpose were selecting the indices to be weighted and determining the minimum probability required to declare a product alternative to be significantly less polluting than the others. In certain cases this will still be insufficient as decision support. In such cases, a highly subjective step has to be added. This will be done in the next subsection.

8.1.5 Preferred sets of weighting triples

Decision makers using LCA in internal applications for everyday product improvements or governmental bodies using it for regulatory purposes may need a tool that provides them with an unequivocal ranking of alternatives for the cases where there is not just one alternative that is dominant for all possible weighting sets. In these cases, it is suggested that a so-called preference field (or space in the case of a tetrahedron) be identified, which includes all weighting sets which are considered by the decision makers to be reasonable given the context in which they operate, i.e., the company's board of directors or the government's environmental policy.

Figure 8.4 suggests such a field assuming that the unknown damage will get a weight of less than 40%, human health a weight of at least 25%, and ecological health a weight of between 25% and 55% (These numbers have been chosen to just illustrate the procedure and are by no means to be taken as a suggestion.) These percentages are directly applied to the damage units in our case. The preference fields in our fictive example result in a clear preference for product B (area *f*). There is only a small probability that any alternative may be significantly dominant (area *g*).

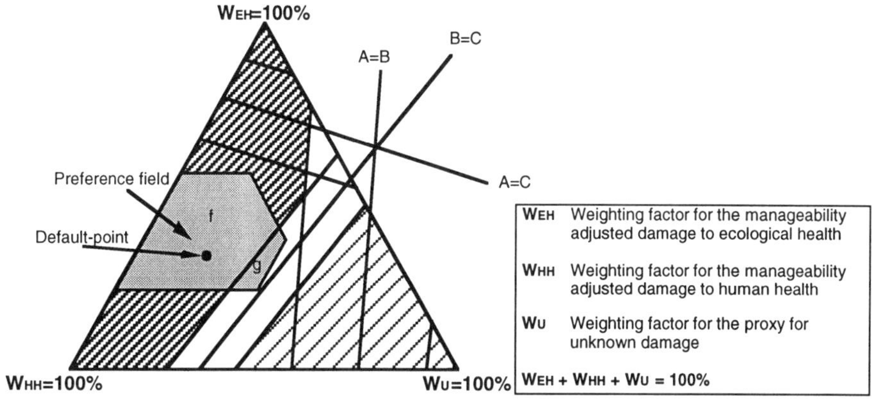

Fig. 8.4: Mixing triangle supplemented with a subjectively chosen preference field and a default weighting point (based on Braunschweig *et al.* 1997).

The value of this procedure as a decision support is significantly increased and facilitated if the decision makers themselves or an other authoritative body is able to fix a weighting point. Such a 'consensus weighting point' can be an arithmetic average of a set of weighting triples preferred by individuals, the result of a consensus process in the group of decision makers, or the preference of a single decision maker. In all cases, the weighting process should be supported by additional information on the meaning and size of the indicators[3]. The largest benefit of setting such a (default) weighting point is the possibility of performing a contribution analysis, i.e., to analyse where the total damage comes from, which effects and substances are responsible for it, and which processes or phases of the product life are responsible for the dominant emissions.

The procedure for a graphical dominance analysis presented here for three indices is applicable in analogy to the case where four indices[4] are used to measure the environmental impact of products. In this case, areas rather than lines represent the change of dominance and spatial blocks represent those weighting quadruples which have the identical ranking order. It is recommendable to program the tetrahedron directly into the LCA-software tool that is used and to do this in such a manner that the tetrahedron can be turned in order to present it in the most informative position possible.

The example has used three product alternatives, but the procedure is applicable as well to between two and *n* alternatives, where *n* can in principle be very large. Anyway, it may well be that only one or two products show up in the dominance

---

[3] Additional information on panel procedures in LCIA has already been given in Subsection 1.3.4; see also Hofstetter (1996b:138-141) and Brunner (1998).

[4] If more than four indices have to be weighted, one still can use the algorithm to identify the weighting sets for which a certain product alternative dominates the others. However, the graphical representation will then become unclear.

analysis as has been suggested before. The advantage of using such a graphical representation is maintained even if a large number of alternatives is compared.

8.1.6 Final remarks

The tools for graphical dominance analysis that have been presented here will be very powerful if and when they are implemented in commercial LCA software. The criticism towards the final weighting step (ISO 1998) can be partly circumvented by this procedure and much information is added explicitly instead of staying hidden.

In the case that the four indices are highly dependent on each other, the most subjective weighting step would have no or only little influence on the ranking of the alternatives as such. Such a finding would indicate that it is possible to develop powerful simplified/streamlining tools focusing on only one of the four indices.

A practical implementation of this approach requires the specification of procedures to measure the indices to be weighted and to identify the preference field and a consensus weighting point, if necessary. Further guidance and programming support can be found in Braunschweig *et al.* (1997).

8.2 Compatible value choices reduce the uncertainty in LCA

This section will show that value choices are not only a necessary element within the life cycle impact assessment, as shown so far, but also within both the goal and scope definition and the inventory analysis. In both cases they can be modelled by Cultural Theory as well. Before proceeding with this demonstration, it is necessary to differentiate uncertainty due to value judgements from "technical uncertainty", a task that will be undertaken in Subsection 8.2.1.

8.2.1 The different types of uncertainty

Sources of uncertainty, when one adopts a broad understanding of this concept, are the following: imprecise measurement, variability, linguistic imprecision, approximations, subjectivity, and disagreements.

Some degree of uncertainty, in principle, enters into the procedure with each number or item which is part of the LCA-model. Imprecise measurements and variability can be treated with classical uncertainty analysis: one uses distributions instead of single values and one applies sensitivity analysis or Monte Carlo simulations. Comprehensive concepts are available for this (SETAC 1994) even though they have rarely been implemented so far. In this book we have used, where appropriate, estimates for lognormal distributions of values. The mainly multiplicative linkage of the values has made it possible to calculate resulting distributions by arithmetic means (see Appendix 6.8).

Linguistic imprecision, which may enter in the weighting phase, could be dealt with through fuzzy-set theory (Pohl *et al.* 1996a/b).

Approximations, subjectivity and the content of scientific disagreements can in principle be dealt with through classical uncertainty analysis, but only at the price of high margins of uncertainty. All elements in LCA are affected by these types of uncertainty:

- the definition of the functional unit and the measurement of the utility of a product,
- the scope of the analysis,
- the definition of safeguard subjects and the way damage to them is measured,
- the choice between the use of marginal or average analysis and whether dynamic aspects and future developments will be included or not,
- the way the separation and allocation is made between the product system to be studied and the rest of the technosphere,
- the design of scenarios for the use and the disposal phases (e.g., expected life-time, change of electricity production during use phase, future waste disposal technologies, assumptions concerning leakage from disposal sites, etc.), and
- all the value choices within the impact assessment identified in this book.

The philosophy of the framework suggested in this book is that we can use the model of the valuesphere to support coherent choices in all the situations listed above. Therefore, each of these value choices should be made separately for each of the active archetypes. Schwarz *et al.* (1990) call this type of uncertainty 'structural uncertainty' in order to distinguish it from the technical uncertainty.

8.2.2 Cultural perspective within uncertainty assessment

Cultural Theory can be used to deal consistently with sources of uncertainty such as approximations, subjectivity and scientific disagreements, i.e., the value choices involved can be based on archetypal world views and management styles. Chapters 4 through 7 have demonstrated the usefulness and the practicability of this approach for the modelling of the ecosphere. We have chosen two items from the list of value choices given above with which to illustrate applications of this approach in the modelling of the technosphere:

- Leakage from disposal sites: in the life of waste disposal sites, one can differentiate between at least four ways of considering emissions: (1) during the controlled phase which lasts some decades and where contaminated water that leaks is purified; (2) during the uncontrolled, but unproblematic phase, where the concentration of pollutants in the leaking water is below thresholds; (3) during the break-through phase, where, e.g., large amounts of heavy metals are washed out because of acidification in the deposit body below pH 4. This process can start centuries after the site has been closed; (4) the potential emission of all pollutants stored in the deposit body. The question now is which concept of emissions should be used for the accounting in a specific case study where landfilling is used as the disposal technique? Based on the characteristics given in Table 3.1, a first guess would be that: the egalitarians will either count the emissions of the first three phases without discounting those that occur in the future or even choose to consider the whole emission potential (4); the individualist would probably look at the controlled phase (1), take only into account emissions which exceed thresholds, and apply a high discount factor to future emissions; the hierarchists would also look at the controlled phase (1) and include, by expert judgement, the probability that a break-through (3) has to be expected and, if at all, apply a moderate discount rate.
- Open loop recycling: According to the law of mass preservation, materials do not just disappear after the use phase of products and can potentially be used for the production of new goods. Let us assume that a virgin plastic is used to construct a refrigerator and can, in principle, be reused after the technical lifetime of the refrigerator. How should the environmental effects from its production and the later recycling process be allocated to the refrigerator and the next product? The market price of the recycled material gives some guidance as to the value of the recycled material. However, the attribution of the environmental impacts is to some extent a value judgement. Individualists may argue that, as long as there is a market demand for recycled plastic, the environmental impacts from the initial production can be allocated to some extent to the whole product cascade. Hierarchists may agree with this procedure only for products with short life times because they consider the development of the recycling market as too uncertain in the long run. Egalitarians would argue that those that use virgin material should

carry the whole responsibility for all the environmental impacts caused by its production because the hypothetical re-use is too uncertain.

We suggest here that all the parameters in an LCA, i.e., in all phases of the LCA study, should be checked for their dependence on value judgements and that they should be characterised for each archetype. This approach results in three alternative routes through the models of the technosphere and the ecosphere. The results of these routes will finally vary less than in the case where only a technical uncertainty analysis is made because the former is not a worst/best case analysis and because the routes make sense in themselves, i.e., the consistency of the alternative routes is higher than of any other chosen combination of parameters (Figure 8.5). This procedure has been suggested and practised already for integrated assessment and proved to be supportive for decision making (van Asselt *et al.* 1996a/b).

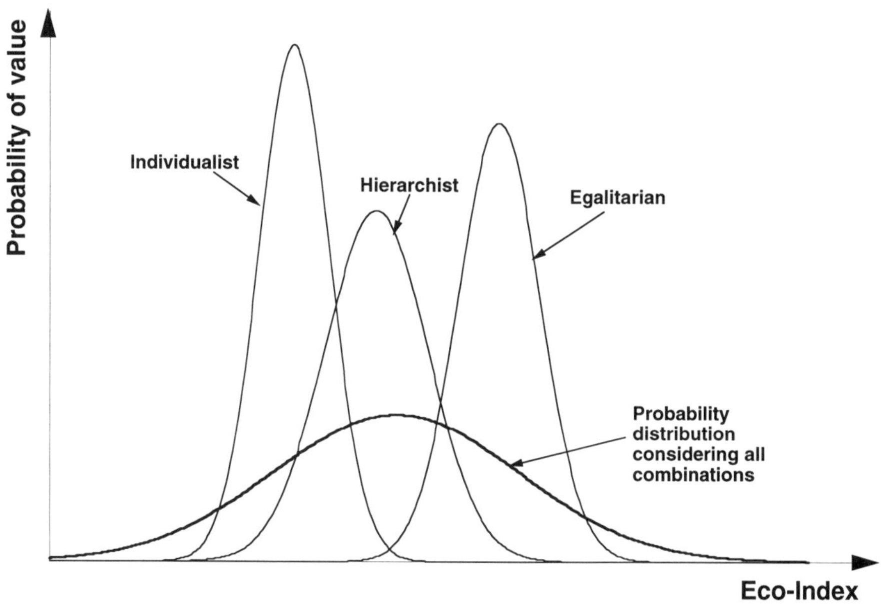

Fig. 8.5: Comparison of the probability distribution treating structural uncertainty like technical uncertainty with the probability distributions considering only compatible combinations of value choices for the structural uncertainty.

We will still have to apply classical uncertainty analysis for the technical uncertainties which are independent of cultural perspectives. This combination of classical, cultural, (and fuzzy) uncertainty analyses will lead to distributions for the value of the eco-index that are different for each of the alternative routes. The results will appear in the form of either a probability distribution (see Figure 8.5), or of an upper and lower value, or of an average value with its standard deviation.

8.2.3 Is the uncertainty really reduced?

The section title suggests that it is possible to reduce the uncertainty by the introduction of compatible value choices. Uncertainty can be reduced if more reliable data becomes available or if available information is evaluated in a more reasonable way. We add information on viable ways of life and their corresponding world views and management styles with the modelling of value choices supported by Cultural Theory. This information allows for a more sensible structuring of the available information. This reduction of uncertainty has been indicated in Figure 8.5. The range between the lowest estimate for the eco-index by the individualist and the highest estimate for it by the egalitarian is smaller than the range when considering all possible combinations.

The range of uncertainty is reduced once more if one looks only at the distribution of one of the archetypes. However, this reduction in uncertainty is bought at the price of an additional value choice in the decision process, i.e., the choice of the appropriate cultural perspective. In the case of a single decision maker this may add no additional uncertainty, but in group decisions it will. A proposal of how to deal within LCA with all three outcomes at the same time will be made in the next subsection.

We can conclude this discussion with the statement that uncertainty is really reduced by the modelling of value choices with Cultural Theory and that it can be further reduced if decision makers feel comfortable with one of the three archetypes.

8.2.4 Cultural dependence of the ranking

Nothing has been said in Section 8.1 about the cultural dependence of the choice of the preference field and of the consensus weighting point. It is obvious that their settings depend on world view and on management style and that, therefore, they have to be set according to the cultural perspectives of decision makers. However, the results cannot be marked in the same triangle or tetrahedron because the manageability adjusted damages are dependent on the cultural perspectives as well.

If decision makers themselves do not agree on just one cultural perspective, but are interested in the robustness of the outcome when using several perspectives, they may choose the mixing triangle presented in Figure 8.6. The corners represent a weighting of 100% for the three active cultural perspectives of the egalitarians, the hierarchists and the individualists, respectively. All combinations of these three archetypes are represented by the points within the triangle.

We have calculated the eco-index for all product alternatives for all three perspectives with the help of the archetype-dependent default weighting point. With reference to Figure 4.12, it is assumed here that egalitarians will weight unknown damage higher than hierarchists and individualists. Based on these data, it is possible in Figure 8.6 to visualise that if egalitarians make up more than 80% of the population of decision makers, then product C will be considered best, and if egalitarians are less than 60% of the population, product B will be superior to the other product alternatives.

In principle, it is possible to determine the shares of a country's people which show the highest affinity to any one of the cultural perspectives (Subsection 3.2.5). This "country mix" could be identified in Figure 8.6. However, as stated already in Subsection 3.2.5, such a mix has little to do with the decisions at hand. Nor, in most cases, does the decision making processes reflect a proportional representation of views.

The question of the shares of cultural perspectives will become obsolete if it can be shown that either one of the following two preconditions fails to be met in reality (see Subsection 8.1.1):

- the three manageability adjusted damages and the unknown damage are independent of each other, and
- not just one product will dominate all the others independent of the weightings of the indices that are used.

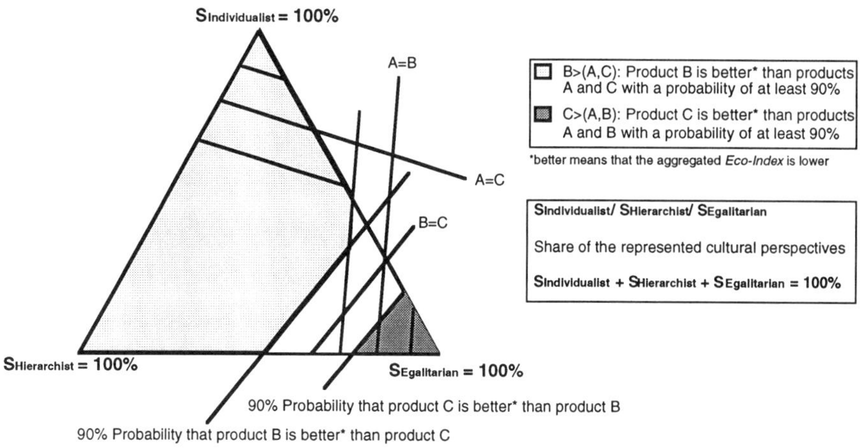

Fig. 8.6: Dominance analysis for product alternatives dependant on the cultural perspective underlying the assessment

This would mean that the result of all assessments will support the same ranking of product alternatives as long as value judgements are made consistently and in a manner that is compatible with one world view. This finding would represent an important step in the development of robust decision support systems and render unnecessary the graphical dominance analysis. However, it would be especially important for product comparisons, but not for the improvement assessment (see Section 9.5).

8.3 The framework as meta-method

The framework that has been developed and presented in this book is not directly a further development of one of the methods for LCIA that already exist and that have been mentioned in Section 1.3. The framework's basis is the modelling of the ecosphere with three submodels which are of different importance, dependent on the cultural perspective chosen and the combination of the three spheres.

None of the known methods for LCIA separates all three submodels as has been suggested here. It is therefore tempting to use this framework to try to group the existing methods. The result of such a positioning exercise is presented in Figure 8.7 for those methods that have been mentioned in Section 1.3. The result is comparable to the grouping already undertaken in Table 1.1. A first group of methods is effect-oriented and covers a range reaching from policy theme assessments to damage assessments. The second group is intervention or exposure-oriented and suggests proxies for environmental impacts rather than for damage assessments. The methods using abatement costs are difficult to be grouped according to this scheme because abatements costs are used as a proxy for environmental impacts, but also represent aspects considered within the model for manageability (i.e., ease of damage reduction). Kortman *et al.* (1994) have shown that expert panels also tend to consider aspects of manageability if they are asked to rank environmental problems according to their harm.

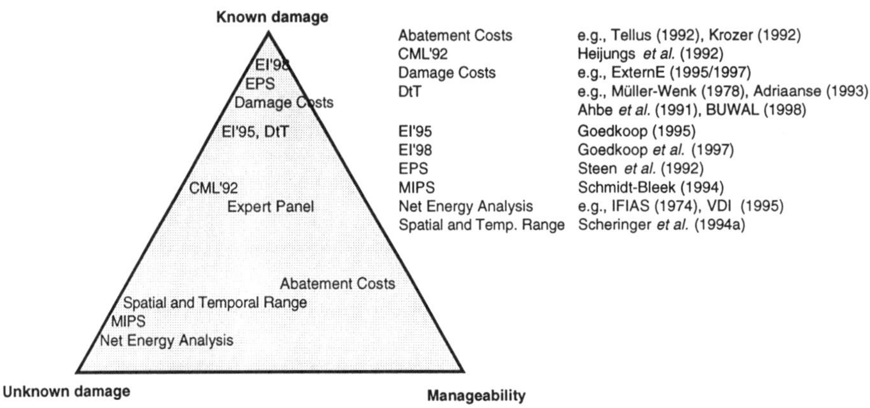

Fig. 8.7: Positioning of a selection of methods for impact assessment used in LCA according to the three submodels of the ecosphere suggested in this book

Figure 8.7 and the short discussion make it obvious that none of the already existing methods covers explicitly all three of the submodels of the ecosphere. When discussing new methods it may be useful to position them within this triangle and to ask how they could be combined with other methods to cover all characteristics constituting the ecosphere. This way of formulating the problem also makes it clear that the framework suggested in Chapter 4 could be based on existing methods, i.e., spatial and temporal range, MIPS, or net energy analysis for the modelling of unknown damage, and a damage cost approach or EI'98 for the modelling of known damage.

However, there is so far no approach available for manageability apart from the proposal made in Section 4.5.

In Section 4.6 we suggested that egalitarians will be more attracted by holistic models of the ecosphere which can be located in the corner of unknown damage (Figure 8.7). Individualists will attribute the most importance to an assessment of proven damages while hierarchists will tend to follow expert opinion and may consider all three of the submodels to some extent. These considerations serve not only to position existing LCIA methods, but also help explain why certain groups will prefer certain types of methods.

The 'less is better' approach can be located between the corners of known and unknown damage while the 'only above threshold' approach is a typical demand from the pure damage assessment approach. Egalitarians will therefore tend to prefer a 'less is better' approach and disagree with individualists or hierarchists who are likely to prefer the 'only above threshold' approach. These predictions made here suggest that consensus is hardly possible on the question whether a 'less is better' or an 'only above threshold' approach should be chosen (White *et al.* 1995). Making transparent the different philosophies behind the methods is an important step forward in choosing appropriate models for the decisions at hand.

9 Results and Discussion

This discussion of results begins with another visual summary of the structure of the framework. It brings together all its elements, but is shorn of many of the details that have been discussed in earlier chapters in order to highlight its essence (Section 9.1). Then follows a discussion and comparison of the results from the two case studies of 'carcinogenic' and of 'respiratory effects' (Section 9.2). In Section 9.3, we attempt to step back somewhat from the role of author in order to look from a different point of view self-critically at the framework proposed in this book. Then follow some additional thoughts on the lack of validation and verification of the framework (Section 9.4) and the final section will focus on the consequences of using this approach as decision support.

9.1 The structured aggregation procedure

'The structured aggregation procedure' worked out in Chapter 4 and completed in Section 8.1 is here presented graphically in Figure 9.1.

Its basic elements are: the model of the product systems within the technosphere, the three submodels for the ecosphere to derive the indices for known damage, unknown damage, and manageability, a further aggregation step, and finally a dominance analysis supported by a graphical interpretation tool. As the figure indicates, there are three parallel layers to the framework, one for each of the world views modelled by the cultural perspective that are identified in Cultural Theory (model of the valuesphere). The structure of the procedure is the same for all three world views, but individual elements and their aggregation themselves are dependent on the cultural perspective that is applied.

The framework and its elements proposed here may appear to be definitive and fixed, but they are not. Especially the final selection of the three submodels for the ecosphere can still be modified and, with it, the composition and aggregation of the indices quantified with just these models of the ecosphere. It is essential that in the near future the framework as such, and the meaning and understanding of its sub-elements, will be worked through and tested by involving potential decision makers. The experience thus gained should serve as the base for further improvement (see also Section 9.4).

Figure 9.1 already suggests how to group the elements for which intermediate results can be presented and at which level this is to occur. But only empirical work will show whether decision makers will be interested in more details than this will provide or if they will be satisfied with the tool of the tetrahedron, completed as it may be with a preference space or even with a consensus weighting quadruple.

The framework is, for the time being, best characterised as a box full of elements which can be revised and their purpose and position determined and then fixed. However, there is one restriction guiding this process besides the requirements of logic and feasibility: the general structure should be kept the same for the three cultural perspectives whenever possible. This will ease the operationalisation *and* the understanding of differences between the three assessment systems[5].

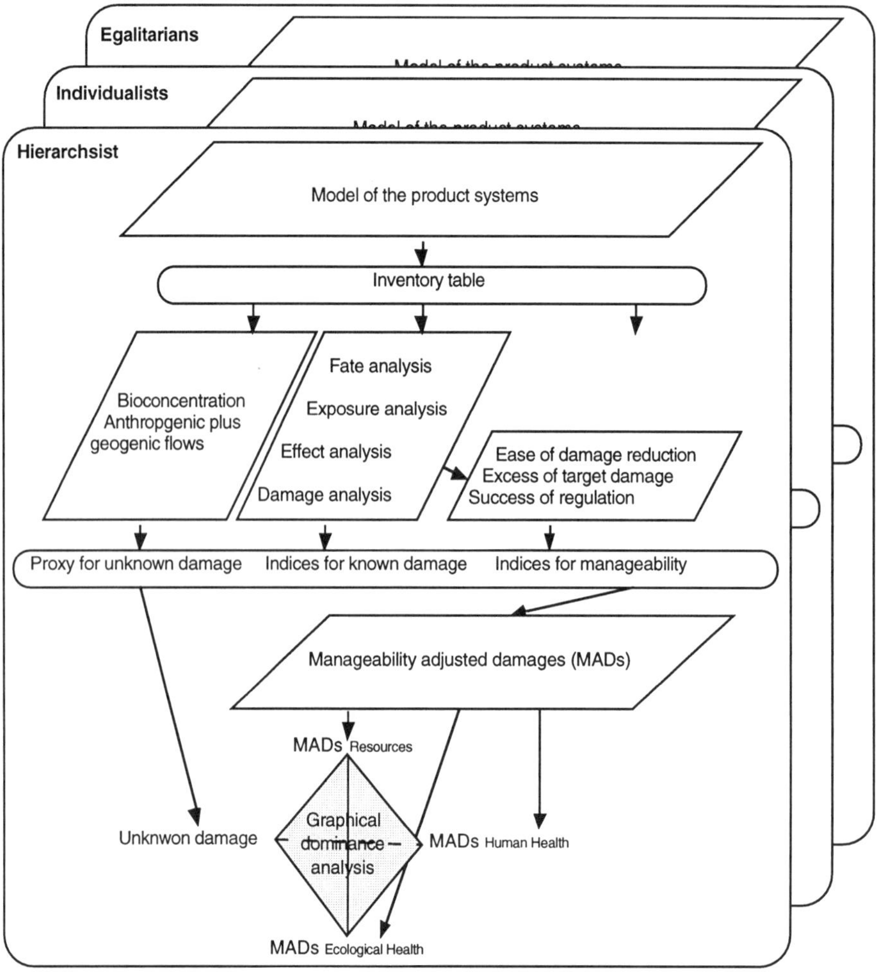

Fig. 9.1: The structured aggregation procedure with a final dominance analysis as suggested in this book.

[5] This restriction can be met by setting to zero the weight of an element from the framework whenever it is not used by a perspective.

9.2 Results from the case studies

The reasons to choose respiratory and carcinogenic effects in human beings for case studies have already been given in Subsection 4.3.6. This choice turned out to be a good one because a lot of information has been found to be available that was of good use for the fate, effect, and damage analyses. This volume of information made it possible to calculate for both cases the damage factors in terms of disability adjusted life years (DALYs) per kilogram emission to air or water. In addition, the manageability factor could be assessed based on first guesses for both effect types.

Some major assumptions behind the results for the known damage and for manageability will be highlighted once more in the two following subsections in order to provide the correct perspective for interpreting the results.

9.2.1 Known damage

A detailed discussion of the results for known damage has been undertaken in Sections 6.5 and 7.5 and the conclusions to be drawn from them can be found in Sections 6.7 and 7.7. Here, we will highlight the more important assumptions behind both case studies, and present and compare their central results.

Relevant assumptions for and limitations of the case studies are:

- The averages for Western Europe for meteorological conditions, geographical factors, exposure conditions including intake parameters, and emission patterns have been chosen as representative for all emissions to be assessed in LCIA. The population density was modelled per substance by assuming that the emission source lies within Europe and that the emissions will disperse over less populated regions for larger atmospheric residence times. Substances with very short lifetimes will mainly cause exposures at the point of emission. This point often lies within densely populated areas and the assumption of a high population density may therefore be justified. Meteorological conditions and background emission pattern are especially relevant for photochemical ozone formation, but also for the formation of secondary particles, i.e., nitrates and sulphates. The height of the atmospheric mixing layer is dependent on the latitude and the climate. Exposures through food and drinking water depend on the source of drinking water and on the geographical origin of the food and of the diet that are typical for a given area. These are some of the main reasons why the findings of this damage assessment cannot be validly generalised for non-European regions.
- The fate modelling has turned out to be one important source of uncertainty for some of the substances. The fate modelling for all heavy metals, primary particles, and carbon monoxide had to be based on poor or inappropriate models or information. Heavy metals are major contributors to cancer and particles to respiratory diseases. The fate modelling for these two substance groups should be improved by using either more sophisticated models or by basing them on reliable measurements of emissions and of changes in ambient concentrations. The fate factors for heavy metals are so uncertain that the damage factors can only be given within very wide ranges.

- For both respiratory and carcinogenic effects it has been assumed that no threshold behaviour occurs at the usual ambient concentrations. This assumption only holds true on a societal level where human beings with very different sensitivities and pre-existing disabilities are considered. In the case of carcinogenity, it was necessary to extrapolate the slope factor for low doses from information about the effects of high doses. This extrapolation leads in most cases to upper estimates.
- Information on the slope of the dose-response functions that have been derived from epidemiological studies always suffer from the risk that not all confounding factors have been controlled for. We spend about 22 hours per day indoors and important confounding factors in this case include active and passive smoking and other sources of indoor pollution. It may well be that these factors are not yet adequately taken into account.
- Knowledge about acute or short-term health damages due to exposure to pollutants are derived more easily and are based on a higher degree of evidence than knowledge about chronic, long-term, or delayed effects. However, the chronic effects contribute most to the total damages in both of the cases studied.
- The concept of disability adjusted life years (DALYs) has not been developed for what it has been used here for, namely the measurement of human health damages due to environmental pollutants. Therefore, the information on disability weights, years life lost, and the average duration of disabilities was either unavailable for the endpoints identified in epidemiological studies or were just an average over all risk factors. This meant that, although we use DALYs as the common damage indicator, we could not fully base them on what might be called the "bible" of DALYs (Murray *et al.*, 1996a/b).
- Each of the long list of damage factors presented in Chapters 6 and 7 may induce the reader to think that they are complete or comprehensive. They are not, as we have pointed out in Subsections 6.3.4 and 7.1.2. Several hundreds of substances could have been included in the list for carcinogenity, but the set has been restricted to just those substances presented in Figure 6.7 in order to limit the effort for the fate modelling. In the case of respiratory effects, we had decided to choose the epidemiological instead of the toxicological approach. This is the reason that only those substances which are measured by the many existing air monitoring systems could be included in the analysis that is based on epidemiological studies. For instance, aldehydes are not included in the analysis presented in Chapter 7 even though Victorin *et al.* (1996) mention them as respiratory irritants.

The result of the damage assessments are the lists with damage factors for respiratory and carcinogenic effects that are contained in Appendices (6.16), (6.17) and (7.4). Below, we evaluate and discuss these results.

Carcinogenic effects

The damage factors for those carcinogenic substances classified by IARC in Groups 1 or 2 lie within a range of 10^{-7} to 10^{3} DALYs per kg emission to air or water. These ten orders of magnitude make clear that the substances have very different potencies per mass unit (Figure 9.2). Another important insight is that the potency of the substances does not decrease or increase with their IARC classification. The

IARC grouping indicates the degree of evidence for the substances' carcinogenity to humans and not their potency per mass unit.

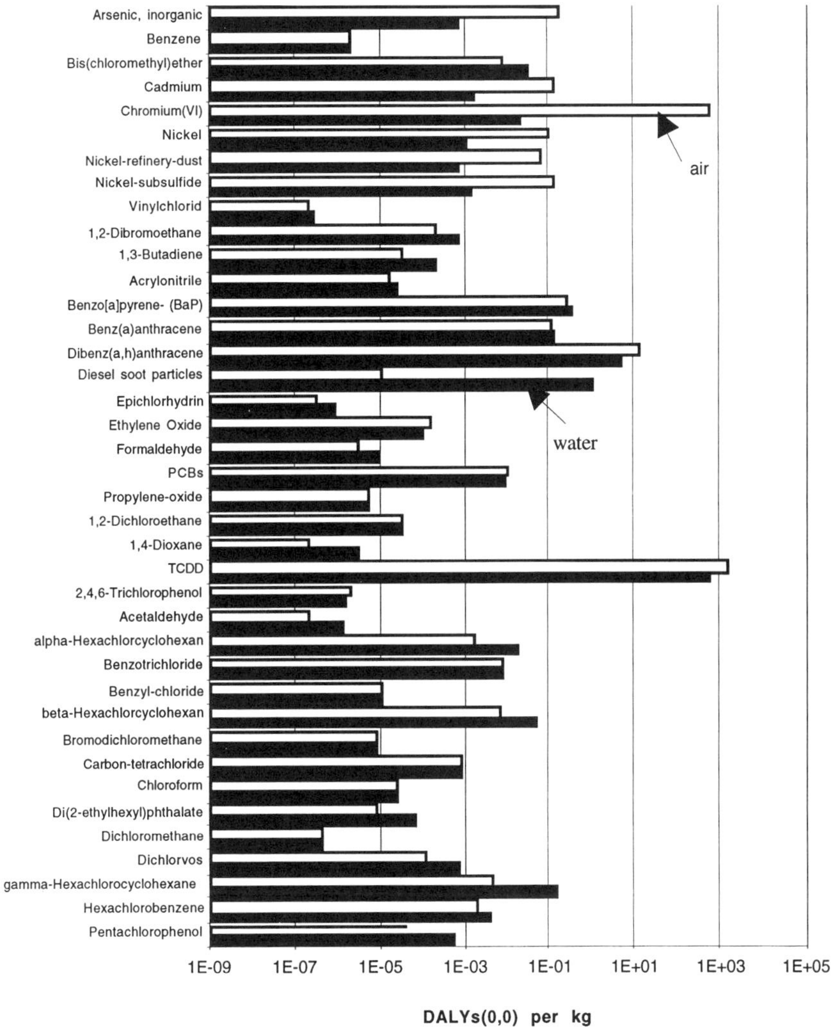

Fig. 9.2: Damage factors for emissions to air and water leading to carcinogenic effects in human beings plotted for the hierarchist's perspective.

However, the yearly emissions of the listed substances vary by many orders of magnitude as well. Emissions into air in 1990 in Europe were 300'000 t/a for benzene and 0.11t/a for dioxins (UBA/TNO 1997). This is a difference of six orders of magnitude. The potential steady-state damages due to environmental carcinogenics in Europe can be assessed by a simple multiplication of the damage factors with the European emissions. Such an extrapolation has been made in Appendix (9.1) and the results are presented in Figure 9.3. These results have to be regarded with caution. They are calculated by taking the mean of the damage factors for the egalitarian perspective and the emissions are rough estimates or adaptations from sources in the available literature. An estimate for the squared geometric standard deviation factor for the emission estimates may well be about $\sigma_g^2 = 10$. All substances for which no emission estimate could be found have been omitted from the table of results in Appendix (6.16). The substances in Figure 9.3 for which no bar is visible have a total damage that is too small to be shown within the resolution of the figure.

Only eight of the 28 substances included are responsible for over 98% of the total DALYs per year due to carcinogenic effects caused by environmental factors. About 80% of the DALYs are caused by heavy metals, precisely those substances for which the estimated contributions are based on preliminary fate models. There are two interpretations for this dominance of heavy metals:

- The best estimates of damage factors used for the heavy metals are in reality too high due to an inappropriate fate modelling[6] and inappropriate extrapolations for oral slope factors[7].
- The high persistence of the heavy metals (and also of the dioxins and of carbon-tetrachloride) leads to very high exposure when steady state modelling is used, i.e., integration over an infinitely long time horizon is assumed.

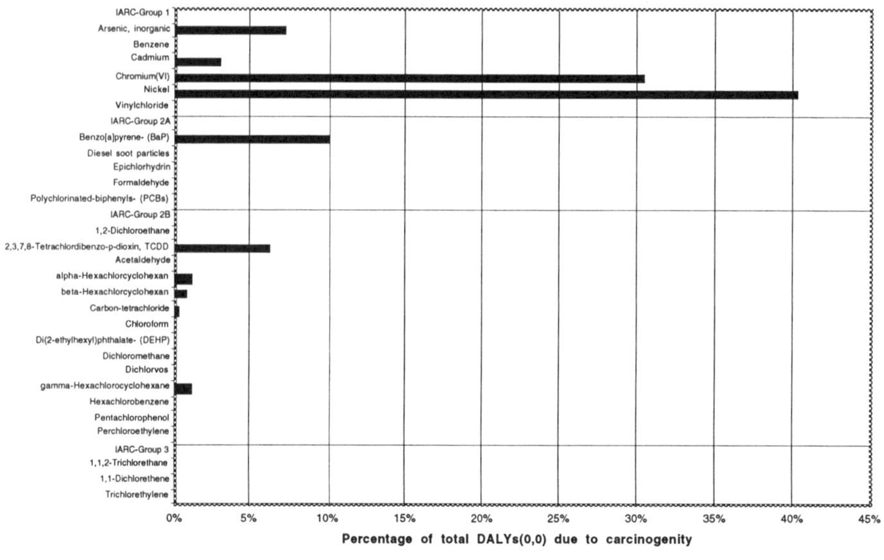

Fig. 9.3: Contributions of the selected carcinogenic substances to the total European damage to human health due to air emissions causing carcinogenic effects. Damage factors for the egalitarian perspective, data from Appendix (9.1).

[6] As discussed in Section 6.2, the fate model that has been used has not been designed for modelling heavy metals. Fate and exposure are therefore highly uncertain.

[7] Potential extrapolation factors were introduced in Subsection 6.3.6 to estimate the unit risk factors for oral intake for a long list of substances.

The damage factors would have to be corrected accordingly if the fate modelling or/and the extrapolation prove to lead to an overestimation. However, if the second interpretation holds true, then the results presented in Figure 9.3 are a very important finding. The importance of carcinogenic damages due to persistent substances would, in this case, have been underestimated so far because extrapolations are mainly based on actual environmental concentrations instead of integrating the damages over a time horizon that is similar to the immobilisation time of the substances.

The total amount of around 2.7 million DALYs per year in Europe (Appendix 9.1) can be compared with the roughly 18 million DALYs due to carcinogenic effects in Europe[8]. Between 1%-5% of the cancer cases are caused by environmental pollution (Doll *et al.* 1981) which adds up to between 0.18 and 0.9 million DALYs. Our best estimate is 3 to 15 times higher than this number from the literature. The interpretation given above suggests that the literature data underestimates the integrated damages. In order to improve the reliability of our own estimates, it would be necessary to improve the fate modelling by making use of more appropriate fate models and by reviewing the estimated slope factors for oral intake.

Respiratory effects

The damage factors presented in Subsection 7.5.3 are summarised in Figure 9.4 (without lower and upper confidence interval) for the three active perspectives identified by Cultural Theory. The main message of this figure is that primary and secondary particles are the dominant causal factors. Hydrocarbons and carbon monoxide do not contribute to particle formation. Their damage factors are therefore very small and do not show up in Figure 9.4 due to the limited resolution of that figure. The numbers for individualists are lower because they apply age-weighting (years lost at high age are less serious than when lost at a middle age) and because they think that the evidence for some causal relationships is too weak to be considered by them as establishing causality in the first place.

In Figure 9.5 we present for respiratory effects an extrapolation to Europe assuming an egalitarian perspective as we have done for carcinogenic substances. The findings from Figure 9.4 are confirmed here. Primary particles and substances forming secondary particles are the dominant cause of respiratory effects with a combined share of more than 98%. Secondary particles together appear to be more important than primary particles alone, a finding which would be altered with an individualistic perspective. Individualists do not consider as causal the relation between nitrates and respiratory effects.

Figure 9.5 is based on Table 7.21. The best estimate for total DALYs is 6.1 millions DALYs per year. Murray *et al.* (1996a) calculated for the established market economies a yearly loss of DALYs of about 160 millions. Again, it is assumed that about 62.5% of these DALYs can be attributed to Europe. This makes that the respiratory effects calculated in the extrapolation have a share of about 6%. Considering the high share of respiratory diseases as a cause of death (Section 5.2), this calculated percentage appears to be reasonable. The upper estimates of 146

[8] It is assumed that 62.5% of the 29 million DALYs lost per year in established market economies due to carcinogenic effects reported by Murray *et al.* (1996a) occur in Europe.

million DALYs per year presented in Table 7.21 is obviously to high, i.e., it should not be used within the damage assessment.

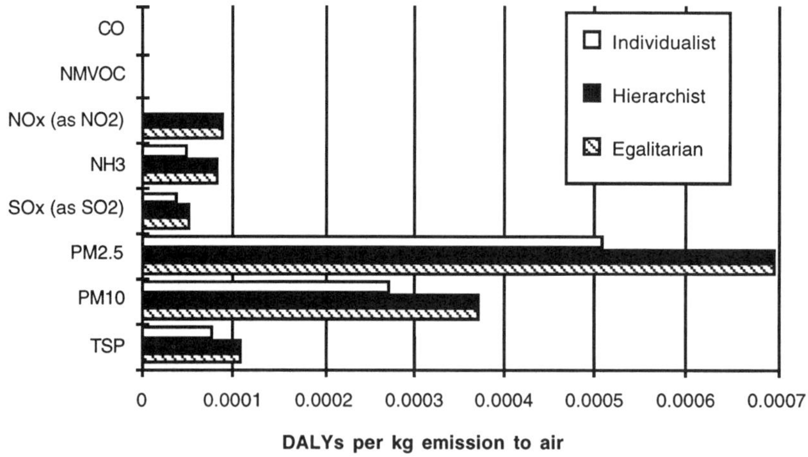

Fig. 9.4: Damage factors for emissions to air leading to respiratory effects in human beings plotted for all three active perspectives. The values for CO are zero for individualists and hierarchists and those for NMVOC are non-zero but small.

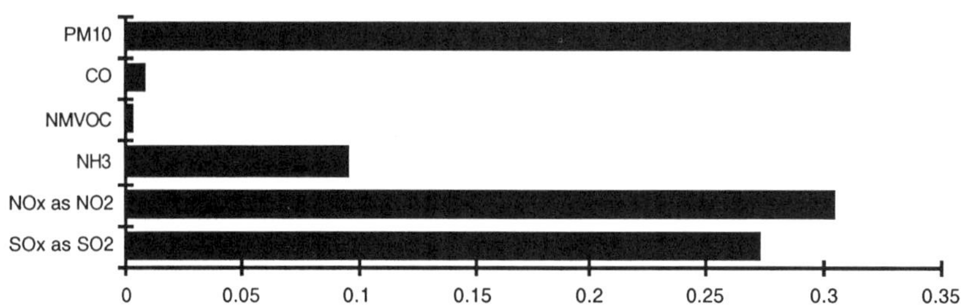

Fig. 9.5: Contributions of single substances to the total European damage to human health due to air emissions causing respiratory effects [-]. Damage factors for the egalitarian perspective, data from Table 7.21.

The analysis of this case study allows the formulation of two recommendations for the inventory analysis:

- Emissions of particles have to be inventoried with a high priority and should be measured either as PM2.5 or PM10. Reliable damage assessments are possible only once such measurements become available (see Berdowski *et al.* (1997) for a first data base).
- It is advisable to differentiate between summer and winter time emissions of hydrocarbons and of NOx because of their potential to contribute to the formation of summer smog. The damage factors listed in Appendix (7.4) assume that this

differentiation cannot be made, i.e., only half of the damage slope in summer is assumed as average for the yearly average.

These recommendations may have a decisive influence on the result of product comparisons if particles of different sizes are emitted in alternative life cycles and if summer smog is a decisive impact mechanism and seasonal differences for the emissions exist. This is the case, for example, for heating systems that run primarily in winter while air conditioning is used primarily in summer during potential smog days.

Comparisons

If one compares the results for carcinogenic effects (Appendix 6.16) with the results for respiratory effects (Appendix 7.4), some additional insights are worth to be noted:

- Looking at them on an European scale and accepting the extrapolations made for Figures 9.3 and 9.5 that are based on Appendix (9.1) and Table 7.21, we see that the importance of the persistent carcinogenics such as heavy metals and dioxins (with the exception of benzo(a)pyrene) lies in the range of the damages due to respiratory effects of ammonia. All other carcinogenics have effects that are comparable to the damages due to respiratory effects of single hydrocarbons. Ranking the substances from high to low results in the following order of importance: primary particles, secondary particles, persistent carcinogenics plus benzo(a)pyrene, other hydrocarbons.
- The best estimate for the effects from cancer due to the emission of 1 kg diesel soot particle is 9.8 E-6 DALYs(0,0). The impact from respiratory effects due to the emission of 1 kg PM2.5 (that is closest to diesel soot) is 7 E-4 or about 100 times higher. Diesel soot is even smaller than 2.5 μm and may present an even higher respiratory risk. This means that the only relevant effects for particles are the ones on the respiratory system; the cancer risk can be neglected. The problem of counting respiratory effects and cancer cases twice, for instance in the case of diesel soot particles, is therefore negligibly small.
- This situation is different for many of the hydrocarbons. The indirect respiratory effects from the formation of ozone (Appendix 7.4) are, in general, of the same order of magnitude as the cancer risks listed in Appendix (6.16). For benzene and chloroform, carcinogenity is the dominant effect, but for acetaldehyde and trichlorethene it's respiratory effect. For formaldehyde, about 25% of the health effect is due to respiratory effects and 75% due to carcinogenity. Both effects therefore have to be considered.
- One can assume that many of the carcinogenic effects will show up in the distant future because of the accumulation of persistent substances in the biota. It is therefore important to notice that the carcinogenic effects will, on average, show up much later than the respiratory ones in the case of both categories of substances being emitted now.

Tab. 7.21 and Appendix (9.1) show that the actual total number of DALYs in Europe, based on the best estimates for the damage factors and European emissions, amount to about 8.8 million DALYs which is about 5 to 10% of the total DALYs due to all causes[9]. This share is in the upper range of estimates from other sources (see Section 5.2). Partly, this higher number results from the comprehensive approach chosen to include all pathways and to assume steady state exposure and is therefore justified. However, the damage factors should be recalculated when new data for the fate, exposure, effect, or damage analyses become available. For the time being, it is advisable to assess potential damages to human health by considering the given lognormal distribution instead of just taking the best estimate.

9.2.2 Index for manageability

The multiplication of the indicators for the 'ease of damage reduction', for 'excess of target damage', and for 'regulatory success' produces the manageability factor. The values for these indicators and for the factor are presented in Figure 9.6.

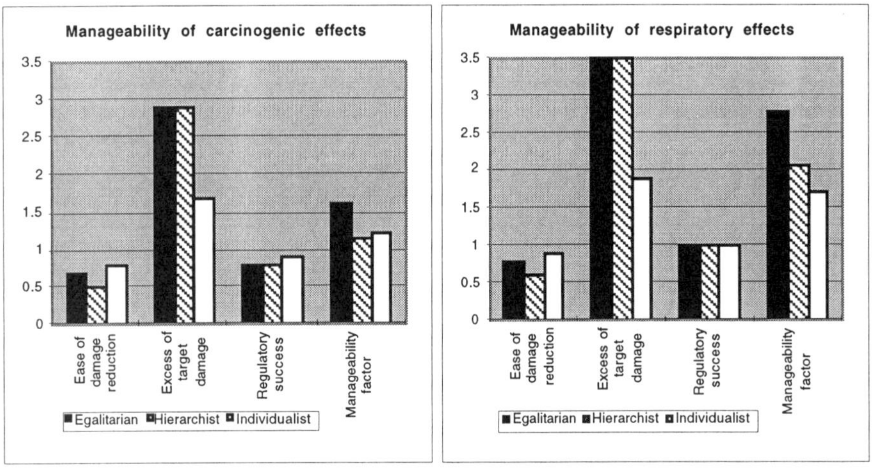

Fig. 9.6: Comparison of the indicators and of the manageability factor for the two case studies of carcinogenic and of respiratory effects for each of the three active cultural perspectives

A comparison of the results for carcinogenic and for respiratory effects reveals a higher manageability for the former (lower values means higher manageability). In addition, we see that the egalitarian perspective scores highest in both cases, but for respiratory diseases, the lowest score is achieved by the individualist perspective while for carcinogenic effects it is the hierarchist that scores lowest. As we lack the possibility to validate these results with actual decision makers, we can only ask if these results seem plausible. In order to answer this question, we have to go back to the individual indicators:

- The two indicators for 'ease of damage reduction' and for 'excess of target damage' dominate the manageability factor for both impact categories.

[9] The number of exposed persons by European emissions was not calculated and the Murray *et al.* (1996a) only give numbers for the established market economies as a total. Therefore, no precise share can be given.

- The indicator for 'ease of damage reduction' does not address the ease of emission reduction, but the easiness with which health damages can be reduced at given background concentrations. The advanced stage of cancer research and the emerging knowledge on suppressers to stop the multistage process of the onset of cancer make it seem plausible that the damage reduction is somewhat larger for carcinogenity than for respiratory effects. However, one could also argue that less research effort has been directed so far towards reducing the consequences of respiratory effects than of carcinogenity and that therefore new insights could be obtained at lower costs in the former than in the latter case. This may be true, but these insights are coming too late for the many persons that are exposed to air pollutants today, at least for all the acute endpoints.
- The indicator for the target damage excess is larger for respiratory effects than for carcinogenity. This is reflected in the death rates that are estimated on the basis of today's emissions to be at least 2 times higher for the former than for the latter. This makes it seem plausible that this indicator is larger for respiratory effects than for carcinogenity.

Adding up the indices of manageability over all the impact categories representing harm to human health will increase the importance of respiratory compared to carcinogenic effects by more for the index of manageability than for the index of magnitude of damage.

It seems plausible that the manageability problems are larger for respiratory effects than for cancer given the structure of the index. However, empirical work with decision makers may reveal that manageability should incorporate the ease of *emission* reduction – excluded from the present version of the index of manageability – if the index is going to be adopted for everyday use. A difference between the intrinsic understanding and meaning of an indicator *and* its effective meaning, implied by its structure, is a serious drawback and a correction may in that case be considered in a further development of the index's structure.

The feasibility of constructing the index has been demonstrated at the price of having had to make rough estimates. The plausibility of the comparison with the index of manageability of carcinogenity is apparent if one argues on the level of single indicators. The problems that arise due to the difference between the everyday meaning of manageability and the meaning given to this concept in this study have, however, at least been identified.

9.2.3 Final remarks

It was stated in the introduction to this section that the selection of cases was a lucky choice thanks to the wide array of available information. However, the applicability of the damage assessment is not restricted to the cases chosen for the Chapters 6 and 7. Studies estimating damage costs due to environmental interventions have included many more causal relationships than have been considered here and may therefore serve as a valuable starting point for the operationalisation of the submodel of the ecosphere of known damage (ExternE 1997, ESEERCO 1995).

The list of references given in Appendix (9.2) is a good starting point for such an operationalisation. Additional useful information is available in books on environmental medicine and in databases that are increasingly made available directly on the Internet[10].

Readers which are primarily interested in the use of the data derived in Chapters 6 and 7 should keep in mind, that:

- The inventory analysis should, whenever possible, differentiate between different particle sizes and report diesel soot, PM2.5, PM10, and TSP separately.
- Emissions of NOx and VOCs do not cause the same damages in summer as in winter time. If they occur especially in winter *or* in summer time, then this information should be provided by the inventory analysis.
- Due to the many assumptions required and the estimates made to calculate the damage factors (average European conditions, approximate fate modelling, extrapolated effect data, estimated damage data), it is essential that the damage factors are understood as probability distributions rather than single values.

The damage assessment presented here will be extended to other effects and the fate modelling will be updated in the course of the ongoing update of the LCIA method 'EcoIndicator'95' (Goedkoop 1995)[11].

Nothing has been said so far about the operationalisation of the index for unknown damage. Indeed, Table 4.9 in Section 4.4 presents the only attempt to apply the suggested calculation procedure to a first set of substances. For its calculation based on an inventory table resulting from the analysis of a product system, additional data have to be collected or assessed and the calculation procedure has to be interpreted for environmental interventions which do not yet fit the assumptions made. The contribution to the index of unknown damage has to be calculated for each environmental intervention independent from the fact that its damages may also be included in the index for known damage.

[10] No addresses are provided here due to the fast development of this area and the frequent change of addresses. Valuable starting bases are the homepages of the European Environmental Agency (EEA) [http://www.eea.dk] and the U.S. Environmental Protection Agency (EPA) [http://www.epa.gov].

[11] Information on the publication of results will become available on http://www.pré.nl.

9.3 Evaluation of the framework

9.3.1 Evaluation criteria

The evaluation of frameworks is largely dependent on the goals to be satisfied by this framework, but it is dangerous to evaluate one's own framework with one's own list of criteria. For this reason we will not use the comprehensive list of criteria and requirements defined in Hofstetter (1996b:134f), but choose instead a list which had been developed for the evaluation of environmental impact assessment tools with respect to their applicability as decision support. Hyman *et al.* (1988:158) defined seven evaluation criteria for this purpose (Table 9.1).

	Less preferable	**More preferable**
	Attributes of natural systems:	
1.	Treats impacts as deterministic	Explicitly recognises risk probabilities
2.	Examines direct effects only	Examines indirect and feedback effects in addition to direct effects
3.	Assumes relationships are static	Considers dynamic aspects or changes in relationships over time
	Characteristics of planning and of decision-making attributes	
4.	Emphasises a single objective	Adopts a multiple-objective approach
5.	Blurs facts and values	Clearly separates facts from values
6.	Relies on expert judgements only	Encourages public participation
7.	Uses money, time, and resources inefficiently	Uses money, time, and resources efficiently

Tab. 9.1. Evaluation criteria for environmental impact assessment tools (Hyman *et al.* 1988:158)

The relevance of these criteria for the evaluation of LCA models will be discussed in the next subsection together with the results from using these criteria to judge the framework proposed in this book. For the moment, however, it is important to see that criterion 7 conflicts with most other criteria and that the preference for more complexity (criteria 2,3, and 4) will make public participation more difficult (criterion 6).

9.3.2 Application of the criteria

The evaluation of the framework based on the criteria listed in Table 9.1 will be given here criterion by criterion. The question of the criterion's importance for LCA will be addressed at the same time.

1. This first criterion is important for all environmental tools because causal relationships in natural systems are probabilistic. The damage assessments presented in Chapters 6 and 7 fulfil this requirement.

2. LCA as such is concerned with indirect effects and LCIA should therefore fulfil this requirement as well. The framework fulfils this criterion to a large extent thanks to an extended fate modelling that includes the secondary formation of toxics. The consideration of feedback is limited due to the limited scientific knowledge that is available.

3. The possibilities to consider dynamic aspects in LCA are very limited due to the compressed way LCA deals with time. However, the submodel of the 'manageability' of the ecosphere is an attempt to complement the merely static modelling with change-oriented information.

4. The requirement hidden behind the fourth criterion was initially thought to be irrelevant when developing the framework. To the contrary, the aim was to end up with as few incommensurable indices as possible. The set of indices offered here and the multi-objective approach chosen can be expected to fit well with strategic and regulatory decision processes. However, a single objective might be more appropriate for the use of LCA in daily product design and improvement. It is essential to recognise that the structured aggregation procedure offers information on all levels. It can therefore be seen as a transparent multi-objective approach that contains guidance on the composition and the aggregation of this information.

5. Criterion five is only partly met – and this on purpose. Value choices are made transparent wherever they occur and Cultural Theory has been used to explicitly consider the world views of different archetypes. However, the framework has not been split into a part dealing with facts and another one dealing with values. Facts and values are – after making them explicit – both integrated within the models.

6. So far, the framework relies on expert judgements only and it therefore scores low on this sixth criterion. However, the framework with its structured aggregation procedure can be validated and challenged by involvement of potential decision makers. However, the complexity of the framework may discourage decision makers from participating in such an effort.

7. The question of efficiency can only be answered when the increase in insight is be compared with the effort needed to gain it. It is still too early for such a final assessment. However, two aspects should be kept in mind: the LCA analysts will not need more time for the impact assessment once the framework is operationalised and computerised than they do today. But they will get more information out of it, and, as already suggested in Section 8.1 and further discussed in Section 9.5, there is a fair chance that the complete development of this tool will allow the development of simplified, but still robust impact assessment systems.

9.3.3 Appraisal

The framework developed in this book fits rather well with the criteria developed earlier for a similar purpose. However, this self-confirmation should be judged critically. The suggested framework is a kind of Rolls-Royce and its operationalisation may need many compromises that could weaken its strength.

The main advantage compared to other methods is that different model philosophies are integrated and can be weighted according to the decision makers' world view and management style. The framework presented here introduces even more sophistication at a time when many LCA analysts and decision makers ask for simplified and streamlined methodologies. However, we are convinced that this higher degree of sophistication is either needed for a reliable decision support tool or necessary to be able to later make justified simplifications with known consequences.

9.4 Validation and empirical work

This section will provide no validation and present no results of empirical work, but discuss their position and the future need for validation and empirical work.

9.4.1 What is the status of the framework and its models?

The question raised in this subsection's title is directed towards the degree of validation and the empirical evidence given for the framework.

A radical and self-critical review could come to the following conclusion:

The framework is based on the author's subjective view of the world and its functioning. In order to hide arbitrariness, an empirically unproven theory has been chosen to represent the wide spectrum of decision makers which themselves have been excluded from its development. The need for three submodels of the ecosphere and especially for those that have been chosen for development is unproven and their combination arbitrary. The models for manageability and for unknown damage can not be validated per se. The model for known damage has been based on models for risk assessment and public health, but the assumptions were chosen in such a way that no actual and observable damages can be modelled. Therefore, the framework is not more than a couple of untested hypotheses and of unverifiable models.

A more friendly review might state:

In the absence of real decision makers, the author acknowledges the value dependence of the framework. The framework is therefore developed not only for the traditional hierarchic standpoint of scientists, but additionally for two other, rather different archetypes, the egalitarians and the individualists. These three perspectives are not invented ad hoc, but are based on Cultural Theory which has already proven itself of use in the past in explaining standpoints and developments. The requirements for the model of the ecosphere have been derived from the published experience in risk perception and empirical work done elsewhere on the weighting of impact scores in the valuation step of LCIA.

The model for the known damage can be built on the basis of available data and models developed and used in other fields of science. Minor adaptations have been necessary to harmonise the models and to bring them in line with the requirements of life-cycle approaches: The damage indicators are based on models of WHO and the World Bank; the fate modelling is based on a widely used system to evaluate new substances, which has been, in the mean time, both adapted and adopted for use as an European standard, and on a dispersion model that is used to inform policy; the effect data is based on information reviewed by governmental organisations and by a large community of health experts; and the results compare reasonably well with other assessments.

The model for unknown damage is based on a thorough review of the available literature. The new proposal is based on adequate reasoning and makes use of information that is or can be made available.

The model to calculate the index of manageability has been developed from scratch. There is no evidence for its validity and reliability besides the arguments made in its favour and the fact that it has been successfully operationalised.

The overall assessment may therefore be phrased as follows: The framework and its models are based, to a large extent, on knowledge and models derived from other fields of science. The testing of the hypotheses that have been used and the validation of value judgements can be done in the course of the further development thanks to the transparent structure of the proposed approach.

Both reviews make it clear that further validation is necessary before the framework can become an important tool in decision support.

9.4.2 Problems of validation

The very constructivistic touch of the whole framework and its use in decision situations as such[12] make a proper validation difficult. Additionally, LCA is used at the micro level and the changes its use brings about are per definition small, i.e., hardly measurable. Furthermore, LCIA is built on a compressed view of time and place. All this makes it impossible to measure changes caused by decisions based on LCA because the decision's effects are spread over time and are difficult to be located.

The arguments in favour of this orientation of LCA have been discussed and mostly settled in Section 1.2 where LCA *sensu stricto* has been defined, but one consequence of those choices is that it is difficult to validate the whole framework by the traditional means of experiments.

The introduction of the submodels for unknown damage and for manageability further increases the problems of validation. The submodel for unknown damage has been introduced in order to assess unknown effects and is therefore, *per se,* untestable. The submodel for manageability is directed to consider damage attributes which influence the perception of the damages including dynamic aspects. Natural scientific experiments will contribute little to the validation of these attributes.

The problems mentioned so far by no means imply that it is impossible to improve the validation of the framework. We suggest proceeding in the following manner:

- that the structure, the arguments in its favour, and the properties to be modelled will be validated by use of panels of decision makers or of representatives of society,
- that the elements used in the submodels for the ecosphere either represent the state-of-the art in the respective sciences or will be validated, and
- that the appropriate elements already approved by national or international bodies will be used.

The first point to improve the framework's validation will be further discussed in the next subsection. The use of validated elements to build the model of the ecosphere

[12] Decision situations are here to change the way things have been working so far. Implementation of decisions will therefore change the "test environment" and lead to new decisions. (This iterative procedure is indicated in Figure 1.3.) Under normal circumstances it is therefore impossible to make an experiment by comparing the world's developments with two different kinds of decisions taken in parallel.

and the use of approved information have already been implemented as far as possible and one should continue further in this direction in the course of the framework's development (see also Subsection 9.4.4).

9.4.3 Replacing the model of the valuesphere with the decision makers' world views

In the absence of decision makers or stakeholder groups, the requirements for decision support systems have been derived from the few experiences with panels in the field of LCIA and the related field of risk perception. The insights gained from these experiences and the modelling philosophy that has been used here, i.e., to describe the same decision support problem from three different points of view encompassing distinct world views and management styles, made it possible to develop a framework without actual interaction with decision makers.

This elegant solution to work with hypothetical archetypes rather than real persons helped in finding a structure that may be of value to a range of different stakeholder groups and decision makers. However, the translation within the framework's structure of the archetypical views into value choices should be validated by real decision makers. This validation should start with the meaning and the nature of the three submodels of the ecosphere and should later proceed to the details of the submodels used. A first example for the validation at the level of submodels is given in Appendix (4). The appropriateness of the indicators that have been chosen for manageability and the concrete attribution of parameters assumed to be dependent on the cultural perspective have to be evaluated as well.

The idea to present three systems for impact assessment should be adhered to at least in the first phase of the validation. It should be tested whether it is indeed possible to find subgroups of decision makers which are attracted most by one of the three systems. In a next step, one could then see whether these groups have the characteristics that are predicted by Cultural Theory. If they do, it is important to form a kind of focus groups because individuals may come up with inconsistent answers if they change their social context during the empirical study (Subsection 3.2.4).

Cultural Theory as the initial model for the valuesphere may better be dropped if one of two developments occur during its validation: (i) the grouping suggested by Cultural Theory cannot be found within the chosen groups of decision makers or of stakeholder representatives; or (ii) their identification with one of the three formulations of the model turns out to be weak. In both of these cases, Cultural Theory can be said to have been helpful for building such a three-layered model, but can now be dropped for guiding its refinement and validation by real decision makers. But decision makers that nonetheless feel comfortable with one of the three shapes of the framework have the leeway in this case to define their own labels for the modelling paths. The pre-settings for the value choices can then be validated by these decision makers, either through anonymous panel procedures or in focus groups.

For the time being, it is assumed that the large range of decision makers and stakeholder groups will prefer the split into three perspective-dependent models proposed here rather than one consensus model. This assumption is based on the observation that very different methods have been developed (Section 8.3) and that no consensus has emerged so far on what is the most appropriate method.

9.4.4 Legitimation and scientific character

Many of the elements suggested in this book will not be accessible to verification/ falsification as shown by the epistemological foundation touched upon in Subsection 1.2.2 and the simplifying modelling assumption required for LCA *sensu stricto* and summarised in Subsection 1.2.6. However, most of the little pieces that are put together to form the proposed framework are elements that have been verified within the sciences from where they originate.

The less a framework can be validated by classical empirical methods the more important its legitimating and scientific character becomes. Legitimation of a tool for decision support is achieved best if it is fully worked out and definitely approved by both governmental and non-governmental organisations and used by companies. However, the framework is not yet developed to that point. One can therefore look out for the legitimation of sub-elements and the support of the provisional framework by researchers. The elements used and further developed within the damage assessment are either already used by national and international organisations like EPA, Worldbank, and WHO, or they are commissioned for further development by, e.g., the Dutch government that finances the update of the Eco-Indicator method (Goedkoop *et al.* 1997). The European Commission supports projects to develop and apply damage assessment and uses their results (ExternE 1997, IER/ETSU/EdM 1997). The close relationship between many of the elements and established risk assessment procedures additionally increases the legitimation of the damage assessment. Even the more speculative elements such as the model for unknown damage are already partly supported by recent governmental statements (see, e.g., Anonymous 1997).

The support given by researchers to at least individual elements of the framework has been ascertained through extensive discussions and appropriate review procedures, both of which are documented by the acknowledgements recorded in the preface. The framework has also been presented and discussed at international congresses. This generated support, in principal, of this work and has already begun to influence future research in LCIA.

The scientific quality will be assured – although the falsification by experiments is missing – by consistent deduction, careful evaluation and comparison of methods that are available for use as elements of the framework, and by checks and verifications with real world data wherever appropriate. Finally, the explicit and pragmatic (reductionistic) nature of the book's suggestions are a sign of scientific quality in itself.

This positive evaluation of the legitimation for the framework and its scientific position should not divert attention from the fact that only its future operationalisation by science and its extensive use for decision support will be able to generate a high degree of legitimation and allow for (and justify) further research to improve the scientific qualities of its elements and the framework as a whole. Especially the link of the valuesphere with the ecosphere is based solely on the author's interpretation of empirical studies carried out within other contexts. This link therefore has to be replaced in the future, using a more appropriate procedure (see previous subsection).

9.5 Dependent or not? – Consequences

Here we will think about the consequences the proposed framework has for the decision maker. Will decision makers indeed have to chose one of the perspectives and to specify their weighting quadruple in the tetrahedron as suggested in Figure 9.1? Or, will the observation concerning the dependence of the indices made at several places in Chapter 8 lead to a much simpler assessment system?

The second possibility should be taken seriously because there are arguments in favour of some kind of dependence and because this would be a way to satisfy a need of decision makers for a simplified or streamlined life cycle assessment. The arguments in favour of this hypothesis of dependency are the following:

- For the time being, all three perspectives base their assessments on the same inventory analysis. Several entries in the inventory table are already dependent, e.g., use of fossil energies and CO_2 emissions.
- The indices for known damage to human health and to ecological health are dependent because they are based on the same inventory table and use the same fate modelling. In addition, toxicological data relevant for human toxicity is sometimes extrapolated from laboratory tests with animals. These may be used for ecotoxicity as well and may therefore be partly dependent. The input- and the output-oriented environmental interventions listed in the inventory table are dependent as mentioned in the previous point. Therefore, the damage indicators for human and for ecological health may well depend on the indicator for resource use.
- The proxy for unknown damage again starts with the same inventory table. If the known damage due to substances is approximately proportional to the unknown damage, and if the chosen model for unknown damage reflects this, then the proxy is dependent on the index for known damage.
- The index for manageability is partly based on the index for known damage. Although the manageability factor is independent from the index for known damage, it may not be discriminant enough to counteract this dependence of the two indices.
- If all indices are dependent on each other and if the product alternatives show different environmental performances, then one can expect a stable and robust ranking of the alternatives, i.e., one of the alternatives will dominate all others in all respects. In that case, the weighting of known *versus* unknown damages becomes unimportant and the cultural perspective behind this choice is obsolete.

If this chain of arguments holds up, the decision support would be very stable because it would mean that just one product alternative dominates the others. Further work could then be directed towards finding that index (or proxy) which still allows for a stable result, but requires a minimal effort for the inventory analysis. This is the basis for the drive to develop simplified or streamlined LCA methodologies.

However, most of these arguments are just hypotheses until they are tested. The following arguments suggest that such tests will reveal a high dependence on the cultural perspective applied:

- In the completely worked out framework the inventory analysis as well will be based on cultural perspectives and thus would provide three distinct inventory tables.
- The damage indicators are again dependent on the cultural perspective. While some of the perspectives take as a given the causality for some substances, others deny that these substances cause damage due to a lack of evidence for the existence of a relation. The suggested dependence of emissions on resource use may hold true for fossil energy, but not for all the other resources.
- The proxy for unknown damage is constructed in such a way that it is not also a proxy for the known damage. It is especially the weighting by the reciprocal value of the total anthropogenic and geogenic emissions that prevents such a dependency.
- It may be that the independent elements of the index for manageability, i.e., the ease of damage reduction and the success of regulation, will average out over the different environmental problems which are added-up. But even in this case the cultural dependency of the index will be maintained.
- If the indices are not dependent on each other, then one can expect to encounter real cases where more than one product alternative dominates the others depending on the weighting of the indices used. The magnitudes of the indices will be different for each cultural perspective for all but for the proxy of unknown damage. Therefore, it can be assumed that the dominance spaces in the tetrahedron are shaped differently for each cultural perspective, i.e., not only the weightings of the indices, but also the dominance spaces as such will differ from each other.

In the absence of empirical support for the dependency hypothesis, we should be ready to accept that the ranking of alternatives is dependent on the cultural perspective, i.e., in general, no inter-perspective dominance of one alternative can be expected.

In this general case, decision makers either have to make an explicit selection of the perspective(s) relevant for their decision or they will have to work out alternatives which are not dominated. The solution of choice is, of course, that products can be improved in such a way that afterwards they score best on all criteria.

This other function of LCA, i.e., to improve products instead of just comparing them with competing alternatives has so far been overlooked in this discussion. The LCA of a product is dominated in many cases by energy transformation and transport processes which may show a high interdependence between, e.g., damages to human health and to ecological health. However, the improvement assessment may well identify other processes to show the best cost-benefit ratio, e.g., the replacement of the solvent in paintings or the optimised use of pesticides. This points out that there probably exist a large number of processes which score either primarily on the damage to human health or to ecological health. This is an important argument to stay with all the indices suggested in Section 4.6 and that a relative weighting of these indices is necessary to prevent a shift of problems from one safeguard subject to another. The assessment of product improvements will therefore be dependent on the world view applied, i.e., it may well come up with perspective dependent assessments.

But is it really such a problem if decision makers have to choose one perspective? Living in a country with a tradition of direct democracy suggests that the answer is a resounding no. To belong to or to sympathise with a political party can be compared to the task of selecting one cultural perspective as basis for the decision support. Being attracted by a group or being member of a group means, to some extent, that decisions are made together and that one adopts the group's perspective on these decisions. The existence of fashions may be taken as another example for the ease with which we adopt distinct perspectives.

Boards of companies sometimes explicitly choose a certain company image which is also reflected in the type of products sold and the way they are advertised or they set down company guidelines which are supposed to help individual employees to act in accordance with the company's philosophy. In most cases, the dominance of one cultural perspective is not made explicit, but can be assessed from looking at the company structure, the type of persons employed and promoted, or the way a company behaves in its contacts with citizens and the government.

Therefore, a final unproven hypothesis is that decision makers, regardless of whether consumers, designers, or managers, usually know quite well what (mix of) cultural perspective(s) best fits the decision at hand and its context[13].

It is a big step forward to accept that not only decisions, but also decision support is policy driven and that the differences in world views and management styles justify different decisions.

[13] An important question in this case is whether environmental assessments need a higher level of legitimation than the decision makers' view. It may be more appropriate to ask authoritative bodies to do the assessment as environmental effects do not primarily concern the decision makers as such, but rather society as a whole. Throughout this book we have assumed that LCA is used voluntarily as decision support. Decision makers using LCA seem therefore concerned that environmental aspects are reflected in decision making. It is the decision makers' perception influenced by their world views which guides the selection of criteria and their assessment. This is not different from the selection of other criteria relevant in the decision making. This freedom of individual perception therefore also has to be catered to when it comes to the selection of environmental criteria.

10 Conclusions

10.1 The perspectives

The book's main title 'Perspectives in Life Cycle Impact Assessment' had been chosen because of the many meanings in which the concept of perspectives is appearing in and made use of in this book:

- *The LCA-perspective of the world:* LCA has a very special view of the world. Its aim is to reduce the environmental damages per service gained from products, i.e., to improve the environmental efficiency of the processes in the technosphere. But in trying to do so, hardly any temporal and spatial resolution is provided, i.e., past, present, and future impacts are compressed and treated as if they would occur today and spatial differentiation is avoided by assuming a unit world approximated in our case by average parameter values for the whole of Western Europe. This way of dealing with time and place enables the tool to analyse environmental interventions of product systems and their impacts over the whole product life cycle.

  The LCIA-perspective assumes that the environmental interventions will cause changes in the ecosphere which, if they influence representative characteristics of the ecosphere that are called 'safeguard subjects', are assessed as damages. The safeguard subjects have been chosen as the measuring endpoints although their change will in turn cause alterations in the ecosphere and influence the state of other safeguard subjects.
- *The perspective of three spheres:* In this book, LCA is understood as the art of modelling and combining the valuesphere, the ecosphere, and the technosphere. This new perspective was adopted in order to better understand the weaknesses of the present approach and to gain a platform on which to structure further developments at the same time. The definition of the three spheres has not been informed by a wish to separate subjective from objective elements or to purge strong value judgement from science – something that seems to be the case for many other authors. The main purpose behind this approach is a wish to give all three spheres the same position and to focus on their integration, composition, and linkage.
- *The cultural perspectives:* Cultural Theory has been chosen in Chapter 3 as the theory to model the valuesphere. Cultural Theory identifies five viable ways of life, calling them cultural perspectives. Only three of them are relevant in decision making given the make-up of their adherents – called archetypes, i.e., the individualists, the egalitarians, and the hierarchists. Fatalists do not believe in their power to change things through decisions and hermits are a very small group which excludes itself from decision making. These three active cultural perspectives and their archetypes' world views and management styles are used throughout the book wherever value choices and judgements had to be made. A specific impact assessment system has been developed for each of the three archetypes, at

least in principle. However, the framework has been designed in such a way that the three impact assessment systems fit into the same structure.

This procedure of a threefold modelling is motivated by the possibility of arriving at impact assessment systems where the value choices inherent in assessment are made compatible with the world views and management styles of a small number of archetypes.

- *The perspectives for future developments:* This book offers a comprehensive, but not readily applicable method for impact assessment in LCA. It does identify perspectives on where to go from here by opening up the playing field for more than one model of the ecosphere. The three submodels suggested here open up new possibilities for further developments and proposals for their further operationalisation have been made. This means concretely that the impact assessment of environmental interventions can be based on their causal damages, a proxy for unknown damages, or dynamic aspects called 'manageability' in this book. Such a threefold structure not only offers new perspectives on the understanding and the positioning of developments in LCIA up till now, but also on the requirements for methods to be developed in the future.

While the LCA-perspective mentioned as a first point provides the frame for the developments, the perspective of three spheres opens the possibilities for new developments. The cultural perspective can be seen as one element of the offered solution and the fourth perspective looks to the future. These four interrelated perspectives are important elements of the new framework which has been developed in order to solve the main problems identified in Chapter 2 which will be re-evaluated in Section 10.4.

10.2 Propositions revisited

Five propositions had been stated and justified in Section 2.2. We admitted already then that a verification of all of them will not be possible on the basis of the research that we have presented here. In this section, we will discuss each proposition and check whether it is supported by the data and discussion presented in Chapters 3 through 9 or if it has to be adapted or even withdrawn.

1. *The combination of models for the three spheres – technosphere, ecosphere and valuesphere – and their interfaces form the LCA tool.*

The verification of this proposition is difficult because it has the character of a definition. In Chapter 3 we explored why the valuesphere and its modelling is a decisive element in LCA and a prerequisite for defining and modelling both the eco- and the technosphere. Cultural Theory, as a basis to model the valuesphere, was not chosen only because of its ability to capture values through its grid/group analysis, but also because of the predictions it makes about world views and management styles. These are the two elements which form the interfaces between, and thus enable the linkage of, the spheres. The three submodels that have been used to model the ecosphere meet the requirements that the archetypes attribute to them and that have been identified in the valuesphere. The modelling of the technosphere has not been a subject of this book. A set of principles to be followed for it in "our" LCA *sensu stricto* has nonetheless been given in Subsection 1.2.6 and detailed model descriptions of the technosphere can be found in Frischknecht *et al.* (1994), Heijungs (1994c), Heijungs (1998), and Frischknecht (1998). While the outcome of the modelling, the so-called inventory table, provides the required interface with the ecosphere, the model of the technosphere itself is not yet embedded in the valuesphere to the extent that seems desirable. We have given some examples in Section 8.2 where such a harmonisation is needed and how it could be done.

To conclude, one can say that two of the three spheres have been modelled here and the interfaces between all spheres could be established.

2. *The potential damages due to substances causing carcinogenic and respiratory effects in human beings can be assessed by a structured multi-step approach. The damage can be expressed in the same unit for all substances and can be assessed in a site-independent manner.*

The character of this second proposition is more akin to a feasibility claim. The basis to verify this claim has laid with the introduction of an index to measure damage to human health. Disability adjusted life years (DALYs) have been identified to fulfil the many requirements for such a measurement. They could easily be adapted to the limitations set by LCA (Chapter 5). Section 4.3 and Chapters 6 and 7 set up a methodology similar to the state-of-the art in calculating damage costs and in risk assessment. The causal chain from emissions, via fate, exposure, effect to damage has been modelled as a multi-step procedure making use of theories, models, and data developed or provided by such disciplines as environmental chemistry, toxicology and preventive medicine. Two examples in the form of carcinogenic and respiratory effects were chosen to demonstrate, for a total of more than 150 substances, how these damage factors could be calculated. The chosen examples are characterised by a comfortable data availability and negligible threshold behaviour.

For other mechanisms, less data may be available or more sophisticated averaging may be necessary to calculate generic damage factors. This last remark is relevant because site-independent damage factors were calculated. However, it was assumed that the emission and receptor sites show meteorological conditions and population densities comparable to those conditions found on average in Western Europe. Different population densities, especially, would lead to damage factors much different from those calculated and this is important where mainly non-urban areas are concerned.

In summary, it can be said that the feasibility claim can be met quite well by the comprehensive modelling undertaken in Chapters 5 through 7 and their results.

3. *Decision makers like to be informed not only about results of the damage assessment, but prefer to get complementary information through other indices for attributes of known and unknown damage.*

This third proposition can not be verified in the absence of empirical work with decision makers, something which could not be undertaken thus far. However, empirical evidence from risk analysis and research in risk perception support this proposition (Fischhoff *et al.* 1978, Slovic *et al.* 1980/1983, Marris *et al.* 1996b). They support the need for damage attributes. There is also some evidence from within LCA for this proposition. An expert panel on the weighting of environmental problems has revealed that criteria other than harm steer experts' valuation (Kortman *et al.* 1994). The very different kind of methods which have been developed so far for LCIA are an additional indirect support for this proposition (see Figure 8.7).

No empirical support has been added here to verify the proposition, but the one that is available provides strong evidence in favour of the statement. The three submodels of the ecosphere developed in this book are a response to this need of decision makers .

4. *The plurality of methods in LCIA and the attitude towards LCA in decision making are caused by different properties of the value perspectives and are due to different intentions in modelling.*

Again no empirical work supports this proposition. However, in Section 8.3 the methods that are available for LCIA could be placed within the three submodels that have been used to model the ecosphere. In Chapter 3 and Section 4.6 it had been claimed that the importance of these three submodels depends on the world view adopted, i.e., on the value perspective. A first analytical proof for the origin of methodological pluralism within LCIA could be provided if the existence of this relation between value perspectives and the differing importance placed on submodels could be shown empirically. The attitudes towards LCA in decision making had been studied earlier by Beentjes *et al.* (1995) and Mengel Jørgensen (1996) and they provide some initial empirical evidence for the existence of this relation.

Many elements can be adduced in favour of this proposition. However, we have not verified all its elements and therefore have not yet verified it.

5. *If LCA is developed and performed based on distinctly different value perspectives, this will significantly influence its recommendations for product development and improvement as well as in comparative assertions.*

This last proposition deals with the consequences of the differentiation between, and of the grouping of, world views that has been introduced into LCIA and points to the implications of this way of proceeding for the modelling of the ecosphere. Section 9.5 has directly addressed this question. The arguments there were that

- supporting empirically the dependence of the decision support on the cultural perspectives and the importance of the submodels for the ecosphere requires a final operationalisation and quantification of the framework according to Figure 4.10 and its application to a large number of cases,
- it may well be that the indices for the three safeguard subjects and the indices for the submodels for unknown damage and manageability depend much more on each other than has been assumed so far because they are all linked to the same inventory table[14] and are partly based on the same toxicity tests, and
- this dependence leads to the same ranking order for all the indices suggested, thus making cultural differences irrelevant for the ranking of product alternatives.

This third point – in fact the opposite to Proposition (5) – cannot, as of yet, be grounded in sufficient empirical work. An attempt to verify/falsify this proposition has to be postponed until a sufficient number of cases have been assessed under the new framework. However, the usefulness of the approach as such, as it has been proposed here, does not have to be questioned even if this fifth proposition will be falsified. The approach proposed is the only way to consistently evaluate such dependencies and to produce sets of compatible value choices within the assessment. But, after a falsification, it would be possible to work out simplified/streamlined methods which could work with proxies that have been proven to generate a robust ranking of alternatives. From Section 9.5 it is clear that Proposition (5) may well hold for product development and improvement, but less for the comparative assertion.

In summarising, we can state that there are arguments that suggest that the proposition could be falsified for product comparisons. But the framework proposed here would, in this case, have proven its worth by making falsification possible and thus laid a sound starting basis for the development of screening and streamlined LCAs.

It has been made clear already in Section 2.2 that a verification of the five propositions was going to be impossible because the empirical work required for testing them is severely lacking. Propositions (3) through (5) especially should be understood as a first attempt that can now serve as a basis for their more precise formulation, subsequent to which, one may then formulate research projects for their verification. However, several new elements have been suggested, developed, and operationalised. These elements are summarised in the next section.

[14] We have suggested in Section 8.2 that the technosphere too should be modelled according to the cultural perspectives. This argument would become moot in that case.

10.3 What is new?

The framework and its operationalisation is largely based on the current literature and little new empirical knowledge has been added. It is therefore sensible to ask which elements have been added to our knowledge through this book. The following list is based on the author's knowledge of the published research literature. The following elements are considered to be new:

Backbones of the framework

- The view of LCA as the art to model and combine the valuesphere, the ecosphere, and the technosphere. This includes the assumption that the technosphere and the ecosphere are embedded in the valuesphere. Values do not just enter when results from the model of the ecosphere have to be interpreted. Values are present from the moment the ecosphere is defined and a model of it built. (And this is true in analogy for the technosphere.)
- The division of the model for the ecosphere into the three submodels for known damage, unknown damage, and manageability. This modelling structure is comprehensive in the sense that it includes all aspects judged to be relevant for the decision support, yet it is simple thanks to the obvious content of the submodels. Lindeijer (1994) has made the only proposal where all these elements are also to some extent considered. (But he did not operationalise them.)
- The explicit modelling of the valuesphere by Cultural Theory. This makes it possible to model the ecosphere and the technosphere in a manner that is compatible with viable ways of life, world views, and management styles. LCAs based on a single perspective allow for a coherent treatment of structural uncertainty and provide therefore, a more reliable decision support. The closest existing and similar application is the uncertainty assessment in the field of integrated assessment. This also makes use of Cultural Theory (van Asselt *et al.* 1996a/b).

New contributions to damage assessment

- The concept of disability adjusted life years (DALYs) that has been developed by the World Bank and WHO (Murray *et al.* 1996a/b) is introduced here to LCA for the assessment of damages to human health. The original concept has been adapted to the needs of LCA and reformulated for its use with cultural perspectives. It is thus fit for further use.
- Comprehensive site-independent damage factors have been calculated for the emission of 55 carcinogenic substances to air and to surface water. The consideration of multi-media fate and exposure analyses and of a tumour-specific assessment of health damages at the level of DALYs is also new. Approaches that have been available so far have used neither a multi-media approach nor a tumour-specific damage analysis or they have used a different valuation endpoint (monetarisation) (Tellus 1992, Steen *et al.* 1992, Goedkoop 1995, ExternE 1995/1997).
- The multi-media model used (USES 1994) has been improved with the introduction of a height for the mixing layer that is variable according to the substance concerned. This adaptation has been necessary in order to arrive at a realistic exposure estimate for substances with a short atmospheric lifetime.

- The problem of uneven population densities was solved by a new model to calculate substance-specific population densities as a function of the substances atmospheric residence time.
- Comprehensive site-independent damage factors have been calculated for 120 substances emitted to air and causing respiratory effects in human beings. The combination of results of the EMEP-model with the results of POCP-calculations have made it possible to calculate the contribution of single VOCs to respiratory effects through the photochemical formation of ozone. This combination and the expression of health damages in DALYs is new and goes beyond the comprehensive assessment in ExternE (1997).

New contributions to the assessment of unknown damages and of manageability

- A proposal for the assessment of unknown damage due to emissions has been developed and made operational for a set of substances. The chosen approach is new and guidance to its more general operationalisation has been developed.
- A model to assess the manageability of environmental problems has been developed and used to assess the manageability of carcinogenic and respiratory effects in human beings. No comparable approach has been available so far.

Graphic decision support

- The use of a mixing triangle or tetrahedron for the visualisation of the dominance analysis is an elegant way to support the final aggregation step without being forced to impose just one weighting set. This procedure has been suggested for the final aggregation for the first time in an updated version of EcoIndicator'95 in Braunschweig *et al.* (1997).

Frame for science policy

- The framework proposed here has been designed to compare environmental impacts of product alternatives or processes, but it can also be used to get a better understanding of the different LCIA methods that have been developed so far. It can also serve to understand problem situations in or for which no conversion of opinions can be observed. The framework can be used at the meta-level to observe and influence science policy in the fields of LCIA and of other environmental decision support systems.

10.4 Problems solved?

The introduction for Chapter 2 identified two main criticisms currently made towards LCA and LCIA especially:

1) LCA is full of subjectivity and does not properly separate objective from subjective elements, and
2) The impact assessment addresses phantoms rather than actual damages.

These two points of criticism had been the basic motivation for making in this book a proposition for a new framework. The first critical point cannot be circumvented skirting around subjective elements or by separating them from objective elements. The desire to find an proactive and transparent way to deal with them has inspired the work, the results of which have been reported here. The framework presented acknowledges that both the ecosphere and the technosphere are relative constructs that are embedded in the valuesphere. It thus acknowledges that LCA cannot be separated into an objective and a subjective subpart. It thus avoids the problem of pseudo-objectivity looked for in other developments (Owens 1998), but inappropriate for the aim of LCA, i.e., to serve as a decision support. A number of other important steps have also been made to reduce the uneasiness expressed in the first point of criticism. The subjective elements are not understood as something that is arbitrary and inconsistent, but as reflections of attitudes which are inspired by distinct characteristics. Cultural Theory is used to model these subjective elements within LCA. This way of modelling differentiates between three different kinds of viable ways of life that incorporate predictable world views and management styles. They are organised around the way individuals organise social relations.

This way of dealing with the first point of criticism does not make it disappear. It does, however, build up a strong and consistent proposition that the subjective elements should not be separated from the objective ones because the objective elements immanently depend on the framing by the subjective settings. We have suggested modelling not only the objective, but also the subjective elements in order to take more of a constructive than relativist position. The hope is that this stance brings more coherence into the value choices and judgements that are unavoidable in any kind of valuation. Hopefully, this book is a constructive contribution to this need to deal with inherent subjectivity.

The second criticism has its roots in several causes. Firstly, the life cycle view builds on an unusual way of dealing with time and place. Both are largely disregarded or mentally thought to be uniform and thus average for all the impacts that are assessed. These simplifications lead to the absurd situation where one knows that the interventions occur in non-sensitive areas and yet they are accounted for as if they did occur in areas with an average sensitivity. This aspect limits the ability of the LCIA models to predict actual impacts. This conundrum is not resolved in this book. Proposals to overcome this situation have been made by, e.g., Udo de Haes (1996) and Potting *et al.* (1997).

Other sources for this criticism is the frequent use of inappropriate models that are either too simplistic or that build on a poor understanding of the mechanisms involved. The choice of simplicity is due to the wish to keep LCIA as simple as possible. Poor understanding simply reflects the very large array of sciences that are involved in the understanding of the problems to be solved within LCA and, in particular, within LCIA. Building up the required international network of experts from the different fields takes time and requires resources. It is therefore just a question of time and money until provisional models have been replaced by more appropriate impact assessments that will consider all the elements of a damage assessment and that are going to be backed by the relevant experts. This book makes a contribution by formalising this procedure for damages to human health in that it suggests a clear definition of the safeguard subject and of the way to measure damage to human health. The procedure suggested and operationalised in Chapters 5 through 7 is, of course, no guarantee against the introduction of phantoms into LCIA, but there exists an in-built barrier in the form of the possibility to compare calculated damages with observed or expected ones, i.e., to check the reliability of the assessment against health statistics. This should do away with a lot of the criticism summarised in Barnthouse *et al.* (1997) and the models should therefore gain wider acceptance.

The improvements made in the modelling in order to overcome the second point of criticism have the disadvantage that only impacts with well understood cause-effect chains can be considered. The consequence is a narrow damage assessment that neglects, to a large extent, all the qualitative information that is available. It is to counter this that the framework models the ecosphere not only with the known damage, but also with both the unknown damage and the manageability of damages.

The power of the framework lies in its two characteristics to make transparent rather than hide subjective elements and to support sound damage assessments without impairing its usefulness for those decision makers with holistic world views.

10.5 Outlook

This book has reviewed and summarised a large amount of published literature in the hope that the reader is spared the task of having to read at least some of them him- or herself. But it is in the nature of a young discipline such as LCA that there will still be a large number of items left that have to be worked out in future research. In order to structure the outlook, we separate this list of items into three sub-lists, one of each being addressed to the groups for which this book should be of interest: LCA researchers, researchers from other fields, and decision makers including their LCA analysts.

Outlook for LCA researchers:

LCA researchers are researchers which work at the further development of LCA (including LCIA) in order to make it meet the needs as a decision support tool. The framework presented here has two major drawbacks.

I) The large amount of assumptions and hypotheses that have been made in the course of the development of the new framework have to be verified with empirical work.

II) The submodels for the ecosphere should be worked out to such an extent that they can be used directly by LCA analysts for a wide range of applications.

Point (I) has to include the validation of the use of Cultural Theory for our purpose and of its predictions that have been used for the modelling of value choices. The claim that the three submodels suggested for the ecosphere fulfil the need of a large range of decision makers also has to be verified. When this is done one should attempt to operationalise the three submodels on the basis of a direct exchange with decision makers and experts. This verification should make use of both non-expert *and* expert panels. Focus groups may be more appropriate for the validation of Cultural Theory and its predictions.

Chapters 5 through 7, and to some extent Section 4.4, can be seen as starting points for making the whole framework operable. However, what is still needed is:

- to define the safeguard subjects for ecological health and for resources,
- to work out the damage category indicators,
- to establish all those causal relationships between interventions and damage indicators which can be quantified and to calculate their damage factors,
- to extend the applicability of the submodels for unknown damages and for manageability to input-oriented effects,
- to derive all manageability factors, and
- to complete the set of proxies for unknown damage for a larger range of environmental interventions.

This is a work program where knowledge has to be integrated from a large range of sciences. It is therefore necessary that the operationalisation is supported by several research groups injecting their competence in different fields. Such a co-operative venture has already succeeded in establishing a comprehensive accounting of damage costs (ExternE 1995/1997) and another one is in the process of doing this for the submodel for the assessment of known damages within LCA (Goedkoop *et al.* 1997, Müller-Wenk 1997/1998).

Outlook for researchers from other fields

The examples given in Chapters 5 through 7 for the damage assessment have revealed the many disciplines that are involved in modelling impact pathways and in assessing damage factors. Subsection 4.3.1 has shown that similar approaches are needed and already in development in green accounting, in the calculation of damage costs, in environmental risk assessment, in risk mapping, and in the setting of thresholds for regulatory purposes. These observations lead to two additional requests for the future:

III) Researchers from environmental chemistry, atmospheric physics, toxicology, preventive medicine, ecology, (resource) economics, the policy sciences, decision theory, and other related disciplines are invited to contribute their latest findings and models. Their support is needed in such a way that it can be used for a generic unit world modelling describing quantitative causalities between interventions and damages or that in can be used for the integration of information and the embedding of LCA in the decision making process.

IV) Researchers developing other environmental tools with assessment phases are invited to share their problems and solutions in order to find common elements and solutions that could be used in several of these tools at the same time.

This networking among disciplines (III) can be very fruitful because tool developers pose new questions and requests and at the same time transform the knowledge available from single disciplines into information that is relevant for decision making. Tool developers can be seen as customers of the scientific disciplines which make sure that oriented research can take place within the disciplines.

In Section 1.5 it had been argued that it can not be the aim of environmental research to develop the one instrument that will cover all the different requests from decision makers (e.g., level of analysis, modelled dimensions, representations of time and of place, procedure *versus* process). Nevertheless, it does not make sense if each community develops *its* tool for environmental decision support and all of them do all the necessary work in parallel. The suggested framework with its three submodels should be able to cover most principle differences in the assessment needs. Aspects such as marginal versus average analysis, the level of detail and the scope of time and place, and legal requirements are the most important aspects to be considered when elements from one tool are adapted to meet the requirements of another.

Outlook for decision makers and their LCA analysts

Finally, decision makers and their LCA analysts are the customers of the development presented in this book. What does the future look like for them? Are their requirements and needs fulfilled by the proposal made here and the operationalisation that is to come? It is difficult to give a clear-cut outlook on these questions without knowing exactly what the new tool will look like and which hypotheses can be validated by the empirical work to come. But assuming that the indices of the submodels suggested are independent enough to produce product rankings that depend on the weighting set that is applied then we can claim that:

V) Decision makers should be educated to the point that they understand the ecosphere and the technosphere as human constructs and that the perception and the models of these two spheres are shaped by their world view and their management style.

VI) LCA analysts should be trained to present results in terms of trade-offs and probabilities rather than point-estimates and they should strive to feed back to the LCA developers their experience with decision makers.

By accepting the claim (V) made above, decision makers will more easily understand other standpoints and better succeed to find compromises by focusing directly on the value choices. They may even learn to accept not only political parties in public policy making, but also archetypes with different world views in LCA.

The capabilities of LCA analysts and their active role in feeding their experiences back to tool developers is essential for the improvement of the tool (VI).

If the hypothesis that the indices of the submodels are largely dependent and rankings based on only one index will already lead to a stable support turns out to be true, then decision makers and LCA analysts can influence the development of simplified tools that make use of proxy indicators. These proxy indicators will be chosen so as to ease, as much as possible, the inventory analysis and yet to support the decision makers with a stable decision support. In that case, the detour via a sophisticated framework would have helped to find simple but stable models.

The following statement should remind the decision makers – as well as everyone who claims LCA to be incomplete – of the principal dilemma behind any decision support and the daily pressure that is exerted to base decisions on improved decision support systems:

Die Notwendigkeit zu entscheiden ist stets grösser als das Mass unserer Erkenntnis.
(The necessity to decide is always larger than the degree of cognition)
Immanuel Kant

APPENDICES

APPENDIX CHAPTER 4:

Derivation of Composition Rules

a) Problem description

The manageability factor proposed in Subsection 4.5.3 is composed of three indicators (R, X, S) and is finally multiplied with the index from the damage assessment (D).

The two main questions are:

- which kind of formula shall be used to combine these indicators, i.e., summing, multiplication, or others, and
- which adjustments or scaling factors are necessary?

Such questions have always to be asked when indices are built out of indicators.

b) Dependent and independent indicators

A first distinction has to be made between dependent and independent indicators. If two indicators depend on each other (or at least one on the other), then the functions of this dependence have to be either known or to be determined. This case is not relevant here, i.e., all indicators are assumed to be independent.

c) Linear and non-linear indicators

If, in addition, the indicators are independent and linear in their relevant sectors, then the number of formulas to be considered is small. Simple weighted sums or a simple multiplication with a scaling factor are enough.

However, the example of target damage excess will show that we are confronted here with an indicator that does not show linear behaviour, i.e., the value of the indicator does not linearly increase with the increase in the ratio of today's damage to the target damage.

Therefore, the indicators (or at least the indicator for target damage excess) may have to be transformed by non-linear factors.

d) The procedure to solve the problem

The general procedure to solve the problem at hand involves five steps (it is assumed that the indicators are already defined in quantitative terms)[15]:

1. Minimum, mean, and maximum results for each indicator are derived or estimated by an expert group.

[15] This procedure was developed after a discussion round where Dr. Olaf Tietje (ETHZ) made a similar proposal.

2. A panel with potential decision makers, stakeholders, or representatives of society (dependent on the purpose of the index) is selected. The different indicators are introduced and the values from step (1) presented. As an option, the panel may now be asked to skip over indicators which are either irrelevant or already covered by others or to suggest additional indicators which will then be defined and quantified by experts and included in the matrix of step (1).
3. The panel is confronted with a matrix where all possible combinations of the minimum, mean, and maximum values for all indicators n are given (in total $3{\cdot}2(n\text{-}1)+n = 7n\text{-}6$). For each combination, the panel is now forced to give an estimate of the "desired" overall score for the index. This subjective step is only meaningful if it is absolutely clear what should be measured by the index and what is measured by the indicators.
4. The panel and the experts discuss the nature of the indicators, i.e., whether they are independent and linear or not. If not, they may make first guesses of the type of functions to be used.
5. Numerical methods are used to fit the principal formulas suggested in step (4) to the predictions in step (3).

The formula with the best and most meaningful fit will be chosen. The parameters determined in this way reflect the most adequate weighting set.

e) The example of manageability

We will use the index of manageability as an example to demonstrate the proposed procedure and to get guidance on the linkage problem. However, no panel is available and only a small set of alternatives will be tested.

Step 1: Minimum, mean and maximum values

The attribution of values is largely based on the definitions in Subsection 4.5.3 and the examples in Sections 6.6 and 7.6. All values will be given for an egalitarian world view and management style.

The minimum value for R is theoretically zero. However, in practice, no example can be given for such a behaviour. Therefore, we assume a 50% reduction at most. The mean value for R is estimated to be 0.7 based on the examples in Sections 6.6 and 7.6 and lies well between the extreme reductions of 0 % and of 50 %. The maximum value for X is assumed to be caused by respiratory effects. Therefore, the value derived in Section 7.6 is taken. If the excess is smaller than 1, the environmental problem would probably not be included in the damage assessment. The mean of 10 may well represent the average target damage excess from all the problems that have been included (first estimate). The values for S are given in Table 4.11.

Thanks to these assumptions we can assume the following values:

	Maximum value (lowest manageability)	Mean value	Minimum value (highest manageability)
Ease of reduction (*R*)	1	0.7	0.5
Excess of target damage (*X*)	500	10	1
Success of regulation (*S*)	1	0.8	0.7

Tab. A4.1: Max, mean, and min values for the three indicators according to Subsection 4.5.3 and expert judgement

Step 2: Evaluation of indicators

This step is skipped due to the lack of a panel.

Step 3: Prediction of index values mpc

In the absence of a panel, we will present our own predictions for a selection of scenarios and for the egalitarian's perspective. There are 15 possible combinations (3 indicators), but we will give estimates for only three of them.

$$Mp,c = Rp,c \cdot Xp,c \cdot Sp,c \cdot Dp,c = mp,c \cdot Dp,c \tag{A4.1}$$

$$\text{with} \quad mp,c = Rp,c \cdot Xp,c \cdot Sp,c \tag{A4.2}$$

It is assumed that a mean manageability should be equal to $m = 1$, i.e., the index for manageability is identical with the index for damage. Furthermore, we assume that the index should discriminate between the smallest and the largest index by a factor of nine and that the distribution is lognormal. Therefore, we conclude that the maximum $m = 3$ and the minimum $m = 0.33$. One should be aware that this is a subjective step and should be backed by a panel composed of representatives relevant to the decision at hand.

	Maximum value (lowest manageability)	Mean value	Minimum value (highest manageability)
Ease of reduction (*R*)	max (=1)	mean (=0.7)	min (=0.5)
Excess of target damage (*X*)	max (=500)	mean (=10)	min (=1)
Success of regulation (*S*)	max (=1)	mean (=0.8)	min (=0.7)
Manageability factor *m*	3	1	0.33

Tab. A4.2: Estimated manageability for a min, mean, and max scenario.

Step 4: Functions to be tested

It is assumed that the three indicators are independent. This assumption is only partly true as we have to assume some correlation between *X* and *S*. However, as we intend that the indicators reflect different aspects they are treated as independent.

We can further assume that *R* and *S* have a linear shape while *X* is strongly non-linear, i.e., the uncertainty for $X = 500$ is not 50 times higher than for $X = 10$.

General functions to be chosen for a fit may be:

$$mpc = a \cdot Rp,c^{b} + c \cdot Xp,c^{d} + e \cdot Sp,c^{f} \text{ or} \qquad (A4.3)$$

$$mpc = a \cdot Rp,c^{b} \cdot Xp,c^{c} \cdot Sp,c^{d} \qquad (A4.4)$$

We decided to make three calculations[16]. First, we assumed a linear and additive behaviour:

$$mp,c = a \cdot Rp,c + b \cdot Xp,c + c \cdot Sp,c \qquad (A4.5)$$

Second, we assumed a non-linear multiplicative behaviour:

$$mp,c = a \cdot Rp,c \cdot Xp,c^{b}\ Sp,c^{c} \qquad (A4.6)$$

And finally, we assumed that only X is non-linear, that the linkage is multiplicative, and that no scaling is necessary:

$$mp,c = Rp,c \cdot Xp,c^{a} \cdot Sp,c \qquad (A4.7)$$

If a panel is available other relationships should be tested as well.

Step 5: Numerical fit

Thanks to the information provided in step (3), it is possible to calculate the variables a, b and c for Function (A4.5) with a simple algebraic resolution of a 3x3 equation system. The following fit was derived:

$$m_{Ec} = 4.65 \cdot R_{Ec} + 0.0024 \cdot X_{Ec} - 2.85 \cdot S_{Ec} \qquad (A4.8)$$

This fit does not convince at all because the success of regulation (S) is considered to be negatively correlated with the index for manageability. This outcome can be explained with the missing consideration of the non-linear behaviour of X.

The fit with Function (A4.6) was only possible with the help of numerical approximation and resulted in:

$$m_{Ec} = 3 \cdot 10^{23} \cdot R_{Ec} \cdot X_{Ec}^{-8.525} \cdot S_{Ec}^{148.543} \qquad (A4.9)$$

This outcome is interesting because it correctly reflects the non-linear behaviour of X. However, at the same time S is corrected by a tremendous exponent and the whole function by a very large scaling factor. As the values of S vary only from 0.7 to 1, it is clear that small deviations of X from an exponential distribution have to be corrected by such high coefficients. These make the calculations very sensitive to the choice between $S = 1$ (with the exponent it also stays one) or $S = 0.7$ or 0.8 (in both cases the factor amounts to about 10^{-23}). This is clearly not intended and the adding of additional equations in step (3) would correct this outcome.

Confronted with the situation that with only three equations from step (3) no meaningful function could be found so far, we used the following function:

$$m_{Ec} = R_{Ec} \cdot X_{Ec}^{0.2} \cdot S_{Ec} \qquad (A4.10)$$

---

[16] We had to restrict the number of variables to three because only three equations were derived from step (3) in this example.

We can now compare the results with Table A4.2. The case R = max, X = max, and S = max leads to 3.5 (instead of 3), R = mean, X = mean, and S = mean leads to 0.9 (instead of 1), and R = min, X = min, and S = min leads to 0.35 (instead of 0.33).

Taking into account that the given predictions for m were rough estimates, we identify a good fit with the simplest formula possible, i.e., with only one additional parameter which makes the indicator X linearly combinable.

f) Appraisal

The question of the rule to combine indicators to indices is often not explicitly put. The developer has a composition in mind and shapes the indicators accordingly. That is a source for implicit value choices because the developer may perceive the indicators in a different manner than decision makers will or intends that the index is used for something other than what it will actually be used for. It is therefore recommended that the suggested five step procedure be executed together with a panel.

This procedure also makes it possible to consider cultural biases. It prevents qualifying the parameters suggested by the model developers as purely technical ones.

No panel was available for the determination of the index for manageability and we failed to produce a meaningful function by numerical fitting. However, the suggested Function (A4.10) approximates in a simple manner the intended meaning of the indicators and the index. Therefore, this function will be chosen as the working hypothesis until the time when empirical tests are available.

APPENDICES CHAPTER 6

Substance-name	CAS-Number	DT50 Photo-degradation in air	DT50 Hydrolysis in water	DT50 Biodegrad. in water	DT50 Bio-deg. in soil	D_H	log K_{ow}	Source
Unit		d	d	d	d	Pa·m³/mol	-	
1,2-Dichloroethane	107-06-2		400					Rippen (1996)
1,3-Butadiene	106-99-0	0.32	D	28	28			Howard *et al.* (1991)
2,3,7,8-Tetrachlordi-benzo-p-dioxin	1746-01-6	D	D					
2,4,6-Trichlorophenol	88-06-2	21.7	D			1.021	log D_{ow} = 2.81	Rippen (1996)
Acrylonitrile-	107-13-1	3.9	D					Rippen (1996)
Aldrin-	309-00-2	0.3	D					Howard *et al.* (1991)
Arsenic, inorganic	7440-38-2		D					
Benzene-	71-43-2		D					
Benzotrichloride-	98-07-7	D	D					
Benzo[a]pyrene- (BaP)	50-32-8		D					
Benzyl-chloride-	100-44-7		D					
Cadmium-	7440-43-9		D					
Carbon-tetrachloride-	56-23-5	10000 §	14965				2.77	Rippen (1996)
Chloroform, Trichloromethane	67-66-3		D					
Chromium(VI)	18540-29-9		D					
Di(2-ethylhexyl)-phthalate- (DEHP)	117-81-7		D					
Dibutyl-phthalate-	84-74-2	1.8	3650					Rippen (1996)
Dichloromethane-	75-09-2		D					
Dichlorvos-	62-73-7	D	62					Rippen (1996)
Dieldrin-	60-57-1	1.7	D					Howard *et al.* (1991)
Formaldehyde-	50-00-0	35	D					Rippen (1996)
gamma-Hexachlorcyclohexane	58-89-9	1.6	D					Rippen (1996)
Hexachlorobenzene-	118-74-1		D					
Hexachlorobutadiene-	87-68-3	D	D					
Nickel-subsulfide-	12035-72-2		D					
Pentachlorophenol-	87-86-5	4	D			0.138	log D_{ow} = 2.99	Rippen (1996)
Perchlorethylen	127-18-4		D					
Polychlorinated-biphenyls- (PCBs)	1336-36-3	D	D					
Propylene-oxide-	75-56-9	D						
Trichlorethylene	79-01-6		D					
Trifluralin-	1582-09-8	D						
Vinylchlorid	75-01-4	2.75	D					Rippen (1996)

App. 6.1: Changes to the substance data given in Guinée *et al.* (1996), blanks mean that the value in Guinée *et al.* (1996) was not changed, § means the maximum score allowed in USES, D for DT50 photodegradation in air is the default in USES and is set to 160 days, D for DT50 hydrolysis is the default in USES and is set to 1'000'000 days.

Substance-name	CAS	Molecular weight	Melting Point	Vapour pressure	log K_{OW}	Water solubility	DT50 Photo-deg. in air	DT50 Hydro-lysis in water	Readily bio-degradable
		g/mol	°C	Pa	-	mg/l	d	d	
1,1,1,2-Tetrachlorethane	630-20-6	167.85	-70.2	1580	3.03	1100	700	40	no
1,1,2,2-Tetrachlorethane	79-34-5	167.85	-36	793	2.39	2962	700	60	no
1,1,2-Trichlorethane	79-00-5	133.41	-36.3	16500	2.49	1495	35	360	no
1,1-Dichlorethene	75-35-4	96.94	-122.1	80500	2.13	3344	0.5	700	no
1,2-Dibromoethane	106-93-4	187.86	9.79	10400		4152	50	700	no
1,4-Dioxane	123-91-1	88.11	11.8	5000	-0.27	1 E+06	1	7	no
3-Methylcholanthrene	56-49-5	268.36	178	1.03E-06	6.42	0.0019	0.3	1 E+06	no
Acetaldehyde (R)	75-07-0	44.05	-123	100600	0.5	1 E+06	1	1 E+06	yes
alpha-Hexachlorcyclohexan (R)	319-84-6	290.83	159	0.0053	3.77	1.59	1.6	1 E+06	no
Benz(a)anthracene	56-55-3	228.3	160	2.80E-05	5.91	0.011	7	60	no
beta-Hexachlorcyclohexan (R)	319-85-7	290.83	312	4.30E-05	3.85	0.32	1.6	1 E+06	no
Bis(2-chlorethyl)ether	111-44-4	143.02	-46.8	4000	-0.38	22000	1	21	no
Bis(chloromethyl)ether BCME	542-88-1	114.96	-41.5	4000	-0.38	22000	1	21	no
Bromodichloromethane	75-27-4	163.8	-57.1	6670	2.1	4500	20	20	no
Chloromethane, Methyl Chloride	74-87-3	50.49	-97.73	1.00E+06	0.91	5235	700	30	no
Dibenz(a,h)anthracene	53-70-3	278.36	267	3.70E-10	6.75	0.0006	7	60	no
Epichlorhydrin	106-89-8	92.53	-57.21	2400	0.3	65800	4	8	yes
Ethylene Oxide	75-21-8	44.05	-111	145855	-0.3	1 E+06	211 (R)	14	no
Hexachloroethane	67-72-1	236.74	186.1	50	3.93	50	700	60	no
Styrene	100-42-5	104.14	-30.6	880	3.05	300	0.2	7	yes
Tribromomethane	75-25-6	252.75	-8.3	727	2.38	3100	60	60	no

App. 6.2: Substance data for the additionally entered substances, if no source is mentioned the data is taken from Mackay *et al.* (1993), an R means that the source is Rippen (1996), 1 E+06 for vapour pressure, solubility and DT50 hydrolysis in water are the upper limits accepted by USES (1994)

Substance-name	CAS-Number	1000 kg/d emitted to air			1000 kg/d emitted to surface water		
		Concen-tration air	Concen-tration drinking water	Human dose by food	Concen-tration air	Concen-tration drinking water	Human dose by food
IARC-Group 1		mg/m^3	mg/l	mg/kg/d	mg/m^3	mg/l	mg/kg/d
Arsenic, inorganic	7440-38-2	3.8E-08	2.0E-05	6.1E-04	5.1E-18	1.7E-05	2.6E-07
Benzene	71-43-2	2.5E-06	3.2E-09	3.6E-11	1.6E-06	2.5E-06	5.2E-09
Bis(chloromethyl)ether BCME	542-88-1	4.0E-07	3.5E-08	1.8E-10	3.1E-07	1.3E-05	3.6E-11
Cadmium	7440-43-9	5.5E-08	8.8E-05	1.6E-04	1.1E-17	1.6E-05	5.1E-07
Chromium(VI)	18540-29-9	5.1E-08	1.4E-06	1.8E-02	2.5E-18	2.2E-06	2.8E-07
Nickel	12035-72-2	3.0E-08	3.4E-05	3.5E-04	4.8E-18	2.5E-05	1.6E-06
Nickel-refinery-dust	12035-72-2	3.0E-08	3.4E-05	3.5E-04	4.8E-18	2.5E-05	1.6E-06
Nickel-subsulfide	12035-72-2	3.0E-08	3.4E-05	3.5E-04	4.8E-18	2.5E-05	1.6E-06
Vinylchlorid	75-01-4	1.1E-06	9.1E-10	6.0E-11	1.1E-06	3.9E-06	2.1E-10
IARC-Group 2A							
1,2-Dibromoethane	106-93-4	2.0E-05	9.9E-08	3.0E-09	2.0E-05	4.1E-06	1.8E-08
1,3-Butadiene	106-99-0	1.3E-07	1.4E-08	2.4E-10	1.0E-07	1.5E-05	1.1E-08
Acrylonitrile	107-13-1	1.6E-06	2.2E-08	0.0E+00	9.1E-07	5.7E-06	1.0E-10
Benzo[a]pyrene (BaP)	50-32-8	5.5E-07	5.3E-05	1.7E-04	7.0E-10	2.7E-06	7.8E-05
Benz(a)anthracene	56-55-3	7.0E-07	5.1E-05	1.9E-04	2.4E-08	2.8E-08	7.3E-05
Dibenz(a,h)anthracene	53-70-3	5.5E-07	5.3E-05	1.2E-03	9.3E-11	1.0E-06	1.7E-04
Epichlorhydrin	106-89-8	1.6E-06	1.3E-07	2.7E-09	1.8E-07	7.3E-06	4.4E-10
Ethylene Oxide	75-21-8	5.1E-05	9.8E-06	6.6E-08	2.6E-05	2.3E-05	3.2E-08
Formaldehyde	50-00-0	3.2E-07	2.4E-07	1.4E-07	3.0E-10	1.3E-05	2.5E-10
Polychlorinated-biphenyls- (PCBs)	1336-36-3	1.1E-05	4.2E-05	1.5E-04	4.0E-06	1.5E-05	9.1E-05
Propylene-oxide	75-56-9	3.8E-05	3.0E-06	2.5E-08	1.1E-05	9.2E-06	7.1E-09
IARC-Group 2B							
1,2-Dichloroethane	107-06-2	3.2E-05	1.7E-07	3.7E-09	3.2E-05	4.1E-06	7.9E-09
1,4-Dioxane	123-91-1	4.0E-07	8.9E-07	6.8E-09	1.7E-08	1.8E-05	3.2E-10
2,3,7,8-Tetrachlordibenzo-p-dioxin, TCDD	1746-01-6	9.2E-07	6.6E-05	1.9E-03	1.0E-07	7.3E-06	2.3E-04
2,4,6-Trichlorophenol	88-06-2	6.9E-06	1.1E-06	9.4E-07	4.6E-07	1.3E-05	1.0E-07
Acetaldehyde	75-07-0	4.0E-07	4.7E-08	5.4E-10	8.6E-08	1.1E-05	3.7E-10
alpha-Hexachlorcyclohexan	319-84-6	6.4E-07	1.7E-06	9.4E-07	5.0E-07	1.6E-04	7.4E-06
Benzotrichloride	98-07-7	6.5E-05	2.2E-09	4.1E-07	6.4E-05	1.9E-06	1.1E-06
Benzyl-chloride	100-44-7	1.7E-06	2.0E-13	8.6E-11	1.1E-06	2.5E-06	7.4E-09
beta-Hexachlorcyclohexan	319-85-7	5.4E-07	4.0E-05	1.5E-05	6.5E-08	5.8E-04	3.2E-05
Bromodichloromethane	75-27-4	8.1E-06	7.4E-08	1.7E-09	6.9E-06	3.7E-06	8.1E-09
Carbon-tetrachloride	56-23-5	3.9E-03	4.0E-06	2.7E-07	3.9E-03	5.9E-06	7.5E-03
Chloroform	67-66-3	3.2E-05	2.4E-07	6.1E-09	3.2E-05	4.3E-06	1.8E-08
Di(2-ethylhexyl)phthalate- (DEHP)	117-81-7	4.1E-07	2.4E-08	2.4E-06	1.0E-07	4.9E-07	1.1E-05
Dichloromethane	75-09-2	2.3E-05	1.7E-07	3.0E-09	2.3E-05	4.3E-06	2.5E-09
Dichlorvos	62-73-7	1.8E-06	5.0E-05	1.3E-06	5.2E-08	1.5E-04	1.2E-07
gamma-Hexachlorocyclohexane (lindane)	58-89-9	5.2E-07	1.3E-05	1.4E-05	9.2E-08	6.6E-04	2.1E-04
Hexachlorobenzene	118-74-1	4.6E-06	6.6E-06	1.5E-05	3.5E-06	3.5E-06	2.6E-05
Pentachlorophenol	87-86-5	1.3E-06	1.5E-05	1.9E-06	6.5E-07	6.7E-04	5.7E-06
Perchloroethylene	127-18-4	1.9E-05	2.3E-08	4.2E-09	1.9E-05	3.9E-06	1.5E-07
Styrene	100-42-5	8.1E-08	1.5E-10	5.0E-11	3.9E-08	2.0E-06	3.3E-08
IARC-Group 3							
1,1,1,2-Tetrachlorethane	630-20-6	2.7E-04	2.5E-06	2.8E-07	2.5E-04	5.1E-06	3.1E-07
1,1,2,2-Tetrachlorethane	79-34-5	2.3E-04	1.1E-05	3.6E-07	2.1E-04	2.2E-05	3.5E-07
1,1,2-Trichlorethane	79-00-5	1.4E-05	2.3E-08	7.8E-10	1.4E-05	3.9E-06	1.9E-08
1,1-Dichlorethene	75-35-4	2.0E-07	2.0E-10	9.9E-12	2.0E-07	3.9E-06	7.7E-09
3-Methylcholanthrene	56-49-5	5.4E-07	5.1E-05	4.8E-04	2.5E-09	1.5E-06	1.1E-04
Aldrin	309-00-2	1.2E-07	2.8E-08	2.3E-06	4.5E-08	4.3E-07	8.0E-05
Bis(2-chlorethyl)ether	111-44-4	4.0E-07	2.9E-08	1.4E-10	3.2E-07	1.2E-05	6.4E-11
Dibutyl-phthalate	84-74-2	6.8E-07	3.2E-08	2.1E-05	1.1E-08	3.0E-06	3.0E-02
Dieldrin	60-57-1	6.6E-07	1.3E-05	4.2E-04	2.1E-08	1.9E-06	1.0E-04
Hexachlorobutadiene	87-68-3	6.5E-05	9.4E-08	7.9E-07	6.0E-05	1.8E-06	2.0E-05
Hexachloroethane	67-72-1	2.7E-04	2.6E-06	1.8E-06	2.5E-04	5.2E-06	2.1E-06
Chloromethane, Methyl Chloride	74-87-3	2.8E-04	6.9E-08	0.0E+00	2.6E-04	3.6E-06	0.0E+00
Trichlorethylene	79-01-6	1.4E-06	3.4E-09	1.2E-10	1.4E-06	4.0E-06	1.5E-08
Trifluralin	1582-09-8	4.5E-05	1.4E-05	4.5E-05	1.1E-06	3.4E-07	1.5E-06

App. 6.3: Results from multimedia calculations derived with the model USES (1994) and adaptations made in Guinée *et al.* (1996) as well as Appendix (6.1), and (6.2).

Substance-name	CAS-Number	$F_{air,air}$	$F_{air,water}$	$F_{air,food}$	$F_{water,air}$	$F_{water,water}$	$F_{water,food}$
IARC-Group 1		m^2a/m^3	m^2a/l	$m^2a/(kg·d)$	m^2a/m^3	m^2a/l	$m^2a/(kg·d)$
Arsenic, inorganic	7440-38-2	3.7E-07	1.9E-04	6.0E-03	4.9E-17	1.6E-04	2.5E-06
Benzene	71-43-2	2.5E-05	3.2E-08	3.5E-10	1.5E-05	2.5E-05	5.0E-08
Bis(chloromethyl)ether BCME	542-88-1	3.9E-06	3.4E-07	1.7E-09	3.0E-06	1.2E-04	3.5E-10
Cadmium	7440-43-9	5.3E-07	8.6E-04	1.6E-03	1.0E-16	1.6E-04	5.0E-06
Chromium(VI)	18540-29-9	5.0E-07	1.4E-05	1.7E-01	2.4E-17	2.1E-05	2.7E-06
Nickel	12035-72-2	2.9E-07	3.3E-04	3.4E-03	4.6E-17	2.4E-04	1.5E-05
Nickel-refinery-dust	12035-72-2	2.9E-07	3.3E-04	3.4E-03	4.6E-17	2.4E-04	1.5E-05
Nickel-subsulfide	12035-72-2	2.9E-07	3.3E-04	3.4E-03	4.6E-17	2.4E-04	1.5E-05
Vinylchlorid	75-01-4	1.1E-05	8.9E-09	5.8E-10	1.1E-05	3.8E-05	2.1E-09
IARC-Group 2A							
1,2-Dibromoethane	106-93-4	2.0E-04	9.6E-07	3.0E-08	2.0E-04	4.0E-05	1.8E-07
1,3-Butadiene	106-99-0	1.3E-06	1.3E-07	2.3E-09	1.0E-06	1.4E-04	1.0E-07
Acrylonitrile	107-13-1	1.5E-05	2.2E-07	0.0E+00	8.9E-06	5.5E-05	9.8E-10
Benzo[a]pyrene- (BaP)	50-32-8	5.4E-06	5.1E-04	1.6E-03	6.8E-09	2.6E-05	7.7E-04
Benz(a)anthracene	56-55-3	6.8E-06	5.0E-04	1.8E-03	2.3E-07	2.7E-07	7.1E-04
Dibenz(a,h)anthracene	53-70-3	5.4E-06	5.1E-04	1.2E-02	9.1E-10	1.0E-05	1.7E-03
Epichlorhydrin	106-89-8	1.5E-05	1.3E-06	2.6E-08	1.8E-06	7.2E-05	4.2E-09
Ethylene Oxide	75-21-8	5.0E-04	9.6E-05	6.4E-07	2.5E-04	2.3E-04	3.1E-07
Formaldehyde	50-00-0	3.1E-06	2.3E-06	1.4E-06	2.9E-09	1.3E-04	2.4E-09
Polychlorinated-biphenyls (PCBs)	1336-36-3	1.1E-04	4.1E-04	1.5E-03	3.9E-05	1.4E-04	8.9E-04
Propylene-oxide	75-56-9	3.7E-04	3.0E-05	2.5E-07	1.0E-04	8.9E-05	6.9E-08
IARC-Group 2B							
1,2-Dichloroethane	107-06-2	3.2E-04	1.7E-06	3.6E-08	3.1E-04	4.0E-05	7.7E-08
1,4-Dioxane	123-91-1	3.9E-06	8.7E-06	6.6E-08	1.6E-07	1.7E-04	3.1E-09
2,3,7,8-Tetrachlordibenzo-p-dioxin, TCDD	1746-01-6	9.0E-06	6.5E-04	1.8E-02	9.9E-07	7.1E-05	2.2E-03
2,4,6-Trichlorophenol	88-06-2	6.7E-05	1.1E-05	6.3E-06	4.5E-06	1.2E-04	1.0E-06
Acetaldehyde	75-07-0	3.9E-06	4.5E-07	5.3E-09	8.4E-07	1.0E-04	3.6E-09
alpha-Hexachlorcyclohexan	319-84-6	6.2E-06	1.7E-05	9.1E-06	4.9E-06	1.5E-03	7.3E-05
Benzotrichloride	98-07-7	6.3E-04	2.2E-08	4.0E-06	6.2E-04	1.9E-05	1.1E-05
Benzyl-chloride	100-44-7	1.7E-05	1.9E-12	8.4E-10	1.1E-05	2.4E-05	7.2E-08
beta-Hexachlorcyclohexan	319-85-7	5.2E-06	3.9E-04	1.5E-04	6.3E-07	5.6E-03	3.1E-04
Bromodichloromethane	75-27-4	7.9E-05	7.2E-07	1.7E-08	6.8E-05	3.6E-05	7.9E-08
Carbon-tetrachloride	56-23-5	3.8E-02	3.9E-05	2.7E-06	3.8E-02	5.8E-05	7.3E-02
Chloroform	67-66-3	3.2E-04	2.3E-06	6.0E-08	3.1E-04	4.2E-05	1.7E-07
Di(2-ethylhexyl)phthalate- (DEHP)	117-81-7	4.0E-06	2.3E-07	2.4E-05	1.0E-06	4.8E-06	1.0E-04
Dichloromethane	75-09-2	2.3E-04	1.7E-06	2.9E-08	2.2E-04	4.2E-05	2.5E-08
Dichlorvos	62-73-7	1.8E-05	4.9E-04	1.3E-05	5.0E-07	1.4E-03	1.2E-06
gamma-Hexachlorocyclohexane (lindane)	58-89-9	5.1E-06	1.3E-04	1.4E-04	9.0E-07	6.4E-03	2.0E-03
Hexachlorobenzene	118-74-1	4.4E-05	6.5E-05	1.4E-04	3.4E-05	3.4E-05	2.5E-04
Pentachlorophenol	87-86-5	1.3E-05	1.5E-04	1.8E-05	6.3E-06	6.6E-03	5.6E-05
Perchloroethylene	127-18-4	1.9E-04	2.2E-07	4.1E-08	1.9E-04	3.8E-05	1.5E-06
Styrene	100-42-5	7.9E-07	1.5E-09	4.9E-10	3.8E-07	2.0E-05	3.2E-07
IARC-Group 3							
1,1,1,2-Tetrachlorethane	630-20-6	2.6E-03	2.4E-05	2.7E-06	2.4E-03	4.9E-05	3.0E-06
1,1,2,2-Tetrachlorethane	79-34-5	2.3E-03	1.1E-04	3.5E-06	2.1E-03	2.1E-04	3.4E-06
1,1,2-Trichlorethane	79-00-5	1.4E-04	2.2E-07	7.6E-09	1.4E-04	3.8E-05	1.9E-07
1,1-Dichlorethene	75-35-4	2.0E-06	2.0E-09	9.6E-11	2.0E-06	3.8E-05	7.5E-08
3-Methylcholanthrene	56-49-5	5.3E-06	4.9E-04	4.6E-03	2.4E-08	1.4E-05	1.1E-03
Aldrin-	309-00-2	1.2E-06	2.7E-07	2.2E-05	4.4E-07	4.2E-06	7.8E-04
Bis(2-chlorethyl)ether	111-44-4	3.9E-06	2.8E-07	1.4E-09	3.1E-06	1.1E-04	6.3E-10
Dibutyl-phthalate	84-74-2	6.7E-06	3.1E-07	2.1E-04	1.0E-07	3.0E-05	2.9E-01
Dieldrin-	60-57-1	6.4E-06	1.2E-04	4.1E-03	2.1E-07	1.8E-05	9.9E-04
Hexachlorobutadiene	87-68-3	6.3E-04	9.1E-07	7.7E-06	5.8E-04	1.8E-05	2.0E-04
Hexachloroethane	67-72-1	2.6E-03	2.5E-05	1.7E-05	2.5E-03	5.1E-05	2.1E-05
Chloromethane, Methyl Chloride	74-87-3	2.8E-03	6.8E-07	0.0E+00	2.5E-03	3.5E-05	0.0E+00
Trichlorethylene	79-01-6	1.3E-05	3.4E-08	1.1E-09	1.3E-05	3.9E-05	1.5E-07
Trifluralin	1582-09-8	4.4E-04	1.3E-04	4.3E-04	1.1E-05	3.3E-06	1.5E-05

App. 6.4: Interim fate factors for 52 substances modelled in USES (1994) and adaptations made in Guinée *et al.* (1996) as well as Appendix (6.1), and (6.2) according Equation (6.6) (Subsection 6.2.3)

Substance-name	Dilution height #	F''air,air	F' air,water	F' air,food	F' water,air	F' water, water	F' water, food
IARC-Group 1	m	m^2a/m^3	m^2a/l	$m^2a/(kg \cdot d)$	m^2a/m^3	m^2a/l	$m^2a/(kg \cdot d)$
Arsenic, inorganic	241	3.7E-07	1.9E-04	6.0E-03	4.9E-17	1.6E-04	2.5E-06
Benzene	3148	7.9E-06	1.0E-08	1.3E-10	1.1E-06	7.1E-07	3.8E+00
Bis(chloromethyl)ether BCME	1029	3.8E-06	3.3E-07	1.6E-09	6.3E-07	3.6E-06	8.3E+00
Cadmium	303	5.3E-07	8.6E-04	1.6E-03	2.2E-17	4.5E-06	4.6E+00
Chromium(VI)	290	5.0E-07	1.4E-05	1.7E-01	5.2E-18	6.1E-07	1.8E+00
Nickel	210	2.9E-07	3.3E-04	3.4E-03	9.9E-18	7.0E-06	3.0E+00
Nickel-refinery-dust	210	2.9E-07	3.3E-04	3.4E-03	9.9E-18	7.0E-06	3.0E+00
Nickel-subsulfide	210	2.9E-07	3.3E-04	3.4E-03	9.9E-18	7.0E-06	3.0E+00
Vinylchlorid	1908	5.7E-06	4.6E-09	2.2E-10	1.2E-06	1.1E-06	4.6E+00
IARC-Group 2A							
1,2-Dibromoethane	10000	2.0E-05	9.6E-08	1.7E-09	4.2E-06	1.1E-06	2.0E+00
1,3-Butadiene	514	2.5E-06	2.6E-07	4.3E-09	4.2E-07	4.0E-06	8.6E+00
Acrylonitrile	2356	6.5E-06	9.3E-08	4.1E-10	8.1E-07	1.6E-06	6.4E+00
Benzo[a]pyrene- (BaP)	1243	5.4E-06	5.1E-04	1.6E-03	1.5E-09	7.5E-07	9.5E-03
Benz(a)anthracene	1434	6.6E-06	4.9E-04	1.8E-03	4.9E-08	7.8E-07	1.1E-02
Dibenz(a,h)anthracene	1241	5.4E-06	5.1E-04	1.2E-02	1.9E-10	2.9E-07	1.7E-03
Epichlorhydrin	2358	6.6E-06	5.5E-07	1.1E-08	1.7E-07	2.0E-06	9.0E+00
Ethylene Oxide	10000	7.8E-05	1.5E-05	1.0E-07	8.4E-06	5.3E-06	3.8E+00
Formaldehyde	894	3.3E-06	2.5E-06	1.5E-06	6.7E-10	3.7E-06	9.7E+00
Polychlorinated-biphenyls- (PCBs)	10000	4.4E-05	1.6E-04	5.9E-04	3.3E-06	3.6E-06	6.1E-02
Propylene-oxide	10000	5.9E-05	4.7E-06	3.5E-08	3.5E-06	2.4E-06	3.9E+00
IARC-Group 2B							
1,2-Dichloroethane	10000	3.2E-05	1.7E-07	2.7E-09	6.7E-06	1.1E-06	1.4E+00
1,4-Dioxane	1016	3.8E-06	8.5E-06	6.5E-08	3.4E-08	5.0E-06	9.7E+00
2,3,7,8-Tetrachlordibenzo-p-dioxin, TCDD	1696	9.0E-06	6.5E-04	1.8E-02	2.1E-07	2.0E-06	8.8E-03
2,4,6-Trichlorophenol	5795	1.4E-05	2.3E-06	1.3E-06	2.0E-07	3.5E-06	7.8E+00
Acetaldehyde	1026	3.8E-06	4.4E-07	5.0E-09	1.8E-07	3.0E-06	9.2E+00
alpha-Hexachlorcyclohexan	1360	4.6E-06	1.3E-05	6.8E-06	7.8E-07	4.4E-05	3.7E+00
Benzotrichloride	10000	6.3E-05	2.2E-09	4.0E-07	1.3E-05	5.3E-07	2.4E-01
Benzyl-chloride	2496	6.8E-06	7.7E-13	3.5E-10	9.2E-07	6.9E-07	4.0E+00
beta-Hexachlorcyclohexan	1221	5.0E-06	3.7E-04	1.4E-04	1.3E-07	1.6E-04	3.3E+00
Bromodichloromethane	6393	1.2E-05	1.1E-07	3.6E-09	2.3E-06	1.0E-06	3.0E+00
Carbon-tetrachloride	10000	3.9E-03	4.0E-06	3.3E-07	8.4E-04	1.1E-06	1.3E-02
Chloroform-	10000	3.2E-05	2.3E-07	3.9E-09	6.8E-06	1.2E-06	1.4E+00
Di(2-ethylhexyl)phthalate- (DEHP)	1044	3.9E-06	2.2E-07	2.3E-05	2.0E-07	1.4E-07	1.3E-02
Dichloromethane	10000	2.3E-05	1.7E-07	2.4E-09	4.8E-06	1.2E-06	1.9E+00
Dichlorvos	2587	1.7E-05	4.7E-04	1.2E-05	1.0E-07	4.1E-05	9.5E+00
gamma-Hexachlorocyclohexane (lindane)	1204	4.4E-06	1.1E-04	9.3E-05	1.7E-07	1.8E-04	8.1E-01
Hexachlorobenzene	4508	1.0E-05	1.5E-05	3.4E-05	1.7E-06	5.4E-07	3.2E-02
Pentachlorophenol	2109	6.8E-06	7.7E-05	9.7E-06	7.2E-07	1.9E-04	7.7E+00
Perchloroethylene	10000	1.9E-05	2.2E-08	5.1E-09	4.0E-06	1.1E-06	1.6E+00
Styrene	386	2.0E-06	3.8E-09	1.2E-09	2.1E-07	5.7E-07	5.0E+00
IARC-Group 3							
1,1,1,2-Tetrachlorethane	10000	2.8E-04	2.5E-06	2.8E-07	5.4E-05	1.1E-06	2.0E-01
1,1,2,2-Tetrachlorethane	10000	2.7E-04	1.3E-05	4.2E-07	5.4E-05	3.4E-06	5.8E-01
1,1,2-Trichlorethane	9005	1.5E-05	2.4E-08	1.3E-09	3.2E-06	1.1E-06	2.4E+00
1,1-Dichlorethene	675	2.9E-06	3.0E-09	2.7E-11	6.2E-07	1.1E-06	5.9E+00
3-Methylcholanthrene	1225	5.2E-06	4.9E-04	4.6E-03	5.1E-09	4.1E-07	3.6E-03
Aldrin	497	2.4E-06	5.4E-07	4.5E-05	1.9E-07	1.2E-07	1.5E-03
Bis(2-chlorethyl)ether	1029	3.8E-06	2.8E-07	1.4E-09	6.5E-07	3.3E-06	8.1E+00
Dibutyl-phthalate	1414	4.8E-06	2.2E-07	1.5E-04	1.6E-08	8.5E-07	1.7E-01
Dieldrin	1380	5.0E-06	9.7E-05	3.2E-03	3.5E-08	5.3E-07	5.4E-03
Hexachlorobutadiene	10000	6.3E-05	9.2E-08	7.7E-07	1.3E-05	5.1E-07	2.4E-02
Hexachloroethane	10000	2.8E-04	2.6E-06	1.8E-06	5.5E-05	1.2E-06	1.8E-01
Chloromethane, Methyl Chloride	10000	2.8E-04	6.8E-08	6.4E-09	5.4E-05	9.9E-07	1.8E-01
Trichlorethylene	2172	6.2E-06	1.5E-08	1.2E-10	1.3E-06	1.1E-06	4.2E+00
Trifluralin	10000	6.1E-05	1.8E-05	6.1E-05	3.2E-07	1.8E-08	3.0E-02

App. 6.5: Interim fate factors for 52 substances modelled in USES (1994) and adaptations made in Guinée *et al.* (1996) as well as Appendix (6.1), and (6.2) and adapted for the dilution height with the empirical relationship given in Subsection 6.2.4. # = calculated from the data given in Appendix (6.4), for PCB a second iteration lead to 10'000 m

Substance-name	CAS-Number	F'' air,air	F'' air,water	F'' air,food	F'' water,air	F'' water, water	F'' water, food
IARC-Group 1		m^2a/m^3	m^2a/l	$m^2a/(kg{\cdot}d)$	m^2a/m^3	m^2a/l	$m^2a/(kg{\cdot}d)$
Arsenic, inorganic	7440-38-2	8E-06	1.9E-04	6.0E-03	4.9E-17	1.6E-04	2.5E-06
Benzene	71-43-2	2.5E-05	3.2E-08	3.5E-10	1.5E-05	2.5E-05	5.0E-08
Bis(chloromethyl)ether BCME	542-88-1	3.9E-06	3.4E-07	1.7E-09	3.0E-06	1.2E-04	3.5E-10
Cadmium	7440-43-9	1.6E-05	8.6E-04	1.6E-03	1.0E-16	1.6E-04	5.0E-06
Chromium(VI)	18540-29-9	5.3E-06	1.4E-05	1.7E-01	2.4E-17	2.1E-05	2.7E-06
Nickel	12035-72-2	4.5E-06	3.3E-04	3.4E-03	4.6E-17	2.4E-04	1.5E-05
Nickel-refinery-dust	12035-72-2	4.5E-06	3.3E-04	3.4E-03	4.6E-17	2.4E-04	1.5E-05
Nickel-subsulfide	12035-72-2	4.5E-06	3.3E-04	3.4E-03	4.6E-17	2.4E-04	1.5E-05
Vinylchlorid	75-01-4	1.1E-05	8.9E-09	5.8E-10	1.1E-05	3.8E-05	2.1E-09
IARC-Group 2A							
1,2-Dibromoethane	106-93-4	2.0E-04	9.6E-07	3.0E-08	2.0E-04	4.0E-05	1.8E-07
1,3-Butadiene	106-99-0	2.5E-06	2.6E-07	4.3E-09	2.0E-06	1.4E-04	1.0E-07
Acrylonitrile	107-13-1	1.5E-05	2.2E-07	0.0E+00	8.9E-06	5.5E-05	9.8E-10
Benzo[a]pyrene (BaP)	50-32-8	5.4E-06	5.1E-04	1.6E-03	6.8E-09	2.6E-05	7.7E-04
Benz(a)anthracene	56-55-3	6.8E-06	5.0E-04	1.8E-03	2.3E-07	2.7E-07	7.1E-04
Dibenz(a,h)anthracene	53-70-3	5.4E-06	5.1E-04	1.2E-02	9.1E-10	1.0E-05	1.7E-03
Diesel soot particles		1.7E-05					
Epichlorhydrin	106-89-8	1.5E-05	1.3E-06	2.6E-08	1.8E-06	7.2E-05	4.2E-09
Ethylene Oxide	75-21-8	5.0E-04	9.6E-05	6.4E-07	2.5E-04	2.3E-04	3.1E-07
Formaldehyde	50-00-0	3.3E-06	2.5E-06	1.5E-06	3.1E-09	1.3E-04	2.4E-09
Polychlorinated-biphenyls- (PCBs)	1336-36-3	1.1E-04	4.1E-04	1.5E-03	3.9E-05	1.4E-04	8.9E-04
Propylene-oxide	75-56-9	3.7E-04	3.0E-05	2.5E-07	1.0E-04	8.9E-05	6.9E-08
IARC-Group 2B							
1,2-Dichloroethane	107-06-2	3.2E-04	1.7E-06	3.6E-08	3.1E-04	4.0E-05	7.7E-08
1,4-Dioxane	123-91-1	3.9E-06	8.7E-06	6.6E-08	1.6E-07	1.7E-04	3.1E-09
2,3,7,8-Tetrachlordibenzo-p-dioxin, TCDD	1746-01-6	9.0E-06	6.5E-04	1.8E-02	9.9E-07	7.1E-05	2.2E-03
2,4,6-Trichlorophenol	88-06-2	6.7E-05	1.1E-05	6.3E-06	4.5E-06	1.2E-04	1.0E-06
Acetaldehyde	75-07-0	3.9E-06	4.5E-07	5.3E-09	8.4E-07	1.0E-04	3.6E-09
alpha-Hexachlorcyclohexan	319-84-6	6.2E-06	1.7E-05	9.1E-06	4.9E-06	1.5E-03	7.3E-05
Benzotrichloride-	98-07-7	6.3E-04	2.2E-08	4.0E-06	6.2E-04	1.9E-05	1.1E-05
Benzyl-chloride-	100-44-7	1.7E-05	1.9E-12	8.4E-10	1.1E-05	2.4E-05	7.2E-08
beta-Hexachlorcyclohexan	319-85-7	5.2E-06	3.9E-04	1.5E-04	6.3E-07	5.6E-03	3.1E-04
Bromodichloromethane	75-27-4	7.9E-05	7.2E-07	1.7E-08	6.8E-05	3.6E-05	7.9E-08
Carbon-tetrachloride	56-23-5	3.8E-02	3.9E-05	2.7E-06	3.8E-02	5.8E-05	4.3E-06
Chloroform	67-66-3	3.2E-04	2.3E-06	6.0E-08	3.1E-04	4.2E-05	1.7E-07
Di(2-ethylhexyl)phthalate- (DEHP)	117-81-7	4.0E-06	2.3E-07	2.4E-05	1.0E-06	4.8E-06	1.0E-04
Dichloromethane	75-09-2	2.3E-04	1.7E-06	2.9E-08	2.2E-04	4.2E-05	2.5E-08
Dichlorvos	62-73-7	1.8E-05	4.9E-04	1.3E-05	5.0E-07	1.4E-03	1.2E-06
gamma-Hexachlorocyclohexane (lindane)	58-89-9	5.1E-06	1.3E-04	1.4E-04	9.0E-07	6.4E-03	2.0E-03
Hexachlorobenzene	118-74-1	4.4E-05	6.5E-05	1.4E-04	3.4E-05	3.4E-05	2.5E-04
Pentachlorophenol	87-86-5	1.3E-05	1.5E-04	1.8E-05	6.3E-06	6.6E-03	5.6E-05
Perchloroethylene	127-18-4	1.9E-04	2.2E-07	4.1E-08	1.9E-04	3.8E-05	1.5E-06
Styrene	100-42-5	2.0E-06	3.8E-09	1.2E-09	9.9E-07	2.0E-05	3.3E-07
IARC-Group 3							
1,1,1,2-Tetrachlorethane	630-20-6	2.6E-03	2.4E-05	2.7E-06	2.4E-03	4.9E-05	3.0E-06
1,1,2,2-Tetrachlorethane	79-34-5	2.3E-03	1.1E-04	3.5E-06	2.1E-03	2.1E-04	3.4E-06
1,1,2-Trichlorethane	79-00-5	1.4E-04	2.2E-07	7.6E-09	1.4E-04	3.8E-05	1.9E-07
1,1-Dichlorethene	75-35-4	2.9E-06	3.0E-09	2.7E-11	2.9E-06	3.8E-05	7.5E-08
3-Methylcholanthrene	56-49-5	5.3E-06	4.9E-04	4.6E-03	2.4E-08	1.4E-05	1.1E-03
Aldrin	309-00-2	2.4E-06	5.4E-07	4.5E-05	8.8E-07	4.2E-06	7.9E-04
Bis(2-chlorethyl)ether	111-44-4	3.9E-06	2.8E-07	1.4E-09	3.1E-06	1.1E-04	6.3E-10
Dibutyl-phthalate	84-74-2	6.7E-06	3.1E-07	2.1E-04	1.0E-07	3.0E-05	4.9E-05
Dieldrin	60-57-1	6.4E-06	1.2E-04	4.1E-03	2.1E-07	1.8E-05	9.9E-04
Hexachlorobutadiene	87-68-3	6.3E-04	9.1E-07	7.7E-06	5.8E-04	1.8E-05	2.0E-04
Hexachloroethane	67-72-1	2.6E-03	2.5E-05	1.7E-05	2.5E-03	5.1E-05	2.1E-05
Chloromethane, Methyl Chloride	74-87-3	2.8E-03	6.8E-07	0.0E+00	2.5E-03	3.5E-05	0.0E+00
Trichlorethylene	79-01-6	1.3E-05	3.4E-08	1.1E-09	1.3E-05	3.9E-05	1.5E-07
Trifluralin	1582-09-8	4.4E-04	1.3E-04	4.3E-04	1.1E-05	3.3E-06	1.5E-05

App. 6.6: Final fate factors for 55 substances taken from Appendices (6.4) and (6.5), and for diesel soot particles from Subsection 6.2.3

Substance-name	CAS-Number	Group IARC (1993b) USEPA (1990)	Target organ in humans (Vainio *et al.* 1991, Higginson *et al.* 1992)	Oral Slope Factor	Inhalation Unit Risk	Drinking Water Unit Risk
IARC-Group 1				$mg^{-1}kg^{-1}$ day^{-1}	$(\mu g/m^3)^{-1}$	$(\mu g/L)^{-1}$
Arsenic, inorganic	7440-38-2	A, 1, §	Lung, skin (liver)	1.5E+00	1.5E-03	5.0E-05
Asbestos	1332-21-4	A, 1	Lung, pleura, peritoneum		2.3E-01	
Benzene	71-43-2	A, 1, §	Leukaemia, hematopoietic system	2.9E-02	6.0E-06	8.3E-07
Benzidine	92-87-5	A, 1	Bladder	2.3E+02	6.7E-02	6.7E-03
Beryllium-	7440-41-7	B2, 1	Lung	4.3E+00	2.4E-03	1.2E-04
Bis(chloromethyl)ether- (BCME)	542-88-1	A, 1	Lung	2.2E+02	6.2E-02	6.2E-03
Cadmium	7440-43-9	B1, 1	Lung, prostate, kidney		1.8E-03	
Chromium(VI)	18540-29-9	A, 1, §	Lung		4.0E-02	
Coke-oven-emissions	8007-45-2	A, 1			6.2E-04	
Nickel		A, 1, §	Lung		3.4E-04	
Nickel-refinery-dust			Nasal cavity, lung		2.4E-04	
Nickel-subsulfide	12035-72-2	A, 1	Nasal cavity, lung		4.8E-04	
Vinyl chloride	75-01-4	A, 1, £	Liver, blood vessels (brain Lung, lymphatic system		1.0E-06	
IARC-Group 2A						
1,2-Dibromoethane	106-93-4	B2, 2A		8.5E+01	2.2E-04	2.5E-03
1,3-Butadiene	106-99-0	B2, 2A	Lymphatic hematopoietic system		2.8E-04	
Acrylonitrile	107-13-1	B1, 2A	Lung	5.4E-01	6.8E-05	1.5E-05
Benzo[a]pyrene- (BaP)	50-32-8	2A, §	Lung	7.3E+00	8.7E-02	2.1E-04
Benz[a]anthracene	56-55-3	B2, 2A, $			8.9E-04	
Dibenz[a,h]anthracene	53-70-3	B2, 2A, $			1.4E-02	
Diesel soot particles		2A, ç	Lung		3.4E-05	
Epichlorohydrin	106-89-8	B2, 2A	Lung	9.9E-03	1.2E-06	2.8E-07
Ethylene Oxide	75-21-8	B1-B2. 2A, $	Lymphatic and hematopoitic system		1.0E-04	
Formaldehyde	50-00-0	B1, 2A	Nose, nasopharynx		1.3E-05	
n-Nitroso-n-methylurea	684-93-5	B2, 2A, $			8.6E-02	
N-Nitrosodiethylamine	55-18-5	B2, 2A		1.5E+02	4.3E-02	4.3E-03
N-Nitrosodimethylamine	62-75-9	2A		5.1E+01	1.4E-02	1.4E-03
Polychlorinated-biphenyls(PCBs)	1336-36-3	B2, 2A, $	Skin (melanoma), liver		1.2E-03	
Propylene-oxide	75-56-9	B2, 2A		2.4E-01	3.7E-06	6.8E-06
IARC-Group 2B						
1,2-Dibromo-3-chloropropane	96-12-8	B2, 2B, $			6.3E-03	
1,2-Dichloroethane	107-06-2	B2, 2B		9.1E-02	2.6E-05	2.6E-06
1,4-Dioxane	123-91-1	B2, 2B, $		1.1E-02	1.4E-06	3.1E-07
2,3,7,8-Tetrachlordibenzo-p-dioxin, TCDD	1746-01-6	B2, 2B, &	Soft tissue sarcoma, lymphatic and hematopoietic system		1.4E+00	
2,4,6-Trichlorophenol	88-06-2	B2, 2B		1.1E-02	3.1E-06	3.1E-07
2-Nitropropane	79-46-9	B2, 2B, $			2.7E-03	
3,3'-Dichlorobenzidine	91-94-1	2B		4.5E-01		1.3E-05
Acetaldehyde	75-07-0	B2, 2B			2.2E-06	
Acrylamide	79-06-1	B2, 2B		4.5E+00	1.3E-03	1.3E-04
alpha-Hexachlorocyclohexane	319-84-6	2B	Lung	6.3E+00	1.8E-03	1.8E-04
Aramite	140-57-8	2B		2.5E-02	7.1E-06	7.1E-07
Benzotrichloride	98-07-7	2B		13 Ω		3.6E-04
Benzyl-chloride	100-44-7	2B		1.7E-01		4.9E-06
beta-Hexachlorocyclohexane (beta-HCH)	319-85-7	2B	Lung	1.8E+00	5.3E-04	5.3E-05
Bromodichloromethane	75-27-4	2B		6.2E-02		1.8E-06
Carbon-tetrachloride	56-23-5	B2, 2B	Liver	1.3E-01	1.5E-05	3.7E-06
Chlordane	57-74-9	B2, 2B		1.3E+00	3.7E-04	3.7E-05
Chloroform-	67-66-3	B2, 2B		6.1E-03	2.3E-05	1.7E-07
Di(2-ethylhexyl)phthalate (DEHP)	117-81-7	B2, 2B, $		1.4E-02	2.4E-07	4.0E-07
Dichloromethane	75-09-2	B2, 2B		7.5E-03	4.7E-07	2.1E-07
Dichlorvos-	62-73-7	2B		2.9E-01		8.3E-06
gamma-Hexachlorocyclohexane (lindane)	58-89-9	C. 2B, $	Lung		3.8E-04	
Gasoline vehicles POM		2B, $			2.5E-04	

App. 6.7: Unit risk factors for carcinogenic substances, ordered following the IARC classification, Ω = for use with Dietary Intakes, if not other stated unit risks from IRIS (1996), $ = USEPA (1990), £ = WHO (1987), § = WHO (1996a), ç = WHO (1996b). & = LAI (1992), see Subsection 6.34 for further explanations

Substance-name	CAS-Number	Group IARC (1993b) USEPA (1990)	Target organ in humans (Vainio *et al.* 1991, Higginson *et al.* 1992)	Oral Slope Factor	Inhalation Unit Risk	Drinking Water Unit Risk
				$mg^{-1}kg^{-1}day^{-1}$	$(\mu g/m^3)^{-1}$	$(\mu g/L)^{-1}$
Heptachlor-	76-44-8	B2, 2B		4.5E+00	1.3E-03	1.3E-04
Hexachlorobenzene	118-74-1	B2, 2B		1.6E+00	4.6E-04	4.6E-05
Hydrazine/Hydrazine sulfate	302-01-2	B2, 2B		3.0E+00	4.9E-03	8.5E-05
N-Nitroso-di-n-butylamine	924-16-3	B2, 2B		5.4E+00	1.6E-03	1.6E-04
N-Nitroso-N-methylethylamine	10595-95-6	2B		2.2E+01		6.3E-04
N-Nitrosodi-N-propylamine	621-64-7	2B		7.0E+00		2.0E-04
N-Nitrosopyrrolidine	930-55-2	B2, 2B		2.1E+00	6.1E-04	6.1E-05
p,p'-Dichlorodiphenyltrichloroethane (DDT)	50-29-3	B2, 2B	Lung	3.4E-01	9.7E-05	9.7E-06
Pentachlorophenol-	87-86-5	2B		1.2E-01		3.0E-06
Perchloroethylene	127-18-4	B2, 2B, $	Lymphatic and hematopoietic system, urogenital system		5.8E-07	
Styrene	100-42-5	B2, 2B, $	Lymphatic and hematopoietic system		5.7E-07	
technical-Hexachlorocyclohexane- (t-HCH)	608-73-1	2B		1.8E+00	5.1E-04	5.1E-05
Toxaphene	8001-35-2	B2, 2B		1.1E+00	3.2E-04	3.2E-05
IARC-Group 3						
1,1,1,2-Tetrachloroethane	630-20-6	3		2.6E-02	7.4E-06	7.4E-07
1,1,2,2-Tetrachloroethane	79-34-5	C, 3		2.0E-01	5.8E-05	5.8E-06
1,1,2-Trichloroethane	79-00-5	C, 3		5.7E-02	1.6E-05	1.6E-06
1,1-Dichloroethylene	75-35-4	C		6.0E-01	5.0E-05	1.7E-05
1,2-Dichloropropane	78-87-5	C, 3, $			1.8E-05	
1,2-Diphenylhydrazine	122-66-7	B2		8.0E-01	2.2E-04	2.2E-05
2,4,6-Trinitrotoluene (TNT)	118-96-7			3.0E-02		9.0E-07
2,4-/2,6-Dinitrotoluene mixture				6.8E-01		1.9E-05
2,4-Dinitroltoluene	121-14-2	B2,$			8.8E-05	
3-Methylchloanthrene	56-49-5	B2, $			2.7E-03	
4,4'-Methylene bis(N,N'-dimethyl)aniline	101-61-1	3		4.6E-02		1.3E-06
Acephate	30560-19-1			8.7E-03		2.5E-07
Aldrin-	309-00-2	B2, 3		1.7E+01	4.9E-03	4.9E-04
Allyl-chloride	107-05-1	B2, 3, $			5.5E-08	
Aniline-	62-53-3	B2, 3, $		5.7E-03	7.4E-06	1.6E-07
Azobenzene	103-33-3	3		1.1E-01	3.1E-05	3.1E-06
Bis(chloroethyl)ether- (BCEE)	111-44-4	B2, 3	Lung	1.1E+00	3.3E-04	3.3E-05
Bromoform	75-25-2	3		7.9E-03	1.1E-06	2.3E-07
Di(2-ethylhexyl)adipate	103-23-1	3		1.2E-03		3.4E-08
Dibromochloromethane	124-48-1			8.4E-02		2.4E-06
Dibutyl-phthalate	84-74-2			6.0E-01	5.0E-05	1.7E-05
Dieldrin	60-57-1	B2, 3		1.6E+01	4.6E-03	4.6E-04
Dimethipin	55290-64-7			5.1E+01	1.4E-02	1.4E-03
Dinoseb	88-85-7			8.0E-01	2.2E-04	2.2E-05
Folpet	133-07-3			3.5E-03		1.0E-07
Fomesafen	72178-02-0			1.9E-01		5.4E-06
Furmecyclox-	60568-05-0			3.0E-02		8.6E-07
Heptachlor-epoxide	1024-57-3	B2		9.1E+00	2.6E-03	2.6E-04
Hexachlorobutadiene	87-68-3	C, 3		7.8E-02	2.2E-05	2.2E-06
Hexachlorodibenzo-p-dioxin, mixture (HxCDD)	19408-74-3			6.2E+03	1.3E+00	1.8E-01
Hexachloroethane	67-72-1	C, 3		1.4E-02	4.0E-06	4.0E-07
Hexahydro-1,3,5-trinitro-1,3,5-triazine (RDX)	121-82-4			1.1E-01		3.1E-06
Isophorone-	78-59-1			9.5E-04		2.7E-08
Methyl chloride	74-87-3	C, 3, $			3.6E-06	
Methylhydrazine	60-34-4	B2, $			3.1E-04	
N-Nitrosodiethanolamine	1116-54-7			2.8E+00		8.0E-05
N-Nitrosodiphenylamine	86-30-6			4.9E-03		1.4E-07
p,p'-Dichlorodiphenyl dichloroethane (DDD)	72-54-8			2.4E-01		6.9E-06
p,p'-Dichlorodiphenyldichloroethylene (DDE)	72-55-9			3.4E-01		9.7E-06
Prochloraz	67747-09-5			1.5E-01		4.3E-06
Trichlorethylene	79-01-6	B2, 3, §			4.3E-07	
Trifluralin	1582-09-8	3		7.7E-03		2.2E-07

App. 6.7 cont: Unit risk factors for carcinogenic substances, ordered following the IARC classification, if not other stated unit risks from IRIS (1996), $ = USEPA (1990), £ = WHO (1987), § = WHO (1996a), ç = WHO (1996b). & = LAI (1992), see Subsection 6.34 for further explanations

Appendix 6.8: Arithmetic of lognormal distributed random variables

1. Motivation

The lognormal distribution may be converted to a normal distribution if the variable is presented on a log scale. The variable has to be positive and the distribution of the variable's values is oblique. Many processes and models in natural science can be described with and presented in a logarithmic form.

Several reports in the field of risk assessment and impact pathway analysis (SETAC 1995, Rabl 1996, and Meier 1997) have shown that the lognormal distribution seems to be a more realistic approximation for the variability in fate and effect factors than the normal distribution.

For simplicity, we assume here that all variables are independent and lognormally distributed.

The lognormal distribution is not so well known. Some basic relations are therefore derived from the normal distribution and presented here[17]. For more details, see Johnson *et al.* (1994).

2. Properties of Normal Distribution

2.1 Density

The normal distribution has the density function:

$$\varphi(t) = \frac{1}{\sqrt{2\pi\sigma^2}} e^{-\frac{(t-\mu)^2}{2\sigma^2}}$$

where μ expectation value (in many cases estimated by mean or median of a sample)
σ standard deviation

2.2 Additivity

If X and Y are normal distributed with $X \sim N(\mu_1, \sigma_1), Y \sim N(\mu_2, \sigma_2)$ and {X, Y} independent then $X \sim N(\mu_1, \sigma_1), Y \sim N(\mu_2, \sigma_2)$

2.3 Confidence Interval

The probability that x is within a certain interval can be written as:

[17] This appendix profits largely from the input by Verena Gelpke and Olaf Tietje (both ETHZ).

$$P[\mu - r\sigma \leq x \leq \mu + r\sigma] = v \qquad \begin{array}{ll} v = 0.68 & \text{if } r = 1 \\ v = 0.95 & \text{if } r = 1.96 \approx 2 \\ v = 0.99 & \text{if } r = 2.58 \end{array} \qquad \text{(A6.1)}$$

3. Properties of Lognormal Distribution

3.1 Multiplying Lognormal Distributions

U is said to be lognormally distributed if log(U) has normal distribution, i.e., log(U) ~ N (μ, σ)

For practical reasons it is convenient to introduce μg and σg which are simple transformations of μ and σ.

$\mu g = e^{\mu}$ μg = geometric mean, i.e., expectation value

$\sigma g = e^{\sigma}$ σg = geometric standard deviation

If *U* and *V* are independent and each have lognormal distribution with μgu, σgu, μgv, σgv respectively

(i.e., $log(U) \sim N(\mu u, \sigma u)$ $\mu u = log(\mu gu)$, $\sigma u = log(\sigma gu)$

$log(V) \sim N(\mu v, \sigma v)$ $\mu v = log(\mu gv)$, $\sigma v = log(\sigma gv)$)

then $W = U \cdot V$ is lognormally distributed again, with

expectation value $\mu gw = \mu gu \cdot \mu gv$ and

geometric standard deviation $\sigma_{gw} = e^{\sqrt{(\log^2(\sigma_{gu}) + \log^2(\sigma_{gv}))}}$

Illustration: $log(W) = log(U \cdot V) = log(U) + log(V)$

This is a sum of two normally distributed random variables and it is well known (see, e.g., Johnson *et al.* 1994) that this sum is normally distributed with

$\mu z = \mu u + \mu v$, and $\sigma_w = \sqrt{(\sigma_u{}^2 + \sigma_v{}^2)}$

$\Rightarrow \mu gw = e^{\mu w} = e^{\mu u + \mu v} = e^{\mu u} \cdot e^{\mu v} = \mu gu \cdot \mu gv$

$$\sigma_{gw} = e^{\sigma w} = e^{\sqrt{\left(\sigma_u{}^2 + \sigma_v{}^2\right)}} = e^{\sqrt{\left(\log^2(\sigma_{gu}) + \log^2(\sigma_{gv})\right)}}$$

More generally we can show that the product of n independent lognormally distributed random variables Xj $j = 1...n$ with parameters $(\mu gj, \sigma gj)$ $j = 1...n$ is lognormally distributed with expectation value

$\mu g\ tot = \Pi_{(j=1..n}\ \mu gj$ and (A6.2)

geometric standard deviation

$$\sigma_{gtot} = e^{\sqrt{\sum_{j=1}^{n} \log^2(\sigma_{gj})}} \tag{A6.3}$$

3.2 Confidence Interval

from Equation (A6.1) it follows that

$P[\mu g/\sigma g^r \leq u \leq \mu g \cdot \sigma g^r] = v$ for $v = 0.68$ if $r = 1$
$v = 0.95$ if $r = 1.96 \approx 2$
$v = 0.99$ if $r = 2.58$

Illustration: U is lognormally distributed with μg and σg, i.e.,
$X = log\ (U) \sim N\ (\mu, \sigma),\ \mu = log\ (\mu g),\ \sigma = log(\sigma g)$
with (A1) $v = P[\mu - r\ \sigma \leq X \leq \mu + r \cdot \sigma]$
$= P[log\ (\mu g) - r \cdot log(\sigma g) \leq log(U) \leq log\ (\mu g) + r \cdot log(\sigma g)]$
$\Rightarrow P[\mu g/\sigma g^r \leq U \leq \mu g \cdot \sigma g^r]$

4. Discussion

With Formula (A6.2) and (A6.3) we are able to calculate the moments of the distribution functions of lognormally distributed variables, multiplied independently, in an easy, arithmetically closed form. One could now ask what will be the result if lognormally distributed variables are added to or multiplied with normally distributed variables. For these cases, the distribution functions get very complicated and the interval has to be numerically integrated (Johnson *et al.* 1994, p. 217 ff and 247 ff).

It is not advisable anymore to use the arithmetic calculation for these more complicated cases of analysis, but rather to use numerical tools such as Monte Carlo simulation instead. Such a tool (@Risk, Palisade Corporation) has been used in a similar application by Meier (1997) and can very easily be used together with a spreadsheet calculation.

Another way to deal with the calculation of uncertainty ranges in risk assessment is to calculate distinct percentiles for each variable and to perform for each percentile a separate simple calculation (Lühr at al. 1991, Yetergil Kiefer 1997). ESEERCO (1995) used a central, a lower and an upper estimate for each variable and estimated in addition for each values the probability of occurrence, i.e., a simplified distribution density. A simple numerical tool is the Latin Hypercube Method (McKay *et al.* 1979) which is superior to Monte-Carlo simulations. This method divides the distribution function into a small number of segments. For each of these segments, the values and their probabilities are calculated separately with a new (numerical) distribution function as the result. This tool is included in standard risk software (like, e.g., @Risk, Palisade Corporation). Funtowicz *et al.* (1990), and for LCA Pohl *et al.* (1996a/b), are useful sources for a more in-depth discussion of the problem of uncertainty assessment and error analysis.

Substance-name	Population density ρ (emissions to air)	Incidence factor Ti, air, inhalation	Incidence factor Ti, air, drinking water	Incidence factor Ti,air, food	Population density ρ (emissions to water)	Incidence factor Ti, water, inhalation	Incidence factor Ti, water, drinking water	Incidence factor Ti, water, food
IARC-Group 1	persons per m^2	Incidence cases/kg	Incidence cases/kg	Incidence cases/kg	persons per m^2	Incidence cases/kg	Incidence cases/kg	Incidence cases/kg
Arsenic, inorganic	9.44E-05	1.6E-05	1.3E-05	1.2E-02	3.00E-04	3.2E-16	3.5E-05	1.6E-05
Benzene	5.59E-05	1.2E-07	2.1E-11	8.1E-12	6.95E-05	9.2E-08	2.0E-08	1.5E-09
Bis(chloromethyl)ether BCME	1.32E-04	4.6E-04	4.0E-06	7.2E-07	1.50E-04	4.0E-04	1.7E-03	1.6E-07
Cadmium	6.82E-05	2.8E-05	0	0	3.00E-04	8.1E-16	0	0
Chromium(VI)	1.15E-04	3.5E-04	0	0	3.00E-04	4.2E-15	0	0
Nickel	1.24E-04	2.7E-06	0	0	3.00E-04	6.8E-17	0	0
Nickel-refinery-dust	1.24E-04	1.9E-06	0	0	3.00E-04	4.8E-17	0	0
Nickel-subsulfide	1.24E-04	3.8E-06	0	0	3.00E-04	9.5E-17	0	0
Vinylchlorid	8.17E-05	1.3E-08	0	0	8.19E-05	1.3E-08	0	0
IARC-Group 2A								
1,2-Dibromoethane	2.30E-05	1.4E-05	7.9E-07	8.3E-07	2.31E-05	1.4E-05	3.3E-05	5.0E-06
1,3-Butadiene	2.30E-04	2.3E-06	0	0	2.56E-04	2.0E-06	0	0
Acrylonitrile	6.96E-05	1.0E-06	3.3E-09	0	8.97E-05	7.8E-07	1.1E-06	6.7E-10
Benzo[a]pyrene- (BaP)	1.14E-04	7.6E-04	1.8E-04	1.9E-02	3.00E-04	2.5E-06	2.3E-05	2.4E-02
Benz(a)anthracene	1.02E-04	8.8E-06	0	0	3.00E-04	8.9E-07	0	0
Dibenz(a,h)anthracene	1.14E-04	1.2E-04	0	0	3.00E-04	5.4E-08	0	0
Diesel soot particles	7.36E-05	6.1E-07	0	0		0	0	0
Epichlorhydrin	6.95E-05	1.8E-08	3.6E-10	2.6E-10	1.93E-04	6.0E-09	5.5E-08	1.2E-10
Ethylene Oxide	1.63E-05	1.2E-05	0	0	2.10E-05	7.5E-06	0	0
Formaldehyde-	1.54E-04	9.5E-08	0	0	3.00E-04	1.7E-10	0	0
Polychlorinated-biphenyls-(PCBs)	2.89E-05	5.5E-05	0	0	4.55E-05	3.0E-05	0	0
Propylene-oxide	1.81E-05	3.6E-07	5.2E-08	1.5E-08	2.98E-05	1.6E-07	2.6E-07	7.0E-09
IARC-Group 2B								
1,2-Dichloroethane	1.92E-05	2.3E-06	1.2E-09	8.9E-10	1.93E-05	2.2E-06	2.9E-08	1.9E-09
1,4-Dioxane	1.34E-04	1.0E-08	5.1E-09	1.4E-09	3.00E-04	9.7E-10	2.3E-07	1.5E-10
2,3,7,8-Tetrachlordibenzo-p-dioxin, TCDD	8.95E-05	1.6E-02	0	0	2.60E-04	5.1E-03	0	0
2,4,6-Trichlorophenol	3.59E-05	1.1E-07	1.7E-09	3.5E-08	1.25E-04	2.5E-08	6.8E-08	2.0E-08
Acetaldehyde	1.33E-04	1.6E-08	0	0	2.81E-04	7.4E-09	0	0
alpha-Hexachlorcyclohexan	1.06E-04	1.7E-05	4.7E-06	8.7E-05	1.19E-04	1.5E-05	4.7E-04	7.8E-04
Benzotrichloride	1.51E-05	0	1.7E-09	1.1E-05	1.51E-05	0	1.5E-06	3.1E-05
Benzyl-chloride	6.66E-05	0	9.0E-15	1.4E-10	8.24E-05	0	1.4E-07	1.4E-08
beta-Hexachlorcyclohexan	1.16E-04	4.6E-06	3.4E-05	4.4E-04	3.00E-04	1.4E-06	1.3E-03	2.4E-03
Bromodichloromethane	3.35E-05	0	6.2E-10	5.0E-10	3.57E-05	0	3.3E-08	2.5E-09
Carbon-tetrachloride	6.30E-06	5.1E-05	1.3E-08	3.1E-08	6.30E-06	5.1E-05	1.9E-08	5.1E-08
Chloroform	1.92E-05	2.0E-06	1.1E-10	1.0E-10	1.93E-05	2.0E-06	2.0E-09	2.9E-10
Di(2-ethylhexyl)phthalate- (DEHP)	1.31E-04	1.8E-09	1.7E-10	6.2E-07	2.57E-04	8.9E-10	7.1E-09	5.3E-06
Dichloromethane	2.18E-05	3.3E-08	1.1E-10	6.9E-11	2.19E-05	3.3E-08	2.7E-09	5.8E-11
Dichlorvos	6.48E-05	0	3.8E-06	3.4E-06	3.00E-04	0	5.1E-05	1.5E-06
gamma-Hexachlorocyclohexane (lindane)	1.17E-04	3.2E-06	0	0	2.71E-04	1.3E-06	0	0
Hexachlorobenzene	4.29E-05	1.3E-05	1.8E-06	1.4E-04	4.82E-05	1.1E-05	1.1E-06	2.7E-04
Pentachlorophenol	7.57E-05	0	4.7E-07	2.4E-06	1.05E-04	0	3.0E-05	1.0E-05
Perchloroethylene	2.35E-05	3.6E-08	0	0	2.36E-05	3.6E-08	0	0
Styrene	2.90E-04	4.8E-09	0	0	3.00E-04	2.4E-09	0	0
IARC-Group 3								
1,1,1,2-Tetrachlorethane	9.93E-06	2.8E-06	2.6E-09	9.9E-09	1.01E-05	2.6E-06	5.3E-09	1.1E-08
1,1,2,2-Tetrachlorethane	1.03E-05	1.9E-05	9.5E-08	1.0E-07	1.05E-05	1.8E-05	1.8E-07	1.0E-07
1,1,2-Trichlorethane	2.65E-05	8.4E-07	1.3E-10	1.6E-10	2.67E-05	8.3E-07	2.3E-08	4.1E-09
1,1-Dichlorethene	1.85E-04	3.9E-07	1.3E-10	4.3E-11	1.86E-04	3.9E-07	1.7E-06	1.2E-07
3-Methylcholanthrene	1.15E-04	2.3E-05	0	0	3.00E-04	2.8E-07	0	0
Aldrin	2.36E-04	4.0E-05	9.0E-07	2.6E-03	3.00E-04	1.8E-05	8.7E-06	5.7E-02
Bis(2-chlorethyl)ether	1.32E-04	2.5E-06	1.8E-08	2.9E-09	1.49E-04	2.2E-06	8.0E-06	1.5E-09
Dibutyl-phthalate	1.03E-04	4.9E-07	7.8E-09	1.8E-04	3.00E-04	2.2E-08	2.2E-06	1.3E-04
Dieldrin	1.05E-04	4.4E-05	8.6E-05	9.9E-02	3.00E-04	4.1E-06	3.6E-05	6.8E-02
Hexachlorobutadiene	1.51E-05	3.0E-06	4.3E-10	1.3E-07	1.55E-05	2.8E-06	8.8E-09	3.4E-06
Hexachloroethane	9.92E-06	1.5E-06	1.4E-09	3.4E-08	1.01E-05	1.4E-06	2.9E-09	4.2E-08
Chloromethane, Methyl Chloride	9.81E-06	1.4E-06	0	0	1.01E-05	1.3E-06	0	0
Trichlorethylene	7.40E-05	6.1E-09	0	0	7.42E-05	6.1E-09	0	0
Trifluralin	1.71E-05	0	7.1E-09	8.2E-07	8.17E-05	0	8.4E-10	1.3E-07

App. 6.9: Tumour incidence rate Tijk per 1 kg substance emissions to air or water (Equation 6.14), population density calculated with Equation (6.12).

Substance-name	CAS-Number	Group IARC (1987/93) USEPA (1990)	Target organ in humans (Vainio *et al.* 1991, Higginson *et al.* 1992)	Oral Slope Factor	Inhalation Unit Risk	Drinking Water Unit Risk
IARC-Group 1				$mg^{-1}kg^{-1}day^{-1}$	$(\mu g/m^3)^{-1}$	$(\mu g/L)^{-1}$
Arsenic, inorganic	7440-38-2	A, 1, §	Lung, skin, liver	1.50E+00	1.50E-03	5.00E-05
Benzene-	71-43-2	A, 1, §	Leukaemia, hematopoietic system	2.90E-02	6.00E-06	8.30E-07
Bis(chloromethyl)ether BCME	542-88-1	A, 1	Lung	2.20E+02	6.20E-02	6.20E-03
Cadmium-	7440-43-9	B1, 1	Lung, prostate, kidney	**6.30E+00**	1.80E-03	
Chromium(VI)	18540-29-9	A, 1, §	Lung	**1.40E+02**	4.00E-02	
Nickel		A, 1, §	Lung	**1.19E+00**	3.40E-04	
Nickel-refinery-dust			Nasal cavity, lung	**8.40E-01**	2.40E-04	
Nickel-subsulfide	12035-72-2	A, 1	Nasal cavity, lung	**1.68E+00**	4.80E-04	
Vinylchlorid	75-01-4	A, 1, £	Liver, blood vessels (brain lung, Lymphatic system	**3.50E-03**	1.00E-06	**1.00E-07**
IARC-Group 2A						
1,2-Dibromoethane	106-93-4	B2, 2A		8.50E+01	2.20E-04	2.50E-03
1,3-Butadiene	106-99-0	B2, 2A	Lymphatic hematopoietic system	**9.80E-01**	2.80E-04	**2.80E-05**
Acrylonitrile-	107-13-1	B1, 2A	Lung	5.40E-01	6.80E-05	1.50E-05
Benzo[a]pyrene- (BaP)	50-32-8	2A, §	Lung	7.30E+00	8.70E-02	2.10E-04
Benz(a)anthracene	56-55-3	B2, 2A, $		**3.12E+00**	8.90E-04	
Dibenz(a,h)anthracene	53-70-3	B2, 2A, $		**4.90E+01**	1.40E-02	
Diesel soot particles		2A, ç	Lung		3.40E-05	
Epichlorhydrin	106-89-8	B2, 2A	Lung	9.90E-03	1.20E-06	2.80E-07
Ethylene Oxide	75-21-8	B1-B2.2A,$	Lymphatic and hematopoitic system		1.00E-04	
Formaldehyde-	50-00-0	B1, 2A	Nose, nasopharynx	**4.55E-02**	1.30E-05	**1.30E-06**
Polychlorinated-biphenyls- (PCBs)	1336-36-3	B2, 2A, $	Skin (melanoma), liver	**4.20E+00**	1.20E-03	
Propylene-oxide-	75-56-9	B2, 2A		2.40E-01	3.70E-06	6.80E-06
IARC-Group 2B						
1,2-Dichloroethane	107-06-2	B2, 2B		9.10E-02	2.60E-05	2.60E-06
1,4-Dioxane	123-91-1	B2, 2B, $		1.10E-02	1.40E-06	3.10E-07
2,3,7,8-Tetrachlordibenzo-p-dioxin, TCDD	1746-01-6	B2, 2B, &	Soft tissue sarcoma, lymphatic and hematopoietic system	**4.90E+03**	1.40E+00	
2,4,6-Trichlorophenol	88-06-2	B2, 2B		1.10E-02	3.10E-06	3.10E-07
Acetaldehyde	75-07-0	B2, 2B		**7.70E-03**	2.20E-06	**2.20E-07**
alpha-Hexachlorcyclohexan	319-84-6	2B	Lung	6.30E+00	1.80E-03	1.80E-04
Benzotrichloride-	98-07-7	2B		1.30E+01	**3.71E-03**	3.60E-04
Benzyl-chloride-	100-44-7	2B		1.70E-01	**4.86E-05**	4.90E-06
beta-Hexachlorcyclohexan	319-85-7	2B	Lung	1.80E+00	5.30E-04	5.30E-05
Bromodichloromethane	75-27-4	2B		6.20E-02	**1.77E-05**	1.80E-06
Carbon-tetrachloride-	56-23-5	B2, 2B	Liver	1.30E-01	1.50E-05	3.70E-06
Chloroform-	67-66-3	B2, 2B		6.10E-03	2.30E-05	1.70E-07
Di(2-ethylhexyl)phthalate- (DEHP)	117-81-7	B2, 2B, $		1.40E-02	2.40E-07	4.00E-07
Dichloromethane-	75-09-2	B2, 2B		7.50E-03	4.70E-07	2.10E-07
Dichlorvos-	62-73-7	2B		2.90E-01	**8.29E-05**	8.30E-06
gamma-Hexachlorocyclohexane (lindane)	58-89-9	C. 2B, $	Lung	**1.33E+00**	3.80E-04	**3.80E-05**
Hexachlorobenzene-	118-74-1	B2, 2B		1.60E+00	4.60E-04	4.60E-05
Pentachlorophenol-	87-86-5	2B		1.20E-01		3.00E-06
Perchloroethylene	127-18-4	B2, 2B, $	Lymphatic and hematopoietic system, urogenital system		5.80E-07	
Styrene	100-42-5	B2, 2B, $	Lymphatic and hematopoietic system	**2.00E-03**	5.70E-07	**5.70E-08**
IARC-Group 3						
1,1,1,2-Tetrachlorethane	630-20-6	3		2.60E-02	7.40E-06	7.40E-07
1,1,2,2-Tetrachlorethane	79-34-5	C, 3		2.00E-01	5.80E-05	5.80E-06
1,1,2-Trichlorethane	79-00-5	C, 3		5.70E-02	1.60E-05	1.60E-06
1,1-Dichlorethene	75-35-4	C		6.00E-01	5.00E-05	1.70E-05
3-Methylcholanthrene	56-49-5	B2, $		**9.45E+00**	2.70E-03	
Aldrin-	309-00-2	B2, 3		1.70E+01	4.90E-03	4.90E-04
Bis(2-chlorethyl)ether	111-44-4	B2, 3	Lung	1.10E+00	3.30E-04	3.30E-05
Dibutyl-phthalate-	84-74-2			6.00E-01	5.00E-05	1.70E-05
Dieldrin-	60-57-1	B2, 3		1.60E+01	4.60E-03	4.60E-04
Hexachlorobutadiene-	87-68-3	C, 3		7.80E-02	2.20E-05	2.20E-06
Hexachloroethane	67-72-1	C, 3		1.40E-02	4.00E-06	4.00E-07
Chloromethane, Methyl Chloride	74-87-3	C, 3, $			3.60E-06	
Trichlorethylene	79-01-6	B2, 3, §			4.30E-07	
Trifluralin-	1582-09-8	3		7.70E-03	**2.20E-06**	2.20E-07

App. 6.10: Unit risk factors for 55 substances, bold unit risk factors are extrapolated from existing factors and therefore of higher uncertainty, if not otherwise stated unit risks from IRIS (1996), $ = USEPA (1990), £ = WHO (1987), § = WHO (1996a), ç = WHO (1996b). & = LAI (1992), (from Appendix 6.7)

Substance-name	Incidence factor Ti, air, inhalation	Incidence factor Ti, air, drinking water	Incidence factor Ti,air, food	Incidence factor Ti, water, inhalation	Incidence factor Ti, water, drinking water	Incidence factor Ti, water, food
IARC-Group 1	Incidence cases/kg	Incidence cases/kg	Incidence cases/kg	Incidence cases/kg	Incidence cases/kg	Incidence cases/kg
Arsenic, inorganic	1.6E-05	1.3E-05	1.2E-02	3.2E-16	3.5E-05	1.6E-05
Benzene	1.2E-07	2.1E-11	8.1E-12	9.2E-08	2.0E-08	1.5E-09
Bis(chloromethyl)ether BCME	4.6E-04	4.0E-06	7.2E-07	4.0E-04	1.7E-03	1.6E-07
Cadmium	2.8E-05	0	**9.8E-03**	8.1E-16	0	**1.3E-04**
Chromium(VI)	3.5E-04	0	**4.0E+01**	4.2E-15	0	**1.6E-03**
Nickel	2.7E-06	0	**7.3E-03**	6.8E-17	0	**7.8E-05**
Nickel-refinery-dust	1.9E-06	0	**5.1E-03**	4.8E-17	0	**5.5E-05**
Nickel-subsulfide	3.8E-06	0	**1.0E-02**	9.5E-17	0	**1.1E-04**
Vinylchlorid	1.3E-08	**1.0E-12**	**2.4E-12**	1.3E-08	**4.5E-09**	**8.6E-12**
IARC-Group 2A						
1,2-Dibromoethane	1.4E-05	7.9E-07	8.3E-07	1.4E-05	3.3E-05	5.0E-06
1,3-Butadiene	2.3E-06	**2.4E-08**	**1.4E-08**	2.0E-06	**1.5E-05**	**3.7E-07**
Acrylonitrile	1.0E-06	3.3E-09	0	7.8E-07	1.1E-06	6.7E-10
Benzo[a]pyrene- (BaP)	7.6E-04	1.8E-04	1.9E-02	2.5E-06	2.3E-05	2.4E-02
Benz(a)anthracene	8.8E-06	0	**8.3E-03**	8.9E-07	0	**9.5E-03**
Dibenz(a,h)anthracene	1.2E-04	0	**9.5E-01**	5.4E-08	0	**3.5E-01**
Diesel soot particles	6.1E-07	0	0	0	0	0
Epichlorhydrin	1.8E-08	3.6E-10	2.6E-10	6.0E-09	5.5E-08	1.2E-10
Ethylene Oxide	1.2E-05	0	0	7.5E-06	0	0
Formaldehyde	9.5E-08	**7.1E-09**	**1.5E-07**	1.7E-10	**7.3E-07**	**4.7E-10**
Polychlorinated-biphenyls- (PCBs)	5.5E-05	0	**2.6E-03**	3.0E-05	0	**2.4E-03**
Propylene-oxide	3.6E-07	5.2E-08	1.5E-08	1.6E-07	2.6E-07	7.0E-09
IARC-Group 2B						
1,2-Dichloroethane	2.3E-06	1.2E-09	8.9E-10	2.2E-06	2.9E-08	1.9E-09
1,4-Dioxane	1.0E-08	5.1E-09	1.4E-09	9.7E-10	2.3E-07	1.5E-10
2,3,7,8-Tetrachlordibenzo-p-dioxin, TCDD	1.6E-02	0	**1.1E+02**	5.1E-03	0	**4.1E+01**
2,4,6-Trichlorophenol	1.1E-07	1.7E-09	3.5E-08	2.5E-08	6.8E-08	2.0E-08
Acetaldehyde	1.6E-08	**1.9E-10**	**7.7E-11**	7.4E-09	**9.1E-08**	**1.1E-10**
alpha-Hexachlorcyclohexan	1.7E-05	4.7E-06	8.7E-05	1.5E-05	4.7E-04	7.8E-04
Benzotrichloride	**5.1E-04**	1.7E-09	1.1E-05	**5.0E-04**	1.5E-06	3.1E-05
Benzyl-chloride	**7.8E-07**	9.0E-15	1.4E-10	**6.1E-07**	1.4E-07	1.4E-08
beta-Hexachlorcyclohexan	4.6E-06	3.4E-05	4.4E-04	1.4E-06	1.3E-03	2.4E-03
Bromodichloromethane	**6.7E-07**	6.2E-10	5.0E-10	**6.1E-07**	3.3E-08	2.5E-09
Carbon-tetrachloride	5.1E-05	1.3E-08	3.1E-08	5.1E-05	1.9E-08	5.1E-08
Chloroform	2.0E-06	1.1E-10	1.0E-10	2.0E-06	2.0E-09	2.9E-10
Di(2-ethylhexyl)phthalate- (DEHP)	1.8E-09	1.7E-10	6.2E-07	8.9E-10	7.1E-09	5.3E-06
Dichloromethane	3.3E-08	1.1E-10	6.9E-11	3.3E-08	2.7E-09	5.8E-11
Dichlorvos	**1.4E-06**	3.8E-06	3.4E-06	**1.8E-07**	5.1E-05	1.5E-06
gamma-Hexachlorocyclohexane (lindane)	3.2E-06	**8.1E-06**	**3.0E-04**	1.3E-06	**9.4E-04**	**1.0E-02**
Hexachlorobenzene	1.3E-05	1.8E-06	1.4E-04	1.1E-05	1.1E-06	2.7E-04
Pentachlorophenol	0	4.7E-07	2.4E-06	0	3.0E-05	1.0E-05
Perchloroethylene	3.6E-08	0	0	3.6E-08	0	0
Styrene	4.8E-09	**9.1E-13**	**9.7E-12**	2.4E-09	**4.8E-09**	**2.8E-09**
IARC-Group 3						
1,1,1,2-Tetrachlorethane	2.8E-06	2.6E-09	9.9E-09	2.6E-06	5.3E-09	1.1E-08
1,1,2,2-Tetrachlorethane	1.9E-05	9.5E-08	1.0E-07	1.8E-05	1.8E-07	1.0E-07
1,1,2-Trichlorethane	8.4E-07	1.3E-10	1.6E-10	8.3E-07	2.3E-08	4.1E-09
1,1-Dichlorethene	3.9E-07	1.3E-10	4.3E-11	3.9E-07	1.7E-06	1.2E-07
3-Methylcholanthrene	2.3E-05	0	**7.2E-02**	2.8E-07	0	**4.5E-02**
Aldrin	4.0E-05	9.0E-07	2.6E-03	1.8E-05	8.7E-06	5.7E-02
Bis(2-chlorethyl)ether	2.5E-06	1.8E-08	2.9E-09	2.2E-06	8.0E-06	1.5E-09
Dibutyl-phthalate	4.9E-07	7.8E-09	1.8E-04	2.2E-08	2.2E-06	1.3E-04
Dieldrin	4.4E-05	8.6E-05	9.9E-02	4.1E-06	3.6E-05	6.8E-02
Hexachlorobutadiene	3.0E-06	4.3E-10	1.3E-07	2.8E-06	8.8E-09	3.4E-06
Hexachloroethane	1.5E-06	1.4E-09	3.4E-08	1.4E-06	2.9E-09	4.2E-08
Chloromethane, Methyl Chloride	1.4E-06	0	0	1.3E-06	0	0
Trichlorethylene	6.1E-09	0	0	6.1E-09	0	0
Trifluralin	**2.4E-07**	7.1E-09	8.2E-07	**2.8E-08**	8.4E-10	1.3E-07

App. 6.11: Tumour incidence rate Tijk per 1 kg substance emissions to air or water, Appendix (6.9) completed by Tijk based on calculated unit risk factors from Appendix (6.10) (bold numbers)

Substance-name	DALYs (0,0) inhalation	DALYs (0,0) drinking water and food	DALYs (0,0) inhalation	DALYs (0,0) drinking water and food	total DALYs (0,0)	DALYs (0,0) inhalation	DALYs (0,0) drinking water and food	total DALYs (0,0)
	DALYs per incidence case	DALYs per incidence case	DALYs per kg emission to air	DALYs per kg emission to air	DALYs per kg emission to air	DALYs per kg emission to water	DALYs per kg emission to water	DALYs per kg emission to water
IARC-Group 1								
Arsenic, inorganic	16.1	13.1	2.6E-04	1.6E-01	1.6E-01	5.1E-15	6.7E-04	6.7E-04
Benzene	16.5	16.5	2.0E-06	4.8E-10	2.0E-06	1.5E-06	3.6E-07	1.9E-06
Bis(chloromethyl)ether BCME	16.1	13.1	7.4E-03	6.2E-05	7.5E-03	6.5E-03	2.2E-02	2.8E-02
Cadmium	16.1	13.1	4.5E-04	1.3E-01	1.3E-01	1.3E-14	1.8E-03	1.8E-03
Chromium(VI)	16.1	13.1	5.6E-03	5.3E+02	5.3E+02	6.8E-14	2.1E-02	2.1E-02
Nickel	16.1	13.1	4.4E-05	9.5E-02	9.5E-02	1.1E-15	1.0E-03	1.0E-03
Nickel-refinery-dust	12.5	13.1	2.4E-05	6.7E-02	6.7E-02	6.0E-16	7.2E-04	7.2E-04
Nickel-subsulfide	12.5	13.1	4.8E-05	1.3E-01	1.3E-01	1.2E-15	1.4E-03	1.4E-03
Vinylchlorid	16.2	16.2	2.1E-07	5.5E-11	2.1E-07	2.1E-07	7.2E-08	2.8E-07
IARC-Group 2A								
1,2-Dibromoethane	13.1	13.1	1.9E-04	2.1E-05	2.1E-04	1.9E-04	5.0E-04	6.8E-04
1,3-Butadiene	13.1	13.1	3.0E-05	5.0E-07	3.0E-05	2.7E-05	2.0E-04	2.2E-04
Acrylonitrile	16.1	13.1	1.7E-05	4.3E-08	1.7E-05	1.3E-05	1.4E-05	2.6E-05
Benzo[a]pyrene- (BaP)	16.1	13.1	1.2E-02	2.5E-01	2.7E-01	4.1E-05	3.1E-01	3.1E-01
Benz(a)anthracene	13.1	13.1	1.2E-04	1.1E-01	1.1E-01	1.2E-05	1.2E-01	1.2E-01
Dibenz(a,h)anthracene	13.1	13.1	1.6E-03	1.2E+01	1.2E+01	7.1E-07	4.6E+00	4.6E+00
Diesel soot particles	16.1		9.8E-06	0.0E+00	9.8E-06	0.0E+00	0.0E+00	0.0E+00
Epichlorhydrin	16.1	13.1	3.0E-07	8.1E-09	3.0E-07	9.6E-08	7.3E-07	8.2E-07
Ethylene Oxide	13.1	13.1	1.5E-04	0.0E+00	1.5E-04	9.8E-05	0.0E+00	9.8E-05
Formaldehyde	12.5	13.1	1.2E-06	2.0E-06	3.2E-06	2.2E-09	9.6E-06	9.6E-06
Polychlorinated-biphenyls- (PCBs)	3.4	3.4	1.9E-04	8.9E-03	9.1E-03	1.0E-04	8.2E-03	8.3E-03
Propylene-oxide	13.1	13.1	4.7E-06	8.8E-07	5.6E-06	2.2E-06	3.5E-06	5.6E-06
IARC-Group 2B								
1,2-Dichloroethane	13.1	13.1	3.0E-05	2.7E-08	3.0E-05	2.9E-05	4.1E-07	3.0E-05
1,4-Dioxane	13.1	13.1	1.4E-07	8.6E-08	2.2E-07	1.3E-08	3.0E-06	3.1E-06
2,3,7,8-Tetrachlordibenzo-p-dioxin, TCDD	13.1	13.1	2.1E-01	1.5E+03	1.5E+03	6.7E-02	5.3E+02	5.3E+02
2,4,6-Trichlorophenol	13.1	13.1	1.4E-06	4.9E-07	1.9E-06	3.2E-07	1.1E-06	1.5E-06
Acetaldehyde	13.1	13.1	2.1E-07	3.5E-09	2.2E-07	9.7E-08	1.2E-06	1.3E-06
alpha-Hexachlorcyclohexan	16.1	13.1	2.7E-04	1.2E-03	1.5E-03	2.4E-04	1.6E-02	1.7E-02
Benzotrichloride	13.1	13.1	6.6E-03	1.5E-04	6.8E-03	6.5E-03	4.3E-04	7.0E-03
Benzyl-chloride	13.1	13.1	1.0E-05	1.8E-09	1.0E-05	8.0E-06	2.0E-06	1.0E-05
beta-Hexachlorcyclohexan	16.1	13.1	7.4E-05	6.2E-03	6.3E-03	2.3E-05	4.8E-02	4.8E-02
Bromodichloromethane	13.1	13.1	8.8E-06	1.5E-08	8.8E-06	8.0E-06	4.7E-07	8.5E-06
Carbon-tetrachloride	16.2	16.2	8.3E-04	7.1E-07	8.3E-04	8.2E-04	1.1E-06	8.3E-04
Chloroform	13.1	13.1	2.6E-05	2.7E-09	2.6E-05	2.6E-05	2.9E-08	2.6E-05
Di(2-ethylhexyl)phthalate- (DEHP)	13.1	13.1	2.4E-08	8.1E-06	8.1E-06	1.2E-08	7.0E-05	7.0E-05
Dichloromethane	13.1	13.1	4.3E-07	2.4E-09	4.4E-07	4.3E-07	3.7E-08	4.7E-07
Dichlorvos	13.1	13.1	1.8E-05	9.4E-05	1.1E-04	2.3E-06	6.9E-04	6.9E-04
gamma-Hexachlorocyclohexane	16.1	13.1	5.2E-05	4.1E-03	4.1E-03	2.1E-05	1.5E-01	1.5E-01
Hexachlorobenzene	13.1	13.1	1.6E-04	1.9E-03	2.0E-03	1.4E-04	3.6E-03	3.8E-03
Pentachlorophenol	13.1	13.1	0.0E+00	3.7E-05	3.7E-05	0.0E+00	5.2E-04	5.2E-04
Perchloroethylene	13.1	13.1	4.8E-07	0.0E+00	4.8E-07	4.7E-07	0.0E+00	4.7E-07
Styrene	13.1	13.1	6.3E-08	1.4E-10	6.3E-08	3.2E-08	1.0E-07	1.3E-07
IARC-Group 3								
1,1,1,2-Tetrachlorethane	13.1	13.1	3.6E-05	1.6E-07	3.6E-05	3.4E-05	2.2E-07	3.4E-05
1,1,2,2-Tetrachlorethane	13.1	13.1	2.5E-04	2.6E-06	2.6E-04	2.4E-04	3.7E-06	2.4E-04
1,1,2-Trichlorethane	13.1	13.1	1.1E-05	3.9E-09	1.1E-05	1.1E-05	3.6E-07	1.1E-05
1,1-Dichlorethene	13.1	13.1	5.1E-06	2.3E-09	5.1E-06	5.0E-06	2.4E-05	2.9E-05
3-Methylcholanthrene	13.1	13.1	3.1E-04	9.5E-01	9.5E-01	3.6E-06	5.9E-01	5.9E-01
Aldrin	13.1	13.1	5.2E-04	3.4E-02	3.4E-02	2.4E-04	7.5E-01	7.5E-01
Bis(2-chlorethyl)ether	16.1	13.1	4.0E-05	2.7E-07	4.0E-05	3.5E-05	1.1E-04	1.4E-04
Dibutyl-phthalate	13.1	13.1	6.4E-06	2.4E-03	2.4E-03	2.9E-07	1.7E-03	1.7E-03
Dieldrin	13.1	13.1	5.8E-04	1.3E+00	1.3E+00	5.4E-05	8.9E-01	8.9E-01
Hexachlorobutadiene	13.1	13.1	3.9E-05	1.7E-06	4.1E-05	3.7E-05	4.5E-05	8.2E-05
Hexachloroethane	13.1	13.1	2.0E-05	4.7E-07	2.0E-05	1.9E-05	5.9E-07	1.9E-05
Chloromethane, Methyl Chloride	13.1	13.1	1.8E-05	0.0E+00	1.8E-05	1.7E-05	0.0E+00	1.7E-05
Trichlorethylene	13.1	13.1	8.0E-08	0.0E+00	8.0E-08	8.0E-08	0.0E+00	8.0E-08
Trifluralin	13.1	13.1	3.1E-06	1.1E-05	1.4E-05	3.7E-07	1.8E-06	2.1E-06

App. 6.12: Damages to human health measured in DALYs (0,0), i.e., no discounting and no age-weighting, per incidence case and per 1 kg substance emissions to air or water

Substance-name	DALYs (0,1) inhalation	DALYs (0,1) drinking water and food	DALYs (0,1) inhalation	DALYs (0,1) drinking water and food	Total DALYs (0,1)	DALYs (0,1) inhalation	DALYs (0,1) drinking water and food	Total DALYs (0,1)
IARC-Group 1	DALYs per incidence case	DALYs per incidence case	DALYs per kg emission to air	DALYs per kg emission to air	DALYs per kg emission to air	DALYs per kg emission to water	DALYs per kg emission to water	DALYs per kg emission to water
Arsenic, inorganic	10.4	8.5	1.7E-04	1.0E-01	1.0E-01	3.3E-15	4.3E-04	4.3E-04
Benzene	10.4	8.5	1.2E-06	2.5E-10	1.2E-06	9.5E-07	1.9E-07	1.1E-06
Bis(chloromethyl)ether BCME	10.4	8.5	4.8E-03	4.0E-05	4.9E-03	4.2E-03	1.4E-02	1.8E-02
Cadmium	10.4	8.5	2.9E-04	8.3E-02	8.3E-02	8.4E-15	1.1E-03	1.1E-03
Chromium(VI)	10.4	8.5	3.6E-03	3.4E+02	3.4E+02	4.4E-14	1.4E-02	1.4E-02
Nickel	10.4	8.5	2.8E-05	6.2E-02	6.2E-02	7.0E-16	6.6E-04	6.6E-04
Nickel-refinery-dust	10.4	8.5	2.0E-05	4.4E-02	4.4E-02	5.0E-16	4.7E-04	4.7E-04
Nickel-subsulfide	10.4	8.5	4.0E-05	8.7E-02	8.7E-02	9.9E-16	9.4E-04	9.4E-04
Vinylchlorid	10.4	8.5	1.3E-07	2.9E-11	1.3E-07	1.3E-07	3.8E-08	1.7E-07
IARC-Group 2A								
1,2-Dibromoethane	10.4	8.5	1.5E-04	1.4E-05	1.6E-04	1.5E-04	3.2E-04	4.7E-04
1,3-Butadiene	10.4	8.5	2.4E-05	3.2E-07	2.4E-05	2.1E-05	1.3E-04	1.5E-04
Acrylonitrile	10.4	8.5	1.1E-05	2.8E-08	1.1E-05	8.1E-06	9.0E-06	1.7E-05
Benzo[a]pyrene- (BaP)	10.4	8.5	7.9E-03	1.6E-01	1.7E-01	2.6E-05	2.0E-01	2.0E-01
Benz(a)anthracene	10.4	8.5	9.2E-05	7.0E-02	7.0E-02	9.3E-06	8.1E-02	8.1E-02
Dibenz(a,h)anthracene	10.4	8.5	1.3E-03	8.1E+00	8.1E+00	5.6E-07	3.0E+00	3.0E+00
Diesel soot particles	10.4	8.5	6.3E-06	0.0E+00	6.3E-06	0.0E+00	0.0E+00	0.0E+00
Epichlorhydrin	10.4	8.5	1.9E-07	5.2E-09	2.0E-07	6.2E-08	4.7E-07	5.3E-07
Ethylene Oxide	10.4	8.5	1.2E-04	0.0E+00	1.2E-04	7.8E-05	0.0E+00	7.8E-05
Formaldehyde	10.4	8.5	9.9E-07	1.3E-06	2.3E-06	1.8E-09	6.2E-06	6.2E-06
Polychlorinated-biphenyls- (PCBs)	10.4	8.5	5.8E-04	2.2E-02	2.3E-02	3.2E-04	2.1E-02	2.1E-02
Propylene-oxide	10.4	8.5	3.7E-06	5.7E-07	4.3E-06	1.7E-06	2.3E-06	4.0E-06
IARC-Group 2B								
1,2-Dichloroethane	10.4	8.5	2.3E-05	1.8E-08	2.4E-05	2.3E-05	2.6E-07	2.4E-05
1,4-Dioxane	10.4	8.5	1.1E-07	5.5E-08	1.6E-07	1.0E-08	2.0E-06	2.0E-06
2,3,7,8-Tetrachlordibenzo-p-dioxin, TCDD	10.4	8.5	1.7E-01	9.8E+02	9.8E+02	5.3E-02	3.5E+02	3.5E+02
2,4,6-Trichlorophenol	10.4	8.5	1.1E-06	3.2E-07	1.4E-06	2.6E-07	7.4E-07	1.0E-06
Acetaldehyde	10.4	8.5	1.7E-07	2.3E-09	1.7E-07	7.7E-08	7.8E-07	8.5E-07
alpha-Hexachlorcyclohexan	10.4	8.5	1.8E-04	7.8E-04	9.6E-04	1.6E-04	1.1E-02	1.1E-02
Benzotrichloride	10.4	8.5	5.3E-03	9.5E-05	5.4E-03	5.2E-03	2.8E-04	5.5E-03
Benzyl-chloride	10.4	8.5	8.1E-06	1.1E-09	8.1E-06	6.4E-06	1.3E-06	7.7E-06
beta-Hexachlorcyclohexan	10.4	8.5	4.8E-05	4.0E-03	4.1E-03	1.5E-05	3.1E-02	3.1E-02
Bromodichloromethane	10.4	8.5	7.0E-06	9.6E-09	7.0E-06	6.4E-06	3.0E-07	6.7E-06
Carbon-tetrachloride	10.4	8.5	5.3E-04	3.7E-07	5.3E-04	5.3E-04	6.0E-07	5.3E-04
Chloroform	10.4	8.5	2.1E-05	1.8E-09	2.1E-05	2.1E-05	1.9E-08	2.1E-05
Di(2-ethylhexyl)phthalate- (DEHP)	10.4	8.5	1.9E-08	5.2E-06	5.3E-06	9.2E-09	4.5E-05	4.5E-05
Dichloromethane	10.4	8.5	3.4E-07	1.5E-09	3.5E-07	3.4E-07	2.4E-08	3.7E-07
Dichlorvos	10.4	8.5	1.4E-05	6.1E-05	7.5E-05	1.9E-06	4.5E-04	4.5E-04
gamma-Hexachlorocyclohexane	10.4	8.5	3.4E-05	2.6E-03	2.7E-03	1.4E-05	9.7E-02	9.7E-02
Hexachlorobenzene	10.4	8.5	1.3E-04	1.2E-03	1.3E-03	1.1E-04	2.3E-03	2.5E-03
Pentachlorophenol	10.4	8.5	0.0E+00	2.4E-05	2.4E-05	0.0E+00	3.4E-04	3.4E-04
Perchloroethylene	10.4	8.5	3.8E-07	0.0E+00	3.8E-07	3.8E-07	0.0E+00	3.8E-07
Styrene	10.4	8.5	5.0E-08	9.0E-11	5.0E-08	2.5E-08	6.5E-08	9.0E-08
IARC-Group 3								
1,1,1,2-Tetrachlorethane	10.4	8.5	2.9E-05	1.1E-07	2.9E-05	2.7E-05	1.4E-07	2.7E-05
1,1,2,2-Tetrachlorethane	10.4	8.5	2.0E-04	1.7E-06	2.0E-04	1.9E-04	2.4E-06	1.9E-04
1,1,2-Trichlorethane	10.4	8.5	8.7E-06	2.5E-09	8.7E-06	8.6E-06	2.3E-07	8.9E-06
1,1-Dichlorethene	10.4	8.5	4.0E-06	1.5E-09	4.0E-06	4.0E-06	1.6E-05	2.0E-05
3-Methylcholanthrene	10.4	8.5	2.4E-04	6.2E-01	6.2E-01	2.9E-06	3.8E-01	3.8E-01
Aldrin	10.4	8.5	4.1E-04	2.2E-02	2.2E-02	1.9E-04	4.9E-01	4.9E-01
Bis(2-chlorethyl)ether	10.4	8.5	2.6E-05	1.8E-07	2.6E-05	2.3E-05	6.8E-05	9.1E-05
Dibutyl-phthalate	10.4	8.5	5.1E-06	1.6E-03	1.6E-03	2.3E-07	1.1E-03	1.1E-03
Dieldrin	10.4	8.5	4.6E-04	8.4E-01	8.4E-01	4.3E-05	5.8E-01	5.8E-01
Hexachlorobutadiene	10.4	8.5	3.1E-05	1.1E-06	3.2E-05	2.9E-05	2.9E-05	5.9E-05
Hexachloroethane	10.4	8.5	1.6E-05	3.0E-07	1.6E-05	1.5E-05	3.8E-07	1.5E-05
Chloromethane, Methyl Chloride	10.4	8.5	1.5E-05	0.0E+00	1.5E-05	1.3E-05	0.0E+00	1.3E-05
Trichlorethylene	10.4	8.5	6.4E-08	0.0E+00	6.4E-08	6.3E-08	0.0E+00	6.3E-08
Trifluralin	10.4	8.5	2.4E-06	7.0E-06	9.4E-06	2.9E-07	1.1E-06	1.4E-06

App. 6.13: Damages to human health measured in DALYs (0,1), i.e. no discounting but age-weighting, per incidence case and per 1 kg substance emissions to air or water

Substance-name	σg^2 F"air, air	σg^2 F"air, water	σg^2 F"air, food	σg^2 F" water, air	σg^2 F"water, water	σg^2 F"water, food	σg^2 ρ	σg^2 E inha-lation	σg^2 E oral intake	σg^2 E drinking water	σg^2 DALYs
IARC-Group 1	-	-	-	-	-	-	-	-	-	-	-
Arsenic, inorganic	4	40	80	40	20	80	3	2	4	4	1.5
Benzene	2	4	8	6	3	12	3	2	4	4	1.5
Bis(chloromethyl)ether BCME	2	4	8	6	3	12	3	2	4	4	1.5
Cadmium	4	40	80	40	20	80	3	2	20	1	1.5
Chromium(VI)	4	40	80	40	20	80	3	2	20	1	1.5
Nickel	4	40	80	40	20	80	3	2	20	1	1.5
Nickel-refinery-dust	4	40	80	40	20	80	3	2	20	1	2
Nickel-subsulfide	4	40	80	40	20	80	3	2	20	1	2
Vinylchlorid	2	4	8	6	3	12	3	2	20	20	1.5
IARC-Group 2A											
1,2-Dibromoethane	2	4	8	6	3	12	3	3	6	6	1.5
1,3-Butadiene	2	4	8	6	3	12	3	3	20	20	1.5
Acrylonitrile	2	4	8	6	3	12	3	3	6	6	1.5
Benzo[a]pyrene- (BaP)	3	6	12	6	3	12	3	3	6	6	1.5
Benz(a)anthracene	3	6	12	6	3	12	3	3	20	1	1.5
Dibenz(a,h)anthracene	3	6	12	6	3	12	3	3	20	1	1.5
Diesel soot particles	2						3	3	1	1	1.5
Epichlorhydrin	2	4	8	6	3	12	3	3	6	6	1.5
Ethylene Oxide	2	4	8	6	3	12	3	3	1	1	1.5
Formaldehyde	3	6	12	4	2	8	3	3	20	20	2
Polychlorinated-biphenyls- (PCBs)	3	6	12	6	3	12	3	3	20	1	1.5
Propylene-oxide	20	40	80	40	20	80	3	3	6	6	1.5
IARC-Group 2B											
1,2-Dichloroethane	2	4	8	6	3	12	3	5	10	10	1.5
1,4-Dioxane	2	4	8	4	2	8	3	5	10	10	1.5
2,3,7,8-Tetrachlordibenzo-p-dioxin, TCDD	3	6	12	6	3	12	3	5	20	1	1.5
2,4,6-Trichlorophenol	20	40	80	40	20	80	3	5	10	10	1.5
Acetaldehyde	2	4	8	4	2	8	3	5	20	20	1.5
alpha-Hexachlorcyclohexan	3	6	12	6	3	12	3	5	10	10	1.5
Benzotrichloride	20	40	80	40	20	80	3	20	10	10	1.5
Benzyl-chloride	2	4	8	6	3	12	3	20	10	10	1.5
beta-Hexachlorcyclohexan	3	6	12	6	3	12	3	5	10	10	1.5
Bromodichloromethane	2	4	8	6	3	12	3	20	10	10	1.5
Carbon-tetrachloride	2	4	8	6	3	12	3	5	10	10	1.5
Chloroform	2	4	8	6	3	12	3	5	10	10	1.5
Di(2-ethylhexyl)phthalate- (DEHP)	3	6	12	6	3	12	3	5	10	10	1.5
Dichloromethane	2	4	8	6	3	12	3	5	10	10	1.5
Dichlorvos	3	6	12	4	2	8	3	20	10	10	1.5
gamma-Hexachlorocyclohexane	3	6	12	6	3	12	3	5	20	20	1.5
Hexachlorobenzene	3	6	12	6	3	12	3	5	10	10	1.5
Pentachlorophenol	20	40	80	40	20	80	3	5	10	10	1.5
Perchloroethylene	2	4	8	6	3	12	3	5	10	10	1.5
Styrene	2	4	8	6	3	12	3	5	20	20	1.5
IARC-Group 3											
1,1,1,2-Tetrachlorethane	2	4	8	6	3	12	3	10	20	20	1.5
1,1,2,2-Tetrachlorethane	20	40	80	40	20	80	3	10	20	20	1.5
1,1,2-Trichlorethane	2	4	8	6	3	12	3	10	20	20	1.5
1,1-Dichlorethene	2	4	8	6	3	12	3	10	20	20	1.5
3-Methylcholanthrene	3	6	12	6	3	12	3	10	20	1	1.5
Aldrin	2	4	8	6	3	12	3	10	20	20	1.5
Bis(2-chlorethyl)ether	2	4	8	6	3	12	3	10	20	20	1.5
Dibutyl-phthalate	3	6	12	6	3	12	3	10	20	20	1.5
Dieldrin	3	6	12	6	3	12	3	10	20	20	1.5
Hexachlorobutadiene	20	40	80	40	20	80	3	10	20	20	1.5
Hexachloroethane	2	4	8	6	3	12	3	10	20	20	1.5
Chloromethane, Methyl Chloride	2	4	8	6	3	12	3	10	1	1	1.5
Trichlorethylene	2	4	8	6	3	12	3	10	1	1	1.5
Trifluralin	3	6	12	6	3	12	3	20	20	20	1.5

App. 6.14: Squared geometric standard deviations σg^2 for the fate factors, effect factors and DALYs per tumour case. A factor 1 means that no estimate was made because the effect factor was zero.

Substance-name	σg^2 DALYs air, inhalation	σg^2 DALYs air, drinking water	σg^2 DALYs air,food	σg^2 DALYs water, inhalation	σg^2 DALYs water, drinking water	σg^2 DALYs water,food
IARC-Group 1	-	-	-	-	-	-
Arsenic, inorganic	7.0	61.0	114.8	51.0	33.2	114.8
Benzene	4.6	9.8	15.8	9.5	8.3	21.7
Bis(chloromethyl)ether BCME	4.6	9.8	15.8	9.5	8.3	21.7
Cadmium	7.0	48.0	229.5	51.0	24.9	229.5
Chromium(VI)	7.0	48.0	229.5	51.0	24.9	229.5
Nickel	7.0	48.0	229.5	51.0	24.9	229.5
Nickel-refinery-dust	7.6	49.9	236.2	53.1	26.2	236.2
Nickel-subsulfide	7.6	49.9	236.2	53.1	26.2	236.2
Vinylchlorid	4.6	33.2	46.1	9.5	29.9	58.2
IARC-Group 2A						
1,2-Dibromoethane	5.7	12.8	19.8	11.1	11.1	26.6
1,3-Butadiene	5.7	33.2	46.1	11.1	29.9	58.2
Acrylonitrile	5.7	12.8	19.8	11.1	11.1	26.6
Benzo[a]pyrene- (BaP)	7.0	16.3	26.6	11.1	11.1	26.6
Benz(a)anthracene	7.0	8.5	58.2	11.1	5.0	58.2
Dibenz(a,h)anthracene	7.0	8.5	58.2	11.1	5.0	58.2
Diesel soot particles	5.7					
Epichlorhydrin	5.7	12.8	19.8	11.1	11.1	26.6
Ethylene Oxide	5.7	6.1	10.9	11.1	5.0	15.6
Formaldehyde	7.6	41.5	60.5	9.0	28.2	48.0
Polychlorinated-biphenyls- (PCBs)	7.0	8.5	58.2	11.1	5.0	58.2
Propylene-oxide	29.9	71.2	131.2	55.9	39.7	131.2
IARC-Group 2B						
1,2-Dichloroethane	8.2	18.8	27.6	14.6	16.6	36.0
1,4-Dioxane	8.2	18.8	27.6	11.3	14.5	27.6
2,3,7,8-Tetrachlordibenzo-p-dioxin, TCDD	9.7	8.5	58.2	14.6	5.0	58.2
2,4,6-Trichlorophenol	36.5	90.3	161.9	66.1	52.2	161.9
Acetaldehyde	8.2	33.2	46.1	11.3	26.9	46.1
alpha-Hexachlorcyclohexan	9.7	23.2	36.0	14.6	16.6	36.0
Benzotrichloride	81.1	90.3	161.9	133.5	52.2	161.9
Benzyl-chloride	26.9	18.8	27.6	39.7	16.6	36.0
beta-Hexachlorcyclohexan	9.7	23.2	36.0	14.6	16.6	36.0
Bromodichloromethane	26.9	18.8	27.6	39.7	16.6	36.0
Carbon-tetrachloride	8.2	18.8	27.6	14.6	16.6	36.0
Chloroform	8.2	18.8	27.6	14.6	16.6	36.0
Di(2-ethylhexyl)phthalate- (DEHP)	9.7	23.2	36.0	14.6	16.6	36.0
Dichloromethane	8.2	18.8	27.6	14.6	16.6	36.0
Dichlorvos	29.9	23.2	36.0	33.2	14.5	27.6
gamma-Hexachlorocyclohexane	9.7	39.7	58.2	14.6	29.9	58.2
Hexachlorobenzene	9.7	23.2	36.0	14.6	16.6	36.0
Pentachlorophenol	36.5	90.3	161.9	66.1	52.2	161.9
Perchloroethylene	8.2	18.8	27.6	14.6	16.6	36.0
Styrene	8.2	33.2	46.1	14.6	29.9	58.2
IARC-Group 3						
1,1,1,2-Tetrachlorethane	14.5	33.2	46.1	23.2	29.9	58.2
1,1,2,2-Tetrachlorethane	52.2	133.5	229.5	90.3	81.1	229.5
1,1,2-Trichlorethane	14.5	33.2	46.1	23.2	29.9	58.2
1,1-Dichlorethene	14.5	33.2	46.1	23.2	29.9	58.2
3-Methylcholanthrene	16.6	8.5	58.2	23.2	5.0	58.2
Aldrin	14.5	33.2	46.1	23.2	29.9	58.2
Bis(2-chlorethyl)ether	14.5	33.2	46.1	23.2	29.9	58.2
Dibutyl-phthalate	16.6	39.7	58.2	23.2	29.9	58.2
Dieldrin	16.6	39.7	58.2	23.2	29.9	58.2
Hexachlorobutadiene	52.2	133.5	229.5	90.3	81.1	229.5
Hexachloroethane	14.5	33.2	46.1	23.2	29.9	58.2
Chloromethane, Methyl Chloride	14.5	6.1	10.9	23.2	5.0	15.6
Trichlorethylene	14.5	6.1	10.9	23.2	5.0	15.6
Trifluralin	29.9	39.7	58.2	39.7	29.9	58.2

App. 6.15: Total squared geometric standard deviations σg^2 for the damage factors calculated from Appendix (6.14) by Formula (A6.3) given in Appendix (6.8).

Substance-name	DALYs(0,0), air-2.5%	DALYs(0,0), air-mean value	DALYs(0,0), air-97.5%	DALYs(0,0), water-2.5%	DALYs(0,0), water-mean value	DALYs(0,0), water-97.5%
IARC-Group 1	a/kg	a/kg	a/kg	a/kg	a/kg	a/kg
Arsenic, inorganic	1.4E-03	1.6E-01	1.8E+01	1.6E-05	6.7E-04	4.0E-02
Benzene	4.2E-07	2.0E-06	9.0E-06	2.0E-07	1.9E-06	1.8E-05
Bis(chloromethyl)ether BCME	1.6E-03	7.5E-03	3.5E-02	3.3E-03	2.8E-02	2.4E-01
Cadmium	6.2E-04	1.3E-01	2.9E+01	7.7E-06	1.8E-03	4.0E-01
Chromium(VI)	2.3E+00	5.3E+02	1.2E+05	9.2E-05	2.1E-02	4.9E+00
Nickel	4.2E-04	9.5E-02	2.2E+01	4.5E-06	1.0E-03	2.3E-01
Nickel-refinery-dust	2.9E-04	6.7E-02	1.6E+01	3.1E-06	7.2E-04	1.7E-01
Nickel-subsulfide	5.8E-04	1.3E-01	3.2E+01	6.1E-06	1.4E-03	3.4E-01
Vinylchlorid	4.5E-08	2.1E-07	9.5E-07	2.4E-08	2.8E-07	4.1E-06
IARC-Group 2A						
1,2-Dibromoethane	3.4E-05	2.1E-04	1.4E-03	5.8E-05	6.8E-04	8.6E-03
1,3-Butadiene	5.2E-06	3.0E-05	1.9E-04	8.8E-06	2.2E-04	6.3E-03
Acrylonitrile	2.9E-06	1.7E-05	9.7E-05	2.4E-06	2.6E-05	2.9E-04
Benzo[a]pyrene- (BaP)	1.1E-02	2.7E-01	6.8E+00	1.2E-02	3.1E-01	8.3E+00
Benz(a)anthracene	1.9E-03	1.1E-01	6.3E+00	2.1E-03	1.2E-01	7.3E+00
Dibenz(a,h)anthracene	2.1E-01	1.2E+01	7.3E+02	7.9E-02	4.6E+00	2.7E+02
Diesel soot particles	1.7E-06	9.8E-06	5.6E-05	0.0E+00	0.0E+00	0.0E+00
Epichlorhydrin	5.2E-08	3.0E-07	1.8E-06	7.4E-08	8.2E-07	9.2E-06
Ethylene Oxide	2.6E-05	1.5E-04	8.8E-04	8.9E-06	9.8E-05	1.1E-03
Formaldehyde	1.9E-07	3.2E-06	1.3E-04	3.4E-07	9.6E-06	2.7E-04
Polychlorinated-biphenyls- (PCBs)	1.8E-04	9.1E-03	5.2E-01	1.5E-04	8.3E-03	4.8E-01
Propylene-oxide	1.7E-07	5.6E-06	2.2E-04	1.2E-07	5.6E-06	2.7E-04
IARC-Group 2B						
1,2-Dichloroethane	3.6E-06	3.0E-05	2.4E-04	2.0E-06	3.0E-05	4.3E-04
1,4-Dioxane	2.1E-08	2.2E-07	2.9E-06	2.1E-07	3.1E-06	4.4E-05
2,3,7,8-Tetrachlordibenzo-p-dioxin, TCDD	2.6E+01	1.5E+03	8.8E+04	9.2E+00	5.3E+02	3.1E+04
2,4,6-Trichlorophenol	4.1E-08	1.9E-06	1.3E-04	2.4E-08	1.5E-06	1.1E-04
Acetaldehyde	2.6E-08	2.2E-07	1.9E-06	5.3E-08	1.3E-06	3.3E-05
alpha-Hexachlorcyclohexan	6.3E-05	1.5E-03	4.5E-02	6.7E-04	1.7E-02	4.7E-01
Benzotrichloride	8.3E-05	6.8E-03	5.6E-01	5.2E-05	7.0E-03	9.4E-01
Benzyl-chloride	3.8E-07	1.0E-05	2.7E-04	3.2E-07	1.0E-05	3.5E-04
beta-Hexachlorcyclohexan	1.9E-04	6.3E-03	2.2E-01	1.9E-03	4.8E-02	1.4E+00
Bromodichloromethane	3.3E-07	8.8E-06	2.4E-04	2.3E-07	8.5E-06	3.3E-04
Carbon-tetrachloride	1.0E-04	8.3E-04	6.8E-03	5.7E-05	8.3E-04	1.2E-02
Chloroform	3.2E-06	2.6E-05	2.2E-04	1.8E-06	2.6E-05	3.8E-04
Di(2-ethylhexyl)phthalate- (DEHP)	2.3E-07	8.1E-06	2.9E-04	1.9E-06	7.0E-05	2.5E-03
Dichloromethane	5.3E-08	4.4E-07	3.6E-06	3.2E-08	4.7E-07	6.9E-06
Dichlorvos	4.0E-06	1.1E-04	3.3E-03	4.7E-05	6.9E-04	1.0E-02
gamma-Hexachlorocyclohexane	7.6E-05	4.1E-03	2.3E-01	2.8E-03	1.5E-01	8.3E+00
Hexachlorobenzene	6.9E-05	2.0E-03	6.9E-02	1.1E-04	3.8E-03	1.3E-01
Pentachlorophenol	2.6E-07	3.7E-05	5.6E-03	8.3E-06	5.2E-04	4.2E-02
Perchloroethylene	5.8E-08	4.8E-07	3.9E-06	3.3E-08	4.7E-07	6.9E-06
Styrene	7.7E-09	6.3E-08	5.3E-07	4.9E-09	1.3E-07	4.5E-06
IARC-Group 3						
1,1,1,2-Tetrachlorethane	2.5E-06	3.6E-05	5.3E-04	1.5E-06	3.4E-05	8.0E-04
1,1,2,2-Tetrachlorethane	4.9E-06	2.6E-04	1.4E-02	2.7E-06	2.4E-04	2.2E-02
1,1,2-Trichlorethane	7.6E-07	1.1E-05	1.6E-04	4.8E-07	1.1E-05	2.6E-04
1,1-Dichlorethene	3.5E-07	5.1E-06	7.4E-05	1.0E-06	2.9E-05	8.8E-04
3-Methylcholanthrene	1.6E-02	9.5E-01	5.5E+01	1.0E-02	5.9E-01	3.4E+01
Aldrin	7.7E-04	3.4E-02	1.6E+00	1.3E-02	7.5E-01	4.4E+01
Bis(2-chlorethyl)ether	2.7E-06	4.0E-05	5.8E-04	5.0E-06	1.4E-04	4.0E-03
Dibutyl-phthalate	4.1E-05	2.4E-03	1.4E-01	2.9E-05	1.7E-03	9.6E-02
Dieldrin	2.2E-02	1.3E+00	7.5E+01	1.5E-02	8.9E-01	5.2E+01
Hexachlorobutadiene	7.6E-07	4.1E-05	2.4E-03	6.1E-07	8.2E-05	1.4E-02
Hexachloroethane	1.4E-06	2.0E-05	3.1E-04	8.2E-07	1.9E-05	4.7E-04
Chloromethane, Methyl Chloride	1.3E-06	1.8E-05	2.7E-04	7.3E-07	1.7E-05	3.9E-04
Trichlorethylene	5.5E-09	8.0E-08	1.2E-06	3.4E-09	8.0E-08	1.9E-06
Trifluralin	2.9E-07	1.4E-05	7.2E-04	4.0E-08	2.1E-06	1.2E-04

App. 6.16: 2.5%, mean value, and 97.5% values of the damages to human health measured in DALYs (0,0), i.e. no discounting and no age-weighting, per 1 kg substance emissions to air or water

Substance-name	DALYs(0,1), air-2.5%	DALYs(0,1), air-mean value	DALYs(0,1), air-97.5%	DALYs(0,1), water-2.5%	DALYs(0,1), water-mean value	DALYs(0,1), water-97.5%
IARC-Group 1	a/kg	a/kg	a/kg	a/kg	a/kg	a/kg
Arsenic, inorganic	9.2E-04	1.0E-01	1.2E+01	1.0E-05	4.3E-04	2.6E-02
Benzene	2.7E-07	1.2E-06	5.7E-06	1.2E-07	1.1E-06	1.1E-05
Bis(chloromethyl)ether BCME	1.0E-03	4.9E-03	2.3E-02	2.1E-03	1.8E-02	1.6E-01
Cadmium	4.0E-04	8.3E-02	1.9E+01	5.0E-06	1.1E-03	2.6E-01
Chromium(VI)	1.5E+00	3.4E+02	7.8E+04	6.0E-05	1.4E-02	3.1E+00
Nickel	2.7E-04	6.2E-02	1.4E+01	2.9E-06	6.6E-04	1.5E-01
Nickel-refinery-dust	1.9E-04	4.4E-02	1.0E+01	2.0E-06	4.7E-04	1.1E-01
Nickel-subsulfide	3.8E-04	8.7E-02	2.1E+01	4.0E-06	9.4E-04	2.2E-01
Vinylchlorid	2.9E-08	1.3E-07	6.1E-07	1.5E-08	1.7E-07	2.4E-06

App. 6.17: The Individualist's Table: 2.5%, mean value, and 97.5% values of the damages to human health measured in DALYs (0,1), i.e., no discounting but age-weighting, per 1 kg substance emissions to air or water

APPENDICES CHAPTER 7

Primary Pollutant	Secondary Pollutant	POCP	Fate Factor	σ_g^2
		%	m^2a/m^3	-
CO	CO		100 E-6	4
TSP	PM10		4.4 E-6	3
PM10	PM10		15 E-6	3
PM2.5	PM2.5		17 E-6	3
SOx (as SO_2)	SO_2		3.0 E-6	2
SOx (as SO_2)	Sulphates		1.3 E-6	2
NH_3	Sulphates		1.7 E-6	2
NH_3	Nitrates		0.6 E-6	2
NOx (as NO_2)	NO_2		2.5 E-6	2
NOx (as NO_2)	Nitrates		3.5 E-6	2
NOx (as NO_2)	O_3		1.5 E-6	4
VOCs				
alkanes				
methane	O_3	0.6	1.5E-08	5
ethane	O_3	12.3	3.1E-07	5
propane	O_3	17.6	4.5E-07	5
butane	O_3	35.2	8.9E-07	5
i-butane	O_3	30.7	7.8E-07	5
pentane	O_3	39.5	1.0E-06	5
i-pentane	O_3	40.5	1.0E-06	5
neopentane	O_3	17.3	4.4E-07	5
hexane	O_3	48.2	1.2E-06	5
2-methyl pentane	O_3	42	1.1E-06	5
3-methyl pentane	O_3	47.9	1.2E-06	5
2,2-dimethyl butane	O_3	24.1	6.1E-07	5
2,3-dimethyl butane	O_3	54.1	1.4E-06	5
heptane	O_3	49.4	1.3E-06	5
2-methyl hexane	O_3	41.1	1.0E-06	5
3-methyl hexane	O_3	36.4	9.2E-07	5
octane	O_3	45.3	1.1E-06	5
nonane	O_3	41.4	1.0E-06	5
decane	O_3	38.4	9.7E-07	5
undecane	O_3	38.4	9.7E-07	5
dodecane	O_3	35.7	9.0E-07	5
cyclohexane	O_3	29	7.3E-07	5
alkenes/dienes				
ethene	O_3	100	2.5E-06	5
propene	O_3	112	2.8E-06	5
1-butene	O_3	108	2.7E-06	5
cis 2-butene	O_3	115	2.9E-06	5
trans 2-butene	O_3	113	2.9E-06	5
methyl propene	O_3	62.7	1.6E-06	5
1-pentene	O_3	97.7	2.5E-06	5
cis 2-pentene	O_3	112	2.8E-06	5
trans 2-pentene	O_3	112	2.8E-06	5
2-methyl 1-butene	O_3	77.1	2.0E-06	5
2-methyl 2-butene	O_3	84.2	2.1E-06	5
3-methyl 1-butene	O_3	67.1	1.7E-06	5
1-hexene	O_3	87.4	2.2E-06	5
cis 2-hexene	O_3	107	2.7E-06	5
trans 2-hexene	O_3	107	2.7E-06	5
1,3-butadiene	O_3	85.1	2.2E-06	5
isoprene	O_3	109	2.8E-06	5
alkynes				
acetylene	O_3	8.5	2.2E-07	5

App. 7.1: Fate factors linking emissions of primary pollutants to air with concentrations of inhaled air pollutants causing respiratory effects. The POCP are taken from Jenkin *et al.* (1997), the fate factors are taken from Table 7.11. The squared geometric standard deviations σ_g^2 indicate the flatness of the assumed distribution.

Primary Pollutant	Secondary Pollutant	POCP	Fate Factor	σ_g^2
		%	m^2a/m^3	-
aromatics				
benzene	O_3	21.8	5.5E-07	5
toluene	O_3	63.7	1.6E-06	5
o-xylene	O_3	105	2.7E-06	5
m-xylene	O_3	111	2.8E-06	5
p-xylene	O_3	101	2.6E-06	5
ethyl benzene	O_3	73	1.8E-06	5
n-propyl benzene	O_3	63.6	1.6E-06	5
i-propyl benzene	O_3	50	1.3E-06	5
1,2,3-trimethyl benzene	O_3	127	3.2E-06	5
1,2,4-trimethyl benzene	O_3	128	3.2E-06	5
1,3,5-trimethyl benzene	O_3	138	3.5E-06	5
o-ethyl toluene	O_3	89.8	2.3E-06	5
m-ethyl toluene	O_3	102	2.6E-06	5
p-ethyl toluene	O_3	90.6	2.3E-06	5
3,5-dimethyl ethyl benzene	O_3	132	3.3E-06	5
3,5-diethyl toluene	O_3	130	3.3E-06	5
aldehydes				
formaldehyde	O_3	51.9	1.3E-06	5
acetaldehyde	O_3	64.1	1.6E-06	5
propionaldehyde	O_3	79.8	2.0E-06	5
n-butyraldehyde	O_3	79.5	2.0E-06	5
i-butyraldehyde	O_3	51.4	1.3E-06	5
pentanal	O_3	76.5	1.9E-06	5
ketones				
acetone	O_3	9.4	2.4E-07	5
methyl ethyl ketone	O_3	37.3	9.5E-07	5
2-pentanone	O_3	54.8	1.4E-06	5
3-pentanone	O_3	41.4	1.0E-06	5
methyl i-propyl ketone	O_3	36.4	9.2E-07	5
2-hexanone	O_3	57.2	1.4E-06	5
3-hexanone	O_3	59.9	1.5E-06	5
methyl i-butyl ketone	O_3	49	1.2E-06	5
methyl t-butyl ketone	O_3	32.3	8.2E-07	5
cyclohexanone	O_3	29.9	7.6E-07	5
alcohols				
methanol	O_3	13.1	3.3E-07	5
ethanol	O_3	38.6	9.8E-07	5
n-propanol	O_3	54.3	1.4E-06	5
i-propanol	O_3	14	3.5E-07	5
n-butanol	O_3	61.2	1.6E-06	5
s-butanol	O_3	40	1.0E-06	5
i-butanol	O_3	37.5	9.5E-07	5
t-butanol	O_3	12.3	3.1E-07	5
2-methyl 1-butanol	O_3	40.7	1.0E-06	5
2-methyl 2-butanol	O_3	14.2	3.6E-07	5
3-methyl 1-butanol	O_3	41.2	1.0E-06	5
3-methyl 2-butanol	O_3	36.6	9.3E-07	5
3-pentanol	O_3	42.2	1.1E-06	5
diacetone alcohol	O_3	26.2	6.6E-07	5
cyclohexanol	O_3	44.6	1.1E-06	5
ethane diol	O_3	38.2	9.7E-07	5
propane diol	O_3	45.7	1.2E-06	5

App. 7.1 (cont.): Fate factors linking emissions of primary pollutants to air with concentrations of inhaled air pollutants causing respiratory effects. The POCP are taken from Jenkin *et al.* (1997), the fate factors are taken from Table 7.11. The squared geometric standard deviations σ_g^2 indicate the flatness of the assumed distribution.

Primary Pollutant	Secondary Pollutant	POCP	Fate Factor	σ_g^2
		%	m^2a/m^3	-
esters				
methyl formate	O_3	3.3	8.4E-08	5
methyl acetate	O_3	4.6	1.2E-07	5
ethyl acetate	O_3	21.3	5.4E-07	5
n-propyl acetate	O_3	29	7.3E-07	5
i-propyl acetate	O_3	21.3	5.4E-07	5
n-butyl acetate	O_3	24.1	6.1E-07	5
s-butyl acetate	O_3	26.7	6.8E-07	5
t-butyl acetate	O_3	6.5	1.6E-07	5
carboxylic acids				
formic acid	O_3	3.2	8.1E-08	5
acetic acid	O_3	9.7	2.5E-07	5
propanoic acid	O_3	15	3.8E-07	5
ethers and glycol ethers				
dimethyl ether	O_3	17.4	4.4E-07	5
diethyl ether	O_3	46.7	1.2E-06	5
di i-propyl ether	O_3	47.6	1.2E-06	5
methyl t-butyl ether	O_3	15.2	3.9E-07	5
ethyl t-butyl ether	O_3	21.4	5.4E-07	5
2-methoxy ethanol	O_3	30	7.6E-07	5
2-ethoxy ethanol	O_3	38.7	9.8E-07	5
1-methoxy 2-propanol	O_3	36.8	9.3E-07	5
2-butoxy ethanol	O_3	43.8	1.1E-06	5
1-butoxy propanol	O_3	43.6	1.1E-06	5
halocarbons				
chloromethane (methylchloride)	O_3	0.5	1.3E-08	5
dichloromethane (methylene chloride)	O_3	6.8	1.7E-07	5
trichloromethane	O_3	2.3	5.8E-08	5
methyl chloroform (1,1,1 Trichlororethane)	O_3	0.9	2.3E-08	5
cis 1,2-dichloroethene	O_3	44.7	1.1E-06	5
trans 1,2-dichloroethene	O_3	39.2	9.9E-07	5
trichloroethene	O_3	32.5	8.2E-07	5
tetrachloroethene	O_3	2.9	7.3E-08	5
NMVOC (Derwent *et al.* 1996)	O_3	59.2	1.5E-06	5

App. 7.1(cont.): Fate factors linking emissions of primary pollutants to air with concentrations of inhaled air pollutants causing respiratory effects. The POCP are taken from Jenkin *et al.* (1997), the fate factors are taken from Table 7.11. The squared geometric standard deviations σ_g^2 ndicate the flatness of the assumed distribution.

Endpoint	Affected population group	E-R slope (*)	Cultural bias	σg^2	Baseline mortality/ share of population	DALYs(0,1)/ case	DALYs(0,0)/ case	σg^2
Bronchodilator usage	Adult asthmatics	0.163	E, H, I	16	4.00%	3.3E-04	2.7E-04	2
	Asthm. children	0.078	E, H, I	16	1.00%	2.5E-04	2.7E-04	2
Cough	Adult asthmatics	0.168	E, H, I	6	4.00%	1.7E-04	1.4E-04	2
	Asthm. children	0.133	E, H, I	6	1.00%	1.3E-04	1.4E-04	2
Lower respiratory symptoms (wheeze)	Adult asthmatics	0.061	E, H, I	6	4.00%	1.7E-04	1.4E-04	2
	Asthm. children	0.103	E, H, I	6	1.00%	1.3E-04	1.4E-04	2
Chronic bronchitis	Children	1.61E-03	E, H, I	16	20%	2.4E-02	2.5E-02	3
	Adults	4.90E-05	E, H, I	6	80%	1.8E+00	2.0E+00	3
Chronic cough	Children	2.07E-03	E, H, I	16	20%	2.4E-02	2.5E-02	3
Restricted activity days (RAD)(#)	Adults	0.025	E, H, I	16	80%	2.2E-04	2.7E-04	2
Respiratory hospital admissions	All	2.07E-06	E, H, I	6	100%	8.6E-03	1.1E-02	2
Acute Mortality (AM)	All	0.04%	E, H, I	16	0.00%	4.8E-01	7.5E-01	5
Chronic Mortality (CM)	All	0.386%	E, H, I	16	0.81%	4.2E+00	6.6E+00	3
ERV for COPD	All	7.20E-06	E	36	100%	6.5E-04	8.2E-04	3
ERV for asthma	All	6.45E-06	E	36	100%	9.5E-04	8.2E-04	3
ERV for croup in pre school children	All	2.91E-05	E	36	100%	7.7E-04	8.2E-04	3
Total PM10								
Bronchodilator usage	Adult asthmatics	0.272	E, H, I	16	4.00%	3.3E-04	2.7E-04	2
	Asthm. children	0.129	E, H, I	16	1.00%	2.5E-04	2.7E-04	2
Cough	Adult asthmatics	0.28	E, H, I	6	4.00%	1.7E-04	1.4E-04	2
	Asthm. children	0.223	E, H, I	6	1.00%	1.3E-04	1.4E-04	2
Lower respiratory symptoms (wheeze)	Adult asthmatics	0.101	E, H, I	6	4.00%	1.7E-04	1.4E-04	2
	Asthm. children	0.172	E, H, I	6	1.00%	1.3E-04	1.4E-04	2
Chronic bronchitis	Children	2.69E-03	E, H, I	16	20%	2.4E-02	2.5E-02	3
	Adults	7.80E-05	E, H, I	6	80%	1.8E+00	2.0E+00	3
Chronic cough	Children	3.46E-03	E, H, I	16	20%	2.4E-02	2.5E-02	3
Restricted activity days (RAD)(#)	Adults	0.042	E, H, I	16	80%	2.2E-04	2.7E-04	2
Respiratory hospital admissions	All	3.46E-06	E, H, I	6	100%	8.6E-03	1.1E-02	2
Acute Mortality (AM)	All	0.068%	E, H, I	16	0.00%	4.8E-01	7.5E-01	5
Chronic Mortality (CM)	All	0.643%	E, H, I	16	0.81%	4.2E+00	6.6E+00	3
ERV for COPD	All	1.20E-05	E	36	100%	6.5E-04	8.2E-04	3
ERV for asthma	All	1.08E-05	E	36	100%	9.5E-04	8.2E-04	3
ERV for croup in pre school children	All	4.86E-05	E	36	100%	7.7E-04	8.2E-04	3
Total PM2.5/Sulphates								
Bronchodilator usage	Adult asthmatics	0.163	E, H	36	4.00%	3.3E-04	2.7E-04	2
	Asthm. children	0.078	E, H	36	1.00%	2.5E-04	2.7E-04	2
Cough	Adult asthmatics	0.168	E, H	16	4.00%	1.7E-04	1.4E-04	2
	Asthm. children	0.133	E, H	16	1.00%	1.3E-04	1.4E-04	2
Lower respiratory symptoms (wheeze)	Adult asthmatics	0.061	E, H	16	4.00%	1.7E-04	1.4E-04	2
	Asthm. children	0.103	E, H	16	1.00%	1.3E-04	1.4E-04	2
Chronic bronchitis	Children	1.61E-03	E, H	36	20%	2.4E-02	2.5E-02	3
	Adults	4.90E-05	E, H	16	80%	1.8E+00	2.0E+00	3
Chronic cough	Children	2.07E-03	E, H	36	20%	2.4E-02	2.5E-02	3
Restricted activity days (RAD)(#)	Adults	0.025	E, H	36	80%	2.2E-04	2.7E-04	2
Respiratory hospital admissions	All	2.07E-06	E, H	16	100%	8.6E-03	1.1E-02	2
Acute Mortality (AM)	All	0.04%	E, H	36	0.00%	4.8E-01	7.5E-01	5
Chronic Mortality (CM)	All	0.386%	E, H	36	0.81%	4.2E+00	6.6E+00	3
ERV for COPD	All	7.20E-06	E	36	100%	6.5E-04	8.2E-04	3
ERV for asthma	All	6.45E-06	E	36	100%	9.5E-04	8.2E-04	3
ERV for croup in pre school children	All	2.91E-05	E	36	100%	7.7E-04	8.2E-04	3
Total Nitrates								
Asthma attacks (AA)	All	4.29E-03	E, H, I	36	100%	3.1E-04	2.7E-04	2
Minor restricted activity day (MRAD)(¶)	Adults	9.76E-03	E, H, I	16	80%	1.1E-04	1.4E-04	2
Respiratory hospital admissions	All	3.54E-06	E, H, I	6	100%	8.6E-03	1.1E-02	2
Symptom days	All	0.033	E, H, I	6	100%	1.6E-04	1.4E-04	2
Acute Mortality (AM)	All	0.059%	E, H, I	16	0.84%	4.8E-01	7.5E-01	5
ERV for asthma	All	1.32E-05	E	36	100%	9.5E-04	8.2E-04	3
Total Ozone								
Respiratory hospital admissions	All	2.04E-06	E, H	6	100%	8.6E-03	1.1E-02	2
Acute Mortality (AM)	All	0.072%	E, H	16	0.84%	4.8E-01	7.5E-01	5
Total SO2								
Acute Mortality (AM)	All	0.034%	E	36	0.84%	4.8E-01	7.5E-01	5
Respiratory hospital admissions	All	1.40E-06	E	16	100%	8.6E-03	1.1E-02	2
Total NOx								
Acute Mortality (AM)	All	0.00145%	E	36	0.84%	4.8E-01	7.5E-01	5
Total CO								

App. 7.2: Basic data to calculate health damages due to air pollutants. Exposure-response slope, cultural bias, and squared geometric standard deviation of the E-R slope are all from Table 7.13. The share of the population group concerned is from Table 7.14, baseline mortality without injuries from Table 7.15, DALYs per case from Table 7.17 and 7.18.

Endpoint	$\Sigma\sigma g^2$	DALYs(0,1) low	DALYs(0,1) best estim.	DALYs(0,1) high	DALYs(0,0) low	DALYs(0,0) best estim.	DALYs(0,0) high
Bronchodilator usage	17.4	1.2E-7	2.2E-6	3.7E-5	1.0E-7	1.8E-6	3.1E-5
	17.4	1.1E-8	2.0E-7	3.4E-6	1.2E-8	2.1E-7	3.7E-6
Cough	6.8	1.7E-7	1.1E-6	7.8E-6	1.4E-7	9.4E-7	6.4E-6
	6.8	2.5E-8	1.7E-7	1.2E-6	2.7E-8	1.9E-7	1.3E-6
Lower respiratory symptoms (wheeze)	6.8	6.1E-8	4.1E-7	2.8E-6	5.0E-8	3.4E-7	2.3E-6
	6.8	2.0E-8	1.3E-7	9.1E-7	2.1E-8	1.4E-7	9.8E-7
Chronic bronchitis	19.7	3.9E-7	7.7E-6	1.5E-4	4.1E-7	8.1E-6	1.6E-4
	8.2	8.6E-6	7.1E-5	5.8E-4	9.6E-6	7.8E-5	6.4E-4
Chronic cough	19.7	5.0E-7	9.9E-6	2.0E-4	5.2E-7	1.0E-5	2.0E-4
Restricted activity days (RAD)(#)	17.4	2.5E-7	4.4E-6	7.7E-5	3.1E-7	5.4E-6	9.4E-5
Respiratory hospital admissions	6.8	2.6E-9	1.8E-8	1.2E-7	3.3E-9	2.3E-8	1.6E-7
Acute Mortality (AM)	24.7	0.0E+0	0.0E+0	0.0E+0	0.0E+0	0.0E+0	0.0E+0
Chronic Mortality (CM)	19.7	6.7E-6	1.3E-4	2.6E-3	1.0E-5	2.1E-4	4.1E-3
ERV for COPD	42.4	1.1E-10	4.7E-9	2.0E-7	1.4E-10	5.9E-9	2.5E-7
ERV for asthma	42.4	1.4E-10	6.1E-9	2.6E-7	1.2E-10	5.3E-9	2.2E-7
ERV for croup in pre school children	42.4	5.3E-10	2.2E-8	9.5E-7	5.6E-10	2.4E-8	1.0E-6
Total PM10 Egalitarian	**15.0**	**1.7E-5**	**2.3E-4**	**3.6E-3**	**2.2E-5**	**3.1E-4**	**5.2E-3**
Hierarchist	**15.0**	**1.7E-5**	**2.3E-4**	**3.6E-3**	**2.2E-5**	**3.1E-4**	**5.2E-3**
Individualist	**15.0**	**1.7E-5**	**2.3E-4**	**3.6E-3**	**2.2E-5**	**3.1E-4**	**5.2E-3**
Bronchodilator usage	17.4	2.1E-7	3.6E-6	6.3E-5	1.7E-7	2.9E-6	5.1E-5
	17.4	1.9E-8	3.2E-7	5.6E-6	2.0E-8	3.5E-7	6.1E-6
Cough	6.8	2.8E-7	1.9E-6	1.3E-5	2.3E-7	1.6E-6	1.1E-5
	6.8	4.2E-8	2.9E-7	2.0E-6	4.6E-8	3.1E-7	2.1E-6
Lower respiratory symptoms (wheeze)	6.8	1.0E-7	6.9E-7	4.7E-6	8.3E-8	5.7E-7	3.9E-6
	6.8	3.3E-8	2.2E-7	1.5E-6	3.5E-8	2.4E-7	1.6E-6
Chronic bronchitis	19.7	6.5E-7	1.3E-5	2.5E-4	6.8E-7	1.3E-5	2.7E-4
	8.2	1.4E-5	1.1E-4	9.2E-4	1.5E-5	1.2E-4	1.0E-3
Chronic cough	19.7	8.4E-7	1.7E-5	3.3E-4	8.8E-7	1.7E-5	3.4E-4
Restricted activity days (RAD)(#)	17.4	4.2E-7	7.4E-6	1.3E-4	5.2E-7	9.1E-6	1.6E-4
Respiratory hospital admissions	6.8	4.4E-9	3.0E-8	2.0E-7	5.6E-9	3.8E-8	2.6E-7
Acute Mortality (AM)	24.7	0.0E+0	0.0E+0	0.0E+0	0.0E+0	0.0E+0	0.0E+0
Chronic Mortality (CM)	19.7	1.1E-5	2.2E-4	4.3E-3	1.7E-5	3.4E-4	6.8E-3
ERV for COPD	42.4	1.8E-10	7.8E-9	3.3E-7	2.3E-10	9.8E-9	4.2E-7
ERV for asthma	42.4	2.4E-10	1.0E-8	4.4E-7	2.1E-10	8.9E-9	3.8E-7
ERV for croup in pre school children	42.4	8.8E-10	3.7E-8	1.6E-6	9.4E-10	4.0E-8	1.7E-6
Total PM2.5/Sulphates Egalitarian	**15.0**	**2.7E-5**	**3.8E-4**	**6.0E-3**	**3.5E-5**	**5.1E-4**	**8.6E-3**
Hierarchist	**15.0**	**2.7E-5**	**3.8E-4**	**6.0E-3**	**3.5E-5**	**5.1E-4**	**8.6E-3**
Individualist	**15.0**	**2.7E-5**	**3.8E-4**	**6.0E-3**	**3.5E-5**	**5.1E-4**	**8.6E-3**
Bronchodilator usage	38.5	5.6E-8	2.2E-6	8.3E-5	4.6E-8	1.8E-6	6.8E-5
	38.5	5.1E-9	2.0E-7	7.5E-6	5.5E-9	2.1E-7	8.1E-6
Cough	17.4	6.6E-8	1.1E-6	2.0E-5	5.4E-8	9.4E-7	1.6E-5
	17.4	9.9E-9	1.7E-7	3.0E-6	1.1E-8	1.9E-7	3.2E-6
Lower respiratory symptoms (wheeze)	17.4	2.4E-8	4.1E-7	7.2E-6	2.0E-8	3.4E-7	6.0E-6
	17.4	7.7E-9	1.3E-7	2.3E-6	8.3E-9	1.4E-7	2.5E-6
Chronic bronchitis	42.4	1.8E-7	7.7E-6	3.3E-4	1.9E-7	8.1E-6	3.4E-4
	19.7	3.6E-6	7.1E-5	1.4E-3	4.0E-6	7.8E-5	1.5E-3
Chronic cough	42.4	2.3E-7	9.9E-6	4.2E-4	2.4E-7	1.0E-5	4.4E-4
Restricted activity days (RAD)(#)	38.5	1.1E-7	4.4E-6	1.7E-4	1.4E-7	5.4E-6	2.1E-4
Respiratory hospital admissions	17.4	1.0E-9	1.8E-8	3.1E-7	1.3E-9	2.3E-8	4.0E-7
Acute Mortality (AM)	50.8	0.0E+0	0.0E+0	0.0E+0	0.0E+0	0.0E+0	0.0E+0
Chronic Mortality (CM)	42.4	3.1E-6	1.3E-4	5.6E-3	4.9E-6	2.1E-4	8.8E-3
ERV for COPD	42.4	1.1E-10	4.7E-9	2.0E-7	1.4E-10	5.9E-9	2.5E-7
ERV for asthma	42.4	1.4E-10	6.1E-9	2.6E-7	1.2E-10	5.3E-9	2.2E-7
ERV for croup in pre school children	42.4	5.3E-10	2.2E-8	9.5E-7	5.6E-10	2.4E-8	1.0E-6
Total Nitrates Egalitarian	**34.0**	**7.4E-6**	**2.3E-4**	**8.0E-3**	**9.6E-6**	**3.1E-4**	**1.1E-2**
Hierarchist	**34.0**	**7.4E-6**	**2.3E-4**	**8.0E-3**	**9.6E-6**	**3.1E-4**	**1.1E-2**
Individualist	**34.0**	**0**	**0**	**0**	**0**	**0**	**0**
Asthma attacks (AA)	38.5	3.5E-8	1.3E-6	5.1E-5	3.0E-8	1.2E-6	4.5E-5
Minor restricted activity day (MRAD)(¶)	17.4	4.9E-8	8.6E-7	1.5E-5	6.3E-8	1.1E-6	1.9E-5
Respiratory hospital admissions	6.8	4.5E-9	3.0E-8	2.1E-7	5.7E-9	3.9E-8	2.7E-7
Symptom days	6.8	7.7E-7	5.3E-6	3.6E-5	6.8E-7	4.6E-6	3.2E-5
Acute Mortality (AM)	24.7	9.6E-8	2.4E-6	5.9E-5	1.5E-7	3.7E-6	9.2E-5
ERV for asthma	42.4	3.0E-10	1.3E-8	5.3E-7	2.6E-10	1.1E-8	4.6E-7
Total Ozone Egalitarian		**9.6E-7**	**9.9E-6**	**1.6E-4**	**9.3E-7**	**1.1E-5**	**1.9E-4**
Hierarchist		**9.6E-7**	**9.9E-6**	**1.6E-4**	**9.3E-7**	**1.1E-5**	**1.9E-4**
Individualist		**9.6E-7**	**9.9E-6**	**1.6E-4**	**9.3E-7**	**1.1E-5**	**1.9E-4**
Respiratory hospital admissions	6.8	2.6E-9	1.8E-8	1.2E-7	3.3E-9	2.2E-8	1.5E-7
Acute Mortality (AM)	24.7	1.2E-7	2.9E-6	7.2E-5	1.8E-7	4.5E-6	1.1E-4
Total SO2 Egalitarian		**1.2E-7**	**2.9E-6**	**7.2E-5**	**1.9E-7**	**4.6E-6**	**1.1E-4**
Hierarchist		**1.2E-7**	**2.9E-6**	**7.2E-5**	**1.9E-7**	**4.6E-6**	**1.1E-4**
Individualist		**0**	**0**	**0**	**0**	**0**	**0**
Acute Mortality (AM)	50.8	2.7E-8	1.4E-6	7.0E-5	4.2E-8	2.1E-6	1.1E-4
Respiratory hospital admissions	17.4	6.9E-10	1.2E-8	2.1E-7	8.8E-10	1.5E-8	2.7E-7
Total NOx Egalitarian		**2.8E-8**	**1.4E-6**	**7.0E-5**	**4.3E-8**	**2.2E-6**	**1.1E-4**
Acute Mortality (AM)	50.8	1.2E-9	5.8E-8	3.0E-6	1.8E-9	9.1E-8	4.6E-6
Total CO Egalitarian	**50.8**	**1.2E-9**	**5.8E-8**	**3.0E-6**	**1.8E-9**	**9.1E-8**	**4.6E-6**

App. 7.3: Low, best, and high estimate for DALYs per (yr·person·µg/m^3). $\Sigma\sigma g^2$ is the result of the single geometric standard deviations listed in Appendix (7.2) applying Equation (A6.3) in Appendix 6.8. The lower and higher estimate span a 95% confidence interval. For each cultural perspective the sum per pollutant is calculated. The background data used is given in Appendix (7.2).

Primary Pollutant		Secondary Pollutant	$\Pi\sigma g^2$	DALYs(0,1) low	DALYs(0,1) best estim.	DALYs(0,1) high	DALYs(0,0) low	DALYs(0,0) best estim.	DALYs(0,0) high
			-	a/kg	a/kg	a/kg	a/kg	a/kg	a/kg
CO	E	CO	64				1.1E-8	7.3E-7	4.7E-5
TSP	E, H, I	PM10	19	4.3E-6	8.0E-5	1.5E-3	5.9E-6	1.1E-4	2.0E-3
PM_{10}	E, H, I	PM10	19	1.5E-5	2.7E-4	5.1E-3	2.0E-5	3.7E-4	7.0E-3
$PM_{2.5}$	E, H, I	PM2.5	19	2.7E-5	5.1E-4	9.5E-3	3.8E-5	7.0E-4	1.3E-2
SOx (as SO_2)	E, H	SO_2	27				4.1E-8	1.1E-6	2.9E-5
SOx (as SO_2)	E, H, I	Sulphates	16	2.4E-6	3.9E-5	6.4E-4	3.3E-6	5.4E-5	8.8E-4
NH_3	E, H, I	Sulphates	16	3.1E-6	5.1E-5	8.3E-4	4.3E-6	7.0E-5	1.1E-3
NH_3	E, H	Nitrates	36				4.1E-7	1.5E-5	5.5E-4
NOx (as NO_2)	E	NO_2	54				8.0E-9	4.3E-7	2.3E-5
NOx (as NO_2)	E, H	Nitrates	36				2.4E-6	8.7E-5	3.2E-3
NOx (as NO_2)	E, H, I	O_3	21	5.7E-8	1.2E-6	2.5E-5	6.1E-8	1.3E-6	2.7E-5
NMVOC	E, H, I	O_3	23	5.1E-8	1.2E-6	2.8E-5	5.5E-8	1.3E-6	3.0E-5
VOCs	E, H, I								
alkanes									
methane		O_3	23	5.1E-10	1.2E-8	2.8E-7	5.5E-10	1.3E-8	3.0E-7
ethane		O_3	23	1.1E-8	2.5E-7	5.7E-6	1.1E-8	2.6E-7	6.2E-6
propane		O_3	23	1.5E-8	3.6E-7	8.3E-6	1.6E-8	3.8E-7	8.9E-6
butane		O_3	23	3.0E-8	7.0E-7	1.6E-5	3.2E-8	7.6E-7	1.8E-5
i-butane		O_3	23	2.6E-8	6.2E-7	1.4E-5	2.8E-8	6.6E-7	1.5E-5
pentane		O_3	23	3.4E-8	7.9E-7	1.8E-5	3.6E-8	8.5E-7	2.0E-5
i-pentane		O_3	23	3.4E-8	7.9E-7	1.8E-5	3.6E-8	8.5E-7	2.0E-5
neopentane		O_3	23	1.5E-8	3.5E-7	8.1E-6	1.6E-8	3.7E-7	8.7E-6
hexane		O_3	23	4.1E-8	9.5E-7	2.2E-5	4.4E-8	1.0E-6	2.4E-5
2-methyl pentane		O_3	23	3.7E-8	8.7E-7	2.0E-5	4.0E-8	9.4E-7	2.2E-5
3-methyl pentane		O_3	23	4.1E-8	9.5E-7	2.2E-5	4.4E-8	1.0E-6	2.4E-5
2,2-dimethyl butane		O_3	23	2.1E-8	4.8E-7	1.1E-5	2.2E-8	5.2E-7	1.2E-5
2,3-dimethyl butane		O_3	23	4.7E-8	1.1E-6	2.6E-5	5.1E-8	1.2E-6	2.8E-5
heptane		O_3	23	4.4E-8	1.0E-6	2.4E-5	4.7E-8	1.1E-6	2.6E-5
2-methyl hexane		O_3	23	3.4E-8	7.9E-7	1.8E-5	3.6E-8	8.5E-7	2.0E-5
3-methyl hexane		O_3	23	3.1E-8	7.3E-7	1.7E-5	3.4E-8	7.8E-7	1.8E-5
octane		O_3	23	3.7E-8	8.7E-7	2.0E-5	4.0E-8	9.4E-7	2.2E-5
nonane		O_3	23	3.4E-8	7.9E-7	1.8E-5	3.6E-8	8.5E-7	2.0E-5
decane		O_3	23	3.3E-8	7.7E-7	1.8E-5	3.5E-8	8.3E-7	1.9E-5
undecane		O_3	23	3.3E-8	7.7E-7	1.8E-5	3.5E-8	8.3E-7	1.9E-5
dodecane		O_3	23	3.1E-8	7.1E-7	1.7E-5	3.3E-8	7.7E-7	1.8E-5
cyclohexane		O_3	23	2.5E-8	5.8E-7	1.3E-5	2.7E-8	6.2E-7	1.5E-5
alkenes/dienes									
ethene		O_3	23	8.5E-8	2.0E-6	4.6E-5	9.1E-8	2.1E-6	5.0E-5
propene		O_3	23	9.5E-8	2.2E-6	5.2E-5	1.0E-7	2.4E-6	5.6E-5
1-butene		O_3	23	9.2E-8	2.1E-6	5.0E-5	9.8E-8	2.3E-6	5.4E-5
cis 2-butene		O_3	23	9.8E-8	2.3E-6	5.4E-5	1.1E-7	2.5E-6	5.8E-5
trans 2-butene		O_3	23	9.8E-8	2.3E-6	5.4E-5	1.1E-7	2.5E-6	5.8E-5
methyl propene		O_3	23	5.4E-8	1.3E-6	3.0E-5	5.8E-8	1.4E-6	3.2E-5
1-pentene		O_3	23	8.5E-8	2.0E-6	4.6E-5	9.1E-8	2.1E-6	5.0E-5
cis 2-pentene		O_3	23	9.5E-8	2.2E-6	5.2E-5	1.0E-7	2.4E-6	5.6E-5
trans 2-pentene		O_3	23	9.5E-8	2.2E-6	5.2E-5	1.0E-7	2.4E-6	5.6E-5
2-methyl 1-butene		O_3	23	6.8E-8	1.6E-6	3.7E-5	7.3E-8	1.7E-6	4.0E-5
2-methyl 2-butene		O_3	23	7.1E-8	1.7E-6	3.9E-5	7.7E-8	1.8E-6	4.2E-5
3-methyl 1-butene		O_3	23	5.8E-8	1.3E-6	3.1E-5	6.2E-8	1.4E-6	3.4E-5
1-hexene		O_3	23	7.5E-8	1.7E-6	4.1E-5	8.0E-8	1.9E-6	4.4E-5
cis 2-hexene		O_3	23	9.2E-8	2.1E-6	5.0E-5	9.8E-8	2.3E-6	5.4E-5
trans 2-hexene		O_3	23	9.2E-8	2.1E-6	5.0E-5	9.8E-8	2.3E-6	5.4E-5
1,3-butadiene		O_3	23	7.5E-8	1.7E-6	4.1E-5	8.0E-8	1.9E-6	4.4E-5
isoprene		O_3	23	9.5E-8	2.2E-6	5.2E-5	1.0E-7	2.4E-6	5.6E-5
alkynes									
acetylene		O_3	23	7.5E-9	1.7E-7	4.1E-6	8.0E-9	1.9E-7	4.4E-6

App. 7.4: Damage factors without discounting but with age-weighting (DALYs(0,1)) and without discounting and without age-weighting (DALYs(0,0)) for the emission of 1 kg pollutant to air under European conditions. The $\Pi\sigma g^2$ stands for the cumulated squared geometric standard deviation over all steps and is the basis for the calculation of the lower and upper estimates which span the 95% confidence interval.

Primary Pollutant	Secondary Pollutant	$\Pi\sigma g^2$	DALYs(0,1) low	DALYs(0,1) best estim.	DALYs(0,1) high	DALYs(0,0) low	DALYs(0,0) best estim.	DALYs(0,0) high
		-	a/kg	a/kg	a/kg	a/kg	a/kg	a/kg
aromatics								
benzene	O_3	23	1.9E-8	4.4E-7	1.0E-5	2.0E-8	4.7E-7	1.1E-5
toluene	O_3	23	5.4E-8	1.3E-6	3.0E-5	5.8E-8	1.4E-6	3.2E-5
o-xylene	O_3	23	9.2E-8	2.1E-6	5.0E-5	9.8E-8	2.3E-6	5.4E-5
m-xylene	O_3	23	9.5E-8	2.2E-6	5.2E-5	1.0E-7	2.4E-6	5.6E-5
p-xylene	O_3	23	8.8E-8	2.1E-6	4.8E-5	9.5E-8	2.2E-6	5.2E-5
ethyl benzene	O_3	23	6.1E-8	1.4E-6	3.3E-5	6.6E-8	1.5E-6	3.6E-5
n-propyl benzene	O_3	23	5.4E-8	1.3E-6	3.0E-5	5.8E-8	1.4E-6	3.2E-5
i-propyl benzene	O_3	23	4.4E-8	1.0E-6	2.4E-5	4.7E-8	1.1E-6	2.6E-5
1,2,3-trimethyl benzene	O_3	23	1.1E-7	2.5E-6	5.9E-5	1.2E-7	2.7E-6	6.4E-5
1,2,4-trimethyl benzene	O_3	23	1.1E-7	2.5E-6	5.9E-5	1.2E-7	2.7E-6	6.4E-5
1,3,5-trimethyl benzene	O_3	23	1.2E-7	2.8E-6	6.5E-5	1.3E-7	3.0E-6	7.0E-5
o-ethyl toluene	O_3	23	7.8E-8	1.8E-6	4.2E-5	8.4E-8	2.0E-6	4.6E-5
m-ethyl toluene	O_3	23	8.8E-8	2.1E-6	4.8E-5	9.5E-8	2.2E-6	5.2E-5
p-ethyl toluene	O_3	23	7.8E-8	1.8E-6	4.2E-5	8.4E-8	2.0E-6	4.6E-5
3,5-dimethyl ethyl benzene	O_3	23	1.1E-7	2.6E-6	6.1E-5	1.2E-7	2.8E-6	6.6E-5
3,5-diethyl toluene	O_3	23	1.1E-7	2.6E-6	6.1E-5	1.2E-7	2.8E-6	6.6E-5
aldehydes								
formaldehyde	O_3	23	4.4E-8	1.0E-6	2.4E-5	4.7E-8	1.1E-6	2.6E-5
acetaldehyde	O_3	23	5.4E-8	1.3E-6	3.0E-5	5.8E-8	1.4E-6	3.2E-5
propionaldehyde	O_3	23	6.8E-8	1.6E-6	3.7E-5	7.3E-8	1.7E-6	4.0E-5
n-butyraldehyde	O_3	23	6.8E-8	1.6E-6	3.7E-5	7.3E-8	1.7E-6	4.0E-5
i-butyraldehyde	O_3	23	4.4E-8	1.0E-6	2.4E-5	4.7E-8	1.1E-6	2.6E-5
pentanal	O_3	23	6.4E-8	1.5E-6	3.5E-5	6.9E-8	1.6E-6	3.8E-5
ketones								
acetone	O_3	23	8.1E-9	1.9E-7	4.4E-6	8.8E-9	2.0E-7	4.8E-6
methyl ethyl ketone	O_3	23	3.2E-8	7.5E-7	1.8E-5	3.5E-8	8.1E-7	1.9E-5
2-pentanone	O_3	23	4.7E-8	1.1E-6	2.6E-5	5.1E-8	1.2E-6	2.8E-5
3-pentanone	O_3	23	3.4E-8	7.9E-7	1.8E-5	3.6E-8	8.5E-7	2.0E-5
methyl i-propyl ketone	O_3	23	3.1E-8	7.3E-7	1.7E-5	3.4E-8	7.8E-7	1.8E-5
2-hexanone	O_3	23	4.7E-8	1.1E-6	2.6E-5	5.1E-8	1.2E-6	2.8E-5
3-hexanone	O_3	23	5.1E-8	1.2E-6	2.8E-5	5.5E-8	1.3E-6	3.0E-5
methyl i-butyl ketone	O_3	23	4.1E-8	9.5E-7	2.2E-5	4.4E-8	1.0E-6	2.4E-5
methyl t-butyl ketone	O_3	23	2.8E-8	6.5E-7	1.5E-5	3.0E-8	7.0E-7	1.6E-5
cyclohexanone	O_3	23	2.6E-8	6.0E-7	1.4E-5	2.8E-8	6.5E-7	1.5E-5
alcohols								
methanol	O_3	23	1.1E-8	2.6E-7	6.1E-6	1.2E-8	2.8E-7	6.6E-6
ethanol	O_3	23	3.3E-8	7.8E-7	1.8E-5	3.6E-8	8.3E-7	1.9E-5
n-propanol	O_3	23	4.7E-8	1.1E-6	2.6E-5	5.1E-8	1.2E-6	2.8E-5
i-propanol	O_3	23	1.2E-8	2.8E-7	6.5E-6	1.3E-8	3.0E-7	7.0E-6
n-butanol	O_3	23	5.4E-8	1.3E-6	3.0E-5	5.8E-8	1.4E-6	3.2E-5
s-butanol	O_3	23	3.4E-8	7.9E-7	1.8E-5	3.6E-8	8.5E-7	2.0E-5
i-butanol	O_3	23	3.2E-8	7.5E-7	1.8E-5	3.5E-8	8.1E-7	1.9E-5
t-butanol	O_3	23	1.1E-8	2.5E-7	5.7E-6	1.1E-8	2.6E-7	6.2E-6
2-methyl 1-butanol	O_3	23	3.4E-8	7.9E-7	1.8E-5	3.6E-8	8.5E-7	2.0E-5
2-methyl 2-butanol	O_3	23	1.2E-8	2.8E-7	6.6E-6	1.3E-8	3.1E-7	7.2E-6
3-methyl 1-butanol	O_3	23	3.4E-8	7.9E-7	1.8E-5	3.6E-8	8.5E-7	2.0E-5
3-methyl 2-butanol	O_3	23	3.2E-8	7.4E-7	1.7E-5	3.4E-8	7.9E-7	1.8E-5
3-pentanol	O_3	23	3.7E-8	8.7E-7	2.0E-5	4.0E-8	9.4E-7	2.2E-5
diacetone alcohol	O_3	23	2.2E-8	5.2E-7	1.2E-5	2.4E-8	5.6E-7	1.3E-5
cyclohexanol	O_3	23	3.7E-8	8.7E-7	2.0E-5	4.0E-8	9.4E-7	2.2E-5
ethane diol	O_3	23	3.3E-8	7.7E-7	1.8E-5	3.5E-8	8.3E-7	1.9E-5
propane diol	O_3	23	4.1E-8	9.5E-7	2.2E-5	4.4E-8	1.0E-6	2.4E-5

App. 7.4 (cont.): Damage factors without discounting but with age-weighting (DALYs(0,1)) and without discounting and without age-weighting (DALYs(0,0)) for the emission of 1 kg pollutant to air under European conditions. The $\Pi\sigma g^2$ stands for the cumulated squared geometric standard deviation over all steps and is the basis for the calculation of the lower and upper estimates which span the 95% confidence interval.

Primary Pollutant	Secondary Pollutant	$\Pi\sigma g^2$	DALYs(0,1) low	DALYs(0,1) best estim.	DALYs(0,1) high	DALYs(0,0) low	DALYs(0,0) best estim.	DALYs(0,0) high
		-	a/kg	a/kg	a/kg	a/kg	a/kg	a/kg
esters								
methyl formate	O_3	23	2.8E-9	6.6E-8	1.6E-6	3.1E-9	7.1E-8	1.7E-6
methyl acetate	O_3	23	4.1E-9	9.5E-8	2.2E-6	4.4E-9	1.0E-7	2.4E-6
ethyl acetate	O_3	23	1.8E-8	4.3E-7	1.0E-5	2.0E-8	4.6E-7	1.1E-5
n-propyl acetate	O_3	23	2.5E-8	5.8E-7	1.3E-5	2.7E-8	6.2E-7	1.5E-5
i-propyl acetate	O_3	23	1.8E-8	4.3E-7	1.0E-5	2.0E-8	4.6E-7	1.1E-5
n-butyl acetate	O_3	23	2.1E-8	4.8E-7	1.1E-5	2.2E-8	5.2E-7	1.2E-5
s-butyl acetate	O_3	23	2.3E-8	5.4E-7	1.3E-5	2.5E-8	5.8E-7	1.4E-5
t-butyl acetate	O_3	23	5.4E-9	1.3E-7	3.0E-6	5.8E-9	1.4E-7	3.2E-6
carboxylic acids								
formic acid	O_3	23	2.7E-9	6.4E-8	1.5E-6	3.0E-9	6.9E-8	1.6E-6
acetic acid	O_3	23	8.5E-9	2.0E-7	4.6E-6	9.1E-9	2.1E-7	5.0E-6
propanoic acid	O_3	23	1.3E-8	3.0E-7	7.0E-6	1.4E-8	3.2E-7	7.5E-6
ethers and glycol ethers								
dimethyl ether	O_3	23	1.5E-8	3.5E-7	8.1E-6	1.6E-8	3.7E-7	8.7E-6
diethyl ether	O_3	23	4.1E-8	9.5E-7	2.2E-5	4.4E-8	1.0E-6	2.4E-5
di i-propyl ether	O_3	23	4.1E-8	9.5E-7	2.2E-5	4.4E-8	1.0E-6	2.4E-5
methyl t-butyl ether	O_3	23	1.3E-8	3.1E-7	7.2E-6	1.4E-8	3.3E-7	7.7E-6
ethyl t-butyl ether	O_3	23	1.8E-8	4.3E-7	1.0E-5	2.0E-8	4.6E-7	1.1E-5
2-methoxy ethanol	O_3	23	2.6E-8	6.0E-7	1.4E-5	2.8E-8	6.5E-7	1.5E-5
2-ethoxy ethanol	O_3	23	3.3E-8	7.8E-7	1.8E-5	3.6E-8	8.3E-7	1.9E-5
1-methoxy 2-propanol	O_3	23	3.2E-8	7.4E-7	1.7E-5	3.4E-8	7.9E-7	1.8E-5
2-butoxy ethanol	O_3	23	3.7E-8	8.7E-7	2.0E-5	4.0E-8	9.4E-7	2.2E-5
1-butoxy propanol	O_3	23	3.7E-8	8.7E-7	2.0E-5	4.0E-8	9.4E-7	2.2E-5
halocarbons								
chloromethane (methylchloride)	O_3	23	4.4E-10	1.0E-8	2.4E-7	4.7E-10	1.1E-8	2.6E-7
dichloromethane (methylene chloride)	O_3	23	5.8E-9	1.3E-7	3.1E-6	6.2E-9	1.4E-7	3.4E-6
trichloromethane	O_3	23	2.0E-9	4.6E-8	1.1E-6	2.1E-9	4.9E-8	1.2E-6
methyl chloroform (1,1,1 Trichlororethane)	O_3	23	7.8E-10	1.8E-8	4.2E-7	8.4E-10	2.0E-8	4.6E-7
cis 1,2-dichloroethene	O_3	23	3.7E-8	8.7E-7	2.0E-5	4.0E-8	9.4E-7	2.2E-5
trans 1,2-dichloroethene	O_3	23	3.4E-8	7.8E-7	1.8E-5	3.6E-8	8.4E-7	2.0E-5
trichloroethene	O_3	23	2.8E-8	6.5E-7	1.5E-5	3.0E-8	7.0E-7	1.6E-5
tetrachloroethene	O_3	23	2.5E-9	5.8E-8	1.3E-6	2.7E-9	6.2E-8	1.5E-6
NMVOC	O_3	23	5.1E-8	1.2E-6	2.8E-5	5.5E-8	1.3E-6	3.0E-5

App. 7.4 (cont.): Damage factors without discounting but with age-weighting (DALYs(0,1)) and without discounting and without age-weighting (DALYs(0,0)) for the emission of 1 kg pollutant to air under European conditions. The $\Pi\sigma g^2$ stands for the cumulated squared geometric standard deviation over all steps and is the basis for the calculation of the lower and upper estimates which span the 95% confidence interval.

APPENDICES CHAPTER 9

Name of substance	DALYs(0,0)air, best estimate	World-wide emissions	European emissions 1990	Total potential damage in Europe	Reference for emission data
IARC-Group 1	a	t/a	t/a	DALYs(0,0/a	
Arsenic, inorganic (1)	1.6E-01		1.2E+03	2.0E+05	UBA/TNO (1997)
Benzene	2.0E-06		3.0E+05	6.0E+02	Pruppers 1996
Cadmium	1.3E-01		6.1E+02	8.0E+04	UBA/TNO (1997)
Chromium(VI)	5.3E+02		1.6E+00	8.3E+05	UBA/TNO (1997)
Nickel	9.5E-02		1.2E+04	1.1E+06	UBA/TNO (1997)
Vinylchloride (2)	2.1E-07	2.0E+05	4.0E+04	8.4E+00	Rippen (1996)
IARC-Group 2A					
Benzo[a]pyrene- (BaP) (2)	2.7E-01	5.0E+03	1.0E+03	2.7E+05	Rippen (1996)
Diesel soot particles	9.8E-06		1.1E+03	1.1E+01	20% of Table 7.21
Epichlorhydrin (2)	3.0E-07	2.3E+04	4.6E+03	1.4E+00	Rippen (1996)
Formaldehyde	3.2E-06		9.5E+03	3.0E+01	Schmucki 1996
Polychlorinated-biphenyl- (PCBs)	9.1E-03		1.2E+02	1.1E+03	UBA/TNO (1997)
IARC-Group 2B					
1,2-Dichloroethane (2)	3.0E-05	4.0E+05	8.0E+04	2.4E+03	Rippen (1996)
2,3,7,8-Tetrachlordibenzo-p-dioxin, TCDD	1.5E+03		1.1E-01	1.7E+05	UBA/TNO (1997)
Acetaldehyde (2)	2.2E-07	100000-500000	5.0E+04	1.1E+01	Rippen (1996)
alpha-Hexachlorcyclohexan (2)	1.5E-03	1.0E+05	2.0E+04	3.0E+04	Rippen (1996)
beta-Hexachlorcyclohexan (2)	6.3E-03	1.5E+04	3.0E+03	1.9E+04	Rippen (1996)
Carbon-tetrachloride (2)	8.3E-04	5.0E+04	1.0E+04	8.3E+03	Rippen (1996)
Chloroform (2)	2.6E-05	100000-300000	4.0E+04	1.0E+03	Rippen (1996)
Di(2-ethylhexyl)phthalate- (DEHP) (2)	8.1E-06	10000-150000	2.0E+04	1.6E+02	Rippen (1996)
Dichloromethane (2)	4.4E-07	5.0E+05	1.0E+05	4.4E+01	Rippen (1996)
Dichlorvos (2)	1.1E-04	3.0E+03	6.0E+02	6.6E+01	Rippen (1996)
gamma-Hexachlorocyclohexane (2)	4.1E-03	3.8E+04	7.6E+03	3.1E+04	Rippen (1996)
Hexachlorobenzene	2.0E-03		8.0E+00	1.6E+01	UBA/TNO (1997)
Pentachlorphenol	3.7E-05		1.8E+03	6.7E+01	UBA/TNO (1997)
Perchloroethylene (2)	4.8E-07	6.3E+05	1.3E+05	6.0E+01	Rippen (1996)
IARC-Group 3					
1,1,2-Trichlorethane (2)	1.1E-05	2.0E+04	4.0E+03	4.4E+01	Rippen (1996)
1,1-Dichlorethene (2)	5.1E-06	2.0E+03	4.0E+02	2.0E+00	Rippen (1996)
Trichlorethylene	8.0E-08		2.4E+05	1.9E+01	UBA/TNO (1997)
Total damage to human health				2.7E+06	

App. 9.1: Rough estimate for damages to human health due to carcinogenic air emissions in Europe (egalitarian perspective). Only substances for which emission estimates are available and which are reported in Appendix (6.16) have been included. Graphic interpretation in Figure 9.3.
(1) all As as As inorganic
(2) assumption that world-wide emissions divided by 5 = European emissions (approximately according to the share of GDP)
(3) assumption that 0.1% of Cr is Cr(VI)

Appendix 9.2: Literature for further operationalisation

This book offers damage factors for a selection of substances causing carcinogenic or respiratory effects in human beings. Many other mechanisms will have to be analysed and innumerable causal relationships will have to be established in order to make the whole framework operable.

In order to support this work we list in this appendix a number of references which hopefully facilitate the establishment of these causal relationships, either by the material they contain or by the references to yet other literature in them. The search for and selection has not been made systematically and the list is not comprehensive.

There are some practical hints which have proven of use:

- Start with a review of the actual literature on the assessment of damage costs. They have similar aims and work in a fully quantitative manner.
- Contact directly the leading researchers in the respective fields in order to make sure that you work with the latest modelling results.
- Use the extensive number of databases on the internet.

A broad list of substances of concern for human and ecological health is given in Hoffmann (1993). Most other sources are more specialised. The following table gives a first compilation:

<table>
<tr><td colspan="8">Several impacts on human health: ExternE 1995/1997, ESEERCO 1995, Stanners et al. 1995, Globe 1992</td></tr>
<tr><td colspan="4">Toxicity:
Kuchuk et al. 1997, Bertollini et al. 1996, Ziqiang et al. 1996, Lebret et al. 1996, Pruppers et al. 1996/1997, Pruppers 1996, Pieters et al. 1996, Paustenbach 1989, Kolluru et al. 1996, Hansson 1997, WHO 1994a, WHO 1995a, WHO 1998, Crumb 1984, Renwick et al. 1993, Fishbein 1993, Fishbein et al. 1993, Victorin et al. 1996, SOU 1996a/b, EHC 199X, BUWAL (1993)</td><td rowspan="2">Ozone depletion:
Slaper et al. 1997, Solomon et al. 1992, Müller-Wenk 1997, Wuebbles et al. 1998, Schopka et al. 1995</td><td rowspan="2">Global warming:
IPCC 1996, Mayerhofer et al. 1996, McMichael et al. 1996, Fankhauser 1995, Martens et al. 1995</td><td rowspan="2">Noise:
SOU 1996a/b</td><td rowspan="2">Ionising radiation:
Frischknecht 1998</td></tr>
<tr><td>Pesticides: Baker et al. 1988, Williamson 1997, Whitmore et al. 1994</td><td>Lead: Wallsten et al. 1986</td><td>Endocrine disrupters: Colborn et al. 1994</td><td>Nitrates: Canter 1997</td></tr>
</table>

<table>
<tr><td colspan="7">Several impacts on ecological health: Stanners et al. 1995, Globe 1992</td></tr>
<tr><td>Toxicity:
Klepper et al. 1997a/b, Paustenbach 1989, Vaal et al. 1997a/b, de Vries et al. 1997</td><td rowspan="2">Acidification:
Tickle et al. 1995, Alcamo et al. 1990, Posch et al. 1995, FOEFL 1994, Blau et al. 1995, Clark 1990, Hedin et al. 1997, Sweet et al. 1993</td><td rowspan="2">Nutrification:
Posch et al. 1995, FOEFL 1996</td><td rowspan="2">Desertification:
Hartmann 1997, Clark 1990</td><td rowspan="2">Summer smog:
Posch et al. 1995</td><td rowspan="2">Global warming:
IPCC 1996, NFP 1996, Mayerhofer et al. 1996</td><td rowspan="2">Ionising radiation:
Amiro 1997</td></tr>
<tr><td>Pesticides:
Williamson 1997</td></tr>
</table>

App. 9.2: Selection of some literature sources which can be used to build up additional damage factors

REFERENCES

Bargatzky 1986	Bargatzky, T., *Einführung in die Kulturökologie: Umwelt, Kultur und Gesellschaft*, Dietrich Reimer Verlag, Berlin 1986
Abbey et al. 1995	Abbey D.E., Lebowitz M.D., Mills P.K., Petersen F.F., Lawrence Beeson W., Burchette R.J., Long-term Ambient Concentrations of Particulates and Oxidants and Development of Chronic Disease in a Cohort of Nonsmoking California Residents. *Inhalation Toxicology* 7: 19-34 (1995)
Ackermann 1997	Ackermann I.J., *MADE: Entwicklung und Anwendung eines Aerosol-Dynamikmodells für dreidimensionale Chemie-Transport-Simulationen in der Troposphäre*, Heft 115, Köln 1997
Adams 1995	Adams J., *Risk*, UCL Press, London 1995
Adriaanse 1993	Adriaanse A., *Environmental Policy Performance Indicators*, SDU 1993
Ahbe *et al.* 1990	Ahbe St., Braunschweig A., Müller-Wenk R., *Methodik für Ökobilanzen auf der Basis ökologischer Optimierung*, Schriftenreihe Umwelt Nr.133, Bundesamt für Umwelt, Wald und Landschaft (BUWAL) Bern 1990
Ahrens *et al.* 1981	Ahrens D, Kamm K., Systemanalyse zur Beurteilung der Umweltverträglichkeit von Heizungssystemen. *Staub-Reinhalt. Luft* 41 (5): 157-62 (Mai 1981)
Alcamo *et al.* 1990	Alcamo J., Shaw R., Hordijk L.(Eds.), *The RAINS Model of Acidification; Science and Strategies in Europe*, Kluwer Academic Publishers, Dordrecht 1990
Alderson 1988	Alderson M., *Mortality, Morbidity and Health Statistics*, Stockton Press, New York 1988
Alheit *et al.* 1994	Alheit P., Völker S., Westermann B., Zwick M.M., *Die Kehrseite der "Erlebnisgesellschaft"*, Werkstattberichte des IBL, Universität Bremen 1994
Ames 1990	Ames B., Misconceptions about Environmental Pollution and Cancer. *Journal of the World Energy Council*, December 1990: 34-50
Amiro 1997	Amiro B.D., Radiological Dose Concersion Factors for Generic Non-Human Biota Used for Screening Potential Ecological Impacts. *J.Environ.Radioactivity* 35 (1): 37-51 (1997)
Anderson *et al.* 1996	Andersson H.R., Ponce de Leon A., Bland J.M., *et al.*, Air Pollution and Daily Mortality in London: 1987-92, *BMJ* 312: 665-9 (16 March 1996)
Anonymous 1994	Concensus Reports in Previous Volumes, *Arbete och Hälsa* 30: 68-72 (1994)
Anonymous 1997	Sweden Sets the Agenda for Tomorrow's Chemicals Policy, *ENDS-Report 269*, June 1997, pp.21-25
Arcos *et al.* 1995	Arcos J.C., Argus M.F., Multifactor Interaction Network of Carcinogenesis - A "Tour Guide", in Arcos J.C., Argus M.F., Woo Y. (eds), *Chemical Induction of Cancer; Modulation and Combination Effects*, Birkhäuser Boston 1995, pp.1-20
Arends *et al.* 1997	Arends B.G., Baard J.H., Ten Brink H.M., Trends in Summer Sulphate in Europe, *Atmospheric Environment* 31 (24): 4063-72, 1997
Assies 1994	Assies J., Experts need ... Experts (II), *LCA News, A SETAC-Europe Publication* 4 (1), January 1994
Assies 1997	Assies J.A., *Risk Indicators for Use in Life-Cycle Impact Assessment; An Approach Based on Sustainability*, University of Groningen 1997
Atkinson *et al.* 1994	Atkinson R., Janet A., Atmospheric Chemistry of Gas-phase Polycylic Aromatic Hydrocarbons: Formation of Atmospheric Mutagens, *Environmental Health Perspectives* 102 (Suppl 4): 117-26 (October 1994)
Axenfeld *et al.* 1992	Axenfeld F., Münch J., Pacyna J.M., Duiser J., Veldt Ch., *Test-Emissionsdatenbasis der Spurenelemente As, Cd, Hg, Pb, Zn und der speziellen organischen Verbindungen Lindan, HCB, PCB und PAK für Modellrechnungen in Europa*, UBA-FB 104 02 588, Dornier Friedrichshafen 1992

Axenfeld *et al.* 1994 — Axenfeld F., Münch J., *Bereitstellung einer Emissionsdatenbasis zur grossräumigen Ozonmodellierung (Bezugsjahr 1990)*, Bayerisches Landesamt für Umweltschutz, Dornier Friedrichshafen 1994

Baccini *et al.* 1991 — Baccini P., Brunner P., *Metabolism of the Anthroposphere*, Springer-Verlag, Berlin 1991

Bachárová *et al.* 1996 — Bachárová L., Fandáková, Bratinka M., *et al.*, The Association between Air Pollution and the Daily Number of Deaths: Findings from the Slovak Republic Contribution to the APHEA Project, *J Epidemiol Comm Health* 50 (Suppl 1): S19-S21 (1996)

Bahro 1987 — Bahro R., *Logik der Rettung*, Edition Weitbrecht, Stuttgart 1987

Baker *et al.* 1988 — Baker S.R., Wilkinson C.F., *The Effects of Pesticides on Human Health, Advances in Modern Environmental Toxicology*, Volume XVIII, Princeton Scientific Publishing Co., Princeton 1988

Ballester *et al.* 1996 — Ballester F., Corella D., Pérez-Hoyos S., Hervás A., Air Pollution and Mortality in Valencia, Spain: a Study Using the APHEA Methodology, *J Epidemiol Comm Health* 50: 527-33 (1996)

Ballschmiter 1992 — Ballschmiter K., Transport and Fate of Organic Compounds in the Global Environment, *Angew.Chem., Int. Ed. Engl.* 31 (5): 487-664, 1992

Barnthouse *et al.* 1997 — Barnthouse L., Fava J., Humphreys K., Hunt R. *et al.*, *Life-Cycle Impact Assessment: The State-of-the-Art*, Report of the SETAC North American Workgroup on Life Cycle Impact Assessment, Pensacola 1997

Barrett 1993 — Barrett J.C., Mechanisms of Multistep Carcinogenesis and Carcinogen Risk Assessment, *Environmental Health Perspectives* 100: 9-20 (1993)

Barrett *et al.* 1996 — Barrett K. Berge E. (Eds), *Transboundary Air Pollution in Europe*, Research Report No.32, EMEP/MSC-W, Report 1/96, Oslo 1996

Basler & Hofmann 1974 — Basler & Hofmann Ingenieure und Planer, *Studie Umwelt und Volkswirtschaft, Vergleich der Umweltbelastung von Behältern aus PVC, Glas, Blech und Karton*, Eidgenössisches Amt für Umweltschutz (BUS), Bern 1974

Basler 1971 — Basler E., Umweltprobleme aus der Sicht der technischen Entwicklung, in H. Leibundgut (ed.), *Schutz unseres Lebensraumes*, Symposium an der ETH Zürich vom 10.-12. November 1970, Verlag Huber Frauenfeld 1971, pp.78-87

Bates *et al.* 1990 — Bates DV, Baker-Anderson M., Sizto R., Asthma Attack Periodicity: A Study of Hospital Emergency Visits in Vancouver. *Environ Res* 51: 51-70 (1990).

Bauer 1992 — Bauer B., *Kombinierte Energie-, Luft-, Abgassteuer - thermodynamisch und zugleich marktorientiert bestimmt*, BWK Bd.44 (1992) Nr.1/2

Baumann *et al.* 1992 — Baumann H., Rydberg Th., *Impact Analysis and Valuation in the Life Cycle Assessment of Products: A Comparative Study of Three Methods Illustrated by Reference to LCA Inventory Data for Milk Packaging Systems*, Potsdam 1992

Baumann *et al.* 1993 — Baumann H., Ekvall Th., Erikson E. *et al.*, *Miljömässiga skillnader mellan återvinning/återvanvändning och förbränning/deponiering*, Reforsk 1993 cited in Lindfors L.-G. *et al.*, LCA Nordic; Technical Reports No 10, Nordic Council of Ministers 1995

Baumgartner 1987 — Baumgartner Th., Die Produktlinienanalyse als neue Form der Informationserhebung und -darstellung, in Beckenbach F., Schreyer m., (eds.), *Gesellschaftliche Folgekosten*, Frankfurt 1987, pp.150-69

Becher *et al.* 1995 — Becher H., Steindorf K., Wahrendorf J., *Epidemiologische Methoden der Risikoabschätzung für krebserzeugende Umweltstoffe mit Anwendungsbeispielen*, UBA-Berichte 7/95, Forschungsbericht 116 06 089, Erich Schmidt Verlag, Berlin 1995

Beck *et al.* 1995 — Beck A., Bosshart St., *Umweltanalyseinstrumente im Vergleich*, Diplomarbeit am Laboratorium für Energiesysteme, ETH Zürich, August 1995

Beentjes *et al.* 1995 — Beentjes C., Wrisberg N., Ywema P.E., *The Social Value of Life Cycle Assessment*; financed by SPOLD Brussels, Draft May 1995

Beltrani 1997 — Beltrani G., Safeguard Subjects; The Conflict between Operationalisation and Ethical Justification, *Int.J.LCA* 2 (1): 45-51 (1997)

Bengtsson *et al.* 1997	Bengtsson M., Carlson R., Molander S., Steen B., Handling GIS Information in Life Cycle Assessment Using a Relational Database, in Ale B.J.M., Janssen M.P.M., Pruppers M.J.M. (eds.), *Book of Papers; Risk 97, International Conference Mapping Environmental Risks and Risk Comparison*, 21-24 October, Amsterdam 1997
Berdowski *et al.* 1997	Berdowski J.M.M., Mulder W., Veldt C., *et al.*, *Particulate Emissions (PM10-PM2.5-PM0.1) in Europe in 1990 and 1993*, TNO, Apeldoorn (forthcoming), cited in *Economic Evaluation of Air Quality Targets for Sulphur Dioxide, Nitrogen Dioxide, Fine and Suspended Particulate Matter and Lead*, Instituut voor Milieuvraagstukken, Vrije Universiteit Amsterdam, Amsterdam 1997
Berg *et al.* 1994	Berg M., Scheringer M., Problems in Environmental Risk Assessment and the Need for Proxy Measures, *Fresenius Environmental Bulletin* 3 (8): 487-92
Bertollini *et al.* 1996	Bertollinin R., Lebowitz M.D., Saracci R., Savitz D.A. (eds), *Environmental Epidemiology - Exposure and Disease*, WHO/Lewis Publishers Boca Raton 1996
Beyrich 1997	Beyrich F., Mixing Height Estimation from SODAR Data – a Critical Discussion, *Atmospheric Environment* 31 (23): 3941-53 (1997)
Bickel *et al.* 1995	Bickel P., Friedrich R., *Was kostet uns die Mobilität? Externe Kosten des Verkehrs*, Springer, Berlin 1995
Blasius *et al.* 1989	Blasius J., Winkler J., Eine empirische Überprüfung der Bourdieuschen Theorie, *Kölner Zeitschrift für Soziologie und Sozialpsychologie* 41: 721-28 (1989)
Blau *et al.* 1995	Blau S., Sereviratne S., *Developments and Regionalisation of the Impact Categories 'Euthrophication' and 'Acidification' within LCA Impact Assessment*, Student Thesis, Laboratorium für Energiesysteme, ETH Zürich, July 1995
Boguski *et al.* 1995	Boguski T.K., Franklin W., *A Partial Impact Assessment for Ethylene Glycol and Propylene Glycol Based Antifreeze*, Franklin Assoc., Overheads presented in the SETAC LCA Impact Assessment Work Group, Washington August 16, 1995
Boguski *et al.* 1996	Boguski T.K., Hunt R.G., Cholakis J.M., Franklin W.E., LCA Methodology in Curran M.A. (ed.), *Environmental life-cycle assessment*, McGraw-Hill Companies, New York 1996
Boholm 1996	Boholm Å., *The Many Faces of 'the Cultural Theory of Risk'; An Anthropological Critique*, Society of Risk Analysis, Europe Annual Meeting, Surrey 1996, pp.527-30
Boström *et al.* 1994	Boström C.-E., Almén J., Steen B., Westerholm R., Human Exposure to Urban Air Pollution, *Environmental Health Perspectives* 102 (Suppl 4): 39-47 (October 1994)
Botti *et al.* 1996	Botti C., Comba P., Forastiere F., Settimi L., Casual inference in environmental epidemiology: the role of implicit values, *The Science of the Total Environment* 184: 97-101 (1996)
Bourdieu 1987a	Bourdieu P., *Die feinen Unterschiede; Kritik der gesellschaftlichen Urteilskraft*, Frankfurt 1987
Bourdieu 1987b	Bourdieu P., *Sozialer Sinn; Kritik der theoretischen Vernunft*, Frankfurt 1987
Boustead *et al.* 1979	Boustead I., Hancock G.F., *Handbook of Industrial Energy Analysis*, Ellis Horwood, Chichester 1979
Brain 1996	Brain J., Preface, in Wilson R., Spengler J.D. (eds), *Particles in Our Air: Concentrations and Health Effects*, Harvard University Press 1996
Brandes *et al.* 1996	Brandes L.J., den Hollander L., van de Meent D., *SimpleBox 2.0: a Nested Multimedia Fate Model for Evaluating the Environmental Fate of Chemicals*, Report No. 719101029, Bilthoven 1996
Brändli *et al.* 1997	Brändli O., Künzli N., Inhalierte Staubpartikel: Wie schädlich sind sie für unsere Lungen?, *Neue Zürcher Zeitung*, 13. August 1997: p.53
Braun *et al.* 1992	Braun H., Angrüner B., Ecker P., *et al.*, *Dioxinemissionen bei Feuerungen*, Wien 1992

Braunschweig 1988	Braunschweig A., *Ökologische Buchhaltung als Instrument der städtischen Umweltpolitik*, Dissertation Chur 1988
Braunschweig 1996	Braunschweig A., Relevant Environmental Interventions, in Schaltegger (ed.), *Life Cycle Assessment (LCA) – Quo vadis?*, Birkhäuser 1996, pp.69-79
Braunschweig 1997	Braunschweig A.. *Ionising Radiation as an Impact Category in LCA*, Draft article, 12 pp., IWÖ St.Gallen, August 1997, publication pendent
Braunschweig et al. 1993	Braunschweig A., Müller-Wenk R., Ökobilanzen für *Unternehmungen; Eine Wegleitung für die Praxis*, Bern 1993
Braunschweig *et al.* 1994	Braunschweig A., Förster R., Hofstetter P., Müller-Wenk R., *Evaluation und Weiterentwicklung von Bewertungsmethoden für Ökobilanzen - Erste Ergebnisse*, IWÖ-Diskussionsbeitrag Nr.19, St. Gallen 1994
Braunschweig *et al.* 1996	Braunschweig A., Förster R., Hofstetter P., Müller-Wenk R., *Developments in LCA Valuation*, IWÖ-Diskussionsbeitrag Nr.32, St. Gallen 1996
Braunschweig *et al.* 1997	Braunschweig A, Brunner St., Hofstetter P., Müller-Wenk R., *Umweltliche Bewertung im Automobilbau; Einführung und Weiterentwicklung des Eco-Indicator'95*, ETH Zürich (unpublished)
Brooks 1986	Brooks G., *The Development and Construction of Health Status Measures; an Overview of the Literature*, The Swedish Institute for Health Economics, Lund 1986
Brown *et al.* 1996	Brown M.L., Hodgson T.A., Rise D.P., Economic Impact of Cancer in the United States, in Schottenfeld D., Fraumeni J.F. (Eds), *Cancer Epidemiology and Prevention*, Oxford University Press, New York 1996
Brunekreef *et al.* 1995	Brunekreef B., Dockery D.W., Kryzanowski M., Epidemiological Studies on Short-term Effects of Low Levels of Major Ambient Air Pollution Compounds, *Environmental Health Perspectives* 103 (Suppl.2): 3-13 (March 1995)
Brunner 1998	Brunner St., *Panel Methods and Their Application for Weighting in LCA*, UNS-Working Paper for the Project 'Environmental Prioritizing' within the Framework of the Swiss Priority Programme Environment (SPPU), ETH Zürich 1998
Brusick 1991	Brusick D., A Proposed Method for Assembly and Interpretation of Short-Term Test Data, *Environmental Health Perspectives* 96: 101-11 (1991)
BUA 1985	Beratergremium für umweltrelevante Altstoffe (BUA), *BUA-Stoffberichte*, Gesellschaft Deutscher Chemiker 1 (1985) - 209 (1997), VCH/Hirzel, Stuttgart 1985ff
Busch Spycher 1997	Busch Spycher P., *Methodische Aspekte der ökonomischen Evaluation adjuvanter Brustkrebstherapien*, Inauguraldissertation, Ofko AG, Bern 1997
BUWAL 1984	BUWAL (Hrsg.), *Oekobilanzen von Packstoffen*, Schriftenreihe Umweltschutz Nr.24, Bern 1984
BUWAL 1991	Habersatter K., Widmer F., *Ökobilanz von Packstoffen - Stand 1990*, BUWAL-Schriftenreihe Umwelt Nr. 132, Bern 1991
BUWAL 1993	BUWAL, *Luftverschmutzung und Gesundheit III*, Schriftenreihe Umwelt Nr.211, Bern 1993
BUWAL 1994	BUWAL, *Krebsrisiko von Diesel-und Benzinmotorabgasen*, Schriftenreihe Umwelt Nr.222, Bern 1994
BUWAL 1995	BUWAL, *Vom Menschen verursachte Luftschadstoffemissionen in der Schweiz von 1900-2010*, Schriftenreihe Umwelt Nr.256, Bern 1995
BUWAL 1996a	BUWAL, *Schwebestaub; Messung und gesundheitliche Bewertung*, Schriftenreihe Umwelt Nr.270, Bern 1996
BUWAL 1996b	BUWAL, NABEL; *Luftbelastung 1995*, Schriftenreihe Umwelt Nr.267, Bern 1996
BUWAL 1996c	BUWAL, *Der Einsatz von Ausbreitungsmodellen für die Massnahmenplanung*, Umwelt-Materialien Nr.46, Bern 1996
BUWAL 1996d	BUWAL, *POLLUMET; Luftverschmutzung und Meteorologie in der Schweiz*, Umweltmaterialien Nr.63, Bern 1996

BUWAL 1996e	BUWAL, *Beurteilungswerte von Luftschadstoffen für Ökobilanzen*, Umwelt-Materialien Nr.48, Bern 1996
BUWAL 1998	BUWAL, *Methode der ökologischen Knappheit - Ökofaktoren 1997*, Schriftenreihe Umwelt Nr.297, ÖBU/BUWAL Bern 1998
Cairns *et al.* 1993	Cairns J., McCormick P.V., Niederlehner B.R., A Proposed Framework for Developing Indicators of Ecosystem Health, *Hydrobiologia* 263 (1): 1-44 (1993)
Calow 1993	Calow P., Ecosystem Health - A Critical Analysis of Concepts, in Rapport D.J., Gaudet C.L., Calow P. (eds.), *Evaluating and Monitoring the Health of Large-Scale Ecosystems*, Springer, Berlin 1993, pp.33-41
Canter 1997	Canter L.W., *Nitrates in Groundwater*, Lewis Publishers, Boca raton 1997
Cantor *et al.* 1996	Cantor K.P., Shy C.M., Chilvers C., Water Pollution, in Schottenfeld D., Fraumeni J.F. (Eds), *Cancer Epidemiology and Prevention*, Oxford University Press, New York 1996
Carpenter 1995	Carpenter R.A., Limitations in Measuring Ecosystem Sustainability, in Trzyna Th.C., Osborn J.K., (eds.), *A Sustainable World; Defining and Measurung Sustainable Development*, IUCN/ICEP, Earthscan Sacramento 1995
Cawse 1980	Cawse P.A., Deposition of trace elements from the atmosphere in the U.K., in *Inorganic Pollution and Agriculture*, Ministry of Agriculture, Fisheries and Food, 326, London 1980
CEC 1991	Commision of the European Communities, *CORINE Biotopes Manual: Habitats of the European Community, Data Specification Part 2*, EUR 12587/EN, Luxemburg 1991
Chemla *et al.* 1997	Chemla P., Labouze E., *Ranking Environmental Impacts; Application to Buildings*, Second International Conference Buildings and the Environment, June 1997, Paris, pp.167-73
Christiansen 1997	Christiansen K. (ed.), *Simplified LCA: Just a Cut*, Report of SETAC-Europe Working Group on Screening and Streamlining of LCA, SETAC-Europe, Brussels 1997
Christiansen *et al.* 1990	Christiansen K., Grove A., Hansen L.E., Hoffman L., Jensen A.A., Pommer K., Schmidt A., *Miljövurdering av PVC og udvalgte alternative materialer*, Miljöprojekt 131, Mijöstyrelsen, Copenhagen 1990
Christoffel *et al.* 1996	Christoffel A., Schreyer Ch., *Reversibilität und räumliche Ausdehnung als Hierarchisierungskriterien für verschiedene Umweltprobleme*, Semesterarbeit ETH Zürich, Gruppe Energie-Stoffe-Umwelt, Zürich 1996 (unveröffentlicht)
Clark 1990	Clark W.C., Verantwortliches Gestalten des Lebensraums Erde, *Spektrum der Wissenschaft, Menschheit der Erde*, 1990, pp.4-12
Clift 1995	Clift R., Clean Technology – An Introduction, *Journal of Chemical technology and Biotechnology* 62: 321-26 (1995)
Cody *et al.* 1992	Cody R.P., Weisel C.L., Birnbaum G., Lioy P.J., The Effect of Ozone associated with Summertime Photo-chemical Smog on the Frequency of Asthma Visits to Hospital Emergency Departments. *Environ Res* 58: 184-194 (1992).
Coebergh *et al.* 1995	Coebergh J.W.W., van der Heijden L.H., Janssen-Heijnen M.L.G., *Cancer Incidence and Survival in the Southern Netherlands 1955-1994*, Eindhoven Cancer Registry 1995
Colborn *et al.* 1994	Colborn Th., vom Saal F. S., Soto A.M., Developmental Effects of Endocrine-diruptin Chemicals in Wildlife and Humans, *Envrion Impact Assess Rev* 14: 469-89 (1994)
Colome *et al.* 1992	Colome S.D., Kado N.Y., Jaques P., Kleinman M., Indoor-outdoor Air Pollution Relations: Particulate Matter Less than 10µm in Aerodynamic Diameter (PM10) in Homes of Asthmatics, *Atmospheric Environment* 26A (12): 2173-8 (1992)
Concawe 1995	Gamble J., King D., Stephenson R., Tordoir W., *Air Quality Standard for Particulate Matter*, Concawe-Report No. 95/62, Brussels 1995

Concawe 1996 — Gamble J., King D., Tordoir W., *Review and Critique of the APHEA Project*, Concawe-Report No. 96/61, Brussels 1996

Connell 1990 — Connell D.W., *Bioaccumulation of Xenobiotic Compounds*, CRS Press, Boca Raton 1990

Constanza *et al.* 1992 — Constanza R., Norton B., Haskell B., *Ecosystem Health, New Goals for Ecosystem Management*, Island Press, Washington 1992

Corten *et al.* 1994 — Corten F.G.P, van den Haspel B., Kreuzberg G.J., Sas H.J.W., de Wit G., *Weging van milieu-effecten voor het produktbeleid; Verslag fase 1*, CE Delft 1994

Coughlin *et al.* 1998 — Coughlin R.M., Lockhart Ch., Grid-group Theory and Political Ideology, a Consideration of their Relative Strenghts and Weaknesses for Explaining the Structure of Mass Belief Systems, *Journal of Theoretical Politics* 10 (1): 33-58

Cowell *et al.* 1997 — Cowell S.J., Hohan S., Clift R., Positioning and Applications of LCA, in Udo de Haes H., Wrisberg N. (eds.), *Life Cycle Assessment: State-of-the-Art and Research Priorities*; Results of LCANET, a Concerted Action in the Environment and Climate Programme (DG XII), LCA Documents, Volume 1, Eco-Informa Press, Bayreuth 1997

Cramer *et al.* 1993 — Cramer J., Quakernaat J., Dokter T. *et al.* , *Theory and Practice of Integrated Chain Management* (in Dutch), TNO Apeldoorn 1993

Crumb 1984 — Crumb K.S., A New Method for Determing Allowable Daily Intakes, *Fundamental and Applied Toxicology* 4: 854-71 (1984)

Dab *et al.* 1996 — Dab W., Medina S., Quénel P. *et al.* , Short Term Respiratory Health Effects of Ambient air Pollution: Results of the APHEA Project in Paris, *J Epidemiol Comm Health* 50 (Suppl 1): S42-S46 (1996)

Dake 1991 — Dake K., Orienting Dispositions in the Perception of Risk; An analysis of Contemporary Worldviews and Cultural Biases, *J of Cross-cultural Psychology* 22 (1): 61-82 (1991)

Dake 1992 — Dake K., Myths of Nature: Culture and the Social Construction of Risk, *Journal of Social Issues* 48 (4): 21-37 (1992)

Dake *et al.* 1993 — Dake K., Thompson M., The Meanings of Sustainable Development: Household Strategies for Managing Needs and Resources, in Wright S.D., Dietz Th., Borden R. *et al.* (eds.), *Human Ecology: Crossing Boundaries*, The Society for Human Ecology, Fort Collins 1993, pp.421-36

Daly 1991 — Daly H.E., *Steady-State Economics*, 2nd Edition, with new essays, Island Press, Washington D.C. 1991

de Haes *et al.* 1985 — De Haes J.C.J.M., van Knippenberg F.C.E., *The Quality of Life of Cancer Patients: A Review of the Literature*, *Soc.Sci.Med.* 20 (8): 809-17 (1985)

de Smet *et al.* 1997 — de Smet B., Hemming C., Baumann K., *et al.*, *Life Cycle Assessment and Conceptually Related Programmes*, Working Group Report of SETAC-Europe, Brussels 1997 (in press)

de Vries *et al.* 1997 — de Vries W., Bakker D.J., Groenenberg J.E., Reinds G.J., Bril J., van Jaarsveld J.A., Calculation and Mapping of Critical Loads for Heavy Metals and Persistent Organic Pollutants for Dutch Forest Soils, in Ale B.J.M., Janssen M.P.M., Pruppers M.J.M. (eds.), *Book of Papers; Risk 97, International Conference Mapping Environmental Risks and Risk Comparison*, 21-24 October, Amsterdam 1997, pp.97-103

Derwent *et al.* 1988 — Derwent R.G., Dollard G.J., Metcalfe S.E., On the Nitrogen Budget for the United Kindom and North-west Europe, *Q.J.R.Meteorol.Soc.* 114: 1127-52 (1988)

Derwent *et al.* 1989 — Derwent R.G., Hov O., Asman W.A.H., van Jaarsveld J.A., de Leeuw F.A.A.M., An Intercomparision of Long-term Atmospheric Transport Models; the Budgets of Acidifying Species for the Netherlands, *Atmospheric Environment* 23 (9): 1893-909 (1989)

Derwent *et al.* 1991 — Derwent R.G., Jenkin M.E., Hydrocarbons and the Long-range Transport of Ozone and PAN across Europe, *Atmospheric Environment* 25A: 1661-78 (1991)

Derwent *et al.* 1996	Derwent R.G., Jenkin M.E., Saunders S.M., Photochemical Ozone Creations Potentials for a Large Number of Reactive Hydrocarbons under European Conditions, *Atmospheric Environment* 30 (2): 181-99 (1996)
Destribats 1990	Destribats A.F. *et al.*, Environmental Costs and Resource Planning Consequence: New England Electric's Rating and Weighing Approach in NARUC, *Proceedings of the NARUC National Conference on Environmental Externalities held at Jackson Hole, WY.* Sept.1-3, 1990
DeVita *et al.* 1993	DeVita V.T., Hellmann S., Rosenberg S.A., *Cancer; Principles & Practice of Oncology*, 4th Edition, J.B. Lippincott Company, Pennsylvania 1993
Diekmann *et al.* 1992	Diekmann, A., Preisendörfer, P., Persönliches Umweltverhalten. Diskrepanzen zwischen Anspruch und Wirklichkeit. *Kölner Zeitschrift für Soziologie und Sozialpsychologie* 44: 226-51 (1992)
Dockery *et al.* 1989	Dockery D.W., Speizer F.E., Stram D.O., Ware J.H., Spengler J.D., Ferries B.G. Effects of Inhalable Particles on Respiratory Health of Children. *Am Rev Respir Dis* 139: 587-594 (1989)
Dockery *et al.* 1993	Dockery D.W., Pope C.A., Xu. X, *et al.*, An Association Between Air Pollution and Mortality in Six U.S. Cities, *The New England Journal of Medicine* 329 (24): 1753-9 (1993)
Dockery *et al.* 1994	Dockery D.W., Pope C.A. III, Acute Respiratory Effects of Particulate Air Pollution. *Ann. Rev. Public Health* 15: 107-32 (1994)
Dockery *et al.* 1996	Dockery D., Pope A., Epidemiology of Acute Health Effects: Summary of Time-Series Studies, in Wilson R., Spengler J.D. (eds), *Particles in Our Air: Concentrations and Health Effects*, Harvard Unsiversity Press 1996
Dolan 1996	Dolan P., Modelling Valuations for Health States: the Effect of Duration, *Health Policy* 38: 189-203 (1996)
Dolan *et al.* 1996a	Dolan P., Gudex C., Kind P., Williams A., Valuing Health States: a Comparison of Methods, *Journal of Health Economics* 15: 209-31 (1996)
Dolan *et al.* 1996b	Dolan P., Kind P., Inconsistency and Health State Valuations, *Soc. Sci. Med.* 42 (4): 609-15 (1996)
Doll *et al.* 1981	Doll R., Peto R., The Causes of Cancer: Quantitative Estimates of Avoidable Risks of Cancer in the United States Today, *JNCI* 66: 1191-308
Donnan *et al.* 1997	Donnan P., Hurley F., ExternE: Maintenance of the 'Classical' Pollutants: PM, SO2, NO2, O3, CO; Exposure-response (E-R) Functions for the Acute and Chronic Public Health Effects of Air Pollution, Document 351, Institute of Occupational Medicine (IOM), Edinburgh 1997 to be published in European Commission , *ExternE Project - External Costs of Energy, JOULE Programme, Effects of Air Pollutants on Health, Methodology Report*, 2nd edition, European Commission DGXII, Brussels 1998
Douglas 1982	Douglas M., Cultural Bias, in Douglas M. (ed.), *In the Active Voice*, Routledge and Kegan Paul, London 1982
Douglas *et al.* 1982	Douglas M., Wildavsky A., *Risk and Culture; An Essay on the Selection of Technological and Environmental Dangers*, Berkley 1982
Dunlap *et al.* 1978	Dunlap R.E., Van Liere K.D., The 'new environmental paradigm', *The Journal of Environmental Education* 9 (4): 10-9 (1978)
Dunlap *et al.* 1993a	Dunlap R.E., Gallup G.H., Gallup A.M., International Public Opinion toward the Environment, Part I: Perceived Seriousness of Environmental Problems, *Impact Assessment* 11: 3-25 (Spring 1993)
Dunlap *et al.* 1993b	Dunlap R.E., Gallup G.H., Gallup A.M., International Public Opinion toward the Environment, Part II: Causes and Solutions of Environmental Problems, *Impact Assessment* 11: 113-43 (Summer 1993)
Durkheim 1933	Durkheim E., *The Division of Labour in Society*, Free Press, New York 1933 (first published in 1893)
Durkheim 1951	Durkheim E., *Suicide: a Study in Sociology*, Free Press, Glencoe 1951 (first published in 1897)
Dürrenberger 1994	Dürrenberger G., Klimawandel: Eine Herausforderung für Wissenschaft und Gesellschaft, *ETH-Bulletin* Nr.253: 20-22 (April 1994)

Dusseldorp *et al.* 1995	Dusseldorp A., Kruize H., Brunekreef B., Hofschreuder P., de Meer G., van Oudvorst A.B., Associations of PM10 and Airborne Iron with Respiratory Health of Adults near a Steel Factory. *Am J Respir Crit Care Med* 152: 1932-9 (1995).
ECETOC 1995	ECETOC, *The Role of Bioaccumulation in Environmental Risk Assessment: The Aquatic Environment and Related Food Webs*, Technical Report No.67, Brussels 1995
ECETOC 1996	ECETOC, *Risk Assessment for Carcinogens*, Monograph No.24, Brussels 1996
EEC 1996	EEC, *Technical Guidance Document in Support of Commission Directive 93/67/EEC on Risk Assessment for New Notified Substances and Comission Regulation (EC) No. 1488/94 on Risk Assessment for Existing Substances*, European Commission Luxembourg: Office for Official Publications of the European Communities, 1996 (4 parts)
EHC 199x	Environmental Health Criteria (EHC), *A Series of Reports on Effects per Substance*, WHO, Geneva 199x
Ehring 1997	Ehring D., *Causation and Persistence: A Theory of Causation*, Oxford University Press New York 1997
Eliassen *et al.* 1982	Eliassen A., Hov Ø., Isaksen I.S.A., Saltbones J., Strordal F., A Langrangian Long-range Transport Model with Atmospheric Boundary Layer Chemistry, *J Appl Met* 21: 1645-61 (1982)
Ellis *et al.* 1997	Ellis R.J., Thompson F., Culture and the Environment in the Pacific Northwest, *American Political Science Review* 91 (4): 885-97 (1997)
Ellwanger 1997	Ellwanger G., Die externen Effekte des Verkehrs, *Rail International* 28 (4):10-15 (1997)
EMEP 1997	EMEP/MSC-W, *MSC-W Status Report 1997 Part 1; Emissions, Dispersion and Trends of Acidifying and Eutrophying Agents; Part 2; Numerical Addendum*, Report 1/97, Oslo 1997
EPA 1983	EPA, *Helath Assessment Document for Acrylonitrile*, Final Report No. EPA-600-8-82-007F, Washington 1983
Escher 1995	Escher B., *The Realtionship between Membrane-water Partitioning, Uncoupling, and Inhibitory Activity of Substituted Phenols in Chromatophores of Rhodobacter Sphaeroides*, Dissertation ETH Nr.11283, Zürich 1995
ESEERCO 1995	Empire State Electric Energy Research Corporation (ESEERCO), *New York State Environmetal Externalities Cost Study, Volume 1: Introduction and Methods*, Oceana Publications Inc., New York 1995
Etienne 1996	Etienne R.S., *Operational Uncertainties in SimpleBox; Operational Uncertainty Analysis of the Air-water Concentration Ratio Computed by SimpleBox for 11 Volatile Compounds*, Reports Environmental Studies No. 136, Katholieke Universiteit Nijmegen, Nijmegen 1996
Euro-Styles 1991	Euro-Styles, *Die europoaweite Bevölkerungskarte mit 16 sozio-kulturellen Typen*, Sonderdruck aus Praxis 3/91 Fachinformation ATAG Ernst & Young, Basel
Euro-Styles 1993	Euro-Styles, *Die Zielgruppenanlyse wird noch genauer: Telecontrol-Mitglieder sind neu auch nach Euro-Styles typologisiert*, TeleVison Nr.8/93, AG für das Werbefernsehen
ExternE 1995	ExternE, *Externalities of Energy*, European Commission EUR 16520 EN, Volume 1-6, Luxembourg 1995
ExternE 1997	ExternE Core Project, *Extension of the Accounting Framework; Final Report*, compiled by Mayerhofer P., Krewitt W., Friedrich R., The European Commission, Contract No. JOS3-CT95-0002, Stuttgart 1997 (available on http://www.ExternE.jrc.es)
Fabian 1992	Fabian P., *Atmosphäre und Umwelt: Chemische Prozesse, menschliche Eingriffe*, 4. Aufl., Springer Berlin 1992
Fankhauser 1995	Fankhauser S., *Valuing Climate Change; The Economics of the Greenhouse*, CSERGE, Earthscan London 1995

Fedra 1997 Fedra K., Integrated Risk Assessment and Management: Overview and State-of-the-art, in Ale B.J.M., Janssen M.P.M., Pruppers M.J.M. (eds.), *Book of Papers; Risk 97, International Conference Mapping Environmental Risks and Risk Comparison*, 21-24 October, Amsterdam 1997

Feijtel *et al.* 1997 Feijtel T., Boeije G., Matthies M. *et al.*, Development of a Geography-references Regional Exposure Assessment Tool for European Rivers – GREAT-ER, in Ale B.J.M., Janssen M.P.M., Pruppers M.J.M. (eds.), *Book of Papers; Risk 97, International Conference Mapping Environmental Risks and Risk Comparison*, 21-24 October, Amsterdam 1997

Feldman 1980 Feldman A.M., *Welfare Economics and Social Choice Theory*, Martinus Nijhoff Publishing, Boston 1980

Festinger 1957 Festinger L., *A Theory of Cognitive Dissonance*, Stanford University Press, Stanford 1957

Finnveden 1994 Finnveden G., *Methods for Describing and Characterising Resource Depletion in the Context of LCA*, IVL-Report No. B1141, IVL Stockholm 1994

Finnveden 1996 Finnveden G., *Valuation Methods within the Framework of Life Cycle Assessment*, IVL-Report B 1231, Stockholm 1996

Finnveden 1997 Finnveden G., Valuation Methods within LCA – Where are the Values?, *Int J LCA* 2 (3): 163-9 (1997)

Fischer-Kowalski *et al.* 1994 Fischer-Kowalski M., Haberl H., Payer H., A Plethora of Paradigms: Outlining an Information System on Physical Exchanges between the Economy and Nature, in Ayres R.U., Simonis U.E. (eds.), *Industrial Metabolism: Restructuring for Sustainable Development*, United Nations University Press, Tokyo 1994

Fischhoff *et al.* 1978 Fischhoff B., Slovic P., Lichtenstein S., Read S., Combs B., How Safe is Safe Enough? A Psychometric Study of Attitudes towards Technological Risks and Benefits, *Policy Sciences* 9: 127-52 (1978)

Fishbein 1993 Fishbein L., Sources, Nature and Levels of Air Pollutants, in Tomatis L. (Ed.), *Indoor and Outdoor Air Pollution and Human Cancer*, Springer, Berlin 1993, pp.17-66

Fishbein *et al.* 1993 Fishbein L., Hemminki K., Sources, Nature and Levels of Indoor Air Pollutants, in Tomatis L. (Ed.), *Indoor and Outdoor Air Pollution and Human Cancer*, Springer, Berlin 1993, pp.67-87

FOEFL 1994 FOEFL, *Critical Loads of Acidifity for Forest Soils and Alpine Lakes, Steady State Mass Balance Method*, Environmental Series No.234, Federal Office of Environment, Forests and Landscape, Bern 1994

FOEFL 1996 FOEFL, *Critical Loads of Nitrogen and their Exceedances; Eutrophying Atmospheric Deposition*, Environmental Series No.275, Federal Office of Environment, Forests and Landscape, Bern 1996

Frankena 1963 Frankena W.K., *Ethics*, Prentince-Hall, 1963

Freijer *et al.* 1996 Freijer J.I., Tiktak A., Hassanizadeh S.M., van der Linden A.M.A., *PESTRAS v.3.1: A One-dimensional Model for the Assessment of the Fate of Pesticides in Soil*, RIVM Report No. 715501 007, Bilthoven 1996

Frey *et al.* 1985 Frey R.L., Gysin C.H., Leu R.E., Schmassmann N., *Energie, Umweltschäden und Umweltschutz in der Schweiz*, Basler Sozialökonomische Studien Band 27, Verlag Rüegger, Grüsch 1985

Frey *et al.* 1993 Frey D., Gaska A., Die Theorie der kognitiven Dissonanz, in Frey D., Irle M. (eds.), *Theorien der Sozialpsychologie, Band I: Kognitive Theorien*, 2. Auflage, Hans Huber, Bern 1993

Friedrich *et al.* 1989 Friedrich R., Voss A., Die sozialen Kosten der Elektrizitätserzeugung, *Energiewirtschaftliche Tagesfragen* 39 (10): 640-9 (1989)

Friedrich *et al.* 1990 Friedrich R., Kallenbach U., Thöne E., Voss A., *Externe Kosten der Stromerzeugung*, 2. korrigierte Ausgabe, VWEW Frankfurt am Main 1990

Frischknecht 1997 Frischknecht R., Goal and Scope Definition and Inventory Analysis, in Udo de Haes H., Wrisberg N. (eds.), *Life Cycle Assessment: State-of-the-Art and Research Priorities; Results of LCANET, a Concerted Action in the Environment and Climate Programme (DG XII)*, LCA Documents, Volume 1, Eco-Informa Press, Bayreuth 1997

Frischknecht 1998 Frischknecht R., *Life Cycle Inventory Analysis for Decision Making; Scope-Dependent Inventory System Models and Context-Specific Joint Product Allocation*, PhD Thesis 12599, ETH Zürich 1998

Frischknecht *et al.* (forthcoming) Frischknecht R., Heijungs R., Hofstetter P., Einstein's Lessons for Energy Accounting in LCA, accepted in *Int J LCA*

Frischknecht *et al.* 1994 Frischknecht R., Hofstetter P., Knoepfel I. *et al. Ökoinventar für Energiesysteme - Grundlagen für den ökologischen Vergleich von Energiesystemen und den Einbezug von Energiesystemen in Ökobilanzen für die Schweiz*, Laboratorium für Energiesysteme, ETH Zürich/ PSI Villigen, 1. Auflage, 1994

Fuhrer *et al.* 1995 Fuhrer, U., Kaiser, F. G., Seiler, I., Maggi, M., From Social Representation to Environmental Concern: The Influence of Face-to-face versus Mediated Communication. In U. Fuhrer (Ed.), *Ökologisches Handeln als sozialer Prozess*, Birkhäuser, Basel 1995, pp.61-75

Funtowicz *et al.* 1990 Funtowicz S.O., Ravetz J.R., *Uncertainty and Quality in Science for Policy*, Kluwer, Dordrecht 1990

Ganz 1990 Ganz P.A., Methods of Assessing the Effect of Drug Therapy on Quality of Life, *Drug Safety* 5(4): 233-42 (1990)

Gardner *et al.* 1996 Gardner G.T., Stern P.C., *Environmental Problems and Human Behaviour*, Allyn&Bacon, Needham Heights 1996

Gaskell 1997 Gaskell D., Risk and Reason, *Chemistry in Britain*, July 1997: 36-8

Gebler 1991 Gebler W., Die Ökobilanzierung als Diagnose- und Bewertungsmethode, in Hirtz W., Huber W. (Hrsg.), *Umweltvorsorgeprüfung im Forschungsbereich*, Jül 2553, Jülich November 1991

Gebler 1992 Gebler W., *Ökobilanzen in der Abfallwirtschaft*, Stuttgarter Berichte zur Abfallwirtschaft, Bericht 41, 2. Auflage, Bielefeld 1992

Geddes 1884 Geddes P., An Analysis of the Principles of Economics, in *Proceedings of the Royal Society of Edinburgh* (XII): 943-80 (1884)

GfK o.J. GfK, *Euro-Socio-Styles*, Nürnberg o.J. cited in Schoenheit I., Niedergesäss U., *Lebensstile und Energieberatung*, HEA/imug, Heidelberg 1995

Giegrich 1994 Giegrich J., Modelling Spatial Information for Impact Assessment in Hofstetter P., Schaltegger St., Udo de Haes H. A., *First Working Document on Life Cycle Impact Assessment Methodology*, Zürich September 1994

Giegrich *et al.* 1995 Giegrich J., Mamper U., Duscha M. *et al.*, *Bilanzbewertung in produktbezogenen Ökobilanzen; Evaluation von Bewertungsmethoden, Perspektiven*, UFOPLAN 101 01 103, IFEU Heidelberg 1995

Globe 1992 Globe, *RIVM. The Environment in Europe: a Global Perspective*, Bilthoven 1992

Goedkoop 1995 Goedkoop M., *The Eco-indicator 95, Final Report and Manual for Designers*, Amersfoort 1995

Goedkoop *et al.* 1997 Goedkoop M., Spriensma R., *The Eco-indicator 97: Problem Definition, Starting Document, Phase 1*, Pré Amersfoort 1997

Gold *et al.* 1989 Gold L.S., Slone Th.H., Bernstein L., Summary of Carcinogenic Potency and Positivity for 492 Rodent Carcinogens in the Carcinogenic Potency Database, *Environmental Health Perspectives* 79: 259-72 (1989)

Gold *et al.* 1997 Gold L.S., Zeiger E., *Handbook of Carcinogenic Potency and Genotoxicity Databases*, CRC Press 1997

Graham 1993 Graham J.D., The Economics of Controlling Outdoor and Indoor Air Pollution, in Tomatis L. (Ed.), *Indoor and Outdoor Air Pollution and Human Cancer*, Springer, Berlin 1993, pp.149-62

Greenpeace 1993 Greenpeace-Studien, Luft: *Krebsgefahr in Städten - die tödliche Wirkung des Autoverkehrs* (9/1993) und *Ergebnisse der Luftschadstoff-Messungen in "Kindernasehöhe"* (6/1992), in http://www.greenpeace.de/GP_DOK_30/STU_LANG/C09ST02.htm

Grendstad 1994 Grendstad G., *Classifying Cultures*, Dissertation, University of Bergen, 1994

Grendstad *et al.* 1997a — Grendstad G., Selle P., Cultural Theory, Postmaterialism and Enviornmental Attitudes, in Ellis R.J., Thompson M. (eds.), *Culture Matters. Essays in Honor of Aaron Wildavsky*, Westview Press, Boulder 1997

Grendstad *et al.* 1997b — Grendstad G., Selle P., Strømsnes K., *Myths of Nature and Views of Society*, paper presented at European Consortium for Political Research – Joint Sessions of Workshop, Bern (26th February - 4th March 1997), Bergen 1997

Griffiths *et al.* 1995 — Griffiths R., Cummins C., Kirk A., Stafford K., *Public Health Report 1995*, West Midlands Regional Health Authority, 1995

Grimen (forthcoming) — Grimen H., Sociocultural Functionalism, in Thompson M., Grendstad G., Selle P. (eds.), *Cultural Theory as Political Science*, Routledge, London forthcoming

Guinée 1993 — Guinée J., *Data for the Normalization Step within Life Cycle Assessment of Products*, CML-Paper No.14, Leiden 1993

Guinée 1995 — Guinée J., *Development of a Methodology for the Environmental Life Cycle Assessment of Products with a Case Study on Margarines*, PhD Thesis, Utrecht 1995

Guinée *et al.* 1993 — Guinée J., Heijungs R., A proposal for the Classification of Toxic Substances within the Framework of Life Cycle Assessment of Products, *Chemosphere* 26 (10): 1925-44 (1993)

Guinée *et al.* 1996 — Guinée J., Heijungs R., van Oers L., van de Meent D., Vermeire Th., Rikken M., *LCA Impact Assessment of Toxic Releases*, CML/RIVM, VROM The Hague 1996

GVF 1996 — GVF, *Monetarisierung der verkehrsbedingten externen Gesundheitskosten, Syntheseberіcht*, GVF-Auftrag Nr.272, GS EVED, 1996

Hansson 1997 — Hansson S.O., Critical Effects and Exposure Limits, *Risk Analysis* 17 (2): 227-36 (1997)

Harding *et al.* 1986 — Harding St., Philips D., Fogarty M., *Contrasting Values in Western Europe; Unity, Diversity and Change, Studies in the Contemporary Values of Modern Society*, The Macmillian Press Ltd., London 1986

Harrison *et al.* 1997 — Harrison R.M., Deacon A.R., Jones M.R., Appleby R.S., Sources and Processes Affecting Concentrations of PM10 and PM2.5 Particulate Matter in Birmingham (U.K.), *Atmospheric Environment* 31 (24): 4103-17 (1997)

Hartmann 1997 — Hartmann St., Der Kampf gegen doe Wüstenbildung, *Tages Anzeiger*, 24. September 1997, p.84

Harvard 1996 — Harvard Center for Cancer Prevention, *Harvard Report on Cancer Prevention, Volume 1: Causes of Human Cancer*, Rapid Science Publishers 1996

Hedin *et al.* 1997 — Hedin L.O., Likens G.E., Atmosphärischer Staub und saurer Regen, *Spektrum der Wissenschaft*, April 1997: 52-5

Heijungs 1994a — Heijungs R., *Maatschappelijke weging van milieuproblemen*, CML-notitie 16, Leiden 1994

Heijungs 1994b — Heijungs R., Valuation: a Societal Approach, in Udo de Haes H.A., Jensen A.A., Klöpffer W., Lindfors L.-G., *Integrating Impact Assessment into LCA*, Proceedings of the SETAC-Europe Congress, 11-14 April 1994, Brussels 1994

Heijungs 1994c — Heijungs R., A Generic Method for the Identification of Options for Cleaner Products, *Ecological Economics* 10 (1): 69-81 (1994)

Heijungs 1997 — Heijungs R., *Economic Drama and the Environmental Stage; Formal Derivation of Algorithmic Tools for Environmental Analysis and Decision-support from a Unified Epistemological Principle*, Leiden 1997

Heijungs 1998 — Heijungs R., Towards Eco-efficiency with LCA's Prevention Principle: an Epistemological Foundation of LCA Using Axioms, in Klostermann J.E.M., Tukker A., *Product Innovation and Eco-efficiency*, Kluwer Academic Publishers, 1998, pp.175-85

Heijungs *et al.* 1992	Heijungs R., Guinée J.B., Huppes G., Lankreijer R.M., Udo de Haes H.A., Wegener Sleeswijk A., Ansems A.M.M., Eggels P.G., van Diun R., de Goede H.P., *Environmental Life Cycle Assessment of Products; Backgrounds & Guide*, Leiden 1992
Heijungs *et al.* 1994a	Heijungs R., Guinée J., The Flux-pulse Problem in LCA, *LCA News, A SETAC-Europe Publication* 4 (3), May 1994
Heijungs *et al.* 1994b	Heijungs R., Guinée J., *Using Environmental Multi-media Models in LCA: the Flux-pulse Problem*, CML-Paper 18, September 1994
Heijungs *et al.* 1997	Heijungs R., Guinée J., Huppes G., *Impact Categories for Natural Resources and Land Use*, CML report 138, CML Leiden 1997
Hemminki *et al.* 1994	Hemminki K., Pershagen G., Cancer Risk of Air Pollution: Epidemiological Evidence, *Environmental Health Perspectives* 102 (Suppl 4): 1187-1192 (October 1994)
Herbert *et al.* 1992	Herbert W., Häberle T., Gellner I., *Umweltbewusstsein bei Experten und Bevölkerung*, Zwischenbericht & Abschlussbericht, Forschungsstelle für Gesellschaftliche Entwicklungen (FGE), Universität Mannheim 1992
Herrmann 1984	Herrmann Th., *Lehrbuch der empirischen Persönlichkeitsforschung*, Verlag für Psychologie, 4. Auflage, Göttingen 1984
Hertwich *et al.* 1997	Hertwich E.G., Pease W.S., Koshland, Evaluating the Environmnetal Impact of Product and Production Processes: a Comparision of Six Methods, *The Science of the Total Environment* 196: 13-29 (1997)
Higginson *et al.* 1992	Higginson J., Muir C.S., Munoz N., *Human Cancer: Epidemiology and Environmental Causes*, Cambridge Monographs on Cancer Research, Cambridge 1992
Hill 1965	Hill A.B., The Environment and Disease: Association or Causation? *Proc Roy Soc Med* 58:295-300 (1965)
Hillier *et al.* 1997	Hillier W., Murphy R.J., Dickinson D.J., Bell J.N.B., *The Risk of Life Cycle Impact Assessment for Preservative Treated Timber Products*, WEI Document 2601, WEI-Congrerss 1997, Oslo 1997
Hillmann 1989	Hillmann K.-H., *Wertewandel: Zur Frage soziokultureller Voraussetzungen alternativer Lebensformen*, Darmstadt 1989, cited in: Schoenheit I., Niedergesäss U., *Lebensstile und Energieberatung*, HEA/imug, Heidelberg 1995
Hines *et al.* 1987	Hines J.M., Hungerford H.R., Tomera A.N., Analysis and Synthesis of Research on Responsible Environmental Behaviour: A Meta-analysis, *The Journal of Environmental Education* 18 (2): 1-8 (1987)
Hirsch Hadorn 1997	Hirsch Hadorn G., Die Bedeutung religionswissenschaftlicher und ethischer Überlegungen für die Objektivitätsprobleme der LCA, in Hofstetter P., Scheringer M.(Hrsg.) (1997). *Schutzgüter und ihre Abwägung aus der Sicht verschiedener Disziplinen.* Vorbereitende Unterlagen des 5. Diskussionsforums Ökobilanzen vom 17. Oktober 1997 an der ETH Zürich. Umweltnatur- und Umweltsozialwissenschaften / Gruppe Sicherheit und Umweltschutz, ETH Zürich. pp.21-5
HK 1991	Hamburgisches Krebsregister (HK), *Krebs in Hamburg -Neumeldungen 1988 des hamburgischen Krebsregisters*, Hamburg 1991
Hoffmann 1993	Hoffmann M.R., *Chemical Pollution of the Environment: Past Present and Future, in Environmental Change and Human Health*, Ciba Foundation Symposium 175, Wiley Chichester 1993, pp.23-41
Hofstede 1991	Hofstede G., *Cultures and Organizations; Software of the Mind*, McGraw-Hill Book Company, London 1991
Hofstetter 1991	Hofstetter P., Bewertungsmodelle für Ökobilanzen in *Tagungsband Energie- und Schadstoffbilanzen im Bauwesen*, 7.3.91 an der ETH Zürich (Bestellung HBT, ETH-Hönggerberg, 8093 Zürich)
Hofstetter 1993	Hofstetter P., *Weighing of Different Environmental Problems*, paper presented at the SETAC/UNEP-Workshop, held in Amsterdam 9-10 June 93
Hofstetter 1996a	Hofstetter P., Time in Life Cycle Assessment, in Braunschweig A., Förster R., Hofstetter P., Müller-Wenk R., *Developments in LCA Valuation*, IWÖ Diskussionbeitrag, St. Gallen 1996, pp.98-121

Hofstetter 1996b	Hofstetter P., Towards a Structured Aggregation Procedure, in Braunschweig A., Förster R., Hofstetter P., Müller-Wenk R., *Developments in LCA Valuation*, IWÖ Diskussionbeitrag, St. Gallen 1996, pp.122-211
Hofstetter 1996c	Hofstetter P., Der Spagat zwischen standortspezifischen Fragen und Lebenzyklus-Ansätzen, in *Tagungungsband Ökobilanzen im Städtebau; Konzepte für umweltorientierte Bewertungsverfahren*, 28.-30. März 1996, IBÖ-Wien 1996
Hofstetter *et al.* 1997	Hofstetter P., Scheringer M. (Hrsg.) (1997). *Schutzgüter und ihre Abwägung aus der Sicht verschiedener Disziplinen.* Vorbereitende Unterlagen des 5. Diskussionsforums Ökobilanzen vom 17. Oktober 1997 an der ETH Zürich. Umweltnatur- und Umweltsozialwissenschaften/ Gruppe Sicherheit und Umweltschutz, ETH Zürich
Hogan *et al.* 1996	Hogan L.M., Beal R.T., Hunt R.G., Threshold Inventory Interpretation Methodology: A Case Study of Three Juice Container Systems, *Int J LCA* 1 (3): 159-167 (1996)
Hohmeyer 1992	Hohmeyer O., Adäquate Berücksichtigung der Erschöpfbarkeit nicht erneuerbarer Ressourcen, in Prognos Schriftenreihe: *Identifizierung und Internalisierung externer Kosten der Energieversorgung*, Band 1, Basel April 1992
Holland 1997	Holland A., The Foundations of Environmental Decision-making, *Int J Environment and Pollution* 7 (4): 483-96 (1997)
Holland *et al.* 1996	Holland A., O'Connor M., O'Neill J., *Costing Environmental Damage: A Critical survey of Current Theory and Practice and Recommendations for Policy Implications*, C3ED, Paris & Centre for the Study of Environmental Change, Lancaster 1996
Holling 1973	Holling C.S., Resilience and Stability of Ecological Systems, *Ann Rev Ecol System* 4: 1-23 (1973)
Holling 1977	Holling C.S., Myths of Ecology and Energy, in *Proceedings of the Symposium on Future Strategies for Energy Development*, Oak Ridge 1977 pp.36-49, cited in van Asseslt *et al.* (1995)
Holling 1979	Holling C.S., Myths of Ecological Stability, in Smart G., Stansbury W. (eds.), *Studies in Crisis Management*, Butterworth, Montreal 1979
Holling 1986	Holling C.S., The Resilience of Terrestrial Ecosystems: Local Surprise and Global Change, in Clark W.C., Munn R.E. (eds.), *Sustainable Development of the Biosphere*, Cambridge University Press, Cambridge 1986
Houghton *et al.* 1996	Houghton J.T., Meira Filho L.G., Callander B.A., Harris N., Kattenberg A., Maskell K. (eds.), *Climate Change 1995; The Science of Climate Change*, Cambridge University Press, Cambridge 1996
Howard *et al.* 1991	Howard P.H., Boethling R.S., Jarvis W.F., *et al.*, *Handbook of Environmental Degradation Rates*, Lewis Publisher, 1991
Hunt *et al.* 1974	Hunt R.G. *et al.*, *Resource and Environmental Profile Analysis of Nine Beverage Container Alternatives*, Midwest Research Instituite for U.S. Environmental Protection Agency, Washington D.C., 1974
Huppes 1997	Huppes G., *Impact Analysis and Evaluation in LCA: More Steps Needed*, Handout of the presentation at 7th International Meeting of SETAC-Europe, 6-10 April 1997, CML Leiden
Hurley *et al.* 1997	Hurley J.F. and Donnan P., *An Update of Exposure-Response (E-R) Functions for the Acute and Chronic Public Health Effects of Air Pollution*, Institute of Occupational Medicine (IOM), Edinburgh, UK 1997, Internal paper for ExternE Project
Huybrechts *et al.* 1996	Huybrechts D., Berloznik R., Wouters G., Marion J.-Y., Valenduc G., The Role of Ecobalances in Environmental Decision-Making, *J Cleaner Prod* 4 (2): 111-9 (1996)
Hyman *et al.* 1988	Hyman E.L., Stiftel B., Moreau D.H., Nichols R.C., *Combining Facts and Values in Environmental Impact Assessment; Theories and Techniques*, Social Impact Assessment Series No.16, Westview Press, Boulder 1988
IARC 1993a	IARC/CEC, *Facts and Figures of Cancer in the European Community*, Lyon 1993

IARC 1993b — International Agency for Research on Cancer (IARC), *IARC Monographs on the Evaluation of Carcinogenic Risks to Humans: Lists of IARC Evaluations*, Lyon 1993

IARC 1995 — IARC, *Survival of Cancer Patients in Europe: The EUROCARE Study*, IARC Scientific Publications No.132, WHO/IARC/EC, Lyon 1995

IER 1997 — IER (ed.), ISET, ZEW, DIW, *ExternE National Implementation Germany*, Contracts JOS3-CT95-0010, JOU2-CT-0264, EC, Draft Final Report, Stuttgart 1997

IER/ETSU/EdM 1997 — IER/ETSU/EdM, *Economic Evaluation of the Draft Incineration Directive*, EU DG XI project, IER Stuttgart, ETSU Oxfordshire, Ecole des Mines, Paris, 1997

IFIAS 1974 — International Federation of Institutes for Advanced Study (IFIAS), *Energy Analysis Workshop on Methodology and Conventions*, Guldsmedshyttan, Sweden 1974

ILSI 1996 — ILSI, *Human Health Impact Assessment in Life cycle Assessment: Analyses by an Expert Panel*, ILSI Health and Environmental Sciences Institute, Washington 1996

Inglehart 1977 — Inglehart R., *The Silent Revolution: Changing Values and Political Styles Among Western Publics*, Princeton, NJ 1977, Princeton University Press.

Inglehart 1979 — Inglehart R., Wertwandel in den westlichen Gesellschaften: Politische Konsequenzen von materialistischen und postmaterialistischen Prioritäten, in Klages H., Kmieciak P. (Hg.), *Wertwandel und gesellschaftlicher Wandel*, Campus Verlag, Frankfurt 1979, pp.279-316,

IPCC 1996 — Houghton J.T., Meira Filho L.G., Callander B.A., Harris N., Kattenberg A., Maskell K (Eds), *Climate Change 1995; The Science of Climate Change*, Cambridge University Press, published for IPCC 1996

IRIS 1996 — U.S. EPA, Office of Health and Environmental Assessment, *Integrated Risk Information System (IRIS)* (on-line data base http://www.epa.gov/ngispgm3/iris/), Cincinnati October 1996

ISO 1997 — ISO, *Environmental Management - Life Cycle Assessment - Principles and Guidelines*, EN ISO 14040, Brussels 1997

ISO 1998 — ISO, *Environmental Management - Life Cycle Assessment - Life Cycle Impact Assessment*, ISO/CD 14042.3, ISO/TC 207/SC5/WG4, SMS Sweden, Stockholm 1998

IVM 1997 — Instituut voor Milieuvraagstukken (IVM), *Economic Evaluation of Air Quality Targets for Sulphur Dioxide, Nitrogen Dioxide, Fine and Suspended Particulate Matter and Lead*, Vrije Universiteit Amsterdam, Amsterdam 1997

Jaenicke 1978 — Jaenicke R., Über die Dynamik atmosphärischer Aitkenteilchen, *Ber Bunsenges Phys Chem* 82: 1198-202 (1978)

Jager *et al.* 1997 — Jager W., van Asselt M.B.A., Rotmans J., Vlek C.A.J., Costerman Boodt P., *Consumer Behaviour; A Modelling Perspective in the Context of Integrated Assessment of Global Change*, Globo Report Series No.17, RIVM Report No.461502017, Bilthoven 1997

Jäggi 1993 — Jäggi Ch.J., *Der Bezug des Menschen zur Natur in Islam und Baha'izum*, Arbeitspapiere zur interreligiösen Umweltethik, Nr.2, inter-edition, Meggen 1993

Jäggi 1994 — Jäggi Ch.J., *Der Bezug des Menschen zur Natur in der New Age-Bewegung und in afrikanischen und indianischen Stammesreligionen*, Arbeitspapiere zur interreligiösen Umweltethik, Nr.4, inter-edition, Meggen 1994

Jäggi 1997 — Jäggi Ch.J., Überlegungen zur Ökobilanz aus der Sicht der angewandten Religionswissenschaften, in Hofstetter P., Scheringer M. (Hrsg.) (1997). *Schutzgüter und ihre Abwägung aus der Sicht verschiedener Disziplinen.* Vorbereitende Unterlagen des 5. Diskussionsforums Ökobilanzen vom 17. Oktober 1997 an der ETH Zürich. Umweltnatur- und Umweltsozialwissenschaften / Gruppe Sicherheit und Umweltschutz, ETH Zürich. pp.11-5

Jansen *et al.* 1972 — Jansen P., Jordan S, Schikarski W., *Vergleichende Modelltheorie der atmosphärischen Schadstoffbelastung durch Kernkraftwerke*, Vortrag gehalten am 10. Colloque IRCHA sur les atmosphères polluées, 3.-5- Mai 1972 in Paris, zitiert in Unger H. Atomkraftwerke. Eine umweltfreundliche Energieerzeugung in Alt C., Weber F. (Hrsg.) *Reinhaltung der Luft*, Karlsruhe 1973

Janssen 1996 — Janssen M., *Meeting Targets; Tools to Support Integrated Assessment Modelling of Global Change*, Den Haag 1996

Janssen *et al.* 1994 — Janssen R., van Herwijnen M., *DEFINITE; A System to Support Decisions on a Finite Set of Alternatives*, Kluwer, Dordrecht 1994

Janssen *et al.* 1995 — Janssen M., Rotmans J., Allocation of Fossil CO_2 Emission Rights Quantifying Cultural Perspectives, *Ecological Economics* 13: 65-79 (1995)

Jenkin *et al.* 1997 — Jenkin M.E., Hayman G.D., Derwnt R.D., Saunders S.M., Pilling M.J., *Tropospheric Chemistry Modelling: Improvements to Current Models and Application to Policy Issues*, AEA/RAMP/20150/R001 Issue 1, AEA Culham 1997

Jenkins *et al.* 1996 — Jenkins S., Hay D., Air Poillution, Health and Exercise: a Review, *Energy & Environment* 7 (1): 51-5 (1996)

Jesinghaus 1993 — Jesinghaus J., *Green Accounting and Indicators: An overview*, Working Document of the Working Group 'Statistics of the environment' Joint Eurostat/ EFTA Group, Meeting of 8&9 December 1993, Document ENV/102

Jevons 1965 — Jevons W.S., *The Coal Question; An Inquiry Concerning the Progress of the Nation and the Probable Exhaustion of our Coal-Mines*, 3rd revised Edition, A.M. Kelley, New York 1965

John 1990 — John O.P., The 'Big Five' Factor Taxonomy: Dimensions of Personality in the Natural Language and in Questionnaires, in Pervin L.A. (ed.), *Handbook of Personality: Theory and Research*, The Guildford Press, New York 1990

John *et al.* 1991 — John O.P., Donahue E.M., Kentle R.L., *The Big Five Inventory: Versions 4a and 54, Technical Report*, Institute of Personality and Social Research, University of California, Berkeley 1991

Johnson 1987 — Johnson B.B., The Environmentalist Movement and Grid/Group Analysis: A Modest Critique, in Johnson B.B., Covello V.T. (eds.), *The Social and Cultural Construction of Risk*, 1987, pp.147-75

Johnson *et al.* 1994 — Johnson, Kotz, *Continuous Univariate Distributions*, Vol 1, Wiley 1994

Jolliet 1993a — Jolliet O., Ökobilanz thermischer, mechanischer und chemischer Kartoffelkrautbeseitigung, *Landwirtschaft Schweiz* 6 (11-12): 675-82 (1993)

Jolliet 1993b — Jolliet O., *Life cycle Analysis in Agriculture: Comparison of Thermal, Mechanical and Chemical Processes to Destroy Potato Haulm*, Expert Seminar on Life Cycle Analysis of Food Products, Technical University of Denmark, 22-23.11.1993

Jolliet 1994 — Jolliet O. (1994). Critical Surface-Time: an Evaluation Method for Life Cycle Assessment, in *Integrating Impact Assessment into LCA*, Proceedings of the 4th SETAC-Europe Congress, pp.133-42.

Jolliet 1997 — Jolliet O., personal communication from July, 22 1997, MIT Boston - EPF Lausanne

Jolliet *et al.* 1997a — Jolliet O., Crettaz P., *Critical Surface-time 95; A Life Cycle Impact Assessment Methodology Including Fate and Exposure*, EPFL Lausanne 1997

Jolliet *et al.* 1997b — Jolliet O., Crettaz P., Fate Coefficients for the Toxicity Assessment of Air Pollutants, Int J LCA 2 (2): 104-10 (1997)

Jones 1981 — Jones J.A., *The Estimation of Long Range Dispersion and Deposition of Continuous Releases of Radionuclides to Atmosphere*, National Radiological Protection Board, NRPB-R123, Chilton 1981

Jones-Lee *et al.* 1997 Jones-Lee M., Loomes G., Valuing Health and Safety: some Economic and Psychological Issues, in Nau R. *et al.* (eds.), *Economic and Environmental Risk and Uncertainty*, Kluwer Publishers, Dordrecht 1997, pp.3-32

Jørgensen 1994 Jørgensen S.E., *Fundamentals of Ecological Modelling* (2nd Edition), Developments in Enviornmental Modelling 19, Elsevier, Amsterdam 1994

Jørgensen *et al.* 1991 Jørgensen S.E., Nielsen S.N., Jørgensen L.A., *Handbook of Ecological Parameters and Ecotoxicology*, Elsevier, Amsterdam 1991

Juchler 1995 Juchler M., Zukunftsängste, TA-Media AG, *inside* 2/95, August 1995: 22-9

Jungermann 1976 Jungermann H. (Hrsg.), *Rationale Entscheidungen*, Bern 1976

Jungermann *et al.* 1993 Jungermann H., Slovic P., Die Psychologie der Kognition und Evaluation von Risiko, in Bechmann G. (Hrsg.), *Risiko und Gesellschaft*, Opladen 1993

Kaiser *et al.* (in press) Kaiser F.G., Shimoda T.A., Responsibility as a Predictor of Ecological Behavior, accepted for publication in *Journal of Environmental Psychology*

Kalisvaart *et al.* 1994 Kalisvaart S., Remmerswaal J., The MET-points Method: a New Single Figure Environmental Performance Indicator, in *Integrating Impact Assessment into LCA*, Proceedings of the 4th SETAC-Europe Congress, 11-14 April 1994, Brussels

Karpowicz-Lazreg *et al.* 1993 Karpowicz-Lazreg C., Mullet E., Societal Risk as seen by the French Public, *Risk Analysis* 13: 253-258 (1993)

Katsouyanni *et al.* 1996 Katsouyanni K., Schwartz J., Spix C. *et al.*, Short Term Effects of Air Pollution on Health: a European Approach Using Epidemiologic Time Series Data: the APHEA Protocol, *J Epidemiol Comm Health* 50 (Suppl 1): S12-S18 (1996)

Keeney 1992 Keeney R.L., *Value-Focused Thinking; a Path to Creative Decision-making*, Harvard 1992

Keeney *et al.* 1976 Keeney R.L., Raiffa H., *Decisions with Multiple Objectives: Preferences and Value Tradeoffs*, New York 1976

Keeney *et al.* 1984 Keeney, Renn, von Winterfeldt, Kotte, *Die Wertbaumanalyse; Entscheidungshilfe für die Politik*, HTV Edition, München 1984

Kemp 1992 Kemp R., *The Politics of Radioactive Waste Disposal*, Manchester University Press, Manchester 1992

Kinsley 1995 Kinsley D., *Ecology and Religion; Ecological Spirituality in Cross-Cultural Perspective*, Prentice Hall, New Jersey 1995

Klages 1992 Klages H., Die gegenwärtige Situation der Wert- und Wertwandelforschung – Probleme und Perspektiven, in Klages H., Hippler H.-J., Herbert W., *Werte und Wandel: Ergebnisse und Methoden einer Forschungstradition*, Frankfurt 1992

Klaus *et al.* 1994 Klaus J., Chies L., Ebert W., Reichert F., *Umweltökonomische Berichterstattung*, Band 5 der Schriftenreihe Spektrum Bundesstatistik, Stuttgart 1994

Klein 1995 Klein M., Wieviel Platz bleibt im Prokuristenbett? Wertewandel in der Bundesrepublik Deutschland zwischen 1973 und 1992 gemessen anhand des Inglehart-Index, *Kölner Zeitschrift für Soziologie und Sozialpsychologie* 47 (2): 207-30 (1995)

Klein Goldewijk *et al.* 1995 Klein Goldewijk C.G.M., Battjes J.J., *The IMAGE 2 Hundred Year (1890-1990) Data Base of the Global Environment (HYDE)*, RIVM Report nr. 481507009, Bilthoven 1995

Kleinman 1995 Kleinman A., *Writing at the Margin: Discourse Between Anthropology and Medicine*, University of California Press, Berkeley 1995

Kleinman *et al.* 1996 Kleinman A., Kleinman J., The Appeal of Experience; the Dismay of Images: Cultural Appropriations of Suffering in our Times, *Daedalus* 125 (1):1-23 (1996)

Klepper *et al.* 1997a Klepper O., van de Meent D., *Mapping the Potentially Affected Fraction (PAF) of Species as an Indicator of Generic Toxic Stress*, RIVM-Report no. 607504001, Bilthoven 1997

Klepper *et al.* 1997b Klepper O., Bakker J., Trass T.P., van de Meent D., Mapping the Potentially Affected Fraction (PAF) of Species as a Basis for Comparision of ecotoxicological Risks between Substances and Regions, in Ale B.J.M., Janssen M.P.M., Pruppers M.J.M. (eds.), *Book of Papers; Risk 97, International Conference Mapping Environmental Risks and Risk Comparison*, 21-24 October, Amsterdam 1997

Klöpffer 1989 Klöpffer W., Persistenz und Abbaubarkeit in der Beurteilung des Umweltverhaltens anthropogener Chemikalien, *UWSF - Z Umweltchem Ökotox* 2: 43-51 (1989)

Klöpffer 1994 Klöpffer W., Kriterien zur Umweltbewertung von Einzelstoffen und Stoffgruppen, *UWSF - Z Umweltchem Ökotox* 6 (2): 61-3 (1994)

Kolluru 1996 Kolluru R.V., Risk Assessment and Management, a Unified Approach, in Kolluru R., Bartell St., Pitblado R., Stricoff S. (eds.), *Risk Assessment and Management Handbook*, McGraw-Hill, New York 1996

Kolluru *et al.* 1996 Kolluru R., Bartell St., Pitblado R., Stricoff S. (eds.), *Risk Assessment and Management Handbook*, McGraw-Hill, New York 1996

Kortman *et al.* 1994 Kortman J.G.M., Lindeijer E.W., Sas H., Sprengers M., *Towards a Single Indicator for Emissions - an Exercice in Aggregating Environmental Effects*, IDES Amsterdam 1994

Kraus 1995 Kraus St.J., Attitudes and the Prediction of Behaviour: A Meta-analysis of the Empirical Literature, *Personality and Social Psychology Bulletin, PSPB* 21 (1): 58-75 (1995)

Kretschmer 1925 Kretschmer E., *Körperbau und Charakter; Untersuchungen zum Konstitutionsproblem und zur Lehre von den Temperamenten*, 4. Auflage, Springer Berlin 1925

Krewitt *et al.* 1996 Krewitt W., Friedrich R., Gesundheitsschäden durch Luftschadstoffe – Kritische Diskussion der Ansätze zur Quantifizierung und Bewertung, *VDI Berichte* 1250: 121-35 (1996)

Krewitt *et al.* 1997 Krewitt W., Mayerhofer P., Friedrich R., Marheineke T, Wirkungspfadanalyse: Ein Ansatz zur Wirkungsbilanzierung, dargestellt am Besipiel der Stromerzeugung, in VDI, Ganzheitliche Bilanzierung von Energiesystemen, *VDI-Berichte* 1328: 25-46 (1997)

Krieger 1994 Krieger D.J., *All-Einheit; Der Bezug des Menschen zur Natur im Hinduismus, Arbeitspapiere zur interreligiösen Umweltethik*, Nr.3, interedition, Meggen 1994

Krotschek *et al.* 1994 Krotschek Ch., Naradoslawsky M., The Sustainable Process Index; a New Dimension in Ecological Evaluation, submitted for publication in *Ecological Engineering*, Amsterdam 1994

Krozer 1992 Krozer J., *Decision Model for Environmental Strategies of Corporations (DESC)*, TME, The Hague 1992

Krüger *et al.* 1994 Krüger O., Grassl H., *Unterstützung der EMEP-Modellrechnungen: Europaweite Deposition schwefel- und stickstoffhaltiger Verbindungen als Folge der Emissionen von Schwefel, Stickoxiden und Ammoniak*, GKSS-Forschungszentrum Geesthacht GmbH, Geesthacht 1994

Krupnick *et al.* 1990 Krupnick A.J., Harrington W., Ostro B., Ambient Ozone and Acute Health Effects: Evidence from Daily Data. *J Environ Econ Manage* 18: 1-18 (1990).

Kuchuk *et al.* 1997 Kuchuk A.A., Krzyzanowski, Huysmans K., The Application of WHO's Health and Environment Geographic Information Systems (HEGIS) in Mapping Environmnetal Health Risks for the European Region, in Ale B.J.M., Janssen M.P.M., Pruppers M.J.M. (eds.), *Book of Papers; Risk 97, International Conference Mapping Environmental Risks and Risk Comparison*, 21-24 October, Amsterdam 1997, pp.269-72

Künzli *et al.* 1996 Künzli N., Kaiser R., Rapp R., *Teilbericht Epidemiologie; Monetarisierung der verkehrsbedingten externen Gesundheitskosten*, GVF-Auftrag Nr.273, Institut für Sozial- und Präventivmedizin, Basel 1996

Kwa 1987 Kwa C., Representations of Nature Mediating between Ecology and Science Policy: the Case of the International Biological Programme, *Social Studies of Science* 17: 413-42 (1987)

LAI 1992 Länderausschuss für Immissionsschutz (LAI), *Krebsrisiko durch Luftverunreinigungen, Entwicklung von 'Beurteilungsmassstäben für kanzerogene Luftverunreinigungen' im Auftrage der Umweltministerkonferenz*, MURL Düsseldorf 1992

LAI 1993 Länderausschuss für Immissionsschutz (LAI), *Krebsrisiko durch Luftverunreinigungen, Entwicklung von 'Beurteilungsmassstäben für kanzerogene Luftverunreinigungen' im Auftrage der Umweltministerkonferenz*, MURL Materialienbände I und II, Düsseldorf 1993

LAI 1995 Länderausschuss für Immissionsschutz (LAI), *Übersicht über Immissionen krebserzeugender Luftschadstoffe in der Bundesrepublik Deutschland im Zeitraum 1989 bis 1994 und ihre Bewertung*, Hamburg 1995

Laszlo *et al.* 1996 Laszlo E., Artigiani R., Combs A., Csányi V., *Changing Visions; Human Cognitive Maps: Past, Present and Future*, Praeger, Westprot 1996

Lave *et al.* 1970 Lave L.B., Seskin E.P., Air Pollution and Human Health, *Science* 169: 723-33 (1970)

Lebret *et al.* 1996 Lebret E., Fischer P.H., Staatsen B.A.M., Franssen E.A.M. *et al.*, *Monitoring of Exposures, Body Burdens and Health Effects of Environmental Pollutants in the Netherlands*, RIVM-Report No.529104001, Bilthoven 1996

Leipert 1989 Leipert Ch., *Die heimlichen Kosten des Fortschritts; Wie Umweltzerstörung das Wirtschaftswachstum fördert*, Fischer, Frankfurt am Main 1989

Levi 1986 Levi F., *Survie en cas de cancer dans le canton de Vaud*, Rapport statistic descriptive, Cah Rech Doc IUMSP No. 4, Lausanne 1986

Levi *et al.* 1986 Levi F., Raymond L., Alaili R., Survie en cas de cancer: données récentes dans les cantons de Vaud et de Genève, *Médicine et Hygiène* 44: 395-400 (1986)

Levi *et al.*1989 Levi F., *et al.* , Cancer Survival from the Incident cases of the registry of Vaud, Switzerland, *Tumori* 75: 83-9 (1989)

Lewtas 1993 Lewtas J., Experimental Evidence for the Carcinogenicity of Indoor and Outdoor Air Pollutants, in Tomatis L. (Ed.), *Indoor and Outdoor Air Pollution and Human Cancer*, Springer, Berlin 1993, pp.103-18

Lillelund *et al.* 1987 Lillelund K., de Haar U., Elster H.-J. Elster, Karbe L., Schwoerbel I., Simonis W. (Hrsg.), *Bioakkumulation in Nahrungsketten*, Forschungsbericht der DFG, VCH Weinheim 1987

Lindeijer 1994 Lindeijer E., The Valuation within LCA: Aim, Criteria and Procdure, in Udo de Haes H.A., Schaltegger S., Hofstetter P. (Eds.), *First Working Document on Life-Cycle Impact Assessment Methodology*, Workshop held at ETH Zurich from July 8-9, 1994, pp.163-170

Lindfors *et al.* 1995 Lindfors L.-G. *et al.*, *Nordic Guidelines on Life-Cycle Assessment*, Nord 1995:20, Copenhagen/ Stockholm 1995

Lüdtke 1989 Lüdtke H., *Expressive Ungleichheit. Zur Soziologie der Lebensstile*, Opladen 1989

Luhmann 1995 Luhmann N., *Soziologische Aufklärung 6: Die Soziologie und der Mensch*, Westdeutscher Verlag, Opladen 1995

Lühr *et al.* 1991 Lühr H.-P., Hefer B., Scholz R.W., Das Donator-Akzeptor-Modell (DAM) in E. Bütow (Ed.), *Ableitung von Sanierungswerten für kontaminierte Böden*, IWS-Schriftenreihe, Band 13, E. Schmidt, Berlin 1991, pp.17-53

Luttik *et al.* 1997 Luttik R., Traas T.P., Mensink H., *Mapping the Potentially Affected Fraction of Avian and Mammalian Target Species in the National Ecological Network*, RIVM report No. 707504002, Bilthoven 1997

Lutz 1997 Lutz K.W., Risikobewertung in der chemischen Kanzerogenese, in Mersch-Sundermann V. (Ed.), *Umweltmedizin - Ökologische Medizin*, Georg Thieme Verlag Stuttgart 1997

Mackay 1979 Mackay D., Correlation of Bioconcentration Factors, *Environ Sci Technol*16: 274-8 (1982)

Mackay 1982 Mackay D., Finding Fugacity Feasible, *Environ Sci Technol* 13 (10): 1218-23 (1979)

Mackay 1991 — Mackay D., *Multimedia Environmental Models. The Fugacity Approach*, Lewis, Chelsea 1991

Mackay *et al.* 1993 — Mackay D., Ying Shiu W., Ma K.Ch., *Illustrated Handbook of Physical-Chemical Properties and Environmental Fate for Organic Chemicals*, Volume 1 to 3, Lewis Publishers, Boca Raton 1993

Mackay *et al.* 1996a — Mackay D., Di Guardo A., Paterson S., Kicsi G., Cowan E., Assessing the Fate of New and Existing Chemicals: A Five-stage Process, Environ Toxicol Chem 15 (9): 1618-26 (1996)

Mackay *et al.* 1996b — Mackay D., Di Guardo A., Paterson S., Cowan E., Evaluating the Environmental Fate of a Variety of Types of Chemicals Using the EQC Model, *Environ Toxicol Chem* 15 (9): 1627-37 (1996)

Maibach *et al.* 1996 — Maibach M. *et al.*, *Die vergessenen Milliarden*, Paul Haupt, Bern 1996

Marris *et al.* 1996a — Marris C., O'Riordan T., Simpson A., *Redefining the Cultural Context of Risk Perception*, Society of Risk Analysis, Europe Annual Meeting, Stuttgart 1996, pp.129-152

Marris *et al.* 1996b — Marris C., Langford I., O'Riordan T., *Integrating Sociological and Psychological Approaches to Public Perceptions of Environmental Risks: Detailed Results from a Questionnaire Survey*, CSERGE Working paper GEC 96-07, London 1996

Martens *et al.* 1995 — Martens W.J., *et al.* , Potential Impacts of Global Warming on Malaria Risk, *Environmental Health Perspectives* 103 (5): 458-64 (1995)

Martinez-Ebers 1997 — Martinez-Ebers V., Using Monetary Incentives with Hard-to-reach Populations in Panel Surveys, *International Journal of Public Opinion Research* 9 (1): 77-86 (1997)

Maslow 1954 — Maslow A.H., *Motivation and Personality*, Harper, New York 1954

Mayer 1992 — Mayer Th., *Truth Versus Precision in Economics*, Edward Elgar, Hants 1992

Mayerhofer *et al.* 1996 — Mayerhofer P., Friedrich R., Die Schadenskosten der Klimaänderung; Diskussion vorliegender Abschätzungen, *Energiewirtschaftlicher Tagesfragen* 46 (1/2): 58-64 (1996)

McClure 1996 — McClure P.R., *Evaluation of a Component-based RELA Potency Approach to Cancer Risk Assessment for Exposure to PAHs*, Syracuse Research Corporation, Meryll Lane, Syracuse, New York, 13219, Poster presentation at the Annual Meeting of the Society of Toxicology, Anaheim, California, March 11, 1996

McKay et al. 1979 — McKay M.D., Beckman R.J., Conover W.J., A Comparison of Three Methods for Selecting Values of Input Variables in the Analysis of Output from a Computer Code, *Technometrics* 21 (2): 239-45 (1979)

McMichael *et al.* 1996 — McMichael A.J., Haines A., Sloof R., Kovats S.(eds.), *Climate Change and Human Health*, WHO/EHG/96.7, Geneva 1996

Meadows *et al.* 1992 — Meadows D. *et al.*, *Die neuen Grenzen des Wachstums*, Stuttgart 1992

Mehlman 1990 — Mehlman M.A. (Ed.), *Environmental and Occupational Cancer: Scientific Update*, Princeton 1990

Meier 1997 — Meier M.A., *Eco-Efficiency Evaluation of Waste Gas Purification Systems in the Chemical Industry*, Diss.ETH No. 12259, Zürich 1997

Mengel Jørgensen 1996 — Mengel Jørgensen A.-M., *LCA Stakeholders and Weighing of Environmental Problems; a Theoretical Approach to Differing Valuation Criteria*, Amsterdam 1996

Metcalfe *et al.* 1989 — Metcalfe S.E., Atkins D.H.F., Derwent R.G., Acid Deposition Modelling and the Interpretation of the United Kindom Secondary Precipitation Network Data, *Atmospheric Environment* 23 (9): 2033-52 (1989)

Metroeconomica *et al.* 1996 — Metroeconomica, IFO Institut, IER, Fondazione Mattei *et al.* , *Green Accounting in Europe (GARPI); The Role of Damage Estimation - Four Case Studies*, Dorset 1996

Miser *et al.* 1985 — Miser H.J., Quade E.S. (Ed.), *Handbook of Systems Analysis, Overview of Uses, Procedures, Applications, and Practice*, John Wiley & Sons, Chichester 1985

Miser *et al.* 1988	Miser H.J., Quade E.S. (Ed.), *Handbook of Systems Analysis, Craft Issues and Procedural Choices*, John Wiley & Sons, Chichester 1988
Mix 1986	Mix M.C., Cancerous Diseases in Aquatic Animals and their Association with Environmental Pollutants: A Critical Literature Review, *Marine Environmental Research* 20: 1-114 (1986)
Möller *et al.* 1994	Möller L., Schuetzle D., Autrup H., Future Research Needs Associated with the Assessment of Potential Human Health Risks from Exposure to Toxic Ambient Air Pollutants, *Environmental Health Perspectives* 102 (Suppl 4): 193-209 (October 1994)
Monn *et al.* 1996	Monn Ch., Fuchs A., Högger D. *et al.*, *Particulate Matter <10mm (PM10) and Fine Particles < 2.5mm (PM2.5): Relationship between Indoor, Outdoor and Personal Concentrations*, Institut für Hygiene und Arbeitsphysiologie, ETH Zürich 1996 (submitted)
Müller 1992	Müller H.-P., *Sozialstruktur und Lebensstile. Der neuere theoretische Diskurs über soziale Ungleichheit*, Frankfurt am Main 1992, cited in: Schoenheit I., Niedergesäss U., *Lebensstile und Energieberatung*, HEA/imug, Heidelberg 1995
Müller-Wenk 1978	Müller-Wenk R., *Ökologische Buchhaltung*, Campus-Verlag, Frankfurt 1978
Müller-Wenk 1980	Müller-Wenk R., Ökologische Buchhaltung, in Udo Ernst Simonis, *Ökonomie und Ökologie, Auswege aus einem Konflikt*, Karlsruhe 1980, pp.13-30
Müller-Wenk 1994a	Müller-Wenk R., Criteria for valuation, and how to include them into a valuation factor, in Udo de Haes H.A., Schaltegger S., Hofstetter P. (Hrsg.), *First Working Document on Life-Cycle Impact Assessment Methodology*, Workshop held at ETH Zurich from July 8-9, 1994
Müller-Wenk 1994b	Müller-Wenk R., The Ecoscarcity Method as a Valuation Instrument within the SETAC Framework, in *Integrating Impact Assessment into LCA*, Proceedings of the 4th SETAC-Europe Congress, 11-14 April 1994, Brussels
Müller-Wenk 1997	Müller-Wenk R., *Safeguard Subjects and Damage Functions as Core Elements of Life-Cycle Impact Assessment*, IWÖ-Diskussionbeitrag Nr.42, St. Gallen 1997
Müller-Wenk 1998	Müller-Wenk R., *Depletion of Abiotic Resources Weighted on Base of 'Virtual' Impacts of Lower Grade Deposits Used in Future*, IWÖ-Schriftenreihe Nr. 57, St. Gallen 1998 (http://www.unisg.ch/iwoe/index.html)
Murray 1994	Murray C.J.L., Quantifying the Burden of Disease: the Technical Basis for Disability Adjusted Life Years, *Bulletin of the World Health Organization* 72 (3): 429-45 (1994)
Murray 1996	Murray Ch.J.L., Rethinking DALYs, Chapter 1 in Murray Ch.J.L., Lopez A.D. (Eds.), *The Global Burden of Disease*, Volume I, WHO / Harvad School of Public Health / World Bank, Harvard University Press, Boston 1996
Murray *et al.* 1994	Murray C.J.L., Lopez A.D., Quantifying Disability: Data, Methods and Results, *Bulletin of the World Health Organization* 72 (3): 481-94 (1994)
Murray *et al.* 1996a	Murray Ch.J.L., Lopez A.D. (Eds.), The Global Burden of Disease, *Volume I of Global Burden of Disease and Injury Series*, WHO / Harvad School of Public Health / World Bank, Harvard University Press, Boston 1996
Murray *et al.* 1996b	Murray Ch.J.L., Lopez A.D., Global Health Statistics, *Volume II of Global Burden of Disease and Injury Series*, WHO/Harvard School of Public Health/World Bank, Harvard University Press, Boston 1996
Murray *et al.* 1996c	Murray Ch.J.L., Lopez A.D., *The Global Burden of Disease*; Summary, WHO / Harvard School of Public Health / World Bank, Summary report on the web: http://www.hsph.harvard.edu/ organizations/bdu
Nagata *et al.* 1995	Nagata K., Fujii Y., Ishikawa M., *Proposing a Valuation Method Based on Panel Data*, Preliminary report (plus study in Japanese), 1995

Nagel *et al.* 1991 — Nagel R., Loskill R. (eds), *Bioaccumulation in Aquatic Systems*, Proceedings of an international workshop, VCH Weinheim 199?

Nelkin 1982 — Nelkin D., Blunders in the Business of Risk, Book Reviews, *Nature* 298: 775-6 (1982)

Newell 1997 — Newell S.A., *Relating Emissions to Concentrations in Environmental Valuation*, internal paper, MIT Boston 1997

NFP 1996 — Programmleitung NFP 31 (Hrsg.), *Klimarisiken – Herausforderung für die Schweizer Wirtschaft; Thesen zu Klimänderungen und Naturkatastrophen*, vdf Zürich 1996

Nriagu *et al.* 1988 — Nriagu J.O., Pacyna J.M., Quantitative Assessment of Worldwide Contamination of Air, Water and Soils by Trace Metals, *Nature* 333: 134-9 (May 1988)

O'Riordan *et al.* 1991 — O'Riordan T., Rayner S., Risk Management for Global Environmental Change, *Global Environmental Change* 1 (2): 91-108 (1991)

Oberdörster 1995 — Oberdörster G., Airborne Polluatnts and Acute Health Effcets, reply on Seaton *et al.* 1995, *Lancet* 345: 799 (March 25, 1995)

Odum 1971 — Odum E.P., *Fundamentals of Ecology*, Philadelphia 1971

OECD 1981 — OECD, *Guidelines for Testing of Chemicals, 305E, Bioaccumulation: Flow-through Fish Test*, Paris 1981

OECD 1991 — OECD, *Environmental Indicators: A Preliminary Set*, Paris 1991

OECD 1994 — OECD, Environmental Indicators: OECD Core Set, Paris October 1994

OECD 1995 — OECD, *The Life Cycle Approach: An Overview of Product / Process Analysis, Technology and Environment*, OECD / GD(95)118, Paris 1995

Olli (forthcoming) — Olli E., Individual Level Rejection of Cultural Biases and Effects on Party Preferences, in Thompson M., Grendstad G., Selle P. (eds.), *Cultural Theory as Political Science*, Routledge, London forthcoming

Ostro 1987 — Ostro B.D., Air Pollution and Morbidity Revisited: A Specification Test. *J Environ Econ Manage* 14: 87-98 (1987)

Ostro *et al.* 1989 — Ostro B.D., Rothschild S., Air Pollution and Acute Respiratory Morbidity: An Observational Study of Multiple Pollutants. *Environ Res* 50: 238-247 (1989)

Ott *et al.* 1994 — Ott W., Dettli R., Heldstab J., *Externe Kosten und kalkulatorische Energiepreiszuschläge für den Strom- und Wärmebereich in der Schweiz, Materialien zu Pacer*, Teilberichte 1-6, Bern 1994

Owens 1995 — Owens J.W., *Layout and Organization of Life-Cycle Impact Assessment*, submitted to ISO TC207/SC5/WG4, 27.9.1995

Owens 1998 — Owens W., Life Cycle Impact Assessment: The Use of Subjective Judgements in Classification and Characterisation, *Int J LCA* 3 (1): 43-6 (1998)

Ozonoff 1994 — Ozonoff D, Conceptions and Misconceptions about Human Health Impact Analysis, *Environ Impact Assess Rev* 14: 499-515 (1994)

Pacyna 1995 — Pacyna J.M., Sources, Particle Size Distribution and Transport of Aerosols, in Koimtzis T., Samara C. (eds.), *Airborne Particulate Matter, Volume 4, Part D, of The Handbook of Environmental Chemistry*, Springer, Berlin 1995, pp.69-97

Pacyna *et al.* 1985 — Pacyna J.M., Long-range Transport of Heavy Metals – Modelling and Measurements, in van Dop H. (ed.), *Air Pollution Modelling and its Application VI*, Plenum Press, New York 1985, pp.367-80

Pagano *et al.* 1996 — Pagano P., de Zaiacomo T., Scarcella E., Bruni St., Calamosca M., Mutagenicity of Total and Particle-Sized Fractions of Urban Particulate Matter, *Environ Sci Technol* 30: 3512-6 (1996)

Panitz *et al.* 1989 — Panitz H.J., Matzerath C., Päsler-Sauer J., *UFOMOD Atmospheric Dispersion and Deposition*, KfK 4332, Kernforschungszentrum Karlsruhe GmbH, Karlsruhe 1989

Päsler-Sauer 1989 — Päsler-Sauer J., *Untersuchung standortspezifischer Ausbreitungsbedingungen*, KfK 4519, Kernforschungszentrum Karlsruhe GmbH, Karlsruhe 1989

Paustenbach 1989	Paustenbach D.J., *The Risk Assessment of Environmental and Human Health Hazards: A Textbook of Case Studies*, John Wiley&Sons, New York 1989
Pearce 1993	Paerce D., *Blueprint 3, Measuring Sustainable Development*, Earthscan, London 1993
Pearce *et al.* 1994	Pearce D., Moran D., *The Economic Value of Biodiversity*, IUCN, London 1994
Pedroni *et al.* 1990	Pedroni G., Zweifel P., *Wie misst man Gesundheit?* Studien zur Gesundheitsökonomie 14, Pharma Information, Basel 1990
Perkins 1997	Perkins St., *Bringing Monetarisation into Environmental Assessment: The OECD Approach, Determining Monetary Values of Environmental Impacts, Enhancing the Quality of Transport Decision Making*, Conference documentation, Landor Publishing, London 1997
Pershagen *et al.* 1993	Pershagen G., Simonato L., Epidemiological Evidence on Outdoor Air Pollution and Cancer, in Tomatis L. (Ed.), *Indoor and Outdoor Air Pollution and Human Cancer*, Springer, Berlin 1993, pp.135-48
Peters *et al.* 1997	Peters A., Döring A., Wichmann H.E., Koenig W., Increased Plasma Viscosity During an Air Pollution Episode: a Link to Mortality?, *Lancet* 349: 1582-7 (May 31, 1997)
Philp 1995	Philp R.B., *Environmental Hazards and Human Health*, Lewis, Boca Raton 1995
Pictet 1995	Pictet J., *Méthodologie multicritère d'aide à la négatiociation environnementale*, Thèse No. 1372, EPF Lausanne 1995
Pieters *et al.* 1996	Pieters M.N., Kroese E.D., *Dosis-effect relations in de humane risicoschatting: een inventarisatie voor stoffen*, RIVM-Report No. 620133001, Bilthoven 1996
Pilkington *et al.* 1997	Pilkington A., Hurley F., Donnan P., *Health Effects in ExternE Transport: Assessment and Exposure-Response Functions, Institute of Occupational Medicine*, Edinburgh, Draft July 1997
Plewnia *et al.* 1983	Plewnia M., Schmitz J., Huber W., *Vergleich ausgewählter Heizungssysteme unter energetischen, ökonomischen und ökologischen Gesichtspunkten*, Jül-Spez-234/Bd.3, KFA Jülich 1983
Pohl *et al.* 1996a	Pohl Ch., Ros M., Waldeck B., Dinkel F., Imprecision and Uncertainty in LCA, in Schaltegger S. (Ed), *Life Cycle Assessment (LCA) - Quo vadis?*, Birkhäuser Verlag, Basel 1996
Pohl *et al.* 1996b	Pohl Ch., Ros M., Sind Ökobilanzen zu präzise? Zum Einsatz von Fuzzy-Set-Theorie und Fehlerrechnung in LCAs, in Ranze *et al.* (Hrsg.), *Intelligente Methoden zur Verarbeitung von Umweltinformationen*, 2. Bremer KI-Pfingstworkshop, Metropolis Verlag, Marburg 1996
Ponce de Leon *et al.* 1996	Ponce de Leon A., Anderson H.R., Bland J.M., Strachan D.P., Bower J., Effects of Air Pollution on Daily Hospital Admissions for Respiratory Disease in London between 1987-88 and 1991-92, *J Epidemiol Comm Health* 50 (Suppl 1): S63-S70 (1996)
Pönkä *et al.* 1996	Pönkä A., Virtanen M., Asthma and Ambient Air Pollution in Helsinki, *J Epidemiol Comm Health* 50 (Suppl 1): S59-S62 (1996)
Pope *et al.* 1992	Pope C.A., Dockery D.W., Acute Health Effects of PM10 Pollution on Symptomatic and Asymptomatic Children. *Am Rev Respir Dis* 145: 1123-6 (1992)
Pope *et al.* 1995a	Pope C.A., Bates D.V., Raizenne M.E., Reassessment?, *Environmental Health Perspectives* 103 (5): 472-80 (May 1995)
Pope *et al.* 1995b	Pope C.A., Thun M.J., Namboodiri M.M., *et al.*, Particulate Air Pollution as a Predictor of Mortality in a Prospective Study of U.S. Adults, *Am J Respir Crit Care Med* (151): 669-74 (1995)
Pope *et al.* 1996	Pope A., Dockery D., Epidemiology of Chronic Health Effects: Cross-Sectional Studies, in Wilson R., Spengler J.D. (eds), *Particles in Our Air: Concentrations and Health Effects*, Harvard University Press 1996

Posch *et al.* 1995 — Posch M., de Smet P.A.M., Hettelingh J.-P., Downing R.J. (eds.), *Calculation and Mapping of Critical Thresholds in Europe*, Status Report 1995, RIVM-Report No. 259101004, Bilthoven 1995

POST 1996 — Parliamentary Office of Science and Technology (POST), *Fine Particles and Health*, Technical Report 82, June 1996, London

Potting *et al.* 1994 — Potting J., Blok K., Spatial aspects of life-cycle impact assessment, in *Integrating Impact Assessment into LCA*, Proceedings of the 4th SETAC-Europe Congress, 11-14 April 1994, Brussels

Potting *et al.* 1997 — Potting J., Hauschild M., Predicted Environmental Impact and Expected Occurrence of Actual Environmental Impact; Part I: The Linear Nature of Environmental Impact from Emissions in Life Cycle Assessment, *Int J LCA* 2(3): 171-7 (1997); Part II: Spatial Differentiation in Life-Cycle Assessment via the Site-Dependent Characterisation of Environmental Impact from Emissions, *Int J LCA* 2 (4) (1997)

Power 1993 — Power S., Risking it All – Personal and Policy Decisions about Environmental Risks, Review Essay, *Journal of Environmental Psychology* 13: 85-9 (1993)

Power *et al.* 1998 — Power M., Mccarty L.S., A Comparative Analysis of Environmental Risk Assessment / Risk Management Frameworks, *Environmental Science & Technology*, May 1, 1998: 224A-31A

Prognos 1992 — Prognos, *Identifizierung und Internalisierung externer Kosten der Energieversorgung*, Band 1-8, Basel 1992

Prose *et al.* 1991 — Prose F., Wortmann K., *Energiesparen: Verbraucheranalyse und Marktsegmentierung der Kieler Haushalte*, Band I-III, Kiel 1991

Pruppers 1996 — Pruppers M.J.M.(Ed.), *Achtergronddocument bij 'Cumulatie van mileiurisico's voor de mens, geografische verschillen in Nederland'*, RIVM-report No.610127002, Bilthoven 1996

Pruppers *et al.* 1996 — Pruppers M.J.M., van den Hout K.D., Ale B.J.M., Buringh E., Miedema H.M.E., *Cumulatie van mileiurisico's voor de mens, geografische verschillen in Nederland*, RIVM-report No.610127001, Bilthoven 1996

Pruppers *et al.* 1997 — Pruppers M.J.M., Janssen M.P.M., Ale B.J.M. *et al.*, Accumulation of Environmnetal Risks to Human Health: Geographical Differences in the Netherlands, in Ale B.J.M., Janssen M.P.M., Pruppers M.J.M. (eds.), *Book of Papers; Risk 97, International Conference Mapping Environmental Risks and Risk* Comparison, 21-24 October, Amsterdam 1997

Pryor 1998 — Pryor S.C., A Case Study of Emission Changes and Ozone Responses, *Atmospheric Environment* 32 (2): 123-31 (1998)

Putta 1991 — Putta S.N., Methods for Valuing and Incorporating Environmental Costs in Electric Resource Planning and Acquisition, in Hohmeyer O., Ottinger R.L. (Hrsg.), *External Environmental Costs of Electric Power*, Workshop at Ladenburg 1990, Berlin 1991

Rabl 1996 — Rabl A., Air Pollution Damages and Costs: an Analysis of Uncertainties, in *Proceedings of Society of Risk Analysis Europe*, University of Surrey 3-5 June 1996, pp.185-8

Rabl 1997 — Rabl A., Quantifying the Benefits of Air Pollution Control: The Interpretation of Exposure-response Functions for Mortality, in Ale B.J.M., Janssen M.P.M., Pruppers M.J.M. (eds.), *Book of Papers; Risk 97, International Conference Mapping Environmental Risks and Risk Comparison*, 21-24 October, Amsterdam 1997

Rabl *et al.* 1995 — Rabl A., Peuportier B., Impact Pathway Analysis: A Tool for Improving Environmental Decision Processes, *Environ Impact Assess Rev* 15: 421-42 (1995)

Rabl *et al.* 1996a — Rabl A., Spadaro J., Curtiss P.S., *Analysis of Environmental Impacts of Treatment of Industrial Waste: Methodology and Case Study*, Final report for contract EV5V-CT94-0383, Paris 1996

Rabl *et al.* 1996b — Rabl A., Curtiss P.S., Spadaro J. *et al.*, *Environmental Impacts and Costs: the Nuclear and the Fossil Fuel Cycles, Version 3.0*, Final report of the project 'External Costs of Fuel Cycles: Implementation of the Accounting Framework in France', JOU2-CT92-0236, Paris June 1996

Rabl *et al.* 1997a — Rabl A., Eyre N., An Estimate of Regional and Global O_3 Damage from Precursor NO_x and VOC Emissions, submitted to *Environment International*, March 1997

Rabl *et al.* 1997b — Rabl A., Spadaro J.V., McGravan P.D., *Health Risk of Air Pollution from Incinerators: a Perspective*, Ecole des Mines, Paris 1997

Raiffa 1994 — Raiffa H., The Perscriptive Orientation of Decision Making, in Ríos S. (ed.), *Decision Theory and Decision Analysis: Trends and Challenges*, Kluwer Academic Publishers, Boston 1994

Rapoport 1976 — Rapoport A., Sociocultural Aspects of Man-environment Studies, in Rapoport A. (ed.), *The Mutual Interaction of People and their Built Environment; A Cross-cultural Perspective*, Mouton Publishers, The Hague 1976

Raymond *et al.* 1993 — Raymond L., Obradovic M., Fioretta G., Droin N., Bouchardy Ch., *Le cancer à Genève*, Registre genevois des tumeurs, Genève 1993

Rayner 1987 — Rayner St., Risk and Relativism in Science for Policy, in Johnson B.B., Covello V.T. (eds.), *The Social and Cultural Construction of Risk*, 1987, pp.5-23

Rayner 1991 — Rayner S., A Cultural Perspective on the Structure and Implementation of Global Environmental Agreements, *Evaluation Review* 15 (1): 75-102 (February 1991)

Rayner *et al.* 1987 — Rayner St., Cantor R., How Fair is Safe Enough? The Cultural Approach to Societeal Technology Choice, *Risk Analysis* 7 (1): 3-9 (1987)

Reichmuth 1996 — Reichmuth P., *Umwelt- und sicherheitsrelevante Informationen über Chemikalien in Datenbanken an der ETH Zürich*, Semesterarbeit am Laboratorium für Technische Chemie, Gruppe für Sicherheit und Umweltschutz ETH Zürich, Zürich 1996

Renn 1991 — Renn O., Riskiowahrnehmung und Risikobewertung: Soziale Perzeption und gesellschaftliche Konflikte, in Chakraborty S., Yadigaroglu G.(Hrsg), *Ganzheitliche Risikobetrachtungen; Technische, ethische und soziale Aspekte*, TÜV Rheinland, Köln 1991

Renn 1995 — Renn O., Individual and Social Perception of Risk, in Fuhrer U. (Hrsg.), *Ökologisches Handeln als sozialer Prozess*, Basel 1995

Renoux 1996 — Renoux A., L'Aerosol atmosphérique, ses origines; quelques notions sur les principales propriétés physiques des aérosol, in CITEPA, *Les poussières; un polluant de passé... et de l'avenir*, Journée d'études du 17 décembre 1996, Paris 1996

Renwick *et al.* 1993 — Renwick A.G., Walker R., An Analysis of the Risk of Exceeding the Acceptable or Tolerable Daily Intake, *Regulatory Toxicology and Pharamcology* 18: 463-80 (1993)

Reusswig 1994 — Reusswig F., *Lebensstile und Ökologie; Gesellschaftliche Pluralisierung und alltagsökologische Entwicklung unter besonderer Berücksichtigung des Energiebereichs*, sozial-ökologische Arbeitspapiere 43, Frankfurt 1994

Rippen 1996 — Rippen, Handbuch *Umwelt-Chemikalien; Stoffdaten - Prüfverfahren - Vorschriften*, ecomed, 35. Ergänzungslieferung, 8/1996

Roe 1996 — Roe E.M., Sustainable Development and Cultural Theory, *Int J Sustain Dev World Ecol* 3: 1-14 (1996)

Roedel 1992 — Roedel W., *Physik unserer Umwelt - Die Atmosphäre*, Springer Verlag Berlin 1992

Roemer *et al.* 1993 — Roemer W., Hoek G., Brunekreef B., Effect of Ambient Winter Air Pollution on Respiratory Health of Children with Chronic Respiratory Symptoms. *Am Rev Respir Dis* 147: 118-24 (1993)

Roghair *et al.* 1997 — Roghair C.J., Struijs J., des Zwart D., *Measurement of Toxic Potency of Fresh Waters in the Netherlands*, RIVM-Report No.607504004, Bilthoven 1997

Roorda *et al.* 1997 — Roorda A.A.H., van Dokkum H.P., van der Ven B.L., Location Specific Assessment within LCA - a Pilot Study, paper submitted to *Int J LCA* 1997

Rosner 1995 — Rosner W.J., Mental Models for Sustainability, *J Cleaner Prod* 3 (1-2): 107-21 (1995)

Rosser 1983 — Rosser R., Issues of Measurement in the Design of Health Indicators: A Review, in Culyer A.J., *Health Indicators*, St. Martins Press, New York 1983

Rotmans 1995 — Rotmans J (ed.), *TARGETS in Transition*, GLOBO, RIVM, Bilthoven 1995

Rotmans *et al.* 1994 — Rotmans J, van Asselt M.B.A., de Bruin A.J. *et al.*, *Global Change and Sustainable Development; a Modelling Perspective for the Next Decade*, GLOBO Report Series No.4, RIVM-Report No. 461502004, Bilthoven 1994

Rotmans *et al.* 1997 — Rotmans J., de Vries B. (eds.), *Perspectives on Global Change; The TARGETS Approach*, Cambridge University Press, Cambridge 1997

Rubik *et al.* 1992 — Rubik F., Baumgartner Th., *Technological Innovation in the Plastics Industry and its Influenece on the Environmental Problems of Plastic Waste*, MONITOR-SAST Activity, SAST-Project No.7, DGXII/439/92-EN, EUR-14737-EN, Brussels-Luxembourg 1992

Ryder 1990 — Ryder R.A., Ecosystem Health, a Human Perception: Definition, Detection, and the Dichotomous Key, *F Great Lakes Res* 16: 619-24 (1990)

S.G.P. 1994 — S.G.P.Consultants, *Etude relative à la normalisation écologique des emballages en Belgique*, Rapport final, Volume 1 et 2 (700 pages), Novembre 1994

Saaty 1980 — Saaty T.L., *The Analytical Hierarchy Process, Planning, Priority Setting, Resource Allocation*, New York, Mc Graw-Hill, 1980

SAB 1997 — Science Advisory Board (SAB), *Report of the Environmental Engineering Committee's Subcommittee on the TRI Relative Risk-Based Environmental Indicators*, DRAFT 3-12-97, Washington (access via http://es.inel.gov/oeca/sfi)

Sagunski *et al.* 1991 — Sagunski H., Lommel A., Ollroge I., Tesseraux I., Kappos A., Pfadbezogene Risikoabschätzung für ausgewählte chemische Kanzerogene, *VDI Berichte* Nr.888: 829-38 (1991)

Sandnes 1993 — Sandnes H., *Calculated Budgets for Airborne Acidifying Components in Europe*, Technical Report no.109, Det Norske Meteorologiske Institut, EMEP/MSW-W Report 1/1993

SC 1995 — Statistique Canada (SC), *Statistiques canadiennes sur le cancer 1995*, Toronto 1995

Schaber 1997 — Schaber P., Philosophische Reflexionen zur ökonomischen Naturbewertung und rationaler Umweltpolitik, in Hofstetter P., Scheringer M. (Hrsg.) (1997). *Schutzgüter und ihre Abwägung aus der Sicht verschiedener Disziplinen*. Vorbereitende Unterlagen des 5. Diskussionsforums Ökobilanzen vom 17. Oktober 1997 an der ETH Zürich. Umweltnatur- und Umweltsozialwissenschaften / Gruppe Sicherheit und Umweltschutz, ETH Zürich. pp.16-21

Schaefer 1982 — Schaefer H., *Kumulierter Energieverbrauch zum Herstellen von Produkten, Methoden der Ermittlung - Probleme der Bewertung*, BWK 34 (7), 1982

Schaltegger *et al.* 1992 — Schaltegger St., Sturm A., *Ökologieorientierte Entscheidungen in Unternehmen*, Schriftenreihe des Instituts für Betriebswirtschaft, WWZ Basel, Bern 1992

Scheringer 1996 — *Scheringer M., Räumliche und zeitliche Reichweite als Indikatoren zur Bewertung von Umweltchemikalien*, Diss.ETH Nr. 11746, Zürich 1996

Scheringer *et al.* 1994a — Scheringer M., Berg, M., Spatial and Temporal Range as Measures of Environmental Threat, *Fresenius Envir Bull* 3: 493-8 (1994)

Scheringer *et al.* 1994b — Scheringer M., Berg M., Müller-Herold U., Jenseits der Schadensfrage: Umweltschutz durch Gefährdungsbegrenzung in Berg M. *et al.* (Hrsg.), *Was ist ein Schaden? Zur normativen Dimension des Schadensbegriffs in der Risiokowissenschaft*, Zürich 1994

Scheringer *et al.* 1997 — Scheringer M., Hofstetter P., Auswahl, Begründung und Vergleich von Schutzgütern in der Ökobilanz-Methodik - ein offenes Problem, in Hofstetter P., Scheringer M. (Hrsg.) (1997). *Schutzgüter und ihre Abwägung aus der Sicht verschiedener Disziplinen.* Vorbereitende Unterlagen des 5. Diskussionsforums Ökobilanzen vom 17. Oktober 1997 an der ETH Zürich. Umweltnatur- und Umweltsozialwissenschaften / Gruppe Sicherheit und Umweltschutz, ETH Zürich. pp.4-10

Schmalensee 1996 — Schmalensee R., *Council Review of the Clean Air Act Section 812 Retrospective Study Entitled 'The Benefits and Costs of the Clean Air Act, 1970 to 1990'*, EPA-SAB-COUNCIL-LTR-97-001

Schmidt-Bleek 1992 — Schmidt-Bleek F., *Ein universelles ökologisches Mass; Gedanken zum ökologischen Strukturwandel*, Wuppertal 1992

Schmidt-Bleek 1993 — Schmidt-Bleek F., MIPS Re-Visited, *Fresenius Envir Bull* 2: 407-12 (1993)

Schmidt-Bleek 1994 — Schmidt-Bleek F., *Wieviel Umwelt braucht der Mensch? MIPS - Das Mass für ökologisches Wirtschaften*, Berlin 1994

Schmucki 1996 — Schmucki D., *Räumliche und zeitliche Betrachtung von Umwelt-schadstoffen, Berechnungen zum Normalisierungsschritt in Ökobilanzen*, Semesterarbeit ETH Zürich bei Gruppe Energie-Stoffe-Umwelt, Zürich 1996 (unveröffentlicht)

Scholz 1996 — Scholz R.W., *Grenzwerte und Risiko: Probleme der Wahrnehmung und des Handelns*, WaBoLu-Hefte 6/96

Scholz *et al.* 1996 — Scholz R., Bösch S., Koller Th., Mieg H.A., Stünzi J., *Industrieareal Sulzer-Escher Wyss; Umwelt und Bauen: Wertschöpfung durch Umnutzung*, vdf Zürich 1996

Schopka *et al.* 1995 — Schoppka H.-J., Steinmetz M. (Ed.), *Environmental UV Radiation and Health Effects*, Proceedings of the International Syposium, Munich-Neuherberg, Germany, May 4-6, 1993, Fachbereich Strahlenhygiene, Bundesamt für Strahlenschutz, BfS-ISH-171/95, Neuherberg 1995

Schouten *et al.* 1996 — Schouten J.P., Vonk J.M., de Graaf A., Short Term Effects of Air Pollution on Emergency Hospital Admissions for Respiratory Disease: Results of the APHEA Project in Two Major Cities in The Netherlands, 1977-1989, *J Epidemiol Comm Health* 50 (Suppl 1): S22-S29 (1996)

Schüler *et al.* 1997 — Schüler G., Bopp M., *Atlas der Krebsmortalität in der Schweiz 1970-1990*, Birkhäuser Verlag Basel 1997, Band A-D

Schultz *et al.* 1995 — Schultz P.W., Oskamp S., Mainieri T., Who Recycles and when? A Review of Personal and Situational Factors, *Journal of Environmental Psychology* 15: 105-21 (1995)

Schulze 1992 — Schulze G., Die Erlebnisgesellschaft. Kultursoziologie der Gegenwart, Frankfurt am Main 1992, cited in: Schoenheit I., Niedergesäss U., *Lebensstile und Energieberatung*, HEA/imug, Heidelberg 1995

Schümann *et al.* 1989 — Schümann M., Flesch-Janys D., Neus H., Regional Population Risk Evaluation for Multiple Inhalation Hazards, *Exp Pathol* 37: 285-90 (1989)

Schwartz 1993 — Schwartz J., Particulate Air Pollution and Chronic Respiratory Disease. *Environmental Research* 62: 7-13 (1993)

Schwartz 1994 — Schwartz J., Air Pollution and Daily Mortality: a Review and Meta Analysis, *Environmental Research* 64: 36-52 (1994)

Schwartz *et al.* 1991 — Schwartz J., Spix C., Wichmann H.E., Malin E., Air Pollution and Acute Respiratory Illness in Five German Communities. *Environmental Research* 56, 1-14 (1991)

Schwartz *et al.* 1995 — Schwartz J. and Morris R., Air Pollution and Hospital Admissions for Cardiovascular Disease in Detroit, Michigan. *Am J Epidem* 142: 23-35.

Schwartz *et al.* 1996 — Schwartz J., Spix C., Touloumi G. *et al.*, Methodological Issues in Studies of Air Pollution and Daily Counts of Deaths or Hospital Admissions, *J Epidemiol Comm Health* 50 (Suppl 1): S3-S11 (1996)

Schwarz *et al.* 1990 — Schwarz M., Thompson M., *Divided we Stand; Redefining Politics, Technology and Social Choice*, University of Pennsylvania Press 1990

Seaton *et al.* 1995 — Seaton A., MacNee W., Donaldson K., Godden D., Particulate Air Pollution and Acute Health Effects, *Lancet* 345: 176-8 (January 21, 1995)

Seidel 1996 — Seidel H.J., *Umweltmedizin*, Georg Thieme Verlag, Stuttgart 1996

SETAC 1991 — SETAC, *A Technical Framework for Life-Cycle Assessments*, Workshop Vermont, 18.-23.8.1990

SETAC 1992 — SETAC, *Life-Cycle Assessment*, Workshop Leiden, 2.-3.12.1991, Leiden 1992

SETAC 1993a — SETAC, *A Conceptual Framework for Life-Cycle Impact Assessment*, Workshop Sandestin, 1.-7.2.1992, Pensacola 1993

SETAC 1993b — SETAC, *Guidelines for Life-Cycle Assessment: A 'Code of Practice'*, Workshop Sesimbra, 31.3.-3.4.1993, Brüssel 1993

SETAC 1994 — SETAC, *Life-Cycle Assessment Data Quality: A Conceptual Framework*, Workshop Report October 1992, Wintergreen, Virginia, Pensacola 1994

SETAC 1995 — SETAC, Cowan C.E., Mackay D., Feijtel T.C.J., van de Meent D., Di Guardo A., Davies J., Mackay N., *The Multimedia Fate Model: A Vital Tool for Predicting the Fate of Chemicals*, Pensacola 1995

Shannon 1997 — Shannon J.D., Scales of Sulfur Concentrations and Deposition from the Perspective of the Receptor, *Atmospheric Environment* 31 (23): 3933-9 (1997)

SIMA-PRO 1993 — SIMA-PRO, Eco-factors for the Nethetherlands, personnal communication from Pré Consultancy, Apeldoorn 1993

Simpson 1992 — Simpson D., Long-period Modelling of Photochemical Oxidants in Europe: Model Calculations for July 1985, *Atmospheric Environment* 26A: 1609-34 (1992)

Simpson 1993 — Simpson D., Photochemical Model Calculations over Europe for Two Extended Summer Periods: 1985 and 1989. Model Results and Comparison with Observations, *Atmospheric Environment* 27A (6): 921-43 (1993)

Simpson *et al.* 1997 — Simpson D., Olendrzynski K., Semb A., *et al.*, *Photochemical Oxidant Modelling in Europe: Multi annual Modelling and Source-receptor Relationships*, EMEP/MSC-W, Report 3/97, Oslo 1997

Sjöberg 1996 — Sjöberg L., A Discussion of the Limitations of the Psychometric and Cultural Theory Approaches to Risk Perception, *Radiation Protection Dosimetry* 68 (3/4): 219-25 (1996)

Sjöberg 1997 — Sjöberg L., Explaining Risk Perception; An Empirical Evaluation of Cultural Theory, *Risk, Decision and Policy* 2 (2): 113-30 (1997)

SK 1994 — Schweizerische Krebsliga (Hrsg.), *Krebs in der Schweiz, Häufigkeit, Sterblichkeit und Überlebensraten*, Bern 1994

SL 1991 — Statistisches Landesamt Saarland, *Morbidität und Mortalität an bösartigen Neubildungen im Saarland 1988*, Sonderhefte 157/1991, Saarbrücken

Slaper *et al.* 1997 — Slaper H., Velders G.J.M., Ozone Depletion and Skin Cancer Incidence: A Source Risk Approach, in Ale B.J.M., Janssen M.P.M., Pruppers M.J.M. (eds.), *Book of Papers; Risk 97, International Conference Mapping Environmental Risks and Risk Comparison*, 21-24 October, Amsterdam 1997

Slovic *et al.* 1980 — Slovic P., Fischhoff B., Lichtenstein S., Facts and Fears: Unterstanding Perceived Risk, in Schwing R.C., Albers W.A. (eds), *Societal Risk Assessment; How Safe is Safe Enough?*, Plenum Press, New York 1980, pp.181-214

Slovic *et al.* 1983 — Slovic P., Fischhoff B., How Safe is Safe Enough? Determinants of Perceived and Acceptable Risk, in Walker C.A., Gould L.C., Woodhouse E.J.(eds.), *Too Hot to Handle?* Yale University Press, New Haven 1983, pp.112-50

Solomon *et al.* 1992 — Solomon S., Albritton D.L., Time-dependent Ozone Depletion Potentials for Short- and Long-term Forecast, *Nature* 357: 33-7 (May 7, 1992)

SOU 1996a — SOU, Commission on Environmental Health Stockholm, *Environment for Sustainable Health Development – an Action Plan for Sweden*, Swedish Official Reports Series 1996:124, Stockholm 1996

SOU 1996b — SOU, *Miljörelaterade hälsoriker, Bilaga 1 till mijöhälsoutredningen*, Statens offentliga utredningar 1996:124, Stockholm 1996

Spadaro (forthcoming)	Spadaro J., Air Pollution: Simplified Approaches for Estimating Respiratory Health Impacts, to be submitted to *Atmospheric Environment*
Spash *et al.* 1995	Spash C.L., Hanley N., Preferences, Information and Biodiversity Preservation, *Ecological Economics* 12: 191-208 (1995)
Spengler *et al.* 1996	Spengler J.D., Wilson R., Emissions, Dispersion, and Concentration of Particles, in Wilson R., Spengler J.D. (eds), *Particles in Our Air: Concentrations and Health Effects*, Harvard University Press 1996
Spilker *et al.* 1996	Spilker B. *et al.*, Quality of Life, Bibliography and Indexes, *Medical Care* 28 (Suppl 12): D51-77
Spix *et al.* 1996	Spix C., Wichmann H.E., Daily Mortality and Air Pollutants: Findings from Köln, Germany, *J Epidemiol Comm Health* 50 (Suppl 1): S52-S58 (1996)
Stanners *et al.* 1995	Stanners D., Bourdeau Ph., *Europe's Environment; The Dobrís Assessment*, European Environment Agency, Copenhagen 1995
Stat. Jahrbuch 1996	*Statistisches Jahrbuch der Schweiz, 104. Jahrgang*, Verlag NZZ, Zürich 1996
Stauth *et al.* 1993	Stauth R., Sowman M., Grindley S., The Panel Evaluation Method: an Approach to Evaluating Contorversial Resource Allocation Proposals, *Environ Impact Assess Rev* 13: 13-35 (1993)
Steen 1996	Steen B., *EPS-Default Valuation of Environmental Impacts from Emission and Use of Resources*; Version 1996, IVL-Report 111, Göteborg 1996
Steen *et al.* 1992	Steen B., Ryding S.-O., Swedish Environmental Research Institute, Federation of Swedish Industries, *The EPS Enviro-accounting Method*, Göteborg 1992
Stern 1992	Stern, P.C., Psychological Dimensions of Global Environmental Change. *Annual Review in Psychology* 43: 269-302 (1992)
Stern 1993	Stern P.C., *Der unbekannte Konsument, Konsumstile in den neuen Bundesländern*, Hamburg 1993, cited in: Schoenheit I., Niedergesäss U., *Lebensstile und Energieberatung*, HEA/imug, Heidelberg 1995
Stern *et al.* 1992	Stern, P.C., Young, O. R., & Druckman, D. (Eds.), *Global Environmental Change: Understanding the Human Dimension*, National Academy Press, Washington 1992
Stern *et al.* 1993	Stern, P.C., Dietz, T., Kalof, L., Value Orientations, Gender, and Environmental Concern. *Environment and Behavior* 25 (3): 322-48 (1993)
Stern *et al.* 1994	Stern, P.C., Dietz, T., The Value Basis of Environmental Concern. *Journal of Social Issues* 50 (3): 65-84 (1994)
Stern *et al.* 1995a	Stern, P.C., Dietz, T., Guagnano, G., The New Ecological Paradigm in Social-psychological Context. *Environment and Behavior* 25: 123-43 (1995)
Stern *et al.* 1995b	Stern, P.C., Dietz, T., Kalof, L., Guagnano, G. A., Values, Beliefs, and Proenvironmental Action: Attidude Formation Toward Emergent Attitude Objects. *Journal of Applied Social Psychology* 25 (18): 1611-36 (1995)
StFV 1995	Arbeitsgruppe 'Beurteilungskriterien' der Eidgenössischen Kommisiion für AC-Schutz, *Beurteilungskriterien zur Störfallverordnung StFV; Beurteilung der Schwere von Schädigungen, Beurteilung der Tragbarkeit des Risikos*, Entwurf vom Juni 1995, BUWAL 1995
Stinchcombe 1968	Stinchcombe A.L., *Constructing Social Theories*, Harcourt, Brace & World, New York, 1968
Sunyer *et al.* 1993	Sunyer J., Saez M., Murillo C., Castellsague J., Martinez F., Ant J.M., Air Pollution and Emergency Room Admissions for Chronic Obstructive Pulmonary Disease: A 5-year Study. *Am J Epid* 137: 701-5 (1993)
Sunyer *et al.* 1996	Sunyer J., Castellsagué J., Sáez M., *et al.*, Air Pollution and Mortality in Barcelona, *J Epidemiol Comm Health* 50 (Suppl 1): S76-S80 (1996)
Suter 1993	Suter G.W., A Critique of Ecosoystem Health Concepts and Indexes, *Environmental Toxicology and Chemistry* 12 (9): 1533-40 (1993)
Suter *et al.* 1989	Suter P., Hofstetter P., *Die ökologische Rückzahldauer; Ein Instrument der Umwelttechnik*, SIA Nr.49, 7.12.1989

SUVA 1996	SUVA: *Tabellen 1-18 betreffend Integritätsschaäden*, Medizinische Abt. der Schweizerischen Unfall-Versicherungs-Anstalt (SUVA), Loseblattordner Stand 1996, Luzern 1996
Sweet *et al.* 1993	Sweet J., Markham A., Kerr A., Agren Ch., *Meeting Critical Loads for Sulphur; A Study of Energy Use and Emission Reduction Strategies in Europe*, Gland 1993
Tal 1997	Tal A., Assessing the Environmental Movement's Attitudes Toward Risk Assessment, *Environmental Science & Technology* 31 (10): 470A-6A (1997)
Talabardon 1995	Talabardon M. (1995). *Calcul de la durée de remanence et du volume de dilution des polluants atmosphèriques*. Travail de séminaire de génie rural, EPFL
Tellus 1992	Tellus Institute, *CSG / Tellus Packaging Study; Assessing the Impacts of Production and Disposal of Packaging and Public Policy Measurements to Alter its Mix*, Boston 1992
Teufel *et al.* 1991	Teufel D., Bauer P., Beker G. *et al.*, *Ökologische und soziale Kosten der Umweltbelastung in der Bundesrepublik Deutschland im Jahr 1989*, UPI-Bericht Nr.20, Heidelberg 1991
Thalmann-Graf 1991	Thalmann-Graf W.R., *Ökobilanzen im Verpackungsbereich*, European Packaging Federation, Berlin 1991
Thompson 199?	Thompson M., *Making Ends Meet, in the Household and on the Planet*, The Musgrave Institute, London, undated
Thompson 1992	Thompson M., The Dynamics of Cultural Theory and their Implications for the Enterprise Culture, in Heap S.H., Ross A. (eds.), *Understanding the Enterprise Culture; Themes in the work of Mary Douglas*, Edinburgh University Press, Edinburgh 1992
Thompson 1997	Thompson M., *Physical Flows and Moral Positions; an Essay in Memory of Aaron Wildavsky*, Working paper of IFF (Institut für interdisziplinäre Forschung und Fortbildung der Universitäten Insbruck, Klagenfurt und Wien), Vienna 1997
Thompson *et al.* 1990	Thompson M., Ellis R., Wildavsky A., *Cultural Theory*, Westview Print Boulder 1990
Thompson *et al.* 1998	Thompson M., Rayner St., Cultural Discourses, in Rayner St., Malone L. (eds.), *Human Choice and Climate Change*, Vol.1, Batelle Press, Columbus Ohio 1998
Tickle *et al.* 1995	Tickle A., Fergusson M., Drucker G., *Acid Rain and Nature Conservation in Europe, A Preliminary Study of Protected Areas at Risk from Acidification*, WWF Gland 1995
Tietje *et al.* 1996	Tietje O., Scholz R.W., Heitzer A., Weber O., *Mathematical Evaluation Criteria*, UNS Working Paper 14, ETH Zürich 1996
Till 1991	Till J.E., Quality of Life Measurement, *Cancer Treatment* 11: 189-204 (1991)
Timmermann 1986a	Timmermann P., Myths and Paradigms of Intersections between Development and Environment, in Clark W.C., Munn R.E. (eds.), *Sustainable Development of the Biosphere*, Cambridge University Press, Cambridge 1986
Timmermann 1986b	Timmermann P., Mythology and Surprise in the Sustainable Development of the Biosphere, in Clark W.C., Munn R.E. (eds.), *Sustainable Development of the Biosphere*, Cambridge University Press, Cambridge 1986
Tolle 1997	Tolle D.A., Regional Scaling and Normalization in LCIA, Int J LCA 2 (4): 197-208 (1997)
Tomatis *et al.* 1993	Tomatis L., Fishbein L., Outdoor and Indoor Air Pollution and Cancer: An Old and New Problem, in Tomatis L. (Ed.), *Indoor and Outdoor Air Pollution and Human Cancer*, Springer, Berlin 1993, pp.3-16
Törnqvist 1994	Törnqvist M., Is Ambient Ethene a Cancer Risk Factor?, *Environmental Health Perspectives* 102 (Suppl 4): 157-60 (October 1994)

Törnqvist *et al.* 1994 — Törnqvist M., Ehremberg L., On Cancer Risk Estimation of Urban Air Pollution, *Environmental Health Perspectives* 102 (Suppl 4):173-81 (1994)

Touloumi *et al.* 1994 — Toulomi G., Pocock S.J., Katsouyanni K., Trichopoulos D., Short-term Effects of Air Pollution on Daily Mortality in Athens: a Time-series Analysis, *International Journal of Epidemiology* 23 (5) 957-67 (1994)

Touloumi *et al.* 1996 — Toulomi G., Samoli E., Katsouyanni K., Daily Mortality and 'Winter Type' Air Pollution in Athens, Greece – a Time Series Analysis within the APHEA Project, *J Epidemiol Comm Health* 50 (Suppl 1): S47-S51 (1996)

Trichopoulos *et al.* 1996 — Trichopoulos D., Li F.P., Hunter D.J., Ursachen für Krebs, in *Spezial 5: Krebsmedizin, Spektrum der Wissenschaft*, Sondernummer 1/96, Heidelberg 1996

Trisoglio *et al.* 1997 — Trisoglio A., Swart R., Thompson M., Rormans J., Dowlatabadi H., Rahmen A., de Vries B., *Scenarios of Climate Change: Making the Human Factor Explicit*, an input into the SOAR project, not published 1997

Tukker 1994 — Tukker A., Iso-utility Functions as a Tool for Valuation in LCA, in Udo de Haes H.A., Schaltegger St., Hofstetter P., *First Working Document on Life-Cycle Impact Assessment Methodology*, ETH Zürich 1994

UBA 1994 — Schmitz St., Oels H.-J., Tiedemann A., *Ökobilanz für Getränkeverpackungen*, Fassung vom 7. Juni 1994 mit Ergänzung vom 10. August für den Workshop vom 22./23.9.1994

UBA/TNO 1997 — UBA/TNO, *The European Atmospheric Emission Inventory of Heavy Metals and Persistent Organic Pollutants for 1990*, UBA-Forschungsbericht 104 02 672/03/TNO, Berlin/Apeldoorn 1997

Udo de Haes 1993 — Udo de Haes H., Application of Life Cycle Assessment: Expectations, Drawbacks and Perspectives, *J Cleaner Prod* 1 (3-4): 131-7 (1993)

Udo de Haes 1996 — Udo de Haes (ed.), *Towards a Methodology for Life Cycle Impact Assessment*, SETAC-Europe Working Group on Impact Assessment, Brussels 1996

Udo de Haes 1998 — Udo de Haes H., New Developments in Life Cycle Impact Assessment, in Hofstetter P., Tietje O. (eds.), *Ökobilanz-Bewertungsmethoden; State-of-the-art, Neuentwicklungen 1998, Perspektiven*, Nachbearbeitung des 6. Diskussionsforums Ökobilanzen vom 12. März 1998, UNS-ETH Zürich 1998

Udo de Haes *et al.* 1994 — Udo de Haes H.A., Schaltegger S., Hofstetter P. (Hrsg.), *First Working Document on Life-Cycle Impact Assessment Methodology*, Workshop held at ETH Zurich from July 8-9, 1994

Udo de Haes *et al.* 1997 — Udo de Haes H., Wrisberg N. (eds.), *Life Cycle Assessment: State-of-the-Art and Research Priorities; Results of LCANET, a Concerted Action in the Environment and Climate Programme (DG XII)*, LCA Documents, Volume 1, Eco-Informa Press, Bayreuth 1997

UNEP 1996 — UNEP, Life Cycle Assessment; What It Is and How To Do It, Paris 1996

UNESCO 1996 — UNESCO, *Statistical Yearbook 1996*, UNESCO Publishing & Bernan Press 1996

United Nations 1991 — United Nations - Economic Commission for Europe, *Protocol to the Convention on Long-range Transboundary Air Pollution Concerning the Control of Emissions of Volatile Organic Compounds or their Transboundary Fluxes*, Geneva 1991

United Nations 1996 — United Nations - Economic Commission for Europe, *The State of Transboundary Air Pollution*, Air Pollution Studies No.12, New York and Geneva 1996

USEPA 1986 — USEPA, *Guidelines for Carcinogen Risk Assessment*, Fed. Regist, 33992-34003, 1986

USEPA 1990 — USEPA, *Cancer Risk from Outdoor Exposure to Air Toxics*, EPA-450/1-90-004a, September 1990

USES 1994 — Jager D.T., Visser C.J.M. (Eds), *Uniform System for the Evaluation of Substances (USES)*, The Hague 1994

Vaal *et al.* 1997a — Vaal M., van der Wal J.T., Hermens J., Hoeckstra J., Pattern Analysis of the Variation in the Sensitivity of Aquatic Species to Toxicants, *Chemosphere* 35 (6): 1291-309 (1997)

Vaal *et al.* 1997b — Vaal M., van der Wal J.T., Hoeckstra J., Hermens J., Variation in the Sensitivity of Aquatic Species in Relation to the Classification of Environmental Pollutants, *Chemosphere* 35 (6): 1311-27 (1997)

Vainio *et al.* 1991 — Vainio H., Coleman M., Wilbourn J., Carcinogenicity Evaluations and Ongoing Studies: The IARC Databases, *Environmental Health Perspectives* 96: 5-9 (1991)

van Asselt *et al.* 1995 — Asselt van M., Rotmans J., den Elzen M., Hilderink H., *Uncertainty in Integrated Assessment Modelling; a Cultural Perspective-based Approach*, GLOBO Report Series No.9, RIVM Report No. 461502009, Bilthoven 1995

van Asselt *et al.* 1996a — van Asselt M.B.A., Rotmans J., Uncertainty in Perspective, *Global Environmental Change* 6 (2): 121-57 (1996)

van Asselt *et al.* 1996b — van Asselt M.B.A., Beusen A.H.W., Hilderink H.B.M., Uncertainty in Integrated Assessment: A Social Scientific Perspective, *Environmental Modelling and Assessment* 1: 71-90 (1996)

van de Meent 1995 — van de Meent D., Prediction of Soil / Air Concentration Ratios for Calculating Critical Concentrations in Air Aimed at Soil Protection, RIVM-Report No.719101 020, Bilthoven 1995

van der Wurff 1992 — van der Wurff R., *Sustainable Development – a Cultural Approach*, FAST, Theme C, Global Perspective 2010 – Tasks for Science and Technology, Vol.21, FOP 336, Commission of the European Community, Belgium 1992

van Jaarsveld 1995 — van Jaarsveld J.A., *Modelling the Long-term Atmospheric Behaviour of Pollutants on Various Spatial Scales*, RIVM-Report No.722501005, Bilthoven 1995

van Kessel *et al.* 1992 — van Kessel A.W.D., Kreis I.A., *Air Pollution, Industrial Activity and Lung Cancer Mortality in the Netherlands; an Ecological Analysis*, RIVM-report No.527801001, Bilthoven 1992

van Loveren *et al.* 1993 — van Loveren H., Rombout P.J.A., Fischer P.H., Lebret E., Van Bree L., *Effects of Oxidant Air Pollution on Resistance to Respiratory Infection*, a Review, RIVM-Report No.619002003, Bilthoven 1993

van Pul *et al.* 1997 — van Pul W.A.J., de Leeuw F.A.A.M., van Jaarsfeld J.A., Sliggers C.J., The Potential for Long-range Atmospheric Transport: An Item in Risk Assessments of Substances, in Ale B.J.M., Janssen M.P.M., Pruppers M.J.M. (eds.), *Book of Papers; Risk 97, International Conference Mapping Environmental Risks and Risk Comparison*, 21-24 October, Amsterdam 1997

VDI 1991 — Verein Deutscher Ingenieure (VDI), *Krebserzeugende Stoffe in der Umwelt: Herkunft, Messung, Risiko*, Minimierung: Kolloquium Mannheim, 23. bis 25. April 1991 / Kommission Reinhaltung der Luft im VDI und DIN, VDI-Berichte Nr. 888, Düsseldorf 1991

VDI 1995 — Verein Deutscher Ingenieure (VDI), *Kumulierter Energieaufwand: Begriffe, Definitionen, Berechnungsmethoden*, Entwurf zu VDI 4600, Düsseldorf Mai 1995

VDI 1996 — Verein Deutscher Ingenieure (VDI), *Externe Kosten von Energieversorgung und Verkehr*, Tagungsbericht Stuttgart vom 5./6. März 1996, VDI Düsseldorf 1996

Veith *et al.* 1983 — Veith G.D., Kosian P., Estimating Bioconcentration Potential from Octanol / Water Partition Coefficients, in Mackay D., Paterson S., Eisenreich S.J., Simons M.S. (eds), *Physical Behaviour of PCBs in the Great Lakes*, Ann Arbor Science Publishers, Ann Arbor, pp.269-82.

Verhoeff *et al.* 1996 — Verhoeff A.P., Hoek G., Schwartz J., van Wijnen J.H., Air Pollution and Daily Mortality in Amsterdam. *Epidemiology* 7: 225-30 (1996)

Vermeire *et al.* 1997 — Vermeire T.G., van Veen M.P., Janssen M.P.M., Smetsers R.C.G.M., *De schatting van de lootstelling van de mens aan stoffen en straling*, Report No.601132002, Bilthoven 1997

Vester 1983 — Vester F., *Ballungsgebiete in der Krise; Vom Verstehen und Planen menschlicher Lebensräume*, dtv Sachbuch, München 1983

Vester 1984	Vester F., *Neuland des Denkens; Vom technokratischen zum kybernetischen Zeitalter*, dtv Sachbuch, München 1984
Vester 1985	Vester F., Ökologisches Systemmanagement; Die Unternehmen am Scheideweg zwischen Mechanistik und Biokybernetik, in Probst G.J.B., Siegwart H. (eds.), *Integriertes Managament: Bausteine des system-orientierten Management*; Festschrift zum 65. Geburtstag von Prof.Hans Ulrich, Haupt, Bern 1985
Vester 1988	Vester F., *Leitmotiv vernetztes Denken: füer einen besseren Umgang mit der Welt*, Heyne Muenchen 1988
Vester et. al 1993	Vester M. *et al.*, *Soziale Milieus im gesellschaftlichen Strukturwandel, zwischen Integration und Ausgrenzung*, Köln 1993, cited in: Schoenheit I., Niedergesäss U., *Lebensstile und Energieberatung*, HEA/imug, Heidelberg 1995
Victorin *et al.* 1996	Victorin K., Hogstedt C., Kyrklund T., Eriksson M., Setting Priorities for Environmental Health Risks in Sweden, in *Proceedings of Society of Risk Analysis Europe*, Stockolm 1996, pp.211-23
Vigon *et al.* 1995	Vigon B.W., Tolle D.A., *Challenges in Classification and Equivalency Characterisation*, Batelle, Overheads presented in the SETAC LCA Impact Assessment Work Group, Washington August 16, 1995
Vigotti *et al.* 1996	Vigotti M.A., Rossi G., Bisanti L., Zanobetti A., Schwartz J., Short Term Effects of Urban Air Pollution on Respiratory Health in Milan, Italy, 1980-89, *J Epidemiol Comm Health* 50 (Suppl 1): S71-S75 (1996)
Viscusi 1993	Viscusi W.K., The Value of Risks to Life and Health, *Journal of Economic Literature* XXXI: 1912-46 (December 1993)
VNCI 1991	VNCI, Association of the Dutch Chemical Industry, *Integrated Substance Chain Management*, 1991
Voigt 1995	Voigt K., Information über Information. CD-ROM und On-line Datenbanken im Bereich Umweltschutz, *Cogito* 6: 12-5 (1995)
Voigt *et al.* 1995	Voigt K., Brüggemann R., An Evalution of Online Databases by Methods of Latice Theory, *Chemosphere* 31 (7): 3585-94 (1995)
Volkwein *et al.* 1996a	Volkwein St., Klöpffer W., The Valuation Step in LCA: Part I: General Principles, *Int J LCA* 1(1): 36-9 (1996)
Volkwein *et al.* 1996b	Volkwein St., Gihr R., Klöpffer W., The Valuation Step within LCA: Part II: A Formalized Method of Prioritization by Expert Panels, *Int J LCA* 1 (4): 182-92 (1996)
Wackernagel *et al.* 1993	Wackernagel M., McIntosh J., Rees W.E., Woolard R., *How big is our Ecological Footprint? A Handbook for Estimating a Communities Appropriated Carrying Capacity*, University of British Columbia, Vancouver 1993
Waeber *et al.* 1997	Waeber R., Braun-Fahrländer Ch. (Eds.), *Bericht über die thematischen Workshops 'Lufthygiene und Atemwege' und 'Kanzerogene Luftschadstoffe'*, Diskussionsforum Lufthygiene und Gesundheit, SPPU, Zürich/Basel 1997
Wahrendorf *et al.* 1993	Wahrendorf J, Becher J., *Riskiomodelle und quantitative Risikoabschätzung*, in LAI (1993)
Wallsten *et al.* 1986	Wallsten T.S., Whitfield R.G., *Assessing the Risks to Young Children of Three Effects Associated with Elevated Blood-lead Levels*, Argonne National Laboratory, Energy and Environmnetal Systems Division, Argonne 1986
Weber 1995	Weber M., Wissenschaftskommunikation und Umweltprobleme, in U. Fuhrer (ed.), *Ökologisches Handeln als sozialer Prozess*, Birkhäuser, Basel 1995
Weidema 1994a	Weidema B., Product Life Cycle Impact Assessment as a Communication Issue, in Udo de Haes H.A., Schaltegger St., Hofstetter P., *First Working Document on Life-Cycle Impact Assessment Methodology*, ETH Zürich 1994
Weidema 1994b	Weidema B.P., Qualitative and Quantitative Parameters in Product Impact Assessment, in Udo de Haes H.A., Jensen A.A., Klöpffer W., Lindfors L.-G., *Integrating Impact Assessment into LCA*, Proceedings of the SETAC-Europe Congress, 11-14 April 1994, Brussels 1994

Wenstøp *et al.* 1997	Wenstøp F., Carlsen A.J., Bergland O., Magnus P., Valuation of Environmental Goods with Expert Panels, in Climaco J. (Ed), *Multicriteria Analysis*, Springer Berlin 1997
White *et al.* 1995	White P., De Smet B., Udo de Haes H., Heijungs R., LCA Back on Track; But is it One Track or Two?, *LCA News, A SETAC-Europe Publication* 5 (3), Brussels May 1995
Whitmore *et al.* 1994	Whitmore R.W., Immerman F.W., Camann D.E., Bond A.E., Lewis R.G., Schaum J.L., Non-Occupational Exposures to Pesticides for Residents of Two U.S. Cities, *Arch Environ Contam Toxicol* 26: 47-59 (1994)
Whittemoreet *al.* 1980	Whittemore A.S., Korn E.L., Asthma and Air Pollution in the Los Angeles Area. *Am J Public Health* 70: 687-96 (1980)
WHO 1947	WHO, The Constitution of the World Helath Organization, *WHO Chronical* 1: 29 (Geneva 1947)
WHO 1987	WHO, *Air Quality Guidelines for Europe*, Geneva 1987
WHO 1992a	WHO, *Global Health Situation and Projections*, WHO/HST/92.1, Geneva 1992
WHO 1992b	WHO, *Acute Effects on Health of Smog Episodes*, Report on a WHO meeting, WHO Regional publications, European Series No.43, Copenhagen 1992
WHO 1993	WHO, *International Statistical Classification of Diseases and Related Health Problems - ICD-10*, Tenth Revision, Geneva 1993
WHO 1994a	WHO, *Concern for Europe's Tomorrow; Health and the Environment in the WHO European Region*; Summary, WHO Regional Publications, European Series No.53, Copenhagen 1994
WHO 1994b	WHO, *Assessing Human Health Risks of Chemicals: Derivation of Guidance Values for Health-based Exposure Limits*, Environmental Health Criteria 170, Geneva 1994
WHO 1995a	WHO, *Concern for Europe's Tomorrow; Health and the Environment in the WHO European Region*; WHO Europe, Wissenschaftliche Verlagsgesellschaft mbH, Stuttgart 1995
WHO 1995b	WHO, *World Health Statistics Annual 1994*, Geneva 1995
WHO 1996a	WHO, *Revised WHO Air Quality Guidelines for Europe 1996*, European Centre for Environment and Health - Bilthoven Division, 1996
WHO 1996b	WHO, *Diesel Fuel and Exhaust Emission*, Environmental Health Criteria 171, Geneva 1996
WHO 1996c	WHO, *Environment and Health 1; Overview and Main European Issues*, WHO Regional Publications, European Series No.68, EEA Environmental Monograph No.2, Copenhagen 1996
WHO 1996d	Briggs D., Corvalàn C., Nurminen M., *Linkage Methods for Environmental and Health Analysis*; General Guidelines, UNEP/USEPA/WHO, Geneva 1996
WHO 1998	WHO, *Air Quality Guidelines for Europe*, Geneva 1998 (forthcoming)
WHO/UNEP 1992	WHO/UNEP, *Urban Air Pollution in Megacities of the World*, Blackwell, Oxford 1992
Williamson 1997	Williamson A.R., POPPIE–A National Scale System for Prediction of Pollution of Surface and Groundwaters by Pesticides, in Ale B.J.M., Janssen M.P.M., Pruppers M.J.M. (eds.), *Book of Papers; Risk 97, International Conference Mapping Environmental Risks and Risk Comparison*, 21-24 October, Amsterdam 1997, pp.77-81
Wilson 1971	Wilson C., *Man's Impact on the Global Environment: A Study of Critical Environmental Problems*, MIT Press, Cambridge 1971
Wilson 1996	Wilson R., Introduction, in Wilson R., Spengler J.D. (eds), *Particles in Our Air: Concentrations and Health Effects*, Harvard University Press 1996
Wilson *et al.* 1994	Wilson B., Jones B., *The Phosphate Report*, Landbank Environmental Research and Computing, London 1994

Wojtyniak *et al.* 1996 — Wojtyniak B., Piekarski T., Short Term Effect of Air Pollution on Mortality in Polish Urban Populations – What is Different?, *J Epidemiol Comm Health* 50 (Suppl 1): S36-S41 (1996)

Wordley *et al.* 1997 — Wordley J., Walters S., Ayres J.G., *Short Term Variations in Hospital Admissions and Mortality and Particulate Air Pollution* (in press).

World Bank 1993 — World Bank, *World Development Report 1993; Investing in Health,* Published for the World Bank, Oxford University Press, New York 1993

Wrisberg et al. 1998 — Wrisberg N., Gameson T. (Eds.), *CHAINET Definition Document,* European Network on Chain Analysis for Environmental Decision Support, CML Leiden 1998

Wuebbles *et al.* 1998 — Wuebbles D.J., Jain A.K., Patten K.O., Connell P.S., Evaluation of Ozone Depletion Potentials for Chlorobromomethane (CH_2ClBr) and 1-Bromo-propane ($CH_2BrCH_2CH_3$), *Atmospheric Enviornment* 32 (2): 107-13 (1998)

Wynne 1992 — Wynne B., Uncertainty and Environmental Learning, *Global Environmental Change* 2: 111-27 (1992)

Yelokhin *et al.* 1996 — Yelokhin A.N., Kozlov E.A., Chernoplekov A.N., Burdakov N.I., Yelokhina T.B., The Criteria of Acceptable Risk in Russia, in *Proceedings of Society of Risk Analysis Europe*, Stockolm 1996, pp.211-23

Yetergil Kiefer 1997 — Yetergil Kiefer Z.D., *Externe Kosten von Krebserkrankungen durch kanzerogene Luftschadstoffe: Eine Abschätzung für die Schweiz mit besonderer Berücksichtigung von Benzol, polyzyklischen aromatischen Kohlenwasserstoffen und Dieselrusspartikeln*, Dissertation Nr. 12308, ETH Zürich 1997

Yetergil Kiefer *et al.* 1997 — Yetergil Kiefer D., Schüler G., Schelbert H., *Soziale Kosten von Lungenkrebs*, BAG, Schweizerische Krebsliga: Broschüre Lungenkrebs, April 1997

Zionts 1997 — Zionts St., Decision Making: Some Experiences, Myths and Observations, in Fandel G., Gal Th., Hanne Th. (eds.), *Multiple Criteria Decision Making*, Proceedings of the Twelfth International Conference, Hagen, Springer Verlag, Berlin 1997

Ziqiang *et al.* 1996 — Ziqiang P., Yongxing Z., Zhuzhou C. *et al.* , Outline of a Public Health Risk Assessment Method, *Int J Environment and Pollution* 6 (4-6): 428-39 (1996)

Zmirou *et al.* 1996 — Zmirou D., Barumandzadeh T. Balducci F. *et al.* , Short Term Effects of Air Pollution on Mortality in the City of Lyon, France, 1985-90, *J Epidemiol Comm Health* 50 (Suppl 1): S30-S35 (1996)

Zwick 1996 — Zwick M.M., *Stilorientierung und Umwelteinstellungen*, Manuskripr zu Handen ETH Zürich, Akademie für Technikfolgenabschätzung in Baden-Würtemberg, Stuttgart 1996

SUBJECT INDEX